T0294960

OESOPHAGOGASTRIC SURGERY

Seventh Edition

A Companion to Specialist Surgical Practice

Series Editors
O. James Garden
Simon Paterson-Brown

Seventh Edition

OESOPHAGOGASTRIC SURGERY

Edited by

Peter J. Lamb, MBBS, MD, FRCS(Gen), FRCS(Ed)
Consultant Upper Gastrointestinal Surgeon, Department of Upper GI Surgery,
Royal Infirmary of Edinburgh, Edinburgh, UK

Graeme W. Couper, MD, MBChB, FRCS
Consultant Upper Gastrointestinal Surgeon, Department of Upper GI Surgery,
Royal Infirmary of Edinburgh, Edinburgh, UK

For additional online content visit eBooks+

ELSEVIER

First edition 1997
Second edition 2001
Third edition 2005
Fourth edition 2009
Fifth edition 2014
Sixth edition 2019
Seventh edition 2024

Notices

Practitioners and researchers must always rely on their own experience and knowledge in evaluating and using any information, methods, compounds or experiments described herein. Because of rapid advances in the medical sciences, in particular, independent verification of diagnoses and drug dosages should be made. To the fullest extent of the law, no responsibility is assumed by Elsevier, authors, editors or contributors for any injury and/or damage to persons or property as a matter of products liability, negligence or otherwise, or from any use or operation of any methods, products, instructions, or ideas contained in the material herein.

ISBN: 978-0-443-10945-4

Content Strategist: Alexandra Mortimer
Content Project Manager: Arindam Banerjee
Design: Ryan Cook
Art Buyer: Muthukumaran Thangaraj
Marketing Manager: Deborah Watkins

Printed in India

Last digit is the print number: 9 8 7 6 5 4 3 2 1

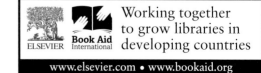

Contents

Series Editors' preface

The *Companion to Specialist Surgical Practice* series has now reached its Seventh Edition and continues to remain popular for both surgeons in training as well as consultant surgeons in independent practice. The strength of this series has always been founded on contemporary, evidence-based information on the subspecialist areas relevant to their general surgical practice and this Seventh Edition has followed this plan.

This Edition continues to keep abreast of increasing sub-specialisation in general surgery. The ongoing developments in minimal access and increasingly robotic surgery are discussed, along with the desire of some subspecialities, such as breast and vascular surgery, to separate away from 'general surgery' in some countries. However, all volumes also underline the importance for all surgeons of being aware of current developments in their surgical field. The importance of evidence-based practice and in particular the management of emergency conditions remains throughout, and authors have provided recommendations and highlighted key resources within each chapter. The ebook version of the textbook has also enabled improved access to the reference abstracts and links to video content relevant to many of the chapters.

As in all the previous editions, we are greatly indebted to the volume editors, and contributors, who have all put so much hard work into delivering such a high quality piece of work. We remain grateful for the support and encouragement of the team at Elsevier and we trust that our original vision of delivering an up-to-date, affordable text has been met and that readers, whether in training or independent practice, will find this Seventh Edition an invaluable resource.

We are grateful to Kathryn Rigby and Jonathan Michaels who wrote the guidelines on Evidence-based Practice in Surgery for previous editions of the series. These have been well received and have been retained again for this new edition in order to help guide readers in their assessment of the various levels of evidence discussed in each chapter.

O. James Garden, CBE, BSc, MBChB, MD, DSc(Hon), FRCS (Glas), FRCS(Ed), FRCP(Ed), FRACS(Hon), FRCSC (Hon), FACS(Hon), FCSHK(Hon), FRCSI(Hon), FRCS(Engl)(Hon), FRSE, MAMSE, FFST(RCSEd)
Professor Emeritus, Clinical Surgery, University of Edinburgh, UK.

Simon Paterson-Brown, MBBS, MPhil, MS, FRCS(Ed), FRCS (Engl), FCSHK, FFST(RCSEd)
Honorary Senior Lecturer, Clinical Surgery, University of Edinburgh, UK.

Editors' preface

The Seventh Edition of *Oesophagogastric Surgery* aims to amalgamate contemporary, evidence-based literature with the opinions of world experts on one of the most challenging disciplines in surgery. The authorship is truly international and reflects the global nature of oesophagogastric surgery.

Existing chapters from the Sixth Edition have been extensively updated and additional chapters introduced to cover the expanding breadth of knowledge in oesophagogastric disease. Authors were specifically asked to focus on areas where practice has changed, and to identify up-to-date key references and relevant video links.

We trust that this Seventh Edition truly reflects current surgical practice and meets the needs of both senior trainees and established oesophagogastric surgeons around the world.

ACKNOWLEDGEMENTS

We wish to thank all our contributors for providing their expertise and experience and for remaining true to the ethos of the series. The editors would like to thank Arindam Banerjee and Alexandra Mortimer at Elsevier for all their support, encouragement and forbearance in the preparation of this edition. We would also like to acknowledge and offer grateful thanks for the input of all previous editions' contributors, without whom this new edition would not have been possible. Grateful thanks in particular to the retiring volume editor of the Sixth Edition, Professor Mike Griffin, who has provided unstinting support with all previous six editions.

Peter J. Lamb
Graeme W. Couper
Edinburgh

Evidence-based practice in surgery

Critical appraisal for developing evidence-based practice can be obtained from a number of sources, the most reliable being randomised controlled clinical trials, systematic literature reviews, meta-analyses and observational studies. For practical purposes three grades of evidence can be used, analogous to the levels of 'proof' required in a court of law:

1. **Beyond all reasonable doubt**. Such evidence is likely to have arisen from high-quality randomised controlled trials, systematic reviews or high-quality synthesised evidence such as decision analysis, cost-effectiveness analysis or large observational datasets. The studies need to be directly applicable to the population of concern and have clear results. The grade is analogous to burden of proof within a criminal court and may be thought of as corresponding to the usual standard of 'proof' within the medical literature (i.e. $P < 0.05$).

2. **On the balance of probabilities**. In many cases a high-quality review of literature may fail to reach firm conclusions due to conflicting or inconclusive results, trials of poor methodological quality or the lack of evidence in the population to which the guidelines apply. In such cases it may still be possible to make a statement as to the best treatment on the 'balance of probabilities'. This is analogous to the decision in a civil court where all the available evidence will be weighed up and the verdict will depend upon the balance of probabilities.

3. **Not proven**. Insufficient evidence upon which to base a decision, or contradictory evidence.

Depending on the information available, three grades of recommendation can be used:

Strong recommendation, which should be followed unless there are compelling reasons to act otherwise.

    a. A recommendation based on evidence of effectiveness, but where there may be other factors to take into account in decision-making, for example the user of the guidelines may be expected to take into account patient preferences, local facilities, local audit results or available resources.

    b. A recommendation made where there is no adequate evidence as to the most effective practice, although there may be reasons for making a recommendation in order to minimise cost or reduce the chance of error through a locally agreed protocol.

Evidence where a conclusion can be reached '**beyond all reasonable doubt**' and therefore where a **strong recommendation** can be given.
This will normally be based on evidence levels:

- Ia. Meta-analysis of randomised controlled trials
- Ib. Evidence from at least one randomised controlled trial
- IIa. Evidence from at least one controlled study without randomisation
- IIb. Evidence from at least one other type of quasi-experimental study.

Evidence where a conclusion might be reached '**on the balance of probabilities**' and where there may be other factors involved which influence the recommendation given. This will normally be based on less conclusive evidence than that represented by the double tick icons:

- III. Evidence from non-experimental descriptive studies, such as comparative studies and case–control studies
- IV. Evidence from expert committee reports or opinions or clinical experience of respected authorities, or both.

Evidence that is associated with either a **strong recommendation** or **expert opinion** is highlighted in the text in panels such as those shown above, and is distinguished by either a double or single tick icon, respectively. The references associated with double-tick evidence are listed as Key References at the end of each chapter, along with a short summary of the paper's conclusions where applicable. The full reference list for each chapter is available in the ebook.

The reader is referred to Chapter 1, 'Evaluation of surgical evidence' in the volume *Core Topics in General and Emergency Surgery* of this series, for a more detailed description of this topic.

Contributors

Moath Saleh Al Saqaaby, MD
Diabetes Complications Research Centre
University College Dublin
Dublin, Ireland;
Consultant Diabetes and Obesity Medicine
Obesity, Endocrine and Metabolism Center
King Fahad Medical City
Riyadh, Saudi Arabia

Natalie S. Blencowe, PhD, FRCS
MRC Clinician Scientist
Linder Foundation Associate Professor in Clinical Trials
Honorary Consultant Upper GI Surgeon
University Hospitals Bristol and Weston NHS Foundation
    Trust
Bristol, United Kingdom

Ben E. Byrne, MB BChir, MA (Cantab), FRCS, PhD
Consultant Surgeon
Department of Oesophagogastric Surgery
University Hospitals Bristol and Weston NHS Foundation
    Trust
Bristol, United Kingdom

Graeme W. Couper, MD, MBChB, FRCS
Consultant Upper Gastrointestinal Surgeon
Department of Upper GI Surgery
Royal Infirmary of Edinburgh
Edinburgh, United Kingdom

Stephen Falk, FRCR, FRCP, MD
Consultant Clinical Oncologist
Bristol Cancer Institute
Bristol, United Kingdom

Rebecca C. Fitzgerald, OBE MD, FRCP, FMedSci
Professor of Cancer Prevention
Early Cancer Institute
University of Cambridge
Cambridge, United Kingdom

Matthew Forshaw, MA, MBBChir, MSc, FRCS
Department of Upper GI Surgery
Glasgow Royal Infirmary
Glasgow, United Kingdom

Heike I. Grabsch, MD, PhD, FRCPath
Professor of Gastrointestinal Pathology
Maastricht University Medical Center+
Maastricht, The Netherlands;
Professor in Gastrointestinal Pathology
Pathology and Data Analytics
Leeds Institute of Medical Research at St James's
University of Leeds
Leeds, United Kingdom

Andreas V. Hadjinicolaou, BA, MA, MB BChir(Cantab), MA, DPhil(Oxon), AFHEA, MRCP
Academic Clinical Lecturer in Gastroenterology
Early Cancer Institute
University of Cambridge;
Division of Gastroenterology and Hepatology
Department of Medicine
Cambridge University Hospitals and University of
    Cambridge
Cambridge, United Kingdom

Shiwei Han, MD, PhD
Research Fellow
Thoracic Surgery
Virginia Mason Medical Center
Seattle, Washington, United States

Jordan J. Haworth, BSc
Clinical Physiologist
Gastrointestinal Physiology
The Functional Gut Clinic
Manchester, United Kingdom

James Helman, MD
Assistant Professor
Cardiac Anesthesiology and Pain Medicine
Department of Anesthesiology and Pain Medicine
University of Toronto Temerty Faculty of Medicine
Toronto, Ontario

Anthony R. Hobson, PhD
Clinical Director
Gastrointestinal Physiology
The Functional Gut Clinic
London, United Kingdom

Arjun D. Koch, MD, PhD
Gastroenterologist
Department of Gastroenterology and Hepatology
Erasmus MC Cancer Institute
University Medical Center Rotterdam
Rotterdam, The Netherlands

Sjoerd M. Lagarde, MD, PhD
Upper GI Surgeon
Department of Surgery
Erasmus MC Cancer Institute
University Medical Center Rotterdam
Rotterdam, The Netherlands

Peter J. Lamb, MBBS, MD, FRCS(Gen), FRCS(Ed)
Consultant Upper Gastrointestinal Surgeon
Department of Upper GI Surgery
Royal Infirmary of Edinburgh
Edinburgh, United Kingdom

Carel le Roux, MBChB, MSc, FRCP, FRCPath, PhD
Metabolic Medicine
Diabetes Complications Research Centre
University College Dublin
Dublin, Ireland

Donald E. Low, MD, FACS, FRCS(C), FRCSI(Hon), FRCS(Eng) (Hon)
Head of Thoracic Surgery and Thoracic Oncology
Department of General and Thoracic Surgery
Virginia Mason Medical Center;
Clinical Assistant Professor
Department of Surgery
University of Washington School of Medicine
Seattle, Washington, United States

Andrew Macdonald, BSc, MBBS, MPhil, FRCSEd
Department of Upper GI Surgery
Glasgow Royal Infirmary
Glasgow, United Kingdom

Brijesh Madhok, MBBS, MS, MD, FRCS
Consultant Upper GI and Bariatric Surgeon
Upper GI Surgery
University Hospitals of Derby and Burton NHS Foundation
  Trust
Derby, United Kingdom

Kamal Mahawar, MS, MSc, FRCSEd
Consultant Surgeon
General Surgery
Sunderland Royal Hospital
Sunderland, United Kingdom

Nicholas D. Maynard, BA(Hons) Oxon, MBBS, MS, FRCS, FRCSEd(Ad Hom)
Upper Gastrointestinal Surgeon
Oxford University Hospitals NHS Foundation Trust
Oxford, United Kingdom

Richard P. Owen, DPhil, FRCS
Upper Gastrointestinal Surgeon
Oxford University Hospitals NHS Foundation Trust
Oxford, United Kingdom

Takeshi Sano, MD, PhD, FRCS
Hospital Director
Cancer Institute of JFCR
Tokyo, Japan

Mark Smithers, AM, MBBS, FRACS, FRCSEng, FRCSEd
Mayne Professor
Academy of Surgery
Faculty of Medicine
University of Queensland;
Director
Upper GI/Soft Tissue Unit
Princess Alexandra Hospital
Brisbane, Queensland, Australia

Jimmy Bok-yan So, MBChB, FRCSE, FAMS, MPH
Professor of Surgery
National University of Singapore;
Head
Division of Surgical Oncology and Associate Director
National University Cancer Institute of Singapore (NCIS);
Head
Upper GI Service
Department of Surgery
National University Hospital
Singapore

Shaw Somers, BSc(Hons), MD, FRCS
Consultant Upper GI and Bariatric Surgeon
Department of Upper GI Surgery
Queen Alexandra Hospital
Hampshire, United Kingdom;
Director and Surgeon
Streamline Surgical
Middlesex, United Kingdom

Sarah K. Thompson, MD, PhD, FRCSC, FRACS
Associate Professor
College of Medicine and Public Health
Flinders University
Bedford Park, South Australia, Australia;
Consultant Surgeon
Adelaide Gastrointestinal Specialists
Eastwood, South Australia, Australia

Iain Thomson, MBBS, FRACS
Surgeon
Upper GI/Soft Tissue Unit
Princess Alexandra Hospital;
Senior Lecturer
Academy of Surgery
Faculty of Medicine
University of Queensland
Brisbane, Queensland, Australia

Maria J. Valkema, MD
Medical Doctor
Department of Surgery
Erasmus MC Cancer Institute
University Medical Center Rotterdam
Rotterdam, The Netherlands

J. Jan B. van Lanschot, MD, PhD
Professor
Department of Surgery
Erasmus MC Cancer Institute
University Medical Center Rotterdam
Rotterdam, The Netherlands

**Shajahan Wahed, MD, FRCS, MBChB(Hons),
BSc(Hons)**
Northern Oesophago-Gastric Unit
Royal Victoria Infirmary
Newcastle upon Tyne
England, United Kingdom

**David I. Watson, MBBS, MD, PhD, FRACS,
FRCSEd(Hon), FAHMS**
Matthew Flinders Distinguished Professor of Surgery
College of Medicine and Public Health
Flinders University;
Senior Consultant Surgeon
Oesophago-Gastric Surgery Unit
Flinders Medical Centre
Bedford Park, South Australia, Australia

Richard Welbourn, MD, FRCS
Consultant Upper Gastrointestinal Surgeon
Upper Gastrointestinal and Bariatric Surgery
Musgrove Park Hospital
Somerset, United Kingdom

Pathology of oesophageal and gastric tumours

1

Heike I. Grabsch

INTRODUCTION

Oesophageal tumours can be broadly divided into epithelial, non-epithelial, and heterotopic, based on the cell of origin or into intraluminal, intramural, and extramural based on their location in relation to the oesophageal wall.

Epithelial neoplasms arise from the mucosa and hence can be recognised endoscopically due to mucosal irregularities. The majority of epithelial neoplasms are malignant or premalignant and these include squamous papilloma, squamous or glandular dysplasia, squamous cell carcinoma, adenocarcinoma, and neuroendocrine neoplasms. In contrast, mesenchymal neoplasms arise from the submucosa or deeper within the wall and present endoscopically with an intact normal or reactive mucosa. The majority of non-epithelial mesenchymal neoplasms are benign, such as leiomyoma, granular cell tumour, haemangioma, lipoma, glomus tumour, etc. Importantly, in a patient presenting clinically with dysphagia, non-neoplastic (tumour-like) lesions such as duplication cysts, inflammatory polyps, and heterotopia need to be considered in the differential diagnosis.

Gastrointestinal stromal tumours, primary melanoma, lymphoma, germ cell tumours, and secondary tumours (metastases) are rare in the oesophagus and will not be discussed here. The molecular pathology of oesophageal tumours will be covered in more depth in Chapter 2.

OESOPHAGUS

BENIGN TUMOURS AND TUMOUR-LIKE LESIONS OF THE OESOPHAGUS AND THE GASTRO-OESOPHAGEAL JUNCTION

Benign oesophageal tumours and tumour-like lesions represent approximately 20% of oesophageal neoplasms found at autopsy[1] but constitute only about 1% of all clinically symptomatic oesophageal lesions.[2] These lesions are usually small, and bleeding due to a benign oesophageal tumour is rare and mostly related to secondary ulceration of the luminal surface.

Squamous cell papillomas are rare (less than 1% of all benign oesophageal tumours) but nevertheless represent the most common benign epithelial tumour of the oesophagus. They are most commonly located in the lower third of the oesophagus, exophytic with a warty surface, sessile or partly pedunculated, well demarcated and usually measure less than 5 mm in diameter. Related to its endoscopic/macroscopic appearance, the differential diagnosis of a verrucous squamous cell carcinoma may need to be excluded

histologically. Squamous cell papillomas have been related to chronic mucosal irritation such as gastro-oesophageal reflux and possibly to human papilloma virus (HPV) infection.

Leiomyoma is a smooth muscle (e.g. mesenchymal) tumour and is the most common benign intramural oesophageal neoplasm with virtually no risk of progression to leiomyosarcoma. Leiomyomas are twice as frequent in males as in females and are usually asymptomatic. Leiomyomas most commonly arise from the muscularis propria and are typically located in the distal or mid oesophagus. Most occur as solitary lesions, are less than 3 cm in size, form a firm white-greyish mass, and may be calcified. In contrast to gastrointestinal stromal tumours, leiomyomas are immunoreactive for desmin and smooth muscle actin and negative for c-KIT (CD117), DOG1 (Discovered On GIST 1) and CD34.

Developmental cysts and duplications are congenital anomalies resulting from aberrant posterior division of the embryonic foregut at 3–4 weeks gestation and represent the second most common benign lesion of the oesophagus. Inclusion cysts are located within the oesophageal wall nearby the tracheal bifurcation and may cause compression of the neighbouring respiratory tract. They are lined with ciliated columnar or stratified squamous epithelium and contain clear fluid. Duplication cysts share the muscularis propria with the oesophagus and can be lined by oesophageal or gastric mucosa. Although they are located extramurally and usually do not communicate with the oesophageal lumen, symptoms and complications may occur due to ulceration, haemorrhage, and perforation requiring surgical intervention.

Fibrovascular polyps account for up to 1% of all benign oesophageal lesions. They are slow-growing tumours arising from the submucosal mesenchymal tissue and are usually located intraluminal in the upper oesophagus near the level of the cricopharyngeus. Histologically, they are composed of loose or dense fibrous tissue, adipose tissue, and vascular structures and are covered by normal squamous epithelium. They are often 7 cm or longer when they become symptomatic. To prevent possible complications such as regurgitation or even fatal asphyxia, fibrovascular polyps are usually surgically removed. Careful morphological investigation together with MDM2 FISH analyses and immunohistochemistry are needed to exclude the possibility of a liposarcoma or gastrointestinal stromal tumour.

Granular cell tumours of the gastrointestinal tract represent 5–10% of all granular cell tumours in the human body, the majority of which are located in the oesophagus. Despite their low overall frequency, oesophageal granular cell tumours are the second most common oesophageal mesenchymal tumour after leiomyoma. Most tumours arise in the distal third of the oesophagus, are less than 1cm in size, and

Table 1.1 Comparison of selected features between oesophageal squamous cell carcinoma and adenocarcinoma

Histological phenotype	Squamous cell carcinoma	Adenocarcinoma
Tumour location in the oesophagus	Upper and middle third	Lower third, gastroesophageal junction
Incidence worldwide (2020)	512,500 (85%)	85,700 (14%). Note that the two numbers don't add up to 100% as there are 'other types' as well
Geographical distribution	Dominant subtype in South Africa and Eastern and South Central Asia ('oesophageal cancer belt')	Most common in Northern and Western Europe, North America, Australia
Ethnicity affected	Black > White	White > Black
Main risk factors	Chewing areca nuts or betel quid, cigarette smoking, alcohol, thermal injury (hot beverages), low intake of fruit and vegetables, low socioeconomic status	Cigarette smoking, acid or bile reflux, obesity, low intake of fruit and vegetables
Associated conditions	Achalasia,[3] coeliac disease,[4] Plummer–Vinson syndrome,[5] Tylosis[6] previous ingestion of corrosive substances,[7] Zenker's diverticulum,[8] after ionising radiation,[9] polymorphisms in *ALDH1B1* and *ALDH2*.[10]	Barrett's oesophagus

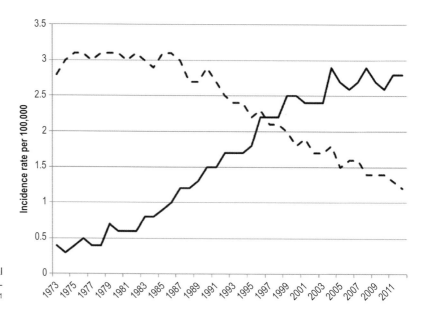

Fig. 1.1 Incidence rates per 100.000 for oesophageal adenocarcinoma (solid line) and oesophageal carcinoma (dashed line) in US SEER 9 registries, 1973–2012.[11]

are located in the submucosa endoscopically visible as pale yellow sessile or polypoid lesions covered by normal mucosa. Histologically, the tumour cells show neuroectodermal differentiation with uniformly large, plump cells with eosinophilic granular cytoplasm which are positive for periodic acid-Schiff (PAS) and S100. The covering squamous epithelium is often thickened and can show pseudoepitheliomatous hyperplasia, which may be misdiagnosed as squamous cell carcinoma if only superficial biopsies are taken.

MALIGNANT TUMOURS OF THE OESOPHAGUS AND THE GASTRO-OESOPHAGEAL JUNCTION

EPIDEMIOLOGY
544,076 people died from oesophageal cancer in 2020 worldwide and it has been estimated that this number will rise to 880,000 deaths/year in 2040.

Oesophageal cancer consist of two main entities with similar clinical symptoms, treatment options, and poor survival rates but differences in the geographical distribution, risk factors, tumour location, tumour histological phenotype, and prognosis (Table 1.1).

The incidence of both squamous cell cancer and adenocarcinomas is higher in males than females; 70% of all patients with oesophageal cancer worldwide are male. For both sexes, the incidence of oesophageal cancer increases with age, 60% of cases are older than 65 years at the time of diagnosis.

There has been a dramatic shift in the incidence of oesophageal cancer subtypes in Western populations with a steep increase of adenocarcinoma (see Fig. 1.1). Population-based studies in the USA and Europe indicate that the incidence of oesophageal adenocarcinoma, adenocarcinoma of the gastro-oesophageal junction, and proximal stomach has doubled between the 1970s and late 1980s, and continues to increase by 5% every year.[12,13] Countries with the highest incidence of oesophageal adenocarcinoma are the UK, Australia, the Netherlands, and the US.

AETIOLOGY
The aetiology of oesophageal cancer is multifactorial and strongly population-dependent. Low socioeconomic

Table 1.2 Aetiological factors for oesophageal and gastric cancer

	Smoking	Alcohol	Dietary influences	Socioeconomic status	*H. pylori*
SCC	++	++	++	++	−
Oesophageal/OGJ ACA	−	+	++	+	+
Gastric ACA	++	+	++	++	++

ACA, Adenocarcinoma; *OGJ*, oesophagogastric junction; *SCC*, squamous cell carcinoma.

status, poverty, and poor oral hygiene have been linked to an increased risk of squamous cell cancer in particular (Table 1.2). Foods containing N-Nitroso compounds are carcinogenic and have been implicated in the development of squamous cell cancer. Alcoholic beverages and other foods can contain or be metabolized to acetaldehyde, a class 1 carcinogen. Most epidemiological studies have confirmed alcoholic beverages as a risk factor for squamous cell cancer although the carcinogenic effects vary with the degree of consumption. There is no evidence to suggest that alcohol consumption increases the risk of oesophageal adenocarcinoma. Interestingly, increased body mass index has been associated with lower risk of squamous cell cancer but increased risk of adenocarcinoma; underlying biological mechanisms for these differences are not clear. The current evidence of an association between squamous cell carcinoma and HPV infection is still inconclusive.

Patients with gastric atrophy seem to have two- to threefold increased risk of developing oesophageal squamous cell cancer and gastric cancer but decreased risk of developing oesophageal adenocarcinoma.[14]

Oesophageal squamous cell cancer and adenocarcinoma genetics are discussed in detail in Chapter 2.

SQUAMOUS CELL CARCINOMA

Squamous cell dysplasia – the precursor lesion of squamous cell carcinoma

Oesophageal squamous cell carcinoma development is believed to be a multistep process from normal squamous epithelium via intraepithelial neoplasia (synonym: dysplasia) to invasive carcinoma based on findings in high-risk populations where dysplasia predates the development of carcinoma by approximately 5 years.[15,16] Squamous cell dysplasia is generally asymptomatic and endoscopically only visible using topical Lugol iodine or advance imaging methods like narrow band imaging.

The histological diagnosis of dysplasia requires the presence of cytological (nuclear enlargement, pleomorphism, overlapping) and architectural atypia (abnormal epithelial maturation towards the surface). Squamous cell dysplasia is classified as 'low-grade' when architectural and cytological abnormalities are seen in the basal half of the squamous epithelium with preserved maturation of the upper half. High-grade squamous cell dysplasia is diagnosed when more than the bottom half shows architectural and cytological abnormalities. Note that high-grade squamous cell dysplasia includes the group of lesions classified as 'carcinoma in situ'.

Large Chinese studies suggest that progression from squamous dysplasia to squamous cell cancer is relatively slow even in a high-risk population, offering ample opportunity for intervention.

Squamous cell carcinoma is per definition a neoplasm with squamous cell differentiation characterised by keratinocyte-like cells with intercellular bridges and/or keratinisation which at least penetrates the epithelial basement membrane into the lamina propria.

The aetiology and predisposing factors for oesophageal squamous cell carcinoma vary significantly among different regions in the world.[17] Tobacco-smoking, alcohol, and hot beverages such as hot mate tea are major risk factors for oesophageal squamous cell carcinoma.[12,18]

Oesophageal squamous cell carcinomas are found in the upper, middle, and lower third of the oesophagus in a ratio of approximately 1:5:2. The native (untreated) macroscopic appearance of the tumour depends on the depth of tumour invasion and is classified into four different types according to the Japanese Esophageal Society,[19] which is similar to the macroscopic classification of gastric cancer (Fig. 1.2). Approximately 60% of squamous cell carcinomas show an exophytic or fungating growth pattern (Fig. 1.3), 25% are ulcerative and 15% are infiltrative.

Squamous cell carcinomas can grow horizontally and vertically. In the West, 60% of patients have carcinomas that have invaded beyond the muscularis propria and have regional lymph node metastases at the time of diagnosis. In contrast, in Japan, up to 40% of all resected oesophageal carcinomas are superficial or early carcinomas involving mucosa and submucosa only.[21] The frequency of lymph node metastases is related to the depth of tumour invasion in the wall (5% for carcinomas in the superficial submucosa [sm1 cancers] versus up to 55% for carcinomas in the deep submucosa [sm3 cancers]). Although tumours located in the upper third of the oesophagus are more likely to spread to cervical and upper mediastinal lymph nodes, a significant proportion will also spread to perigastric lymph nodes.

Tumours located in the middle and lower oesophagus can spread to upper mediastinal as well as perigastric nodes and patients with lymph node metastases on both sides of the diaphragm have been shown to have a poorer prognosis.[22–24]

Distant metastases due to haematogenous spread are most commonly found in liver, lung, adrenal gland and kidney.[25]

Histologically, squamous cell carcinomas are characterised by keratinocyte-like cells, which show a variable degree of keratinisation. Depending on the extent of mitotic activity, nuclear atypia, and degree of squamous differentiation including degree of keratinisation, squamous cell carcinomas are graded as well, moderately, or poorly differentiated[26] (Fig. 1.4).

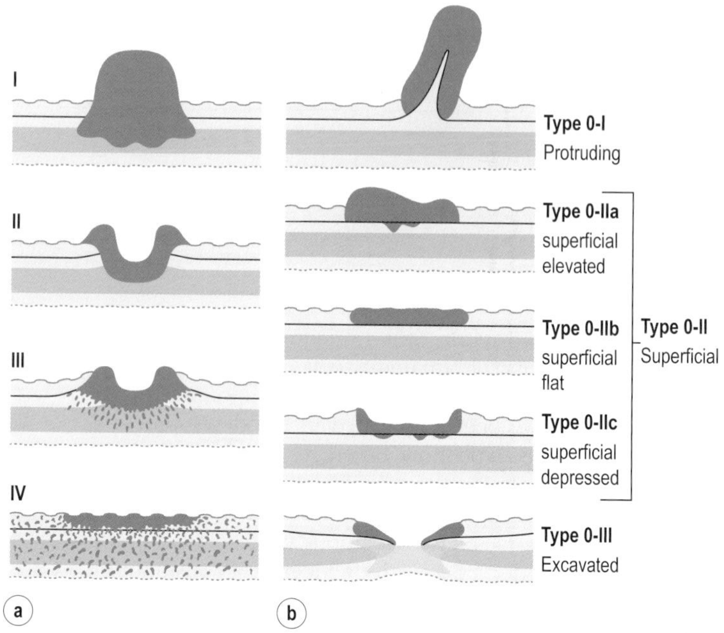

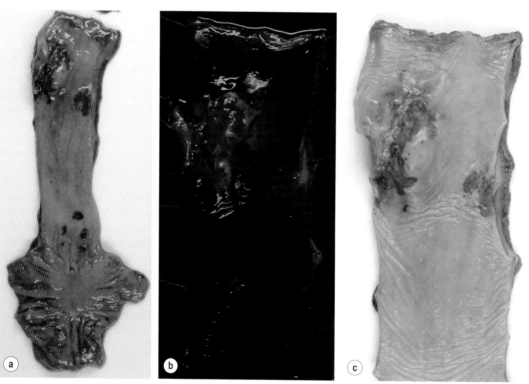

Fig. 1.2 **(a)** Borrmann classification for advanced oesophageal and gastric cancers. Type I: polypoid with a broad base, may be superficially ulcerated. Type II: excavated ulcerated lesion with elevated borders, sharp margin with no definitive infiltration into adjacent mucosa. Type III: ulcerative, diffusely infiltrating base. Type IV: diffusely infiltrative thickening of the wall (linitis plastica). **(b)** Murakami classification for early cancers. (Modified from Japanese Gastric Cancer Association. Japanese classification of gastric carcinoma, 3rd English edition.[20])

Type 0-I
Protruding

Type 0-IIa
superficial
elevated

Type 0-IIb
superficial
flat

Type 0-II
Superficial

Type 0-IIc
superficial
depressed

Type 0-III
Excavated

Fig. 1.3   Oesophageal squamous cell carcinoma located in the middle oesophagus. **(a)** Fresh oesophagectomy specimen with a polypoid exophytic tumour growth and a smaller flat (red-coloured) mucosal abnormality. **(b)** Lack of (dark) iodine staining in the abnormal areas. **(c)** Same specimen after fixation. (Courtesy of Dr Tomio Arai, Tokyo, Japan.)

Three main variants of squamous cell carcinoma have been described:[26]

1. **Verrucous carcinoma** of the oesophagus is a rare, slow-growing, locally aggressive tumour, which is more common in males and arises in the setting of chronic mucosal injury. Macroscopically, the tumour has an exophytic papillary appearance and is most frequently located in the lower third of the oesophagus. Tumours are usually very large before they become clinically apparent. Microscopically, the tumour is very well differentiated with minimal atypia. Superficial endoscopic biopsies can be insufficient to distinguish between a squamous papilloma, pseudoepitheliomatous hyperplasia, and verrucous carcinoma.[10]

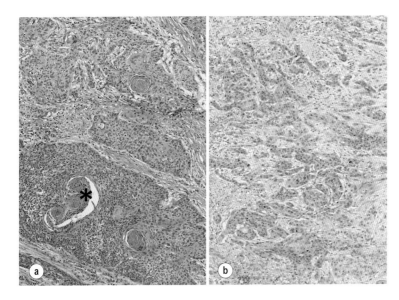

Fig. 1.4 Histological images of squamous cell carcinoma. **(a)** Moderate to well-differentiated squamous cell carcinoma showing evidence of keratinisation (* indicates area with keratinisation). **(b)** Poorly differentiated squamous cell carcinoma with small islands and strands of tumour cells within desmoplastic stroma without evidence of keratinisation.

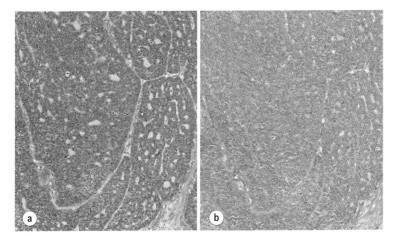

Fig. 1.5 Histology of basaloid squamous cell carcinoma. **(a)** Haematoxylin/eosin-stained section showing a tumour with a solid growth pattern and small gland-like structures. **(b)** PAS stained section of the same tumour showing light pink coloured material in the gland-like lumen.

2. **Spindle cell squamous cell carcinoma** (also known as carcinosarcoma, sarcomatoid carcinoma, and metaplastic carcinoma) is a polypoid tumour located in the middle or lower third of the oesophagus. Histologically, the tumour is biphasic with an epithelial element (well to moderately differentiated squamous cell carcinoma) and a spindle cell component, which is usually of high grade and can show osseous, cartilaginous, or skeletal muscle differentiation.[27] Spindle cell carcinomas are highly aggressive carcinomas with 5-year survival rates of 10–15%.[28]

3. **Basaloid squamous cell carcinoma** accounts for approximately 5% of all oesophageal cancers and needs to be distinguished from 'pure' squamous cell carcinoma, adenoid cystic carcinoma, and neuroendocrine tumours using appropriate immunohistochemical marker. It is a highly aggressive carcinoma with a very poor prognosis. Histologically, this tumour shows the characteristic basaloid cells together with a mucoid hyaline-like PAS positive substance (Fig. 1.5).

It can be difficult to distinguish between poorly differentiated squamous cell carcinomas and poorly differentiated adenocarcinoma based on the routine haematoxylin/eosin stained tissue section alone. In this context, an immunohistochemical marker panel is used in routine clinical practice to establish the diagnosis. Squamous cell cancers are usually immunopositive for CK5/6, CK14, p63, or p40 and negative for CK7, CK20, and CDX2.

To date, there are no molecular markers established in routine clinical practice in patients with squamous cell carcinoma to predict prognosis or response to chemotherapy. However, in the research setting, a number of genomic changes have been described which are discussed in more detail in Chapter 2.

ADENOCARCINOMA

Adenocarcinoma is histologically defined as a malignant epithelial tumour with glandular and/or mucinous differentiation that has at least infiltrated into the lamina propria.

Barrett's oesophagus-the precursor lesion of adenocarcinoma

The normal oesophagus is lined with squamous epithelium with a sharp transition to gastric cardia-type mucosa at the Z line. Moersch et al.[29] and Hayward[30] were the first to suggest that the columnar lining of the oesophagus might be an acquired condition/adaptive response to recurrent injury of the squamous mucosa due to gastro-oesophageal reflux. In response to the damaging effect of reflux, the squamous epithelium changes

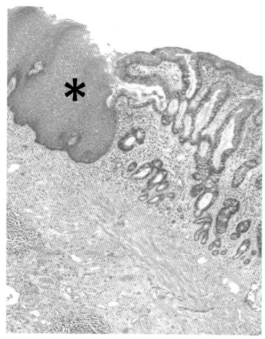

Fig. 1.6 Histology of Barrett's oesophagus. Haematoxylin/eosin-stained tissue section showing normal squamous epithelium on the left (*) and directly adjacent metaplastic intestinal-type mucosa with goblet cells as can be seen in Barrett's oesophagus. No evidence of dysplasia.

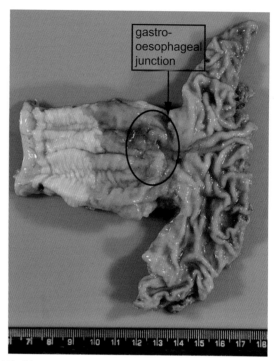

Fig. 1.7 Macroscopy of a distal oesophagectomy with Barrett's oesophagus and adenocarcinoma. An irregular, partly ulcerated tumour *(black circle)* is located at the gastro-oesophageal junction. Between the proximal edge of the tumour and the squamous lined oesophagus is metaplastic columnar epithelium. The squamocolumnar junction (border between the pale-appearing squamous epithelium and brownish-appearing metaplastic epithelium) is located at least 2.5 cm proximal to the gastro-oesophageal junction. (Courtesy of Dr B. Disep, Newcastle, UK.)

to a non-goblet columnar epithelium similar to gastric cardia type epithelium. Over time, this newly formed epithelium can differentiate into parietal and chief cells or develop goblet cells and Paneth cells. Barrett's oesophagus is defined as presence of metaplastic columnar epithelium in the oesophagus and is considered a precancerous lesion. For a histological illustration of Barrett's oesophagus, see Fig. 1.6.

Barrett's oesophagus is defined as an oesophagus in which any portion of the normal distal squamous lining has been replaced by metaplastic columnar epithelium, which is clearly visible endoscopically above the gastro-oesophageal junction and confirmed histopathologically.[31] In the UK, presence of intestinal metaplasia is considered highly corroborative but not specific for a diagnosis of Barrett's oesophagus. Ninety-five per cent of oesophageal adenocarcinomas are associated with Barrett's oesophagus, which has been identified as the single most important risk factor.

Further details about Barrett's oesophagus, including the proposed metaplasia–dysplasia–adenocarcinoma sequence and molecular pathology findings, can be found in Chapter 2.

Barrett's oesophagus-associated adenocarcinomas are located almost exclusively in the distal third of the oesophagus and often infiltrate into the proximal stomach (Fig. 1.7). The macroscopic appearances of a locally advanced adenocarcinoma are similar to that of squamous cell carcinoma or gastric adenocarcinoma (see Fig. 1.2). Histologically, oesophageal adenocarcinoma can be classified as having tubular, papillary, mucinous, or signet-ring cell patterns and are graded as well, moderately, or poorly differentiated according to the proportion of tumour that is composed of glands (see also gastric adenocarcinoma).[26] Approximately 10% of all oesophageal adenocarcinomas are of mucinous or signet-ring cell type.

Most patients present with locally advanced disease, e.g. tumour extension into the peri-oesophageal fat and involvement of regional lymph nodes. Should a patient present with early disease, it is important to remember that a duplication of the muscularis mucosae can be seen in many cases with Barrett's oesophagus. Carcinomas infiltrating between the two layers of the muscularis mucosae are still classified as 'intramucosal' (pT1a) cancers. However, carcinomas that have infiltrated into the double muscularis mucosae have been associated with a higher frequency of lymphoangioinvasion and lymph node metastases.[32]

There is an ongoing debate whether adenocarcinoma in the proximity of the oesophagogastric junction should be classified as oesophageal or gastric carcinoma, as both disease entities are currently treated with different multimodal therapy approaches. One problem is the lack of worldwide consensus on the definition of the 'gastro-oesophageal junction' (see WHO classification of digestive cancer, 4e, 2010).[26] The British Society of Gastroenterology guideline on the diagnosis and management of Barrett's oesophagus recommends using the distal end of the palisade vessels or the proximal end of the gastric folds to identify the gastro-oesophageal junction.[32]

Siewert et al.[34] defined different types of adenocarcinoma of the gastro-oesophageal junction based on the location of the 'tumour epicentre' by combining clinical preoperative findings (radiology, endoscopy) with intra- and postoperative observations:

- Type I: Adenocarcinoma of the distal oesophagus, which may infiltrate the gastro-oesophageal junction from above. This entity is also referred to as 'Barrett's oesophagus'. These adenocarcinomas have their centre within 1 cm to 5 cm above the anatomic gastro-oesophageal junction.
- Type II: 'True carcinoma of the cardia' arising from gastric cardia epithelium or from short segments of metaplastic columnar epithelium at the gastro-oesophageal junction. This entity is also referred to as 'junctional carcinoma'. These adenocarcinomas have their centre within 1 cm above and 2 cm below the anatomic gastro-oesophageal junction.
- Type III: Subcardial gastric carcinoma, which infiltrates the oesophagogastric junction and distal oesophagus from below. This entity is also referred to as 'proximal gastric carcinoma'. These adenocarcinomas have their centre within 2 cm and 5 cm below the anatomic gastro-oesophageal junction.

The TNM classification which is routinely used to stage cancers does not recognize cancers involving the gastro-oesophageal junction as own entity. In the current TNM classification (8th ed.), cancers in this location are classified either as oesophageal (epicentre located within the proximal 2 cm of the cardia) or as gastric (epicentre located within the distal 2 cm of the cardia) cancer.[34]

Rare types of malignant epithelial tumours of the oesophagus

1. **Adenoid cystic carcinoma** is very rare (0.1% of all oesophageal malignancies). These carcinomas are histologically identical to salivary gland-type adenoid cystic carcinoma and occur more frequently in males. These cancers are located in the middle third of the oesophagus and thought to arise from submucosal oesophageal glands and usually form well-circumscribed solid nodules in the submucosa with the overlying squamous epithelium showing no abnormality. Histologically, these tumours show glandular differentiation with epithelial and myoepithelial cells in true glandular and pseudoglandular lumina arranged in cribriform, tubular, or solid architecture.
2. **Adenosquamous carcinoma/mucoepidermoid carcinoma** is equally rare. They are located in the middle and lower oesophagus and are more frequent in males. Histologically they show an admixture of adenocarcinoma and squamous cell carcinoma. Some studies suggest that these cancers are more aggressive than conventional squamous cell carcinomas.

NEUROENDOCRINE NEOPLASMS

Neuroendocrine neoplasms (NEN) are epithelial neoplasms with neuroendocrine differentiation and include well-differentiated neuroendocrine tumours (NETs), poorly differentiated neuroendocrine carcinomas (NEC, small cell type versus large cell type), and mixed neuroendocrine-non-neuroendocrine neoplasms (MiNENs). Neuroendocrine differentiation needs to be confirmed by immunohistochemistry for synaptophysin and chromogranin A. Furthermore Ki67 immunohistochemistry is required to establish the proliferation index for grading (Ki67 index <3% = low grade (G1); 3–20% = intermediate grade (G2), >20% high grade (G3)).

Oesophageal NENs are exceedingly rare (<1% of all gastroenteropancreatic NENs), more frequent in males and

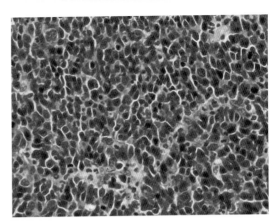

Fig. 1.8 Microscopic image of a neuroendocrine carcinoma.

mostly located in the distal oesophagus. The majority of oesophageal NENs are poorly differentiated neuroendocrine (small cell) carcinomas, which are highly aggressive with a median survival of 6–12 months or less. Histologically, these may appear as homogeneous tumours (Fig. 1.8) or consist of a mixture of squamous and mucoepidermoid elements. The main differential diagnosis of oesophageal small cell NECs are basaloid squamous cell carcinoma and metastasis of small cell carcinoma of the lung.

STOMACH

BENIGN TUMOURS AND TUMOUR-LIKE LESIONS OF THE STOMACH

GASTRIC POLYPS

Gastric polyps are usually found incidentally during endoscopy. According to the cell of origin, polyps can be epithelial, neuroendocrine, lymphohistiocytic (xanthelasma, lymphoid hyperplasia), mesenchymal (gastrointestinal stromal tumour, neural or vascular tumours), or mixed. They can be sporadic or occur as part of a syndrome. The epithelial gastric polyps can be subdivided into surface epithelial-derived polyps and gastric gland derived polyps (see Fig. 1.9).

It is clinically important to not only biopsy/excise the polyp, but also obtain biopsies from the background gastric mucosa at the same time.

Fundic gland polyps are the most common type of gastric polyps and are found in different clinical scenarios: (a) in patients taking proton pump inhibitors,[35] (b) sporadically, and (c) in hereditary polyposis syndromes (familial adenomatous polyposis (FAP),[36] gastric adenocarcinoma proximal polyposis of the stomach (GAPPS),[37] MUTYH-associated polyposis.[38]

Sporadic fundic gland polyps are more common in women and typically measure less than 0.5 cm. Histologically, the polyps show dilated oxyntic glands combined with foveolar hypoplasia. Interestingly, the incidence of fundic gland polyps is very low in patients with *Helicobacter pylori* infection.

✔✔ Seventy-five per cent of FAP-associated fundic gland polyps show an *APC* mutation, whereas sporadic fundic gland polyps are devoid of *APC* mutations and harbour *CTNNB1* (β-catenin) mutations in up to 90%.[39] While low-grade dysplasia is frequent in FAP patients with fundic gland polyps, dysplasia is very rare on sporadic fundic gland polyps.[40]

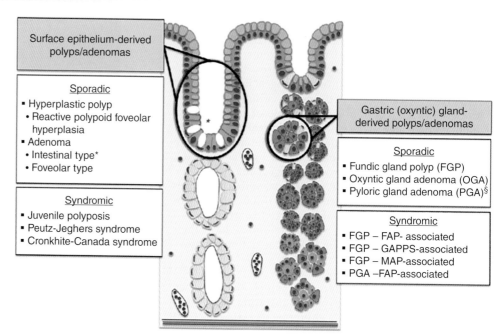

Surface epithelium-derived
polyps/adenomas

Sporadic
- Hyperplastic polyp
  - Reactive polypoid foveolar
    hyperplasia
- Adenoma
  - Intestinal type*
  - Foveolar type

Syndromic
- Juvenile polyposis
- Peutz-Jeghers syndrome
- Cronkhite-Canada syndrome

Gastric (oxyntic) gland-
derived polyps/adenomas

Sporadic
- Fundic gland polyp (FGP)
- Oxyntic gland adenoma (OGA)
- Pyloric gland adenoma (PGA)§

Syndromic
- FGP – FAP- associated
- FGP – GAPPS-associated
- FGP – MAP-associated
- PGA –FAP-associated

Fig. 1.9 Classification of gastric polyps according to the mucosal compartment of origin. (Histopathology 2021, 78, 106–124. https://doi.org/10.1111/his.14275)

Hyperplastic polyps are the second most common type of polyps in adults and the most commonly diagnosed polyp in children. They represent hyper-regenerative epithelium with oedematous lamina propria in response to a chronic inflammatory background. Thus, the background gastric mucosa is likely to show either *H. pylori*-related gastritis, autoimmune gastritis, or reactive gastropathy. Hyperplastic polyps are most frequently found in the antrum. Removal of the underlying injury (such as *H. pylori* infection) resulted in regression of the hyperplastic polyps in 70% of patients.[41] The management of patients with hyperplastic polyps depends on the size of the lesion (risk of malignant transformation increases for lesions > 25 mm),[40] whether dysplasia is detected or not, and presence of preneoplastic changes in the background mucosa.

Adenomatous polyps are subdivided into classic intestinal-type adenomas and non-intestinal-type adenomas such as pyloric gland adenoma, foveolar-type adenoma, and oxyntic gland adenoma. Non-intestinal-type adenomas are very rare and not further discussed here.

Sporadic intestinal-type adenomas are most common in patients over 70 years of age, more frequent in male, and most frequently found at the lesser curve of the antrum. They are usually solitary, less than 2 cm in diameter, and well circumscribed, pedunculated, or sessile. Their prevalence varies widely from 4% in Western countries to 27% in Japan. Adenomatous polyps are morphologically similar to conventional colonic tubular adenomas and there is usually chronic atrophic gastritis in the background. They are direct precursors of gastric adenocarcinomas and 50% of adenomatous polyps > 2 cm harbour an adenocarcinoma.[42]

Other lesions that can endoscopically appear as polyps in the stomach are: inflammatory fibroid polyps which consist of benign submucosal proliferations of spindle cells, small vessels, and inflammatory cells; xanthomas, which consist of aggregates of lipid-laden macrophages embedded in the lamina propria; and lipomas, which are circumscribed masses of adipose tissue without atypia usually located in the submucosa. Pancreatic heterotopia is the presence of

heterotopic pancreatic tissue within the stomach wall. It presents most commonly as a polypoid tumour-like lesion located within few centimetres of the pylorus.

POLYPOSIS SYNDROMES

Hamartomatous polyps are characterized by disorganized growth or normal tissue indigenous to the site. In the stomach they have been found in patients with Peutz–Jeghers syndrome, juvenile polyposis, Cronkhite–Canada syndrome, and Cowden disease. With the exception of Peutz–Jeghers polyps, the histological features of these polyps overlap with those of sporadic hyperplastic polyps. The pathological diagnosis of a 'syndromic polyp' requires knowledge of the clinical context. All patients with aforementioned polyposis syndromes have an increased risk of developing gastric carcinoma, which appears to be highest in patients with Peutz–Jeghers syndrome, at 30%.[43] Up to 80% of patients with Peutz–Jeghers syndrome have a germline mutation of the *STK11/LKB1* gene, which encodes an enzyme responsible for cell division, differentiation and signal transduction. The most common genetic alterations in patients with juvenile polyposis are germline mutation of *SMAD4* or *BMPR1A*, both genes implicated in the TGFbeta signaling pathway. Cowden disease is caused by germline mutations of *PTEN*, resulting in multiple hamartomas involving multiple different organs. Cronkhite–Canada syndrome is a non-inherited polyposis syndrome of unknown pathogenesis.

GASTRIC CARCINOMA

EPIDEMIOLOGY

Despite a steady decline of gastric carcinoma incidence at a rate of approximately 5% per year since the 1950s,[44] gastric carcinoma is still the fifth most common carcinoma in the world, with nearly one million people newly diagnosed per year, representing 8% of all new cancers diagnosed per year in the world. Age-standardised incidence rates of gastric carcinoma are twice as high in males as in females and show prominent geographical variation, ranging from 3.9 per 100 000 males in Northern Africa to 42.4 in Eastern Asia.[45] Approximately 75% of all gastric carcinoma are diagnosed in Asia. Gastric carcinoma is the third leading cause of cancer death in both sexes worldwide, responsible for 10% of all cancer deaths. A male: female ratio of 2:1 has been reported for non-cardia gastric carcinoma in contrast to a male: female ratio of 5:1 for gastric cardia carcinoma.[46] Although distal cancers still predominate in countries with the highest incidence, there has been a decrease in the incidence of mid or distal gastric carcinomas with a progressive increase in cardia carcinomas.

AETIOLOGY AND RISK FACTORS

Many aetiological factors for oesophageal and gastric carcinoma are shared, although their effect varies (Table 1.2). The nutritional effect of salt preservation of foods and vitamin deficiencies (riboflavin, vitamin A and C) are key components of the Correa hypothesis of progression for superficial mucosal inflammation to chronic gastritis and atrophy which increase susceptibility to other carcinogens. The prominent geographic variation in gastric carcinoma incidence suggests that environmental factors, such as *diet*, might play an important aetiological role. However, evidence for fruit and vegetable consumption, vitamin C supplementation, dietary salt, and nitroso compounds as risk factors is still conflicting.[47–49]

A dose-dependent relationship between *smoking* and gastric carcinoma risk has been shown in prospective studies and it has been estimated that 18% of gastric carcinomas in the European population were attributable to smoking.[50] There is currently no conclusive evidence for an association between alcohol consumption and gastric carcinoma.[51] An increased risk of gastric carcinoma after previous gastric surgery for benign peptic ulcer disease has been reported.[52]

Helicobacter pylori

In 1994, the International Agency for Research on Cancer designated *H. pylori* to be a type I carcinogen for gastric carcinoma.[53] Furthermore, there is evidence that *H. pylori* infection is a risk factor for gastric mucosa-associated lymphomas (MALT lymphomas), see later.

✔✔ Although the evidence for *H. pylori* inducing gastric carcinoma is convincing, not all those infected develop the disease. The risk of malignant transformation appears to be enhanced by bacterial virulence and host factors. *H. pylori* with cytotoxin-associated gene A (*cagA*) appears to be associated with the greatest risk.[54]

H. pylori infection increases the risk of gastric carcinoma up to sixfold and represents one of the most important environmental risk factors for the development of gastric carcinoma. Humans are the only known host for *H. pylori*, which can colonise the gastric body and the antrum (Fig. 1.10). The development of gastric carcinoma after *H. pylori* infection has been considered as a multistep process progressing from chronic active pan- or corpus-predominant gastritis to increasing loss of gastric glands (atrophy), replacement of the normal mucosa by intestinal metaplasia, and malignant transformation.[53–55] However, most *H. pylori*-infected individuals will remain asymptomatic and only 1–5% of the infected population will develop gastric carcinoma, a phenomenon that has been attributed to different bacterial strains, host-inflammatory genetic susceptibility, and in particular *H. pylori* virulence factors vacuolating cytotoxin antigen (VacA) and cytotoxin-associated gene A antigen (CagA).[54–56]

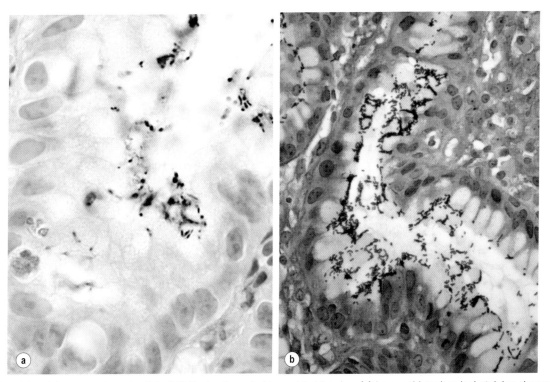

Fig. 1.10 Special staining procedures to detect *Helicobacter pylori* in gastric biopsies. **(a)** Immunohistochemical staining demonstrates the organisms as brown rods in the epithelial surface. **(b)** Warthin-Starry sliver staining shows individual spiral-shaped (black-coloured) organisms densely populating the surface epithelium.

The role of *H. pylori* infection in the aetiology of junctional cancer is unclear but appears to be evolving. It has been suggested that the reduction in acid production secondary to *H. pylori*-induced gastric atrophy could, in association with ammonia production from urea by the bacteria, protect the lower oesophagus by changing the content of the refluxing gastric juice. In countries with an increase in junctional cancer, there has been a corresponding decrease in incidence of *H. pylori* infection.

Epstein-Barr virus

It has been estimated that up to 10% of gastric carcinomas are associated with Epstein–Barr virus (EBV) infection.[57] In contrast to *H. pylori*, which has a role in the early stage of gastric carcinoma development as it can only bind to the surface of the normal gastric epithelial cell but not to the surface of gastric carcinoma cells, EBV is absent in normal or dysplastic gastric epithelial cells but present in gastric carcinoma cells.[58] For unknown reasons, EBV prevalence is higher in males and in gastric stump cancer.[59]

Hereditary cancer syndromes

Ten per cent of gastric carcinomas show familial clustering, but only 1–3% of gastric carcinomas are related to identified inherited gastric carcinoma predisposition syndromes such as hereditary diffuse gastric carcinoma (HDGC), Lynch syndrome, familial adenomatous polyposis (FAP), Peutz–Jeghers syndrome, Li–Fraumeni syndrome, and familial breast and ovarian cancer.[60,61] One of the defining characteristics of HDGC is the presence of a germline *CDH1* (Ecadherin) mutation.[62] The lifetime risk of developing gastric carcinoma in *CDH1* mutation carriers is 67% in males and 83% in females. Recently, a novel autosomal dominant syndrome of fundic gland polyposis and predisposition to gastric cancer of the intestinal type has been described. The syndrome has been termed gastric adenocarcinoma and proximal polyposis of the stomach (GAPPS) reflecting the fundic gland polyposis in the proximal part of the stomach and high risk of gastric carcinoma[40] and is considered to be a variant of FAP.

HDGC and GAPPS will be covered in detail in Chapter 2.

✓✓ Total gastrectomy is recommended for patients diagnosed with HDGC irrespective of tumour location or disease stage. The resection specimen should be worked up and reported according to the recommendations of the International Gastric Cancer Linkage Consortium (IGCLC).[63]

LESIONS PREDISPOSING TO GASTRIC CARCINOMA

Chronic atrophic gastritis and metaplasia

Inflammation of the gastric mucosa is most commonly the result of bacterial infection (most commonly due to *H. pylori* infection), chemical agents (non-steroidal anti-inflammatory drugs (NSAIDS), alcohol, bile reflux), or the consequence of an autoimmune process (i.e. autoimmune gastritis due to parietal cell auto-antibodies). Chronic inflammation can either result in the shrinkage or complete disappearance of the typical gastric glands followed by replacement fibrosis of the lamina propria or the replacement of the native glands by metaplastic glands (i.e. intestinal and/or pseudopyloric metaplasia). Under both conditions, there is 'atrophy' (loss of native gastric glands), but only the presence of metaplastic

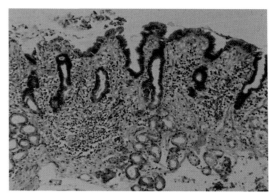

Fig. 1.11 Microscopic image showing gastric atrophy.

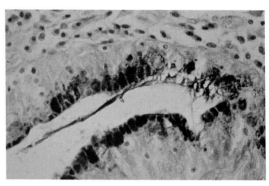

Fig. 1.12 Incomplete intestinal metaplasia (Type III) with sialomucins (blue-greenish) in goblet cells and neutral and sulfomucins (dark brown) in columnar cells. (Alcian blue-high-iron diamine staining technique to differentiate different mucin types).

glands is considered a condition with an increased risk of carcinoma development (Fig. 1.11).

Two main types of intestinal metaplasia have been defined depending on whether the epithelium is similar to small bowel epithelium or large bowel epithelium and on the histochemical characteristics of the mucin. Type I = complete, small bowel type, positive for neutral mucin and sialomucin, negative for sulfomucin; Type II/III = incomplete, large bowel type, positive or negative for neutral mucin, positive for sialomucin and sulfomucin (Fig. 1.12).

International guidelines for the secondary prevention of gastric carcinoma recommend using the OLGA (Operative Link on Gastritis Assessment) staging system to identify patients with low risk (stage 0–II) and high-risk (stage III–IV) gastritis to facilitate patient specific surveillance programmes.[64,65] This system grades the intensity of the inflammatory cells and stages the extent of atrophy in antrum and corpus biopsies separately.

✓ Some but not all studies indicate that there is a positive correlation between gastric carcinoma risk and degree and extent of incomplete intestinal metaplasia.

Chronic gastric ulcer

Chronic gastric ulcers are typically located at the edge of atrophic mucosa. If a chronic gastric ulcer is detected on endoscopy, it should be considered malignant until histology has proven otherwise. Patients with gastric ulcer have an increased risk for gastric carcinoma as gastric ulcer and gastric carcinoma have the same risk factors. Five per cent of endoscopically benign ulcers eventually prove to be malignant.

> **Box 1.1 Vienna classification of epithelial neoplasms of the gastrointestinal tract**
>
> 1. Negative for neoplasia
> 2. Indefinite for neoplasia
> 3. Non-invasive low-grade neoplasia
> 4. Non-invasive high-grade neoplasia:
>   4.1 High-grade adenoma
>   4.2 Non-invasive carcinoma
>   4.3 Suspicious for invasive carcinoma
> 5. Invasive adenocarcinoma:
>   5.1 Intramucosal carcinoma
>   5.2 Submucosal carcinoma or beyond

However, overall, less than 1% of all gastric carcinomas develop in pre-existing peptic ulcers.

Gastric polyps

These are discussed earlier.

Gastric dysplasia

Gastric dysplasia (synonym: intraepithelial neoplasia) can have a flat, slightly depressed or polypoid growth pattern. In Europe and North America, polypoid dysplasia is termed 'adenoma' whereas in Japan, dysplasia with any growth pattern is called 'adenoma'.

The prevalence of gastric dysplasia varies between 20% in high-risk areas in Asia and 4% in Western countries.[66] Dysplasia is more frequent in males and patients over the age of 70 years, and most commonly affects the lesser curve and the antrum. Histologically, dysplasia is characterised by architectural as well as cytological atypia and is stratified into two grades, low-grade dysplasia (LGD) and high-grade dysplasia (HGD). In a recent retrospective multicentre study, only 4.3% of LGD cases progressed to invasive carcinoma (median follow-up: 2.6 years). In 59% of the patients with HGD, GC was diagnosed histologically within 12 months of the initial diagnosis.

The diagnosis of dysplasia shows significant inter-observer variability due to the low specificity of the abnormalities used to establish the diagnosis and in particular the difficulties in distinguishing regenerative atypia from dysplasia and high-grade dysplasia from intramucosal carcinoma. In an attempt to standardise the terminology used to describe the morphological spectrum of lesions, several proposals, including the Padova and Vienna classifications (Box 1.1), have been made.[67–69]

Whilst chromosomal and microsatellite instability, *APC* and *p53* mutations, as well as CpG-island methylation, have all been found in gastric dysplasia, none of these molecular findings is specific enough to establish and support the diagnosis of dysplasia in routine clinical practice.

EARLY AND ADVANCED GASTRIC CARCINOMA

Early gastric carcinoma is defined as adenocarcinoma limited to the mucosa or submucosa with or without regional lymph node metastases.[70] The term 'early' does not refer to the size or age of the lesion. Gastric carcinoma infiltrating into the muscularis propria and beyond is defined as 'advanced'. These two categories of gastric carcinoma differ not only in prognosis but also often with respect to morphology and clinical aspects. Early gastric carcinoma has an excellent prognosis, with a 5-year survival rate exceeding 90% in Japan.[71,72] The 5-year survival rate of advanced gastric carcinomas, the most frequent type in the West, is around 23% when treated by surgery alone and around 36% when treatment includes perioperative cytotoxic chemotherapy.[73] Long-term follow-up studies have shown that the tumour growth rate can differ significantly between early and advanced carcinomas; a doubling time of several years for early carcinoma but less than a year for advanced carcinoma has been estimated.[74,75]

The macroscopic appearance differs between early and advanced gastric carcinoma.

The macroscopic growth pattern of advanced carcinomas is classified according to Borrmann into four major types.[76] Type V is used for unclassifiable cancers. Early gastric carcinomas are macroscopically Borrmann type '0' and classified according to Murakami as protruding, superficial elevated/flat/depressed, and excavated (Figs. 1.2 and 1.13).

The classification of the macroscopic tumour appearance can be used by radiologists, endoscopists, and pathologists alike. Consistent use of this macroscopic classification can greatly improve the communication within the multidisciplinary treatment team. Interestingly, approximately 10% of gastric carcinomas retain their endoscopic and radiologic 'early cancer' appearance as they progress to advanced stage.[77] This may lead to a potential underestimation of the 'true' clinical disease stage at the time of diagnosis.

In Japan, approximately 2% of early gastric carcinoma recur after curative resection. Submucosal invasion, lymph node metastases, and differentiated type histology have been associated with increased risk of recurrence.[78] Differentiated histology is a risk factor for recurrence as cancers with differentiated histology show a higher incidence of haematogenous spread compared to undifferentiated cancers which are more prone to recur in lymph nodes or serosa-lined cavities. The incidence of lymph node metastases is 2–3% for intramucosal carcinomas[79,80] and 20–30% for submucosal carcinomas.[81]

Risk factors for lymph node metastasis in early gastric carcinoma include younger age at time of diagnosis, size greater than 20 mm, depressed macroscopic type, undifferentiated histology, presence of an ulcer or scar, lymphatic invasion, and submucosal invasion by more than 500 µm.[79,81]

For advanced gastric carcinoma, depth of infiltration into the wall (T stage) and number of lymph nodes with metastatic tumour (N stage) remain the strongest prognostic indicators.

MORPHOLOGICAL SUBTYPES OF GASTRIC CARCINOMA

The histology of gastric carcinoma is characterised by marked intra- and inter-tumoural heterogeneity. The variability of the histological appearance seems to increase with increasing depth of infiltration into the wall and increasing patient age at time of diagnosis. As a result of this marked morphological diversity, a number of different classification systems have been advocated by different authors such as Laurén,[82] Ming,[83] Nakamura,[84] Mulligan,[85] Goseki,[86] Carneiro,[87] and the World Health Organisation (WHO).[10] Table 1.3 provides a 'conversion' table between the different histological subtypes.

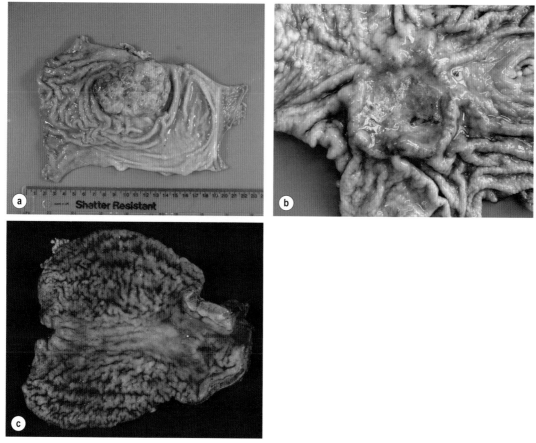

Fig. 1.13 The macroscopic appearances of advanced gastric carcinoma. **(a)** Polypoid (Borrmann type I). **(b)** Ulcerating (Borrmann Type III). **(c)** Linitis plastica (Borrmann Type IV) with diffuse infiltration of the wall of the stomach by tumour and apparent thickening of the rugal folds.

Table 1.3   Comparison of histological types according to different classification systems.

Lauren (1965)	Nakamura et al (1968)	JGCA (2017)	WHO 5th ed (2019)
Intestinal	Differentiated	• Papillary • Well differentiated tubular • Moderately differentiated tubular	• Papillary • Well differentiated tubular • Moderately differentiated tubular
Indeterminate	Undifferentiated	• Poorly differentiated tubular type (solid type)	• Poorly differentiated tubular type (solid type)
Diffuse	Undifferentiated	• Signet-ring cell type • Poorly differentiated non-solid type	• Poorly cohesive, signet-ring cell type • Poorly cohesive, other cell types
Not defined	Not defined	• Mucinous	• Mucinous
Mixed	Not defined	• Description according to proportion of subtype	• Mixed
Not defined	Not defined	Special types: • Adenosquamous • Squamous cell carcinoma • Undifferentiated • Carcinoma with lymphoid stroma • Hepatoid adenocarcinoma • Adenocarcinoma with enteroblastic differentiation • Adenocarcinoma of fundic gland type	Special types: • Adenosquamous • Squamous cell carcinoma • Undifferentiated • Carcinoma with lymphoid stroma • Hepatoid adenocarcinoma • Adenocarcinoma with enteroblastic differentiation • Adenocarcinoma of fundic gland type • Micropapillary adenocarcinoma

✔ The histological classification according to Laurén (intestinal-type versus diffuse-type versus mixed-type), Ming (expanding-type versus infiltrative-type), and WHO (tubular versus papillary versus mucinous versus poorly cohesive including signet-ring versus mixed) are the classifications most commonly used outside of Japan.

In Japan, the recommended histological typing is similar but not 100% identical to the WHO classification.[88] In the West, 60–70% of gastric carcinomas are classified as intestinal-type according to Laurén (Fig. 1.14a). Intestinal-type carcinomas are usually sharply demarcated and have a pushing margin according to Ming's classification. Laurén's diffuse-type is composed of scattered poorly cohesive cells or small clusters of cells and is diffusely infiltrative (Fig. 1.14b). Cells may contain cytoplasmic mucus, which compresses the nucleus to a sickle-like shape and gives the whole cell a 'signet-ring' cell appearance (Fig. 1.14c). Gastric carcinomas that consist of approximately 50% diffuse and 50% intestinal-type, solid type carcinomas, and others that cannot be classified as diffuse or intestinal are called indeterminate, unclassifiable, or mixed according to Lauren classification. Note that the definition of 'mixed-type' according to the WHO 2019 classification is different.[26] The WHO classification defines 'mixed-type' as a cancer that has a poorly cohesive component and a non-poorly cohesive component irrespective of the relative percentages.

Intestinal-type carcinomas are more common in males over 60 years of age and in high-risk countries, are located in the antrum, show a Borrmann Type II growth pattern, and metastasise to the liver. In contrast, diffuse-type carcinomas are more common in younger females, have a similar incidence in most countries, are located predominantly in the proximal body of the stomach, and show a linitis plastica-type growth pattern with transperitoneal metastases.

Gastric carcinomas are graded as well differentiated (more than 90% of the carcinoma consists of well-formed glands), moderately differentiated (intermediate between well and poor), and poorly differentiated (highly irregular glands which may be difficult to recognise as glands). Grading of tumour differentiation is prone to considerable interobserver variation and therefore the value of the histological subtyping and/or tumour grading in predicting patient prognosis is still controversial.

Rare morphological variants of gastric carcinoma

Gastric carcinomas with prominent lymphoid stroma (so called medullary carcinoma) are associated with EBV infection in 80% of cases. Medullary carcinomas are more common in males, predominantly located in the proximal stomach, and more common in the remnant stomach. The prognosis of this subtype is better than conventional gastric carcinoma, with a 5-year survival rate of 75%. Hepatoid and alpha-fetoprotein-producing carcinomas are particular aggressive carcinomas with high AFP serum levels.

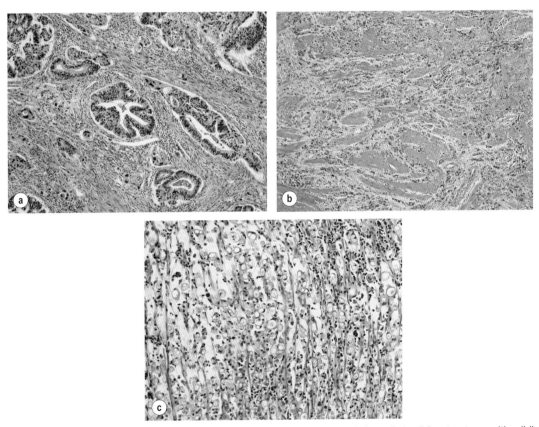

Fig. 1.14 **(a)** Intestinal-type carcinoma tubular subtype composed of irregularly sized and shaped glandular structures with mildly pleomorphic nuclei. However, this tumour is admixed with poorly differentiated tubular structures with large cells and bizarre-shaped nuclei. **(b)** Diffuse-type carcinoma. Poorly cohesive single cells are diffusely infiltrating the smooth muscle wall. **(c)** Signet ring cell carcinoma. The neoplastic cells are characterised by large amount of intracytoplasmic mucin (almost 'clear' cytoplasm) with eccentrically located and mostly flattened nuclei.

Adenosquamous carcinomas consist of at least 25% squamous elements. These tumours are deeply invasive and associated with lymphovascular invasion and poor prognosis.

Molecular pathology of gastric carcinoma will be discussed in detail in Chapter 2

MACROSCOPY AND MICROSCOPY OF EPITHELIAL TUMOURS OF THE OESOPHAGUS AND STOMACH AFTER NEOADJUVANT THERAPY

Neoadjuvant chemo(radio)therapy is standard of care for patients with locally advanced resectable gastric and oesophageal cancer in the West since the publication of landmark trials such as the MAGIC trial, OE02 trial, and CROSS trial. Adjuvant chemotherapy is currently favoured in Asian patients based on the results from ACTS-GC and CLASSIC trial

The macroscopic appearance of epithelial tumours can change dramatically after preoperative chemo(radio)therapy depending on the extent of tumour response. These changes can be asymmetric, thus for the classification of tumours according to the Siewert or TNM classification into oesophageal, junctional, or gastric cancer, it is recommended to use the pre-treatment findings.

Histologically, squamous cell carcinoma and adenocarcinoma appearance can change after neoadjuvant chemo(radio)therapy showing extensive necrosis, inflammation, fibrosis, and foreign body type granulomas around keratin pearls.

✓✓ The regression grading according to Mandard et al.[89] considers the relative proportion of residual viable tumour cells and fibrosis in the primary cancer after neoadjuvant chemo(radio)therapy and is currently the one most commonly used in the UK.

Very recently, a grading system to assess tumour regression in lymph nodes has been proposed and showed prognostic significance in a small series of patients.[90] There is also evidence that lymph node status after preoperative chemotherapy is more relevant for predicting prognosis than primary tumour regression.[91]

NEUROENDOCRINE NEOPLASMS OF THE STOMACH

Neuroendocrine neoplasms (NEN) are epithelial neoplasms with neuroendocrine differentiation and include well-differentiated neuroendocrine tumours (NETs), poorly differentiated neuroendocrine carcinomas (NEC, small cell type versus large cell type) and mixed neuroendocrine-non-neuroendocrine neoplasms (MiNENs). Neuroendocrine differentiation needs to be confirmed by immunohistochemistry for synaptophysin and chromogranin A. furthermore, Ki67 immunohistochemistry is required to establish the proliferation index for NEN grading (Ki67 index < 3% = low grade (G1); 3–20% = intermediate grade (G2), > 20% high grade (G3)).

The gastric mucosa contains several types of neuroendocrine cells, which produce histamine, ghrelin, somatostatin, serotonin, gastrin and other neurotransmitter and releases them into the bloodstream. Histamine-secreting enterochromaffin-like cells are exclusively located in the fundus/body and gastric producing G cells are only found in the antrum.

Gastric NENs arise most commonly from histamine-secreting enterochromaffin-like (ECL) cells located in the corpus/fundus. Hypergastrinaemia due to unregulated hormone release by a gastrinoma or due to hyperplasia of gastrin-producing cells in the antrum secondary to achlorhydria is consistently associated with hyperplasia of the ECL cells.[92]

The incidence of gastric neuroendocrine neoplasms has been increasing about 15-fold over the last decades and accounts for 6% of all gastrointestinal neuroendocrine tumours.[93] For an overview of gastric NENs, their frequency, and clinicopathological features, see Table 1.4.

NET type 1 occur almost exclusively in females, are usually limited to mucosa and submucosa, and metastases are confined to local regional lymph nodes.

NET type 2 occur associated with Zollinger-Ellison syndrome in patients with MEN type 1 disease, and are equally common in males and females. These tumours often extend deep into the muscle wall. The loss of the tumour suppressor gene *MEN1* on chromosome 11q13 is seen in the majority of these tumours, a defect also found in those tumours of the gut, pancreas, and parathyroid associated with MEN1.[94]

NET type 3 are more common in males, tend to be larger, and have a more aggressive behaviour. Serosal infiltration with lymphatic and vascular invasion and liver metastasis with an accompanying carcinoid syndrome are common. Metastases are present in 52% of cases and approximately one-third of the patients will have died within 51 months.

✓✓ Grading of neuroendocrine tumours with a combination of the morphological features and the proliferation fraction (mitotic index or Ki67 index) has shown to be of prognostic value. Grade 1 neuroendocrine tumours typically have a Ki67 index below 3%, whereas grade 3 tumours are poorly differentiated, have a Ki67 index above 20%, show necrosis, and are classified as neuroendocrine carcinomas. Guidelines for the management of gastric neuroendocrine tumours have been updated recently.[95]

Table 1.4   Selected clinicopathological characteristics of gastric neuroendocrine neoplasms

Tumour type	Frequency	Pathogenesis	Multiplicity	Background gastric mucosa	Acid secretion
NET type 1	80–90% of NET	Hypergastrinaemia	Yes	Atrophic gastritis	Low
NET type 2	5–7% of NET	MEN 1 hypergastrininaemia	Yes	Parietal cell hyperplasia	High
NET type 3	10–15% of NET	Sporadic	Uncommon	No specific change	Normal
NEC	Rare	Sporadic	No	No specific change	Normal
MiNEN/ MANEC	Rare	Sporadic	No	No specific change	normal

MEN 1, Multiple endocrine neoplasia type 1; *MiNEN/MANEC*, mixed neuroendocrine-non-neuroendocrine neoplasma; *NEC*, neuroendocrine carcinoma; *NET*, neuroendocrine tumour.

MESENCHYMAL TUMOURS OF THE STOMACH

Non-epithelial tumours such as glomus tumour, inflammatory myofibroblastic tumours, leiomyoma, leiomyosarcoma, schwannoma, synovial sarcoma and Kaposi sarcoma are all rare in the stomach and will not be discussed here.

This chapter will focus on gastrointestinal stromal tumours (GIST), which are the most common primary mesenchymal tumours of the gastrointestinal tract and 60–70% of GISTs occur in the stomach. Most GISTs are sporadic, but 5–10% occur in association with syndromes, namely Carney's triad, Carney-Stratakis syndrome, neurofibromatosis type 1 or can extremely rarely be familial due to germline mutations of the *KIT* and *PDGFRA* genes.

GISTs can occur in any part of the stomach and vary from small nodules in the wall, which are covered by intact mucosa to large masses leading to gastric outlet obstruction. Histologically, GISTs are variable and can show spindle cell morphology or epithelioid histology or mixtures thereof.

GISTs are strongly immunoreactive for KIT (CD117), DOG1 and often also for CD34. Even if all common immunohistochemical markers are unexpectedly negative, it is still legitimate to make the diagnosis of a GIST based on morphology alone. However, those cases should be investigated for relevant mutations. 85% GISTs contain *KIT* or *PDGFRA*-activating mutations. *KIT*-activating mutations are most frequently found in exon 11 and most GISTs with *KIT* mutations are imatinib-sensitive whereas GISTs with *PDGFRA*-activating mutations are usually imatinib-resistant. With the exception of very small tumours, all GISTs have the potential to become malignant. The management of gastric GISTs is discussed in detail in Chapter 10.

✔✔ A combination of site of origin, size and mitotic index has been shown to predict the risk of progressive disease in patients with GISTs (Table 1.5).[96]

LYMPHOMA OF THE STOMACH

Any type of lymphoma can also occur in the gastrointestinal tract, which is the most common extranodal site. Within the gastrointestinal tract, 50–75% of lymphomas are located in the stomach. Five to ten percent of all gastric malignancies are primary lymphomas. The two most common subtypes of primary gastric lymphomas are extranodal marginal-zone lymphoma of the mucosa-associated lymphoid tissue (so called MALT lymphoma) and diffuse large B-cell lymphoma. The incidence of primary gastric lymphoma is similar in males and females.

MALT lymphoma

It is thought that the development of MALT lymphoma is a multistage process initiated by chronic active inflammation due to *H. pylori* infection. Eradication of *H. pylori* with antibiotics has been shown to be associated with MALT lymphoma remission in up to 77% of patients within 12 months. Less than 10% relapse, and this could be due to reinfection with *H. pylori*; in the absence of reinfection, the relapse appears to be self-limiting.

The majority of MALT lymphomas occur in patients over the age of 50 years, with equal sex distribution, who present clinically with either symptoms suggesting a diagnosis of gastritis or peptic ulcer disease or are asymptomatic. The tumours appear macroscopically as an ill-defined thickening of the mucosa with erosions, sometimes ulcerated (Fig. 1.15) and are frequently multifocal. Gastric MALT lymphoma can spread to the regional lymph nodes. MALT lymphoma is composed of neoplastic small B cells, which resemble follicle centre cells and are termed centrocyte-like, whereas other cells show plasma cell differentiation and occasionally there are blast cells. The characteristic lymphoepithelial lesion (Fig. 1.16) is composed of small to medium-sized tumour cells (B cells) with irregular nuclei that infiltrate the pit epithelium. The presence of such a lesion should raise the question of a lymphoma but it is not pathognomonic of a lymphoma and may be seen in *H. pylori*-associated gastritis.

Cytogenetic studies show three major translocations in MALT lymphomas: t(11:18)(q21;q21)/*API2-MALT1* (30–40% of cases), t(14:18)(q32:q21)/*IGH-MALT1* and t(1:14)(p22:q32)/*IGH-BCL10*. Some of the translocations have been related with unresponsiveness to *H. pylori* eradication. Other translocations are associated with the juxtaposition of *BCL10* to the immunoglobulin heavy chain gene resulting in deregulation of the immunoglobulin. In addition, there is loss or mutation of *p53*, *c-MYC* mutation, inactivation of *p15/p16* by hypermethylation and *FAS* gene mutation.

Most low-grade MALT lymphomas are associated with disease confined to the gastric mucosa with slow dissemination. The favourable clinical behaviour may reflect the partial dependence on the *H. pylori* antigenic drive. The progression to the more common high-grade MALT lymphoma is thought to require the acquisition of further genetic

Table 1.5 Prediction of malignant potential of gastrointestinal stromal tumours

Tumour parameters		Risk of progressive disease (metastasis or tumour-related death)			
Mitotic index	Size	Gastric	Duodenum	Jejunum/ileum	Rectum
≤ 5 (in 5 mm²)	≤ 2 cm	None (0%)	None (0%)	None (0%)	None (0%)
	≤ 2 to ≤ 5 cm	Very low (1.9%)	Low (8.3%)	Low (4.3%)	Low (8.5%)
	> 5 to ≤ 10 cm	Low (3.6%)	(Insufficient data)	Moderate (24%)	(Insufficient data)
	> 10 cm	Moderate (10%)	High (34%)	High (52%)	High (57%)
> 5 (in 5 mm²)	≤ 2 cm	(Insufficient data)	(Insufficient data)	High (limited data)	High (54%)
	≤ 2 to ≤ 5 cm	Moderate (16%)	High (50%)	High (73%)	High (52%)
	> 5 to ≤ 10 cm	High (55%)	(Insufficient data)	High (85%)	(Insufficient data)
	> 10 cm	High (86%)	High (86%)	High (90%)	High (71%)

Reproduced from Royal College of Pathologists Dataset for gastrointestinal stromal tumours, published January 2020.

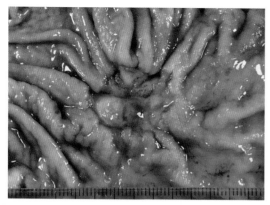

Fig. 1.15 Macroscopic image of stomach with lymphoma.

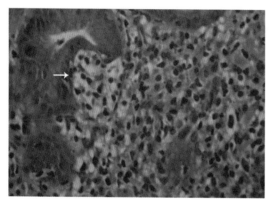

Fig. 1.16 Microscopic image of lymphoepithelial lesion *(white arrow)*.

abnormalities.[97] Gastric MALT lymphoma with the t(11:18)(q21;q21) translocation should be treated with chemotherapy or radiation together with *H. pylori* eradication, as *H. pylori* eradication alone is ineffective. The other lymphomas which are resistant to *H. pylori* eradication are those with abnormalities of the *BCL10* locus or those associated with autoimmune gastritis. These can be identified by strong nuclear staining with anti-BCL10 in the former and in the latter by staining with the product of the *FAS* oncogene. These non-responsive lymphomas can be treated surgically or by surgery in combination with chemoradiotherapy. The 5-year survival for localised cases is 90–100%. Continued follow-up of these patients is recommended as it is now recognised that synchronous and metachronous adenocarcinomas can occur.[98]

DIFFUSE LARGE B-CELL LYMPHOMA

Primary gastric diffuse large B-cell lymphoma is composed of B-cells with a nuclear size equivalent to a macrophage nucleus or at least twice the size of a normal lymphocyte. Similar to MALT lymphoma, the neoplastic cells destroy the gastric glandular architecture. Up to 50% of diffuse large B-cell lymphomas have foci of MALT lymphomas and regression of diffuse large B-cell lymphoma after eradication of *H. pylori* has been reported. Macroscopically, this lymphoma appears as a large ulcerated mass mimicking advanced gastric carcinoma.

Chromosomal translocations involving the immunoglobulin heavy chain gene locus are frequent in diffuse large cell lymphomas resulting in deregulation of *BCL6*, *BCL2* and *MYC*.[99] In the presence of EBV, diffuse large B-cell lymphomas are more likely to be resistant to chemoradiotherapy.[100]

Key points

- Squamous cell dysplasia is regarded as a precancerous condition of the oesophagus. In screened high-risk populations, the finding of dysplasia predates the development of carcinoma by approximately 5 years.
- It is difficult to distinguish between distal oesophageal adenocarcinoma and proximal gastric adenocarcinoma in advanced cancers based on the location of the tumour with respect to the gastro-oesophageal junction. Intestinal metaplasia can indicate the presence of Barrett's oesophagus, but can also occur in the stomach.
- The pathogenesis of gastric carcinoma is complex and multifactorial with several potential precursor lesions including gastric dysplasia.
- Although it is possible to reverse the inflammatory and some of the intestinal metaplastic changes associated with *H. pylori* infection, atrophy and the colonic-type intestinal metaplasia (type III – incomplete metaplasia) are regarded as irreversible. There is continuing controversy as to the value of identifying the colonic-type mucin and its predictive value in identifying patients at risk of developing cancer.
- There are several problems associated with histological interpretation of grades of glandular oesophageal and gastric dysplasia; these include high inter-observer variation, distinguishing regenerative atypia from true dysplasia, the ability to differentiate high-grade dysplasia from intramucosal carcinoma, and a lack of experience due to the relative rarity of dysplasia, especially in low-incidence Western countries.
- There are several classifications for gastric carcinoma, the most widely used being Laurén's classification. The tumours are divided into two main types: those that form glandular structures are known as intestinal-type, while those without glandular structures are referred to as diffuse-type carcinomas. Those with a mixed, solid, or unusual appearance are regarded as unclassifiable/indeterminate.
- The molecular features characterising intestinal-type and diffuse-type gastric carcinoma suggest that the different histological phenotype is related to a different underlying genetic phenotype and most likely different aetiology.
- Abnormalities of the *CDH1* (Ecadherin) gene and aberrant expression of this protein have been found in up to 90% of sporadic gastric carcinomas, especially the diffuse-type. Germline *CDH1* mutations are the defining molecular defect in hereditary diffuse gastric cancer.
- The stomach is the commonest site for gastrointestinal lymphomas which are mostly B-cell non-Hodgkin's lymphomas. The most common lymphoma is low-grade MALT lymphoma thought to be initiated by *H. pylori* infection. Several different chromosomal translocations have been identified, some of them conferring therapy resistance.
- Three subgroups of patients with neuroendocrine tumours (formerly called 'carcinoids') can be identified. Most are benign and associated with overgrowth of the ECL cells. Solitary lesions frequently metastasise.

 References available at http://ebooks.health.elsevier.com/

KEY REFERENCES

[10] WHO Classification of Tumours Editorial Board. Digestive system tumour. Lyon (France): International Agency for Research on Cancer; 2019. WHO classification of tumour series. 5th ed. vol. 1.

[12] Esophageal cancer. epidemiology, pathogenesis and prevention. Nat Clin Pract Gastroenterol Hepatol 2008;5(9):517–26. https://doi.org/10.1038/ncpgasthep1223.

[14] Islami F, Sheikhattari P, Ren JS, Kamangar F. Gastric atrophy and risk of oesophageal cancer and gastric cardia adenocarcinoma–a systematic review and meta-analysis. Ann Oncol 2011;22(4):754–60. https://doi.org/10.1093/annonc/mdq411. Epub 2010 Sep 22. PMID: 20860989.

[19] Praud D, Rota M, Rehm J, et al. Cancer incidence and mortality attributable to alcohol consumption. Int J Cancer 2016;138(6):1380–7. https://doi.org/10.1002/ijc.29890.

[32] Fitzgerald RC, di Pietro M, Ragunath K, et al. British Society of Gastroenterology guidelines on the diagnosis and management of Barrett's oesophagus. Gut 2014;63:7–42. PMID: 24165758.

[40] Abraham SC, Nobukawa B, Giardiello FM, et al. Sporadic fundic gland polyps: common gastric polyps arising through activating mutations in the beta-catenin gene. Am J Pathol 2001;158:1005–10. PMID: 11238048.

[45] GBD 2017 Stomach Cancer Collaborators. The global, regional, and national burden of stomach cancer in 195 countries, 1990-2017: a systematic analysis for the Global Burden of Disease study 2017. Lancet Gastroenterol Hepatol 2020;5(1):42–54. https://doi.org/10.1016/S2468-1253(19)30328-0. [published correction appears in Lancet Gastroenterol Hepatol. 2020 Mar;5(3):e2].

[55] Seeneevassen L, Bessède E, Mégraud F, Lehours P, Dubus P, Varon C. Gastric cancer: advances in carcinogenesis research and new therapeutic strategies. Int J Mol Sci 2021;22(7):3418. Published 2021 Mar 26. https://doi.org/10.3390/ijms22073418.

[60] Sun K, Jia K, Lv H, et al. EBV-positive gastric cancer: current knowledge and future perspectives. Front Oncol 2020;10:583463. Published 2020 Dec 14. https://doi.org/10.3389/fonc.2020.583463.

[63] Blair VR, McLeod M, Carneiro F, et al. Hereditary diffuse gastric cancer: updated clinical practice guidelines. Lancet Oncol 2020;21(8):e386–97. https://doi.org/10.1016/S1470-2045(20)30219-9.

[64] Rugge M, Meggio A, Pravadelli C, Barbareschi M, Fassan M, Gentilini M, et al. Gastritis staging in the endoscopic follow-up for the secondary prevention of gastric cancer: a 5-year prospective study of 1755 patients. Gut 2019;68(1):11–7. https://doi.org/10.1136/gutjnl-2017-314600. Epub 2018 Jan 6. PMID: 29306868.

[72] Huang Q, Zou X. Clinicopathology of early gastric carcinoma: an update for pathologists and gastroenterologists. Gastrointest Tumors 2017;3(3–4):115–24. https://doi.org/10.1159/000456005.

[79] Yamao T, Shirao K, Ono H, et al. Risk factors for lymph node metastasis from intramucosal gastric carcinoma. Cancer 1996;77:602–6. PMID: 8616749.

[81] Tajima Y, Murakami M, Yamazaki K, et al. Risk factors for lymph node metastasis from gastric cancers with submucosal invasion. Ann Surg Oncol 2010;17:1597–604. PMID: 20131014.

[88] Mandard AM, Dalibard F, Mandard JC, et al. Pathologic assessment of tumor regression after preoperative chemoradiotherapy of esophageal carcinoma. Clinicopathologic correlations. Cancer 1994;73:2680–6. PMID: 8194005.

[94] Ramage JK, Ahmed A, Ardill J, et al. Guidelines for the management of gastroenteropancreatic neuroendocrine (including carcinoid) tumours (NETs). Gut 2012;61:6–32. PMID: 22052063.

[95] Miettinen M, Lasota J. Histopathology of gastrointestinal stromal tumor. J Surg Oncol 2011;104:865–73. PMID: 22069171.

2 Genetics and early detection of oesophageal and gastric cancer

Andreas V. Hadjinicolaou | Rebecca C. Fitzgerald

INTRODUCTION

There has been an increase in the incidence of oesophageal and oesophagogastric junctional (OGJ) cancers in many Western countries, especially amongst White males. In contrast, stomach cancer incidence has declined except for proximal cancers in the gastric cardia. Both oesophageal and gastric cancers (GCs) are associated with < 20% survival at 5 years, mainly as a result of late diagnosis at advanced non-curable stages of disease.[1,2] Consequently, there is now a focus on early detection and secondary prevention, with the aim to move towards more personalised screening and surveillance strategies. These efforts have been supported by an increased understanding of the natural history of these cancers including risk factors, cellular and genetic pathology, and the identification of premalignant lesions and cancer precursors. In this chapter, we discuss the early detection of oesophago-GCs and provide evidence-based, practical suggestions for screening, surveillance, diagnosis, and management. Finally, we discuss genetic aberrations and their applications in biomarker discovery.

TYPES OF OESOPHAGEAL CANCER

Oesophageal cancer continues to be classified on the basis of anatomical location and histopathology, although molecular features are starting to inform clinical management. It comprises of two distinct types—oesophageal adenocarcinoma (OAC), including OGJ adenocarcinomas, and oesophageal squamous cell carcinoma (OSCC).

PREMALIGNANT CONDITIONS

BARRETT'S OESOPHAGUS

The risk of OAC associated with gastro-oesophageal reflux disease (GORD) is related to chronic injury of the distal oesophagus[3] and the development of Barrett's oesophagus (BO), now widely accepted as a key precursor to oesophageal and OGJ adenocarcinoma, with BO patients having a relative risk of around 11 compared to the general population.[4,5]

Most adenocarcinomas are diagnosed *de novo* and BO is not always evident histologically, leading to questions about whether all adenocarcinomas do in fact arise from Barrett's metaplasia, or whether Barrett's is a pre-requisite but in some cases the cancer overgrows the precursor.[6] In a meta-analysis from 2018, only 11.8% of patients with OAC had a previous diagnosis of BO.[7]

DEFINITION OF BARRETT'S OESOPHAGUS

The latest British Society of Gastroenterology (BSG) guidelines define BO as an abnormal acquired state in which a segment of squamous epithelium in the distal oesophagus is transformed into columnar epithelium via a process known as metaplasia.[8] While all pathological subtypes are included in the BSG definition, surveillance is limited to cases of intestinal metaplasia ([IM]; and longer segments where sampling bias may have missed focal IM). The American College of Gastroenterology (ACG) guidelines and the more recent position of the European Society of Gastrointestinal Endoscopy (ESGE) necessitate the histological presence of IM in order to make a diagnosis.[9,10]

EPIDEMIOLOGY OF BARRETT'S OESOPHAGUS

Prevalence

Assessing the prevalence of BO is challenging as it often asymptomatic. Therefore, rates are generally extrapolated from endoscopy performed for individuals with reflux symptoms. Overall, it appears that the population prevalence of BO, proved histologically, is around 1–2%.[11] This rises to 5–15% for patients with GORD symptoms.[12] According to a Dutch study of 500,000 medical records, the incidence of BO has been increasing, even when accounting for the number of upper GI endoscopies performed.[13] This is likely to be related to the increase in GORD prevalence, a reduction in *Helicobacter pylori* and rise in obesity, and also increased recognition amongst endoscopists.

According to the Barrett's Esophagus Study, a US-based multicentre consortium of 3643 patients with BO, at index endoscopy 70.1% of the cohort had non-dysplastic BO (ND-BO), 11.5% had low-grade dysplasia (LGD), 5.4% had high-grade dysplasia (HGD), and 5.1% had OAC.[14] The study showed that there has been a significant increase in the prevalence of HGD and OAC, respectively, at index endoscopy over the last 25 years, whereas LGD levels remained stable.

RISK FACTORS FOR BARRETT'S OESOPHAGUS

Gastro-oesophageal reflux disease

A recent meta-analysis evaluating 102 studies and a total of 460 984 adults reported a pooled prevalence of 14.8% for GORD in the general population.[15] Although the prevalence of BO is higher, ranging between 5% and 15%, in those that have a background of reflux symptoms compared to the general population, not all patients with GORD harbour BO or even oesophagitis.[16] Similarly, around half of patients with BO do not report heartburn symptoms.

Other risk factors

Other established risk factors include increasing age, male sex, White race, smoking, and obesity, but more specifically central adiposity.[17,18] A UK-based study looking at 21 899 index endoscopies reported that each additional year from age 20 to 59 led to a 7.4% increase in BO prevalence for male subjects, with similar findings but at 20 years later in life for females.[18] Males between 60 and 70 years of age have a twofold increased likelihood of having BO compared to age-adjusted females.[19] The incidence of BO was approximately five times higher in White compared to Black patients.[20] A meta-analysis of five case-control studies showed that BO cases were significantly more likely to have been in smokers compared to controls, with additional evidence showing 1) a positive correlation between smoking duration and; 2) a synergistic effect between smoking and GORD.[21] A recent pooled analysis[22] from eight case-control studies revealed that waist circumference was associated with risk for BO risk. The latest meta-analysis, studying the impact of obesity, metabolic syndrome, and insulin resistance, included 119 273 subjects from 46 studies and showed that all three were significantly associated with an increased risk for BO.[23]

In addition to environmental factors, there is also a genetic component that influences the development of BO. Familial clustering has been reported in 6–7% of BO/OAC cases in US and Dutch studies,[24,25] a finding consolidated by case-control genome-wide association studies (GWASs). Previous GWASs analysing Western populations have identified multiple genetic variants associated with the development of BO and OAC. A meta-analysis comprising 6 167 BO and 4 112 OAC cases, compared to 17 159 controls, identified 16 independent risk loci for BO and/or OAC, including locations related to the *CFTR*, *Foxf1*, *Foxp1*, *ALDH1A2*, *CTRC1*, *TBX5*, and *GDF7* genes and the major histocompatibility complex (MHC) region.[26] Studies have also shown that the prevalence of GORD, a known risk factor for BO/OAC, has been shown to be higher in the relatives of patients with BO.[27,28] Twin studies have reported an estimated GORD heritability of 30–40%.[29,30] Similar findings have been reported with a high prevalence of BO, ranging between 18% and 28% amongst relatives of patients with BO/OAC.[31,32]

It remains to be determined whether the genetic risk loci can be used as part of a clinical algorithm to identify individuals at risk.

SCREENING

Systemic mass endoscopic screening on a population level is not supported by any guidelines, given that upper GI endoscopy does not fulfil the criteria for a good screening test. Enriching the population for those at highest risk is therefore a serious consideration, and GORD has been generally advocated as the most useful risk factor. The BSG endorses screening in patients with chronic GORD symptoms plus a strong family history of BO or OAC (i.e. first-degree relatives), or chronic GORD symptoms and three other risk factors including male sex, White race, age more than 50 years, and obesity.[8] Similarly, the ACG proposes selective screening in patients who have had GORD for at least 5 years with symptoms at least weekly, plus two or more of the following risks factors: White race, age over

50 years, central obesity, smoking history, or a first-degree relative with BO/OAC.[9] Given that up to 40% of patients with OAC are asymptomatic, even with these criteria a large proportion of patients that might harbour BO/OAC are not screened.[3,33] Furthermore, a recent prospective study of 1 241 patients suggested that available clinical factor-based risk assessment tools, such as HUNT, M-BERET, and Kunzmann, are in fact more accurate than frequency and duration of GORD symptoms in identifying patients at risk of neoplastic BO.[34]

In order to improve precision screening, a three-step approach has been proposed. The first stage enriches at-risk patients within the general population using risk-prediction algorithms. This is followed by triaging using an affordable, minimally invasive test in a primary care setting to find high-risk patients, and finally endoscopy to confirm diagnosis.[35] Various options are currently being investigated for the second step in this screening process.

Non-sedated transnasal endoscopy (TNE) has been shown to have improved patient acceptability and similar clinical effectiveness to traditional upper GI endoscopy in assessing the oesophagus for endoscopic BO and histological IM, respectively.[36,37] TNE has been evaluated successfully for use in travelling vans for community BO screening.[38] The use of TNE is supported in recent BO screening guidelines.

With advances in imaging, oesophageal capsule endoscopy (OCE) is another less invasive, clinic-based alternative that uses a wireless, pill-sized swallowed camera to visualise the oesophagus. However, a meta-analysis from 2009 assessing the original capsule showed poor sensitivity and specificity for BO diagnosis.[39] Newer versions are currently under investigation.

INTRODUCTION OF NON-ENDOSCOPIC SCREENING TRIAGE TOOLS APPLIED TO AN AT-RISK POPULATION

An alternative to endoscopic imaging is the use of non-endoscopic cell sampling devices combined with genetic or cytological biomarker evaluation. The Cytosponge is a mesh-containing capsule attached on a string that can be swallowed by patients in an office-based setting. The capsule dissolves in the stomach about 5–7 minutes post ingestion, which allows the compressed mesh to expand and, while withdrawn by pulling the string, collect up to 1 million cells from the entire length of the oesophagus.[40] These cells are evaluated by immunocytology for Trefoil Factor-3 (TFF3), a protein marker of IM overexpressed in BO to determine whether the test is positive or negative.[41] The BEST1 trial established that this approach is feasible in primary care, with high levels of patient acceptability and encouraging accuracy data.[42] The BEST-2 study recruited 1 100 subjects (647 BO cases vs 463 controls with heartburn symptoms) and reported a sensitivity of 79.9% and a specificity of 92.4% in a per-protocol analysis. When patients with an inadequate sample were offered a repeat Cytosponge, and for cases with circumferential BO segments ≥ 3 cm, sensitivity increased to 89.7% and 87.2%, respectively.[43]

The BEST-3 trial was a randomised trial to determine whether the offer of Cytosponge to patients on medication for heartburn increased the detection of BO compared to usual care, meaning endoscopy referral if the family doctor felt it was indicated. This showed that an offer of Cytosponge-TFF3 led to a tenfold increase in the number of BO diagnoses.[44]

A cost-effectiveness analysis showed that initial Cytosponge-based screening of GORD patients followed by upper GI endoscopy for positive tests was 27–29% less costly compared to endoscopy screening alone.[45] Overall, these data are encouraging and implementation research is underway in the UK (NIHR ID: ISRCTN91655550).

Other investigators have since developed balloon and sponge devices coupled with methylation panels. A multicentre US-based case-control study of 295 patients showed that the EsophaCap, a sponge-on-a-string device, had a sensitivity of 92% and a specificity of 94% for diagnosing BO and was preferred to upper GI endoscopy by 94% of subjects.[46] The test used a total of five methylated DNA biomarkers. The five-biomarker panel did not distinguish between dysplastic and ND-BO, and similar to Cytosponge the test was susceptible to BO length with some short length segments being missed. It is worth noting that, in contrast to the Cytosponge study, this was not an intention-to-treat analysis. A large case-control study using EsophaCap is currently underway (Clinical Trials ID: NCT04214119). EsoCheck is a balloon device deployed via a slim catheter that can be inflated and deflated such that you sample 5–6 cm above the oesophago-gastric junction (OGJ). The cells are analysed using a DNA methylation biomarker panel comprising of VIM and CCNA1 that showed a sensitivity of 90.3% and a specificity of 91.7% for detecting BO in a small pilot trial, despite poor DNA yields.[47] Again, this was not an intention-to-treat analysis. Following device improvements, the use of EsoCheck in combination with the aforementioned two-marker panel for diagnosing BO in an at-risk screening cohort is being evaluated in a 1000-participant US-based study (Clinical Trials ID NCT04293458).

Finally, promising and even less invasive options currently under investigation for use in BO screening include liquid biopsy, looking for cancer-related biomarkers in the blood – particularly microRNAs[48,49] or circulating tumour DNA – as well as breath-sampling devices measuring exhaled volatile organic compounds.[50,51]

DIAGNOSIS OF BARRETT'S OESOPHAGUS

ENDOSCOPIC ASSESSMENT

Endoscopy is currently the gold-standard diagnostic test for BO.

✔✔ All international societal guidelines diagnostic criteria require that the BO columnar epithelium segment is visible endoscopically, at least 1 cm above the OGJ, and for any columnar metaplasia (BSG) and in particular IM (BSG, American Gastroenterological Association [AGA], ESGE) to be confirmed histologically on oesophageal biopsies.[8–10]

In the context of a healthy oesophagus, the top of the gastric fold coincides with the squamo-columnar junction (SCJ), but in the presence of BO the SCJ shifts at least 1 cm proximally to the OGJ, generating a characteristic salmon pink colour and velvety texture easily distinguishable from the pale, glossy appearance of squamous mucosa (Fig. 2.1). An irregular Z-line describes the situation where the SCJ might lie above the OGJ but without any confluence, forming tongues shorter than 1 cm, thus not fulfilling the diagnostic criteria for BO (Fig. 2.2). An irregular Z-line is found in 10–15% of patients undergoing upper GI endoscopy,[52] and despite the fact that it can harbour histological IM in 39–44% of cases,[53,54] its neoplastic potential is low, with

no patients progressing beyond ND-BO in one study[52] and only 4% of patients progressing to BO with LGD and none progressing to HGD/OAC in another study.[54] Therefore, current societal guidelines do not recommend sampling or further evaluation of irregular Z-lines.

BO can be crudely categorised into short- (< 3 cm) and long-segment (≥ 3 cm) disease, with the latter being 3.5-fold more prevalent than the former (6.0% vs 1.6%, respectively).[55] This distinction is relevant, as long-segment BO has a higher probability of harbouring dysplasia (prevalence 31% vs 10%) and a higher risk of neoplastic progression.[2]

Equally important as making an accurate endoscopic diagnosis is the report of endoscopic findings to ensure precise clinical communication and tailored follow-up according to the risk of cancer progression.

✔✔ The Prague C&M endoscopic classification scores the BO extent in terms of its circumference (C) and maximal tongue length (M), both measured in cm from the OGJ (Fig. 2.3).[56] Other islands of columnar-type mucosa above the main Barrett's segment should be reported separately. The Prague classification has good inter-user reliability for BO segments larger than or equal to 1 cm.[56]

Any other visible lesions associated with the BO segment should be described independently according to the Paris classification[57] and have their position mapped based on clock-face circumferential markings and distance from the incisors (Figs. 2.4 and 2.5). Such lesions are often subtle, include ulcers and nodules, and are frequently enriched with dysplastic changes,[58,59] with sessile/depressed lesions more likely to already contain cancer.[60] Additionally, in various studies the presence of endoscopically visible nodules was associated with a higher risk, up to fourfold, of neoplastic progression to HGD/OAC compared to no nodular appearances,[61,62] whereas HGD in the context of an ulcer conferred an enhanced risk of progressing to cancer compared to non-ulcer HGD.[63] With improved magnification and narrow-band imaging (NBI), high-resolution images enable evaluation of the mucosal pit pattern and vessels within the Barrett's segment, and any associated lesions (see Figs. 2.4 and 2.5).[64] Compared with non-metaplastic columnar mucosa, which displays round pits, in BO with IM pits acquire a villous shape, whereas in the presence of dysplasia they have a totally irregular pattern. The microvasculature remains well structured in IM but tends to become disorganised with dilated, irregular, and diffusely distributed vessels not following the normal architecture of the mucosa (i.e. not along or between mucosal ridges) in areas of dysplasia. Complex NBI classification systems, such as Amsterdam and Kansas,[65,66] exist to predict the histologic presence and grade of dysplasia based on vascular and mucosal patterns but are mainly used in specialised, tertiary centres. The steps in evaluating BO endoscopically are summarised in Box 2.1.

BIOPSY ACQUISITION PROTOCOL

Biopsies should be acquired according to the Seattle biopsy protocol originally proposed in 2000.[67–69] Targeted biopsies should be taken from visible lesions and then random biopsies from each of the four quadrants along the oesophageal circumference at least every 2 cm, starting distally at 1 cm above the OGJ and moving proximally to reduce any visual hindrance from biopsy-associated bleeding. Targeted biopsies cannot replace random quadrantic biopsies as lesions can be subtle and up to 20% may be invisible to the eye with

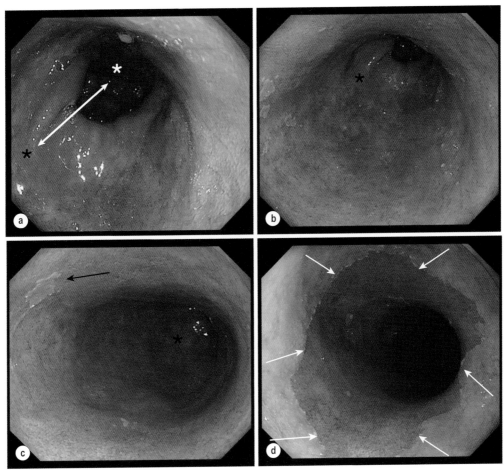

Figure 2.1   White light endoscopy images of a case of long Barrett's oesophagus (BO) with a hiatus hernia and diagnostic landmarks. (a) The distance between the diaphragmatic pinch *(white asterisk)* and the oesophagogastric junction (OGJ), identified as the top end of the gastric folds *(black asterisk)*, is increased and represents the size of the hiatus hernia *(white double arrow)*, a known risk factor for gastro-oesophageal reflux (GORD) and BO. (b and c) Panoramic views of at two levels of the BO segment with the *OGJ (black asterisks)* visible at the bottom end of the BO, where the normal squamous mucosa has been replaced by a salmon-coloured segment of columnar epithelium extending well beyond the OGJ, suggesting the presence of BO. A small island of squamous epithelium is present *(black arrow)*. The squamo-columnar junction (SCJ), i.e. the transition from the squamous mucosa of the oesophagus to the columnar mucosa of the stomach, which coincides with the OGJ in a healthy states, is not visible in this case of BO. (d) Upon further withdrawal of the endoscope, the upper border of the long BO is visible. The SCJ is visible in the mid-oesophagus with transition from the salmon pink columnar Barrett's mucosa to the whitish-pink squamous mucosa of the healthy oesophagus *(white arrows)*. (Courtesy of Dr Massimiliano di Pietro (Senior Clinician Scientist and Consultant Gastroenterologist, Early Cancer Institute, Department of Oncology, University of Cambridge, UK.))

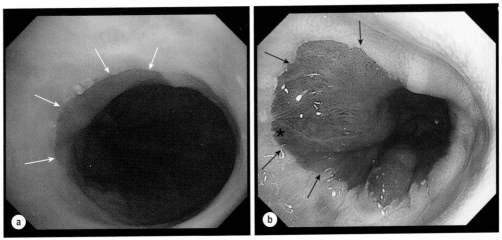

Figure 2.2   Irregular Z-line. (a) On white light endoscopy (WLE), an irregular Z-line *(white arrows)* can easily be mistaken for short Barrett's oesophagus (BO). (b) Narrow-band imaging (NBI) of the same irregular Z-line. NBI allows sharper delination of the squamo-columnar junction (SCJ; *black arrows*) by better visualisation of the gastric folds, here seen at the 9 o'clock position *(asterisk)* extending all the way to the SCJ, suggesting that this should not be diagnosed endoscopically as BO. (Courtesy of Dr Massimiliano di Pietro (Senior Clinician Scientist and Consultant Gastroenterologist, Early Cancer Institute, Department of Oncology, University of Cambridge, UK.))

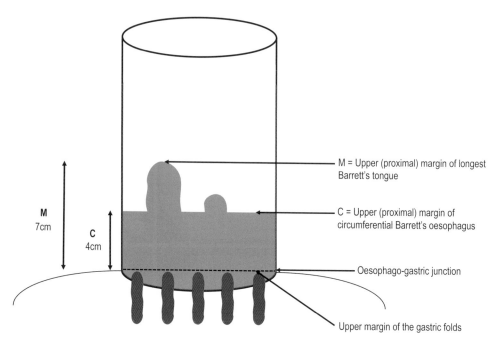

Figure 2.3 The evaluation of Barrett's oesophagus (BO) based on the Prague classification. The oesophagogastric junction is found at the top of the gastric folds, coinciding with the squamo-columnar junction (SCJ) in a healthy oesophagus. This is no longer the case in the presence of BO, as the SCJ is located more proximally. According to the Prague classification, the BO segment is measured based on the circumferential extent *(C)* and the maximal extent *(M)*. In the case showed in this example, the circumferential extent is 4 cm and the maximal extent is 7 cm, hence reported as C4M7.

M = Upper (proximal) margin of longest Barrett's tongue

C = Upper (proximal) margin of circumferential Barrett's oesophagus

Oesophago-gastric junction

Upper margin of the gastric folds

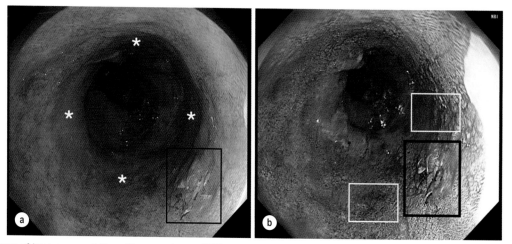

Figure 2.4 A case of long-segment Barrett's oesophagus (BO) with a superficial neoplastic lesion. (a) White light endoscopy image of long-segment BO with a Paris 0–IIb superficial lesion with surface ulceration at the 4 o'clock position *(black box)*. Biopsy histology showed intramucosal adenocarcinoma (IMC). In such a case biopsies should be taken from all four quadrants *(white asterisks)* every 2 cm as well as from the visible lesion. (b) Narrow-band imaging (NBI) reveals that the underlying pathology is more extensive than that seen on WLE, with dysplastic-looking areas at the 3 and 6 o'clock positions *(white boxes)* in addition to the main lesion *(black box)*. (Courtesy of Dr Massimiliano di Pietro (Senior Clinician Scientist and Consultant Gastroenterologist, Early Cancer Institute, Department of Oncology, University of Cambridge, UK.))

white light endoscopy (WLE) alone (Fig. 2.4). The Seattle biopsy protocol minimises sampling error when compared to non-systematic random biopsies, enhancing the detection of LGD and HGD by 17% and 3%, respectively.[70] Unfortunately, it is often poorly adhered to in daily practice.[71] The ACG guidelines from 2016 recommend at least eight random biopsies to be taken from the suspected Barrett's segment in an effort to achieve high diagnostic yield and accuracy.[9] Interestingly, it appears that dysplasia is more likely in the BO segment closest to the OGJ. Highlighting the substantial room for improvement in biopsy practice and endoscopic surveillance, a recent meta-analysis, looking at post-endoscopy oesophageal adenocarcinoma (PEEC) and including 52 studies with 145,000 patients, showed that PEEC accounts for almost one out of four of all HGD/OAC

cases and has a significant inverse association with OAC incidence.[69] Another meta-analysis has shown that missing OAC lesions appear to be more prominent during the first year following a diagnosis of BO.[72]

HISTOLOGICAL ASSESSMENT

All society guidelines agree that IM is a hallmark of BO with malignant potential and that IM must be documented. IM can also be observed within the gastric cardia, and hence it is critical that the location of the biopsy is accurately recorded by the endoscopist and reported to the pathologist. Focal IM may be a variant of normal IM and only confers a very low cancer risk. Grading of dysplasia is based on the Vienna classification system in which the IM of ND-BO progresses to LGD, HGD, and finally to intra-mucosal carcinoma,[73,74]

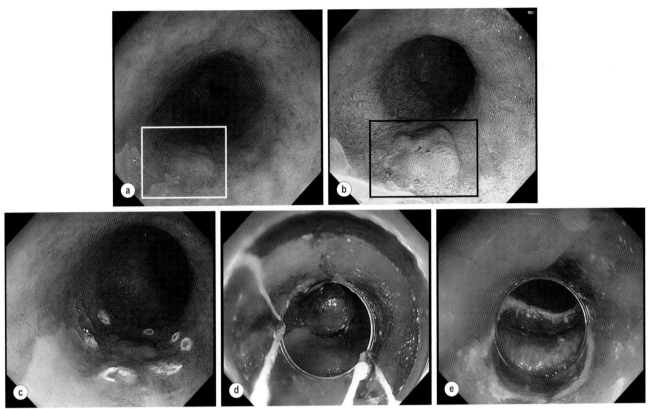

Figure 2.5 Detection, assessment and endoscopic treatment of superficial neoplastic lesion in Barrett's oesophagus (BO). (a) White light endoscopy (WLE) of a BO segment with a superficial, slightly elevated (Paris 0–IIa) lesion at 7 o'clock *(white box)*. (b) Narrow-band imaging of the same area allows better visualisation of the lesion and sharper delination of its margins *(black box)*. Biopsies showed high-grade dysplasia (HGD), and endoscopic mucosal resection (EMR) was decided. (c) WLE imaging showing the markings made around the HGD lesion in preparation for EMR. (d) WLE imaging of the multiband mucosectomy device with the HGD lesion trapped in the rubber band. (e) WLE imaging of the area following EMR resection of the HGD lesion. ((Courtesy of Dr Massimiliano di Pietro (Senior Clinician Scientist and Consultant Gastroenterologist, Early Cancer Institute, Department of Oncology, University of Cambridge, UK.))

Box 2.1 Endoscopic assessment of Barrett's oesophagus

- Identify key landmarks – oesophagogastric junction, squamous-columnar junction, and diaphragmatic pinch
- Evaluate Barrett's segment with white light endoscopy and report according to the Prague C+M classification
- Look carefully for any lesions and characterise them according to the Paris classification
- Evaluate Barrett's segment with narrow-band imaging, looking at pit (round vs villous), mucosal (regular vs irregular), and microvasculature (regular vs irregular) patterns
- Acquire random quadrantic biopsies every 2 cm and targeted biopsies of any lesions or suspected areas

---

although not all steps are necessarily observed. A study comparing the identification of LGD between US-based and European histopathologists showed that the degree of agreement was extremely poor (k = 0.11).[75] Furthermore, a Dutch study proved that expertise in GI histopathology is crucial, as only 27% of specimens originally labelled as LGD by general histopathologists were eventually deemed to be correct by experts, with the rest relegated to ND or ID.[76] Underlining the importance of correctly grading dysplasia, these true LGD cases displayed an annual risk of cancer progression of

9.1%, significantly higher than the demoted ID (0.9%) and ND (0.6%) cases. The risk of progression is even higher in cases with persistent (defined as detected at both first and follow-up endoscopy) LGD.[77] All societal guidelines recommend the confirmation of dysplasia by two expert gastrointestinal pathologists. This is especially important as dysplasia is now an indication for endoscopic therapy.

PROGRESSION TO CANCER (OAC)

BO imposes a substantially increased risk of developing OAC for an individual compared to the general population,[78,79] but only around 5% of patients with OAC actually have a previous diagnosis of BO.[80] The progression of non-dysplastic BO to cancer is low and estimated at around 0.33% per year based on the largest meta-analysis to date involving 11,434 patients from 57 studies.[81] However, this is significantly higher in the context of BO with histological evidence of dysplasia, which is the best established and the only accepted predicting biomarker for BO neoplastic progression.[82]

✅✅ The degree of dysplasia is the primary biomarker determining the risk of neoplastic progression for BO and the surveillance required.[83]

According to meta-analyses, ND-BO, BO with LGD, and BO with HGD have a risk of progression to OAC of 0.3, 0.5 and 6.6 per 100 person-years, respectively.[81,84,85] In cases when cellular atypia features are present but equivocal for inflammation or dysplasia, a diagnosis of indefinite for dysplasia (ID) is made. A recent meta-analysis of eight studies evaluated for the first time the neoplastic potential of BO ID, reporting a pooled annual risk of 11.4% for progression to LGD, 1.5% for progression to HGD/OAC, and 0.6% for progression to OAC only.[82] Since this is similar to the neoplastic progression risk seen in BO with LGD, the authors concluded that BO ID warrants rigorous endoscopic surveillance. In essence, its presence warrants further investigation and effective acid-suppression therapy that may reduce inflammation and aid subsequent histopathological assessment.

In addition to dysplastic changes, the detection of histological IM and the length of the Barrett's segment are key risk factors for progression to cancer.[86] A large population-based study of 8 522 BO cases reported that the presence of IM posed an enhanced annual risk of 0.38% for malignant transformation[87] and was also associated with increased mutational frequency in carcinogenic genes.[88] Long-segment BO, defined as ≥ 3 cm in length,[89] has been shown to have an annual risk of cancer progression of 0.22%, significantly higher than the 0.03% and 0.01% risk reported in the context of short (≥ 1 to ≤ 3 cm) and ultra-short (< 1 cm) segment BO.[2]

✔✔ A systematic review and meta-analysis evaluating studies that reported on predictors of BO neoplastic progression (20 studies, 74 943 patients) identified older age (odds ratio [OR] 1.03), male sex (OR 2.16), and smoking (OR 1.47), in addition to a longer BO segment (OR 1.25) and LGD (OR 4.25), as risk factors for progression, whereas PPIs (OR 0.55) and statins (OR 0.48) were revealed to protect from neoplastic progression.[83]

A recently developed scoring system (Progression in Barrett's Esophagus score) based on male sex, smoking, length of BO, and baseline LGD has shown promise in identifying patients with BO at low, intermediate, and high risk for HGD or OAC.[90] The score is heavily dependent on dysplasia, which remains the main biomarker for progression.

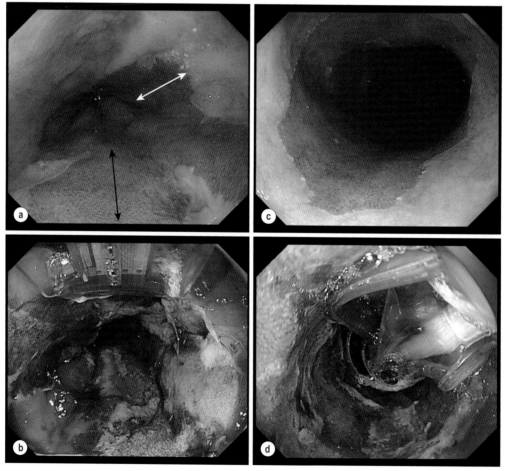

Figure 2.6 Treatment of dysplastic Barrett's oesophagus (BO) with radiofrequency ablation (RFA). (a) White light endoscopy (WLE) of a dysplastic (low-grade) Barrett's segment with significant tongues before RFA. *White and black arrows* denote the segment's circumferential and maximal extent, respectively. (b) WLE of the same Barrett's segment post-RFA with the Halo-90, system which uses an electric pad at the tip of the scope to deliver targeted energy for ablation. Note the white discolouration of the mucosa following RFA as a result of coagulation. (c) WLE of a long Barrett's segment that harboured high-grade dysplasia on biopsies before RFA. (d) WLE of the same Barrett's segment post-RFA with the Halo-360 system, which uses a plastic balloon with electrical coils on its surface attached to the scope tip to deliver energy for circumferential ablation. ((Courtesy of Dr Massimiliano di Pietro (Senior Clinician Scientist and Consultant Gastroenterologist, Early Cancer Institute, Department of Oncology, University of Cambridge, UK.))

MANAGEMENT: SURVEILLANCE AND ENDOSCOPIC TREATMENT

As the management of nodular and non-nodular (flat) BO differs, the first step in surveillance is determining whether there is a visible lesion. In cases where there is any endoscopically visible (flat or nodular) lesion with associated background BO-LGD or BO-HGD, endoscopic resection by endoscopic mucosal resection (EMR) or endoscopic submucosal dissection (ESD) should be carried out at a Barrett's tertiary expert centre for detailed histopathological assessment and staging[10] (Fig. 2.5). If LGD or HGD is confirmed on the resected specimen by two expert GI pathologists, then the residual Barrett's segment should be ablated by radiofrequency ablation (RFA) (Fig. 2.6) or alternatively undergo intense surveillance. These recommendations are mainly based on expert opinion given the limited data available in this context.

NON-DYSPLASTIC BARRETT'S OESOPHAGUS

All societies recommend surveillance for ND-BO based on evidence from retrospective and population-based studies suggesting that surveillance correlates with improved survival when compared to symptomatic diagnosis.[91–95] This was confirmed in a recent systematic review and meta-analysis.[96] The authors reported that regular surveillance was linked to reduced OAC-related (relative risk [RR] 0.60) and all-cause mortality (hazard ratio [HR] 0.75). Furthermore, surveillance-detected OAC showed reduced OAC-related (OR 0.73) and all-cause mortality (HR 0.59) when compared to symptom-based OAC detection.

In an attempt to provide evidence on the efficacy and cost-effectiveness of BO endoscopic surveillance, the BOSS study, a multicentre UK-based randomised controlled trial (RCT), compared 2-yearly endoscopic surveillance against 'at need' endoscopy by randomising 3 400 patients in the two groups followed for 10 years with overall survival as the primary outcome.[97] At the time of writing, this study was pending its report.

According to American guidelines,[4,9,68] ND-BO warrants endoscopic surveillance every 3–5 years. Recommendations for surveillance intervals for ND-BO from BSG 2014 and ESGE 2017 are slightly different as the two societies stratify cases based on the length of the Barrett's segment.[8,10] In cases of an irregular Z-line or tongues of columnar-lined oesophagus < 1 cm (previously known as ultra-short BO) ESGE suggests no endoscopic surveillance, whereas for lengths ≥ 1 cm but < 3 cm and ≥ 3 cm but < 10 cm, 5- and 3-year surveillance intervals are recommended, respectively. BSG guidelines recommend 3–5-year surveillance intervals for BO with IM and segment lengths less than 3 cm and 2–3-year intervals for BO lengths more than 3 cm. However, in cases where the maximum length is < 3 cm but no IM is confirmed histologically, upper GI endoscopy should be repeated to ensure appropriate biopsy acquisition and eliminate sampling errors. If, despite strict adherence to the Seattle protocol there is still no IM on histology, the patient should be considered for discharge. Given the low to average risk of cancer progression, the numbers needed to treat to prevent one case of OAC do not justify any prophylactic endoscopic therapy for ND-BO.[10]

BARRETT'S OESOPHAGUS INDEFINITE FOR DYSPLASIA OR WITH LOW-GRADE DYSPLASIA

According to all the societal guidelines, BO-ID and BO-LGD cases should have their histologic diagnosis confirmed by a second expert GI pathologist. Once confirmed, acid-suppression therapy should be commenced as cellular atypic changes can be difficult to interpret in the context of inflammation.[4,10] Repeat upper GI endoscopy should be performed within 3–6 months.

In the context of an initial BO-ID diagnosis, if no definite dysplasia is found on subsequent biopsies, or if histologically there is again BO-ID, surveillance should revert to that recommended for ND-BO. If genuine dysplasia is identified, then the appropriate surveillance strategy should be followed as discussed in the following.

For an initial BO-LGD diagnosis, in the absence of LGD on subsequent 6-month interval endoscopy, seen in around 30% of single endoscopy LGD cases, a repeat endoscopy can be performed after 12 months. If two back-to-back endoscopies are negative or ID then the surveillance pathway can revert to that for ND-BO.[10,98] On the contrary, if there is indeed LGD again on repeat endoscopy at 6 months, endoscopic ablation should be the next step, usually in the form of RFA provided that there is no visible lesion. These recommendations arose following the results of recent trials that shed light on the natural history of LGD.[9,99]

The efficacy of RFA has been confirmed in two separate meta-analyses. A 2013 meta-analysis evaluated 18 studies with 3 802 cases of dysplastic (any grade) BO reporting complete eradication of IM and dysplasia in 78% and 91% of patients, respectively. Looking specifically at RFA treatment in the context of BO-LGD, a 2018 meta-analysis analysed eight studies with 619 patients. Complete eradication of IM and LGD was seen in 88.2% and 96.7% of cases, respectively (P < 0.001). The pooled recurrence rate was 5.6% for IM and 9.7% for LGD (P < 0.001), whereas progression to HGD/OAC was

significantly less likely compared to the surveillance group (OR 0.07).[100]

The most commonly used ablation technique is RFA, in which a balloon catheter with two electrodes at the tip of the scope delivers damaging levels of heat energy to the targeted BO segment. The Halo90 and Halo360 systems allow the ablative process to be carried out with focus on a specific site or in a circumferential fashion, respectively (see Fig. 2.6). In a recent cost-effectiveness analysis, endoscopic eradication therapy (ETT), which includes RFA, was deemed to be cost effective compared to endoscopic surveillance for LGD-BO and HGD-BO, but not in the context of ND-BO or ID-BO.[101]

Photodynamic treatment using 5-aminolevulinic acid and porfimer sodium, the method that predated RFA, confers no benefit in halting progression to cancer or overall patient survival when compared to RFA, with significantly worse side effects.[102,103] In contrast, argon plasma coagulation (APC), a technique that exploits the ablative properties of ionised argon gas, has shown some promise in eradicating remnant BO post-EMR for HGD-BO/intramucosal carcinoma (IMC), with 78% of cases treated displaying histological remission.[104] Cryotherapy, using either liquid nitrogen or cold carbon dioxide, is an emerging ablative strategy whereby the cryogen drives freezing and thawing-induced apoptosis of diseased BO epithelium followed by the natural healing process that generates neosquamous mucosa. Despite the lack of head-to-head studies against RFA, cryotherapy has been shown thus far to be safe and effective at exterminating dysplastic changes, especially HGD (87% overall, 94–97% for HDG), even following cases of failed ablation with other modalities.[105,106] As with other ablative techniques, there is a risk of oesophageal stricturing (3%) that is amenable to balloon dilatation. It is less expensive than RFA but has a steep learning curve.

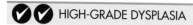
HIGH-GRADE DYSPLASIA

Societal guidelines agree on the management of BO-HGD. First, any visible lesion should be identified as these will require resection (see Fig. 2.5). Flat HGD is not common and occurs in less than 20% of BO-HGD cases,[10] and requires confirmation by two expert GI pathologists and a second high-resolution endoscopy. HGD confirmed by two GI pathologists should be endoscopically ablated, ideally with RFA.[4,8,10,107]

ENDOSCOPIC FOLLOW-UP POST-ERADICATION THERAPY

Complete eradication of Barrett's mucosa might require multiple RFA sessions with or without endoscopic resection of visible lesions at 2–3-month intervals. Surveillance endoscopy guidelines following successful (complete eradication of BO endoscopically and IM histologically) RFA treatment

regimens are mainly driven by expert opinion, as high-quality evidence on the topic remains scarce. The aim of surveillance is not only to detect any buried or recurring metaplasia within the neosquamous epithelium, but also to inform any further treatment that might be necessary. A large systematic review and meta-analysis of 39 studies on eradication treatments including RFA and EMR showed that, even after achieving complete eradication of IM, the pooled incidence rate was 7.5 and 2.8 per 100 person-years for any (IM or dysplasia) recurrence and dysplasia alone, respectively.[108] A recent large study from the Dutch database looking at 10-year outcomes post-eradication showed a lower, but still significant, annual recurrence rate of dysplasia of 1%.[109] This supports previous data from the UK National HALO and US Radiofrequency Ablation Registries that modelled the ideal surveillance endoscopy intervals following successful eradication to ensure that recurrence of unresectable OAC

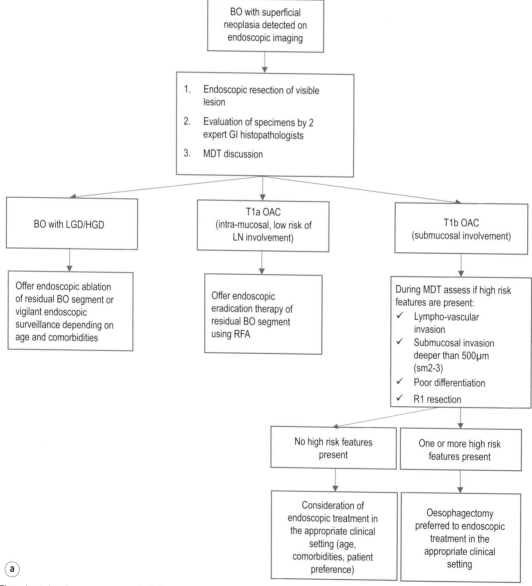

Figure 2.7 Flowchart for the management of Barrett's oesophagus (BO) with (a) and without (b) visible lesions on endoscopy based on the latest societal guidelines. *BO*, Barrett's oesophagus; *CxMx*, circumferential and maximal extent of Barrett's segment; *EMR*, endoscopic mucosal resection; *ESD*, endoscopic submucosal dissection; *GI*, gastrointestinal; *HGD*, high-grade dysplasia; *ID-BO*, Barrett's oesophagus indefinite for dysplasia; *IM*, intestinal metaplasia; *IMC*, intramucosal carcinoma; *LGD*, low-grade dysplasia; *LN*, lymph node; *MDT*, multidisciplinary team; *ND-BO*, non-dysplastic Barrett's oesophagus; *OAC*, oesophageal adenocarcinoma; *RFA*, radiofrequency ablation; *WLE*, white light endoscopy.

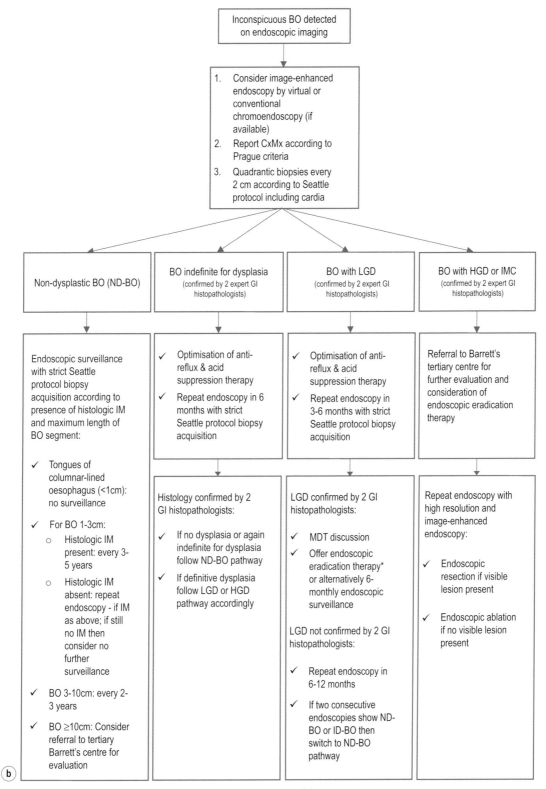

Figure 2.7, cont'd

was less than 0.1%.[110] Based on these predictive models, the latest Barrett's eradication guidelines from the AGA in 2020 recommend initial surveillance endoscopy after successful eradication at 1 and 3 years and every 2–3 years thereafter for baseline diagnosis of BO-LGD. For baseline BO-HGD or IMC diagnosis, surveillance endoscopy is advised at 3, 6, and 12 months followed by annual endoscopy thereafter. Inspection should be done with care and vigilance using high-definition WLE (and ideally also optical chromoendoscopy) to evaluate the neosquamous mucosa and gastric cardia. Random four-quadrant biopsies of the neosquamous mucosa and the gastric cardia and, where appropriate, targeted

oklesion biopsies, should be obtained for histological evaluation. Recurrent disease should be approached in a similar fashion to any initial disease.[111]

✔️✔️ INTRAMUCOSAL CARCINOMA

T1a cancers, also known as IMCs, are confined in the mucosa without spread beyond the muscularis mucosa and without involvement of the lymph nodes or other organs (see Fig. 2.4). Their management is the same as BO-HGD as per societal guidelines.

Endoscopic resection is the first line of treatment as it not only allows for histopathological staging, but in cases with confirmed lack of submucosal involvement, potentially achieves curative treatment. In the context of IMC, ablation of the residual Barrett's segment is supported by evidence of a significant 5-year risk of 14.5% for the development of metachronous neoplastic lesions or recurrence of the original cancer.[112] Based on this, ESGE in fact recommends complete eradication by RFA of all remaining Barrett's epithelium following endoscopic resection of any visible lesion containing any degree of dysplasia or neoplasia.[10]

The treatment of early oesophageal cancers is discussed in more detail in Chapter 7.

It is imperative that all cases of dysplasia or IMC are discussed within a multidisciplinary team setting comprising of gastroenterologists, surgeons, oncologists, and pathologists, as well as discussed with the patient so that decisions are made holistically in a patient-centred fashion.

A practical algorithm for the management of dysplastic and ND-BO with or without visible lesions is presented in Fig. 2.7.

CHEMOPREVENTION

Ideally, methods that prevent the development of dysplasia in BO would be ideal. Case-control studies evaluating proton pump inhibitors (PPIs), non-steroidal anti-inflammatory drugs (NSAIDs), aspirin, and statins as chemopreventative agents in BO have reported contradictory results ranging from no effect to a reduction in neoplastic progression.[113] Acid suppression has some biological rationale based on effects on cell differentiation and proliferation;[114] however, while some studies report reduced neoplastic progression risk,[7,115] others show no benefit.[116,117] The most recent and largest meta-analysis on the topic included 155 769 patients from 12 studies and showed that the use of PPIs is linked to a significantly reduced risk of BO progression to HGD/OAC (OR 0.47; P<0.001).[118] The potential protective mechanisms of aspirin and NSAIDs stems from their inhibition of cyclo-oxygenase (COX).

✔️✔️ The Aspirin and Esomeprazole Chemoprevention in Barrett's metaplasia Trial (AspECT), a UK-based multicentre RCT, recruited 2 557 patients newly diagnosed with BO > 1 cm and split them into four arms to receive high (40 mg twice daily) or low (20 mg once daily) doses of esomeprazole with or without high-dose (300 mg daily) aspirin.[119] High-dose PPI was better at prolonging the time to the endpoint of mortality or HGD/OAC compared to low-dose PPI for over 9 years. Aspirin alone had no significant effects on outcomes, but its addition to PPI had a synergistic effect on reducing neoplastic progression to HGD/OAC.

The multicentric anticancer effects of statins in the context of BO were assessed in a recent large meta-analysis (11 studies, > 18 000 patients with BO) that showed a decreased incidence of BO progression to HGD/OAC (pooled adjusted OR 0.59; P< 0.001).[120] A case-control study evaluating the effects of a combination of statin and aspirin chemoprevention found that regular use of both together reduced the incidence of OAC in a synergistic manner (OR 0.31).[121]

GENETICS AND MOLECULAR BIOMARKERS FOR PREDICTING PROGRESSION AND IMPROVING SURVEILLANCE

A detailed discussion of molecular biomarkers can be found elsewhere,[122] but the salient literature and implications for clinical practice are discussed here. In view of the difficulties inherent in diagnosing dysplasia, additional biomarkers would be helpful to identify patients at high risk of progression and to corroborate the histopathological diagnosis. TP53 and p16 are tumour suppressors that have been known for some time to be commonly inactivated in BO.[123,124] TP53 aberrations, including loss of heterozygosity, and altered DNA copy number or aneuploidy are prominent in dysplastic BO and OAC, such that their early-stage presence might be associated with neoplastic progression from premalignant pathology.[125,128] This was confirmed in a whole-genome sequencing (WGS) study that reported p53 mutations in the majority of BO-HGD (72%) and OAC (69%) of cases but in only 2.5% of ND-BO samples.[129] An exome sequencing study found that TP53 mutations occurred early in the neoplastic process including at the stage of ND-BO, perhaps as an enabling event triggering and followed by polyploidy and the accumulation of oncogene aberrations.[128] Along with p53, SMAD4 aberrations have been identified as an alteration that denotes the transition to invasion; however, the prevalence of SMAD4 mutations is low, limiting its clinical utility.[129] TP53 is the most common gene mutated in OAC, followed by a long tail of mutated genes, including ARID1A and SMAD4 which are also frequently mutated.[130] Recent work comparing paired BO and OAC samples suggested that BO is heavily mutated even in the absence of dysplasia, and also confirmed that the mutational landscape of the two states shows an overlap in line with a common cause.[131] This supports previous findings reporting the accumulation of mutations within BO segments even in the absence of dysplastic changes and linking clonal diversity to increased risk of dysplastic and neoplastic progression.[132] Mutated p53 can be identified by immunohistochemistry as over expression or an absent pattern when compared with wild-type p53. Aberrant TP53 expression is therefore the most well substantiated biomarker and often applied in clinical practice.[133] In a multivariate analysis, even after adjusting for confounders such as histological status, p53 overexpression remained able to predict progression to HGD/OAC better than LGD (HR 6.5 vs 3.6).[134] A meta-analysis of 102 studies looking at various potential biomarkers identified aberrant p53 (loss or mutation) and high levels of Ki-67 as the biomarkers able to predict neoplastic progression in BO.[135] As such, p53 immunostaining is a valuable additive tool to improve diagnostic reproducibility and risk stratification, and is this thus endorsed as an adjunct in routine clinical evaluation of dysplasia in the context of BO by both BSG and ESGE.

Aside from TP53, the molecular landscape is highly heterogeneous with huge variation between patients, making biomarkers more challenging to implement for clinical use.

ADVANCED IMAGING

Given that the Seattle biopsy protocol is laborious and prone to sampling errors, the use of advanced imaging to accurately identify dysplastic areas for more targeted evaluation and biopsy sampling and eradication would be advantageous. Virtual histology via real-time imaging techniques may mean that treatment can be performed in one sitting. High-resolution endoscopy, which allows high-definition magnified visualisation of the mucosa, has higher sensitivity than traditional endoscopy for the recognition of early neoplastic lesions.[136,137]

NBI, already used in daily clinical practice, allows improved visualisation of the mucosa and associated vessels. In a meta-analysis, NBI was found to be extremely specific (94%) and sensitive (96%) at detecting BO-HGD and equally sensitive (95%) but with low specificity (65%) at characterising IM.[138]

Chromoendoscopy, an alternative modality that exploits the absorptive properties of various chemicals, has been shown to highlight areas of suspicious mucosa. In a meta-analysis of nine prospective studies (1 379 patients with BO) comparing acetic acid–based chromoendoscopy to histopathology diagnosis, chromoendoscopy displayed high diagnostic accuracy for detecting HGD/OAC with a pooled sensitivity and specificity of 92% and 96%, respectively. However, the specificity for the detection of specialized intestinal metaplasia (SIM) was low (69%) despite a high sensitivity (96%), suggesting that chromoendoscopy results still require histological verification.[139]

Autofluorescence imaging (AFI) uses short-wavelength light to induce the emission of detectable light of a longer wavelength by tissue. This allows deep tissue mapping including vasculature and flagging up of suspicious areas or lesions. Although studies have shown no benefit of AFI alone compared to high-resolution endoscopy alone for the detection of dysplasia,[136,140] there is some evidence that AFI-targeted biopsies in combination with molecular biomarkers can accurately identify dysplasia[141] and improve predictions of neoplastic progression in BO[125] while reducing the number of biopsies taken.

Confocal laser endomicroscopy (CLE) is a real-time microscopy technique that uses a probe to magnify the field of vision by ×1 000 to achieve histology-like image evaluation. A meta-analysis of 14 studies including 789 patients with 4 047 lesions evaluated the ability of CLE to detect neoplastic changes in the context of BO. The study revealed a sensitivity of 89% and specificity of 83% in the per-patient analysis, with values changing to 77% and 89%, respectively, in the per-lesion analysis.[142]

Finally, optical coherence tomography (OCT) and volumetric laser endomicroscopy (VLE) are advanced imaging techniques that exploit infrared light to obtain high-resolution microscopic views *in-vivo*. A 2019 meta-analysis of 14 studies (721 patients with 1 565 lesions) suggested that targeted biopsies using OCT or VLE could improve the detection of dysplasia and cancer based on pooled sensitivities of 85% and 89% and specificities of 73% and 91%, for VLE and OCT, respectively, in detecting HGC/OAC in BO lesions.[143]

✓✓ The AGA has highlighted that advanced imaging modalities have yielded promising results, and in the hands of expert endoscopists their use is appropriate, but validation in larger cohorts is needed before they can replace WLE and Seattle protocol biopsies.[144] However, the most recent guidelines from the American Society for Gastrointestinal Endoscopy (ASGE) do recommend the use of chromoendoscopy plus Seattle protocol biopsy sampling instead of WLE.[68]

SQUAMOUS OESOPHAGEAL CARCINOMA

PREMALIGNANT PATHOLOGY AND PROGRESSION TO CANCER: SQUAMOUS DYSPLASIA

OSCC is the most common histological subtype worldwide, making up nearly 90% of all oesophageal cancers,[145] although the rising incidence of OAC has led to it overtaking OSCC in prevalence in the Western hemisphere. Squamous cell carcinoma (OSCC) is also often diagnosed late, with 5-year survival rates of 10–15%. Similar to OAC, early-stage OSCC has a significantly better prognosis than late-stage disease, with 5-year survival rates of > 80%.[146] Hence, there is currently a major shift towards early detection of non-invasive or early OSCC and oesophageal squamous dysplasia (SD), also known as squamous intraepithelial neoplasia, the only precursor lesion of OSCC.[147]

SD was first identified as a precursor of OSCC in the 1980s when studies based in China looked at the natural history of the condition in high-risk patients to show that it predicted the development of OSCC with the risk of neoplastic progression increasing with the degree of dysplasia.[148,149]

✓✓ Over a 13.5-year follow-up, OSCC developed in 24%, 50%, and 74% of cases with mild, moderate, and severe dysplasia at baseline, respectively, compared to only 8% in subjects with normal index histology.[150]

The neoplastic potential is so significant that even at the earlier timepoint of 3.5 years of follow-up of the same population, 65% of high-grade SD cases showed progression to OSCC.[148]

EPIDEMIOLOGY OF AND RISK FACTORS FOR SQUAMOUS DYSPLASIA

SD has a worldwide prevalence estimated to be between 3% and 38%,[151] with the large range reflecting the variation in endoscopic methods, histopathological scoring, and the studied populations from high-risk geographic regions such as China and Korea. The prevalence of SD in Western countries is not well known, since it is difficult to diagnose using WLE. A recent Chinese observational study compared 2 925 controls to 402 patients with precancerous dysplastic lesions for OSCC (defined histologically), assessing the effects of known OSCC risk factors.[152] The study showed that smoking (> 20 pack-years), heavy (> 100 mL/day) and prolonged (> 30 years) alcohol consumption, GORD, oesophagitis, and family history of oesophageal or stomach cancer were positively associated with the presence of precancerous lesions and had a synergistic effect. Interestingly, central adiposity showed a negative association with the presence of precancerous lesions.

DIAGNOSIS OF SQUAMOUS DYSPLASIA

SD can regress and relapse spontaneously, making it difficult to follow-up and monitor. It comprises of low-grade and high-grade intra-epithelial neoplastic changes. Although it can manifest with a range of appearances from flat erythematous lesions to nodules, plaques, or erosions, its features are often so subtle that it resembles healthy squamous mucosa and is easily missed on WLE.[153] Even in the context of screening high-risk individuals, less than 60% of early OSCC lesions have been detected by traditional WLE.[154] The sensitivity for SD in high-risk groups was only 7.7% when using biopsies obtained during WLE without enhanced imaging.[155]

In contrast to the localised presence of BO, SD can be present anywhere along the oesophagus, presenting a major challenge for mucosal sampling. Chromoendoscopy with Lugol's iodine is the current gold-standard technique for diagnosis as the dye improves the detection of SD by failing to stain the diseased epithelium and highlighting Lugol voiding lesions (LVLs)[156,157] (Fig. 2.8). In a study of asymptomatic high-risk patients, lesions highlighted by Lugol's iodine had an eightfold increased likelihood of harbouring dysplastic changes compared those without.[158] The size of the stained lesion is crucial, as LVLs > 10 mm showed a 60% probability of harbouring HGD as opposed to only 4% for LVLs < 5 mm.[159] A pink discolouration of the LVL within 3 minutes of staining is another strong sign of the histological presence of HGD or carcinoma.[160] Overall, the sensitivity and specificity of Lugol's solution at detecting early OSCC > 5 mm have been reported at 80–100% and 64–94%, respectively. NBI and CLE have also been evaluated for early OSCC detection, with a reported sensitivity of 82–88% and 94–95.7%, respectively, and specificity of 75–95% and 90%, respectively.[161] Early OSCC and SD appear as areas of brownish discolouration with irregular intra-papillary capillary loops on NBI, the latter also visible on CLE. AFI may also have a role to play in early OSCC detection by highlighting the lesion in a magenta colour within a green background. Although Lugol's chromoendoscopy still is the standard of care for screening, a recent meta-analysis of 18 studies with 1 911 patients has shown that NBI has superior specificity, more accurately distinguishing between neoplastic and benign changes, and equivalent sensitivity to Lugol's.[162] NBI is now readily available and easy to perform (see Fig. 2.8).

 SCREENING

As for BO, a window of opportunity appears to exist for screening, surveillance, and treatment given the significant amount of time needed for dysplasia to progress to cancer.[163] In a trial of patients in Chinese regions where OSCC is endemic, single endoscopy screening by expert endoscopists with Lugol's chromoendoscopy was performed followed by EMR or APC treatment of SD and early cancers and a 10-year follow-up. Screening reduced OSCC incidence and led to a reduction of cancer-associated mortality by one-third compared to non-screening.[164] The current guidelines for screening according to the National Health Commission of the People's Republic of China[165] suggest that individuals should undergo endoscopic screening if they are over 40 years old and also fulfil one of the following criteria:
- Origin from a high incidence of OSCC
- Exhibition of upper GI symptoms
- A family history of OSCC
- A personal history of oesophageal diseases
- The presence of other OSCC risk factors such as smoking or heavy alcohol drinking.

Outside of endemic areas, screening has been found to have a survival benefit compared to symptomatic diagnosis in individuals with primary head and neck cancers, a group that is at high risk of secondary OSCC.[166,167] Although there are no formal societal guidelines on screening programs in the Western world, suggestions[168,169] include:
- Lugol's or NBI-based endoscopy every 6–12 months for 10 years following therapy for head and neck squamous cell carcinoma.
- Annual gastroscopy with/without Lugol's 10–15 years after the onset of achalasia.
- Gastroscopy with quadrantic biopsies for the upper, mid, and lower oesophagus every 1–3 years and starting at 30 years of age for individuals with tylosis (keratosis palmaris et plantaris).
- Gastroscopy every 2–3 years at 10–20 years after suffering a caustic oesophageal injury.

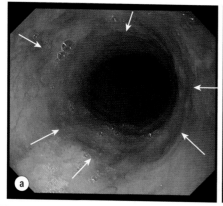 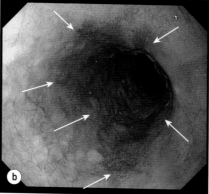 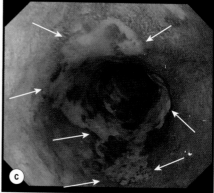

Figure 2.8 Endoscopic diagnosis of oesophageal squamous dysplasia (SD) or early oesophageal squamous cell carcinoma (OSCC). (a) The white light endoscopy image shows areas of red discolouration of flat oesophageal mucosa (arrows), which are not easy to appreciate. (b) Narrow-band imaging (NBI) of the same area allows better visualisation and demarcation of the suspicious oesophageal lesion (arrows), seen as brown discoloration on a background of a grey-green colour representing the normal appearances of healthy oesophageal epithelium. (c) Chromoendoscopy view of the same area using Lugol's iodine (2.5%), which allows the best visualisation and delineation of the mucosal lesion. The SD or early OSCC lesion voids staining by Lugol's iodine and appears unstained, allowing sharp demarcation of its margins (arrows). This imaging modality is ideal during screening endoscopy and essential prior to endoscopic resection. (Courtesy of Dr Massimiliano di Pietro (Senior Clinician Scientist and Consultant Gastroenterologist, Early Cancer Institute, Department of Oncology, University of Cambridge, UK.))

SURVEILLANCE AND MANAGEMENT

The lack of high-quality evidence has prohibited the generation of guidelines from GI societies on how to manage SD. However National Comprehensive Cancer Network (NCCN) guidelines recommend endoscopic eradication treatment of SD and T1a OSCC to prevent progression to more advanced disease.[170] For non-flat lesions, endoscopic resection by EMR (only if < 10 mm) or ideally ESD (certainly if ≥ 10 mm) should be attempted. EMR has been shown to be effective for premalignant and early OSCC lesions.[171] However, ESD has proven to be more superior at achieving curative (R0) resection.[172] The most recent ESGE guidelines recommend ESD as the optimal treatment for early OSCC, whereas ASGE guidelines do not make the choice between EMR and ESD.[173,174] Endoscopic resection can be followed by consideration for RFA in eligible patients to treat any remnant dysplastic lesions[161,175] and surveillance endoscopy every 6 months for 2 years and subsequently at yearly intervals for 3 years to look for metachronous dysplastic/neoplastic disease.[170] A practical algorithm on the management of SD is presented in Fig. 2.9.

RFA has also been evaluated for treating flat, non-invasive intraepithelial squamous or premalignant lesions such as high-grade SD. However, the success of RFA in this context is significantly lower than in BO and is not recommended as part of routine practice in SD and early OSCC.

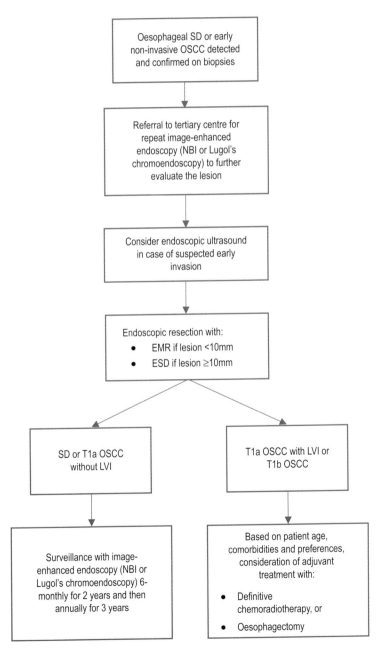

Figure 2.9 Flowchart for the practical management of oesophageal squamous dysplasia. *EMR*, Endoscopic mucosal resection; *ESD*, endoscopic submucosal dissection; *LVI*, lymphovascular invasion; *NBI*, narrow-band imaging; *OSCC*, oesophageal squamous cell carcinoma; *SD*, squamous dysplasia. (Courtesy of Dr Massimiliano di Pietro (Senior Clinician Scientist and Consultant Gastroenterologist, Early Cancer Institute, Department of Oncology, University of Cambridge, UK.))

GENETICS

There is a germline predisposition to OSCC. A large population-based case-control study confirmed familial aggregation of OSCC with an almost twofold increase in risk for the disease in the context of a positive family history of oesophageal cancer.[176] A two-step discovery and replication GWAS comparing OSCC cases with or without family history of upper GI cancers identified 19 significant low-penetrance susceptibility single-nucleotide polymorphisms (SNPs) associated with family history and singled out an intergenic region SNP near the *DLGAP1* gene with potential CTCF binding functions (pooled OR 1.59).[177] Original findings from a GWAS suggested that certain functional variants of *ALDH1B* and *ALDH2* were linked to increased OSCC risk via effects on alcohol and tobacco metabolism.[178] These were supported by polymorphisms in the same genes as well as genes involved in carcinogen detoxification and DNA repair that were identified in a whole-genome sequencing study, suggesting predisposition to OSCC via increased susceptibility to environmental risk factors.[179] The same study also identified the *LRP1B* and *TTC28* genes as those most frequently affected by structural variation and genetic alterations in the PI3K-AKT pathway, which is of critical importance to tumour progression. A Chinese meta-analysis of 2 961 OSCC cases and 3 400 controls identified five significant genome-wide SNPs at 2q33 mapping to the genetic region of *CASP8/ALS2CR12/TRAK2* with a combined OR of 1.29.[180] A subsequent GWAS meta-analysis of 9 654 OSCC cases and 10 058 controls revealed two more OSCC susceptibility loci, a synonymous SNP in *TMEM173* (OR 0.85), and an intronic SNP in *ATP1B2* near *TP53* (OR 0.88) along with a human leukocyte antigen class II region locus (OR 1.33) that was specifically significant in high-risk Chinese patients.[181] The two most recent GWAS meta-analyses looking at all oesophageal cancers[182] or all aerodigestive squamous cancers[183] reported variants in or near the loci of genes such as *ADH1B*, *CDKN1A*, *PTEN*, *TMEM237*, *MDM4*, *HLADQA1*, and *BRCA2*, among others, that were significantly associated with OSCC risk.

In terms of somatic acquired mutations, recent large whole-genome and whole-exome sequencing studies of sporadic OSCC have now identified mutations in TP53, seen in 70–90% cases, which seems to be the most frequently genetically altered gene, as in the case of OAC. Other affected tumour-suppressor genes include *ZNF750* and *FAT1/4*, whereas mutations in or overexpression of cell cycle promoter genes *CCND1* (46.4%), *CDK4/6*, and *MDM2*, as well as mutations in cell cycle–regulating genes *RB1*, *CDKN2A*, and *NFE2L2* and oncogenes *PIK3CA* and *NOTCH1/3* (25–33%), have also been reported.[184–187]

In contrast to GC (see later), there is less scientific support for inherited oesophageal cancer syndromes caused by single gene variants and the majority of cases are sporadic, resulting from acquired somatic mutations relating to environmental risk factors in the context of multiple low-penetrance susceptibility genes. However, OSCC can be associated with tylosis, an autosomal dominant dermatological condition. The link was first described in two distantly related families in Liverpool, England, in which context the risk of OSCC development was calculated at 95% by 65 years of age[188,189] and subsequently identified in other extended families in Europe and the Americas.[190] Linkage analysis and focussed next-generation sequencing identified the genetic cause of the syndrome at the 17q25 locus where missense mutations deactivate the *RHBDF2* gene encoding the iRhom2 protein, an indirect controller of the epidermal growth factor receptor (EGFR) signalling pathway via regulation of the ADAM17 sheddase.[191–193] The 17q25 locus has subsequently been shown to be deleted in the majority (60–70%) of sporadic OSCC and associated with more aggressive tumours with a worse prognosis.[194,195] In line with this, EGFR has been shown to be overexpressed in 60–76% of sporadic OSCC cases and associated with a poor prognosis.[196,197]

GASTRIC CANCER

With a poor overall 5-year survival rate of less than 25%,[198] early detection of GC and the premalignant conditions associated with it is key to improve patient outcomes. The majority of cases are adenocarcinomas and categorised by anatomical location (cardia or non-cardia) and histology (intestinal or diffuse type), with the intestinal-type non-cardia GC being the most common entity.

In this chapter we focus on the early detection of GC and the management of its associated precursor lesions. Guidelines presented in this section are mainly based on recent societal guidelines produced by the ASGE,[199] AGA,[200] BSG,[201] and the updated MAPS (management of epithelial precancerous conditions and lesions in the stomach) consensus, which represents the position of the ESGE amongst other European societies.[202]

PRECANCEROUS LESIONS

Similar to OAC, intestinal-type gastric adenocarcinoma tends to evolve from a background of premalignant conditions, namely chronic gastric atrophy (GA) and gastric intestinal metaplasia (GIM). Intestinal-type gastric adenocarcinoma is thought to evolve according to a stepwise cascade proposed by Correa in 1975.[203] This starts with the development of chronic inflammation (gastritis), progresses to atrophy and then metaplasia and dysplasia, and eventually culminates with the transformation to cancer.[204]

RISK FACTORS

An awareness of risk factors is essential in estimating the possibility of a patient harbouring GA, GIM, or GC. This is indeed the basis of the recent BSG guidelines proposed for the management of individuals at high risk of GC.[201] The main culprit of chronic inflammation is *H. pylori* infection, which has long been considered a major risk factor for GC.[204,205] *H. pylori* eradication is important as part of primary and secondary prevention of GC.

✓✓ The AGA technical review evaluated 22 studies including seven RCTs and three cohort studies to reveal that *H. pylori* eradication conferred a 32% and 33% reduction in incident GC risk and GC-related mortality, respectively.[206]

Another accepted risk factor for GA, GIM, and GC is autoimmune gastritis, a condition where the adaptive immune system targets parietal cells and intrinsic factor to cause pernicious anaemia. A meta-analysis of 27 heterogeneous studies reported that, based on random effects analysis, pernicious anaemia was linked to an overall relative risk of 6.8.[207] High salt intake (OR 2.87) and heavy smoking (OR 2.75) have also been associated with GA and GIM.[208] Epstein-Barr virus (EBV) has been linked to 9% of GC cases, but the changes it incurs do not lead to the development of a recognizable precancerous lesion, providing no options for early detection in this context.[209,210]

Inherited genetic factors are also important for GC, with 10–20% of cases a displaying family history of the disease.[211,212] Some of this risk probably links to familial inheritance, but the rest is likely to relate to genetic effects that render individuals more susceptible to the environmental risk factors of GC. A meta-analysis of 155 studies revealed an OR of 1.98 and 2.20 for the presence of GIM and GA, respectively, in first-degree relatives of GC patients versus controls.[213]

PREVALENCE

✓✓ The prevalence of GA and GIM together ranges between 0% and 8.3% in the Western world but is significantly higher, with a range of 33–84% in high-risk far-Eastern populations.[201]

In a large US-based retrospective study comprising of 810 821 subjects that had undergone upper GI endoscopy with gastric biopsies, the prevalence of GIM was 8.4% and was found more frequently with increasing age in men and East Asian individuals. Despite a historic downward trend in incidence over the last 50 years, likely as a result of effective *H. pylori* eradication and decline in infection rates,[214] worryingly, recent studies from Sweden and the USA have identified an increasing incidence in precancerous stomach conditions and gastric adenocarcinoma, respectively, amongst young White adults less than 50 years of age,[215,216] a trend that is predicted to continue in the future.[1]

ENDOSCOPIC DIAGNOSIS AND HISTOLOGICAL EVALUATION

The endoscopic diagnosis of GA and GIM is challenging, especially when compared to other premalignant conditions such as BO. The change from normal to pathological mucosa is subtle and additional endoscopic signs such as the disappearance of gastric folds can be affected by the degree of air insufflation and the large surface of the stomach. Additionally, premalignant gastric lesions are often patchy and thus easy to miss. Suspicious endoscopic features of GA include loss of gastric folds, vasculature prominence, pallor, and an atrophic border[201] (Fig. 2.10). GIM is challenging to confirm on WLE where the combination of small grey-white plaques and mix of pink and pale mucosal patches give the appearance of an uneven surface. Given this diagnostic challenge, image-enhanced and magnification endoscopy are recommended to improve diagnostic yield (Figs. 2.10 and 2.11). In the gastric body, GIM can then present as a 'groove type' or 'villiform' pattern normally seen in the antrum or intestine, respectively. Characteristic signs such as the light blue crest line and marginal turbid band signs, best seen using NBI, can help in GIM detection (Fig. 2.11). A multicentre, prospective study showed that WLE had a significantly lower sensitivity when compared to WLE plus NBI for both GIM (53% vs 87%) and gastric dysplasia (74% vs 92%), suggesting that WLE alone is not accurate enough for assessing the premalignant stomach.[217]

The Operative Link on Gastritis Assessment (OLGA) and Operative Link on Gastric Intestinal Metaplasia Assessment (OLGIM) were established to standardize the histological evaluation and scoring of GA and GIM on gastric biopsies with the aim of providing quantitative information for the risk for cancer progression.[218,219] Studies have shown that high-stage (III/IV) OLGA and OLGIM are linked to significantly increased risk (OR 2.64 and 3.99, respectively) for developing GC.[220] This suggests that patients with OLGA/OLGIM stages type III/IV should perhaps be considered as high risk and undergo regular surveillance.

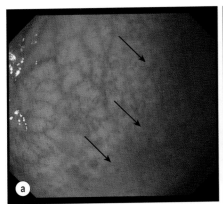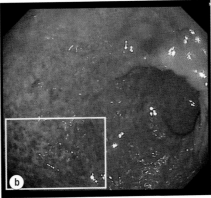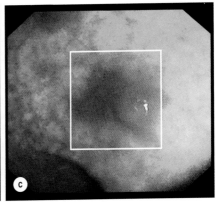

Figure 2.10 Endoscopic diagnosis of gastric atrophy (GA). (a) White-light endoscopy image with pale atrophic mucosa on the left compared to red non-atrophic mucosa on the right. Note the clearly visible atrophic border between the two *(arrows)*. (b) Narrow-band imaging view of pale, atrophic gastric mucosa (again, see the clearly demarcated border between atrophic and normal mucosa) with the presence of small nodular areas of enterochromaffin-like hyperplasia, a precursor lesion of neuroendocrine carcinoma *(box)*. (c) Autofluorescence imaging (AFI) highlighting the presence of GA. The AFI signal from normal healthy gastric mucosa is red (not seen here), but in the presence of GA the signal becomes green due to the thinning of the mucosa. In the case presented here, there is a superficial neoplastic lesion *(box)* with a shift to red-brown signal due to abnormal thickening of the mucosa. (Courtesy of Dr Massimiliano di Pietro (Senior Clinician Scientist and Consultant Gastroenterologist, Early Cancer Institute, Department of Oncology, University of Cambridge, UK.))

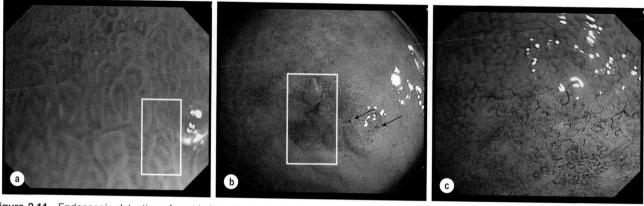

Figure 2.11 Endoscopic detection of gastric intestinal metaplasia (GIM) using magnified narrow-band imaging (NBI). (a) The light blue crest (LBC) sign *(box)* is a blue-white discolouration at the mucosal pit ridges that is pathognomonic of GIM. (b) A Paris IIa–c gastric lesion *(arrow)* on a background of GIM. Note the abnormal loss of pit pattern *(white box)* with microvasculature *(black arrows)*. Histology revealed high-grade dysplasia. (c) A flat gastric lesion with diffuse irregular microvasculature and loss of round mucosal pits. Histology revealed intra-mucosal adenocarcinoma.

The latest BSG guidelines from 2019 recommend that patients at high risk for GC or its premalignant lesions should have a systematic endoscopic evaluation lasting at least 7 minutes, with photographic documentation of the stomach regions.[201] Endoscopic suspicion should trigger the acquisition of a total of five biopsies at minimum according to the modified Sydney protocol. Three of these should come from the distal stomach, with two from the antrum (greater and lesser curvature) and one from the incisura, whereas the last two biopsies should be sampled at the gastric body (greater and lesser curvature).[201,221] These five biopsies should be directed at areas suspicious of GA/GIM and form the basis of the OLGA/OLGIM assessment. WLE suspicion of dysplastic or early neoplastic changes such as mucosal colour change, loss of vascularity, and mucosal elevation, depression, thickening, or nodularity should also be evaluated further using enhanced imaging (Figs. 2.10 and 2.11).

PROGRESSION TO GASTRIC CANCER AND FACTORS AFFECTING NEOPLASTIC TRANSFORMATION

In a recent systematic review, the risk of progression from GA/GIM to GC was reported at approximately 0.1–0.5%.[222] A Dutch study analysing patients (n = 92 250) with a first diagnosis of premalignant gastric lesions reported an annual incidence of GC of 0.1% for GA, 0.25% for GIM, 0.6% for mild/moderate dysplasia and 6% for severe dysplasia within 5 years of follow-up.[223] The distribution of GA and GIM is important, and extensive GA or GIM involving the proximal stomach is associated with higher risk of cancer.[224,225] Practice guidelines from the BSG consider severe forms of GA/GIM affecting the gastric cardia and body as an indication for endoscopic surveillance.[201] In a meta-analysis, incomplete GIM was found to better predict a risk of progression to dysplasia (pooled RR 4.82) and GC (pooled RR 4.96) compared with complete GIM.[226]

Epithelial gastric polyps have a variable link to GC. Fundic gland polyps (FGPs), the most common gastric polyps, generally related to PPI use and found in the proximal stomach, are almost always completely benign with no potential for neoplastic transformation. However, larger FGPs carry a probability of 1.9% to harbour dysplasia and 1.9% to harbour cancer. Hyperplastic polyps, often found next to ulcers, stomas, or gastrectomy regions, are frequently linked to GA/GIM and *H. pylori* gastritis. Although the majority (up to 70%) regress following *H. pylori* eradication, hyperplastic polyps can be dysplastic in 1.9–19% of cases and progress to cancer in 0.6–2.1% of cases.[201] Neoplastic risk is higher if the hyperplastic polyp is larger than 1 cm or in a post-gastrectomy context, and increases dramatically to 6% when dysplastic features are present histologically. Similar to hyperplastic polyps, adenomatous polyps are also linked to the synchronous presence of GA/GIM. They are often found at the antrum or incisura and carry a significant neoplastic risk. Synchronous GC is seen in around 30% of these polyps whereas adenomas larger than 2 cm can harbour adenocarcinoma in 50% of cases.

SCREENING

Early-stage GC has a much better prognosis and endoscopic treatment options in the form of EMR and ESD are available to successfully manage early neoplasia.[227] Japan and South Korea, the countries with established national screening programs, are the most prominent examples of achieving early-stage GC diagnosis, and as such, overall 5-year survival rates are significantly higher (65% and 71.5%, respectively) than the rest of the world (20–25%).[210]

Endoscopic screening by upper GI endoscopy, the only validated screening test for GC, in high-risk populations has been linked to decreased GC mortality and cost-effectiveness. A recent meta-analysis that evaluated 342 -013 Asian subjects showed that endoscopic screening, with the aim of diagnosing GC at an early stage, could reduce GC-related mortality by 40% (Zhang Gastroenterology, 2018). A Chinese multicentre study comparing one-time only endoscopically screened against unscreened individuals reported a reduction of 62% and 42% in non-cardia and cardia GC, respectively.[228] Unfortunately, a meta-analysis of 22 studies revealed that 9.4% of GCs are still missed on endoscopy, suggesting that the quality of the examination has a key role to play.[229] While population screening for GC is not recommended in low- and intermediate-risk populations such as the USA and Europe, societal guidelines suggest consideration of screening in individuals with multiple risk factors.[200,201,202] As an example, the BSG recommends a screening baseline endoscopy in individuals older than 50 years of age with other risk factors such as male sex, smokers, first-degree relatives with GC, or evidence of pernicious anaemia.

In order to improve the cost-effectiveness of screening strategies, especially in areas of low GC incidence, non-invasive testing methodologies have been investigated. Serum pepsinogen, a proenzyme of pepsin, a protease enzyme released in gastric secretions, represents is a serological marker with the potential to act as a triage tool. In a meta-analysis incorporating 31 studies, serum pepsinogen measurement displayed a sensitivity and specificity of 69% and 73%, respectively, for GC, and 69% and 88%, respectively, for GA.[230]

A large population-based Chinese study showed that the combination of five stomach-specific blood markers—pepsinogen I, pepsinogen II, pepsinogen I/II ratio, gastrin-17, and H. pylori IgG serology—was significantly better than traditional risk factors at predicting the presence of premalignant gastric lesions at baseline and the risk of progression to GC during follow-up.[231] Despite these data, the use of serum pepsinogen for large-scale screening in low-risk populations is not yet supported.

MANAGEMENT AND SURVEILLANCE OF GASTRIC ATROPHY AND GASTRIC INTESTINAL METAPLASIA

There is no clear consensus amongst GI societies. While AGA does not consider GA alone an indication for surveillance, the European MAPS (representing the ESGE) and BSG recommend follow-up in specific contexts. They suggest surveillance at 3-year intervals in cases of severe GA in the proximal stomach. However, follow-up for severe GA in the distal stomach is suggested where there is a positive family history or persistent H. pylori infection. The same follow-up is proposed in cases of moderate or severe pangastric GA; i.e. present in both the proximal and distal stomach.

✔✔ In the context of GIM, the AGA and ASGE state that they do not support routine endoscopic surveillance but do make a case for shared decision-making between physicians and patients based on the presence of high-risk factors and features of GIM.[199,200]

Both societies agree that incomplete type GIM, extensive GIM, or a family history of GC are high-risk factors for GC development.[232] All guidelines recommend systematic H. pylori testing and, if needed, eradication in patients with precancerous gastric lesions and those that have had early-stage GC removed endoscopically. This is based on evidence of significant relative risk reduction for incident GC following H. pylori eradication compared to placebo, even when GIM has already developed.[201,206]

ESGE recommendations are based on the evaluation of observational studies that show a reduction in GC risk and benefit in patient outcomes by screening and surveillance of premalignant gastric lesions. In contrast, the AGA does not recommend routine endoscopic surveillance in most premalignant contexts based on the lack of randomised controlled trials to provide evidence of benefit.

A practical algorithm for the endoscopic management of premalignant gastric lesions, based on the latest BSG and ESGE guidelines, is presented in Fig. 2.12. It is worth noting that although there are ways to select high-risk patients based on histological features, e.g. incomplete GIM or highly scoring OLGA/OLGIM, these are still the subject of ongoing research and, despite being mentioned in societal guidelines, not readily used in routine clinical practice.

MANAGEMENT OF DYSPLASIA

According to the latest guidelines from the BSG, LGD or HGD with visible lesions should be treated by endoscopic resection en bloc. To achieve en block resection, EMR is recommended in the context of small lesions ≤ 1 cm in size, whereas for lesions > 1 cm ESD is the preferred modality. Therapy should be followed by annual surveillance using systematic image-enhanced endoscopy.

In the context of non-visible dysplasia picked up on random biopsies, a repeat endoscopy is recommended to evaluate the stomach systematically with enhanced imaging. If non-visible LGD is still detected on the second endoscopy, annual surveillance with systematic image-enhanced endoscopy is recommended. The surveillance interval could be extended to 3-yearly if three consecutive endoscopies show no dysplasia on biopsies.

For non-visible HGD, the recommended surveillance interval following second confirmatory endoscopy is 6 months. If HGD persists without any visible lesions amenable to endoscopic resection, it should be discussed at the regional upper GI multidisciplinary team and referred to a tertiary centre for further evaluation.

MANAGEMENT OF GASTRIC POLYPS

The recent BSG guidelines have addressed the management of gastric polyps. It is imperative that the number and location of the gastric polyps is explicitly documented in the endoscopy report, along with representative photographic evidence. With the exception of FGPs, all other gastric polyps should be biopsied and sent for histological evaluation. In the context of adenomas or hyperplastic polyps, the BSG recommends evaluation of the background gastric mucosa to exclude the presence of GA, GIM, or synchronous dysplasia and cancer. Furthermore, H. pylori should be tested for and, if present, eradicated. Adenomas and hyperplastic polyps > 3 cm should be resected whereas hyperplastic polyps that are either symptomatic, pedunculated or larger than 1 cm should only be resected if H. pylori is absent or if still present on repeat endoscopy following H. pylori eradication. Annual surveillance endoscopy is recommended following complete resection of any adenoma, or of hyperplastic polyps displaying histological dysplasia. FGPs with typical appearances (small, smooth, shiny, with a similar colour to the surrounding mucosa and normal vasculature) warrant no follow-up. However, FGPs should be biopsied or excised if larger than 1 cm, present in the antrum, or display ulceration or other unusual, potentially dysplastic, features. FGPs found in large numbers (n > 20) in a young patient (< 40 years) with dysplastic features should lead to consideration of familial adenomatous polyposis (FAP) syndrome.

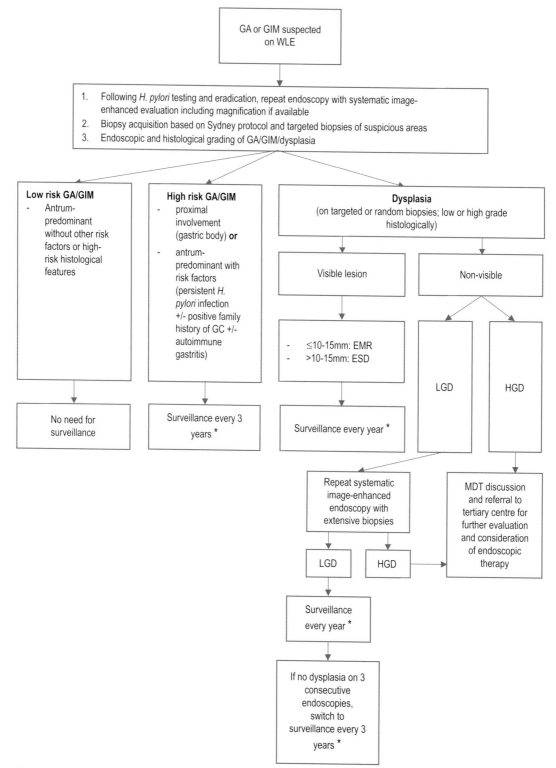

Figure 2.12 Flowchart on the management of gastric atrophy and gastric intestinal metaplasia based on the latest British Society of Gastroenterology (BSG) and European Society of Gastrointestinal Endoscopy (ESGE) guidelines. *EMR*, Endoscopic mucosal resection; *ESD*, endoscopic submucosal dissection; *GA*, gastric atrophy; *GC*, gastric cancer; *GI*, gastrointestinal; *GIM*, gastric intestinal metaplasia; *HGD*, high-grade dysplasia; *LGD*, low-grade dysplasia; *MDT*, multidisciplinary team. *All surveillance should be in the form of systematic, image-enhanced endoscopies with extensive biopsy acquisition.

GENETICS AND INHERITANCE OF GASTRIC CANCER

INHERITED GASTRIC CANCER SYNDROMES

Around 2–5% of patients with GCs occur on the basis of a hereditary syndrome. The best characterised of these is hereditary diffuse GC (HDGC), a cancer syndrome with a high prevalence for diffuse GC and lobular breast cancer (LBC). HDGC is thought to have an incidence of 5–10 per 100 000 births globally.[233] The disease has high penetrance and shows an autosomal dominant inheritance pattern characterised by deleterious (missense or truncating) germline mutations in the tumour-suppressing *CDH1* gene, which encodes for the epithelial (E)-cadherin protein.[234] E-cadherin is a transmembrane protein with a role in the maintenance of cell-cell cohesion.[235,236] *CDH1* mutations are present in approximately 40% of HDGC cases.[237] Carrying a *CDH1* mutation confers a lifetime risk of 42–70% in males and 33–56% in females for developing GC.[211,238] While some families fulfilling the criteria for HDGC do not have the underlying mutation characterised, a small proportion without *CDH1* mutations have a mutation in another junctional adhesion protein called α-catenin encoded by the *CTNNA1* gene.[239]

✓✓ In 2020, the International Gastric Cancer Linkage Consortium (IGCLC) 2015 guidelines for the management of HDGC were updated to reflect the combination of genetic tests becoming readily available in routine clinical practice and the increased understanding of HDGC endoscopic surveillance and post-gastrectomy follow-up.[233]

The major change in the new guidelines is a shift from the purely clinical definition to a new hybrid diagnostic definition based on clinical and genetic features. With the latter, HDGC is denoted by the presence of a pathogenic germline *CDH1* or *CTNNA1* variant and concomitant DGC in an individual or a family with at least one case of DGC among first- or second-degree relatives.[233] A separate HDGC-like category also exists based on the established presence of one DGC case and another GC without the detection of pathogenic *CDH1* or *CTNNA1* variants.

In order for clinicians to recommend genetic testing, specifically for the *CDH1* mutation, at least one of the criteria seen in Table 2.1 must be met:

If clinical criteria are met but no *CDH1* mutations are identified, it is recommended that genetic testing is extended to look for pathogenic *CTNNA1* variants. Where criteria are met, genetic counselling with extensive family history assessment and testing of younger family members should be considered. A multidisciplinary team approach involving geneticists, pathologists, gastroenterologists, and surgeons is of paramount importance when discussing management options, which include endoscopic surveillance and prophylactic total gastrectomy. The 2020 guidelines recommend that individuals carrying pathogenic *CDH1* variants with an established family history of DGC (as described earlier) have HDGC by definition and should be offered a prophylactic total gastrectomy.

Carriers of *CDH1* mutations were found to have positive gastric biopsies with evidence of microscopic signet-ring cell carcinoma (SRCC) in 40–61% of cases compared to < 10% in non-carriers.[240,241] Systematic, vigilant inspection during a dedicated session of at least 30 minutes with repeated inflation

Table 2.1   Clinical criteria to trigger genetic testing for hereditary diffuse gastric cancer

Family history criteria	Individual criteria
2 or more cases of GC, at least 1 being DGC, regardless of age	DGC earlier than 50 years of age
1 or more DGC at any age plus 1 or more LBC earlier than 70 years of age, in distinct members of the family (1st- or 2nd-degree relatives)	DGC in the context of Māori ethnicity or positive family history (1st-degree relative), or cleft lip/palate regardless of age
2 or more cases of LBC in members of the family (1st- or 2nd-degree relatives) less than 50 years old	Presence of both DGC and LBC earlier than 70 years of age or bilateral LBC earlier than 70 years of age
	Presence of signet-ring cells in the stomach either in situ or with pagetoid spread in an individual < 50 years old

and deflation is essential.[242] The Cambridge protocol is recommended in which 28–30 random biopsies are recommended which should include cardia ($n = 3–5$), fundus ($n = 5$), body ($n = 10$), transition zone ($n = 5$), and antrum ($n = 5$).[241,242]

Gastrectomy is not appropriate for individuals fulfilling HDGC criteria without an identified germline mutation. Annual endoscopic surveillance should also be offered to patients with pathogenic *CDH1* variants without a family history of DGC, especially if there is a family history of breast cancer. Although the penetrance of pathogenic *CTNNA1* variants is still under investigation, evidence from gastrectomy specimens of young asymptomatic carriers harbouring intra-mucosal DGC foci suggests that DGC risk might be as significant as for *CDH1* mutations.[243]

Gastric adenocarcinoma and proximal polyposis of the stomach (GAPPS) is a syndrome characterised by GC in the context of hundreds of fundic polyps.[237] It is an autosomal dominant, rare syndrome that was originally thought to be a distinct gastric syndrome but is now thought to be a subset of FAP syndrome (found in 2% of cases) based on evidence of the presence of *APC* gene mutations.[244,245] Another primary GC syndrome is that of familial intestinal gastric cancer (FIGC), which follows autosomal dominant inheritance with high incidence in Portugal and Japan, and is typified by intestinal-type GC.[237]

In addition to the syndromes listed earlier, other cancer syndromes confer high risk for GC development. These include:

- Lynch syndrome – characterised by mutations in the DNA mismatch repair genes, specifically *MLH1*, *MSAH2*, *MSH6*, *PMS1*, and *PMS2*, and a GC lifetime risk of 11–19%.[246–248]
- Juvenile polyposis syndrome – characterised by *SMAD4*, *BMPR1A*, and *ENG* gene mutations and a GC lifetime risk of 21%.[249]
- Peutz-Jeghers syndrome – caused by *STK11* mutations and a GC lifetime risk of 29%.[250]
- Li-Fraumeni syndrome – caused by *TP53* mutations and a GC lifetime risk of 2–3% for carriers.[251]
- Hereditary breast and ovarian cancer syndrome (HBOCS) – caused by *BRCA1* and *BRCA2* genes and a GC lifetime of 5%.[252]

- FAP syndrome – as per GAPPS previously, with a GC lifetime risk of 2% for carriers.

In addition to the hereditary syndromes, 10–20% of sporadic GC cases display familial aggregation confirming the genetic component involved in the pathogenesis of the disease, with early twin studies reporting that up to 28% of GC risk can be attributed to genetic factors.[212,253,254] In line with this, GC has been associated with inherited germline mutations. A volume of accumulating evidence has implicated pathogenic variants of the PALB2 and other genes of the homologous recombination DNA repair pathway (HRDR) in the pathogenesis of both HDGC and sporadic familial GC.[255–257] In combination with BRCA1, BRCA2, and RAD51C, PALB2 forms a protein complex that is responsible for repairing chromosomal breaks during DNA replication. In a study from Iceland, three different variants of ATM, another HRDR gene, were linked to increased risk of GC.[258] Exome sequencing from two distinct studies from The Cancer Genome Atlas (TCGA) confirmed the presence of recurrent germline mutations in HRDR genes such as PALB2, ATM, BRCA1, and BRCA2 in a significant proportion of cases.[259,260] GWAS using WGS assays have shed further light to the genetic variants linked to a high risk for GC. Eight genetic regions containing SNPs conferring high GC risk have been reported. Genes mapped to these regions include ZBTB20 (OR 1.32), PRKAA1 (OR 1.41), POLR3G-4 (OR 1.19), UNC5CL/LRFN2 (OR 1.18), ATM (OR 4.74), MUC1 (OR 1.35), PSCA (OR 1.33), and PLCE1 (OR 1.57).[209,254,261,262] Of interest as to the pathophysiology of GC, MUC1 encodes for a cell surface mucin abundant in the gastric epithelium that is important for cell signalling and protection from H. pylori colonization.

A recent review on the genetic predisposition of GC has concluded that, based on the available evidence for association to GC development, CDH1 and PALB2 should be the only genes considered as tier 1 genes and thus potentially useful in a clinical context, with tier 2 genes comprising of CTNNA1, MSH2, TP53, STK11, ATM, BRCA1, BRCA2, BRIP1, and ATR, and all remaining associated genes (e.g. APC, SMAD4) forming tier 3 genes.[254]

From a somatic mutation standpoint, a major study by TCGA Research Network revealed significant overlap between the driver gene landscape of diffuse and intestinal GC types that led to tumour classification according to four major categories: genomically stable, chromosomal unstable, microsatellite unstable, and EBV positive, with each category characterised by specific genetic anomalies.[209] Somatic mutations were most commonly identified in TP53, KRAS, ARID1A, PIK3CA, ERBB3, PTEN, and HLA-B. Highlighting the gene-environment interaction, in 2020 Bass and colleagues showed that early TP53 inactivation in gastric cells conferred increased susceptibility to premalignant states and progression to dysplasia and cancer.[263] It is worth noting that when evaluating true gastric and true OACs from a molecular perspective, the two are considered to be part of a spectrum, with OGJ adenocarcinomas somewhere between the two.

Genetic changes have also been studied in the context of precancerous gastric lesions. Firstly, the degree of DNA methylation in GIM has been shown to be higher than in GA, suggesting that this might contribute to propagation down the Correa cascade, perhaps triggered by persistent noxious agents such as H. pylori[264,265] Interestingly, GIM cases that eventually regressed displayed normal epigenomic states.[259] TP53 mutations were not as prevalent in GIM as

in paired GC samples, suggesting it might be a late event,[266] whereas microsatellite instability (MSI) might be an early event given that it has been shown to be augmented in GIM areas adjacent to GCs of the MSI subtype.[267]

FUTURE DIRECTIONS

Oesophageal and GCs are both among the top causes of cancer-related deaths worldwide and data suggest that, at least partly due to the ageing population, they will continue to occur frequently. An enhanced understanding of the risk factors, natural history, molecular genetics, and pathophysiology of the diseases has revealed premalignant lesions that can be targeted for early detection and treatment to prevent neoplastic transformation. Identifying cancer precursors or early-stage cancers can have a huge impact on patient outcomes and survival. More work is required to implement systematic clinical programmes to identify individuals at risk and intercept early. Biomarker discoveries continuously push the evolution of predicting which patients with premalignant pathologies will display neoplastic progression in order to guide surveillance. Technological advances in non-invasive screening devices, advanced diagnostic imaging, and endoscopic therapy are likely to shape future detection and management.

Key points

- Oesophageal and gastric cancers display significantly better survival rates when diagnosed at early vs late stages of disease.
- Premalignant, precursor lesions exist for oesophageal adenocarcinoma, oesophageal squamous cell carcinoma, and intestinal-type gastric cancer. These are Barrett's oesophagus, squamous dysplasia, and gastric atrophy/gastric intestinal metaplasia.
- Surveillance and treatment of Barrett's oesophagus is determined by the degree of histological dysplasia. High-grade dysplasia and persistent low-grade dysplasia warrant treatment with radiofrequency ablation ± endoscopic resection if visible lesions are also present.
- Squamous dysplasia and early oesophageal squamous neoplasia can be diagnosed using Lugol's chromoendoscopy or narrow-band imaging and treated with endoscopic mucosal resection, or ideally endoscopic submucosal dissection ± RFA applied to the background mucosa, followed by regular surveillance endoscopy.
- Gastric atrophy and gastric intestinal metaplasia are part of the Correa cascade following chronic inflammation, often as a result of H. pylori infection.
- Surveillance of gastric intestinal metaplasia depends on its location, subtype, extent, degree of histological dysplasia, and other patient risk factors.
- Screening for cancer precursors is not currently indicated in the Western world, unlike certain regions in the East where large, successful screening programs exist, but innovative strategies using non-invasive techniques and biomarkers to identify high-risk groups might change this in the future.
- Genetic studies have confirmed the presence of a hereditary component for both oesophageal and gastric cancer. Specific gene variants interact with environmental factors and there are rare inherited cancer syndromes, for example Hereditary Diffuse Gastric Cancer. It is important to identify patients with a likely inherited cancer syndrome so that their relatives are appropriately evaluated.

References available at http://ebooks.health.elsevier.com/

KEY REFERENCES

[3] Lagergren J, Bergström R, Lindgren A, Nyrén O. Symptomatic gastroesophageal reflux as a risk factor for esophageal adenocarcinoma. N Engl J Med 1999;340(11):825–31.

[8] Fitzgerald RC, di Pietro M, Ragunath K, Ang Y, Kang JY, Watson P, et al. British Society of Gastroenterology guidelines on the diagnosis and management of Barrett's oesophagus. Gut 2014;63(1):7–42.

[9] Shaheen NJ, Falk GW, Iyer PG, Gerson LB. ACG clinical guideline: diagnosis and management of barrett's esophagus. Am J Gastroenterol 2016;111(1):30–50. quiz 1.

[10] Weusten B, Bisschops R, Coron E, Dinis-Ribeiro M, Dumonceau JM, Esteban JM, et al. Endoscopic management of barrett's esophagus: European society of gastrointestinal endoscopy (ESGE) position statement. Endoscopy 2017;49(2):191–8.

[44] Fitzgerald RC, di Pietro M, O'Donovan M, Maroni R, Muldrew B, Debiram-Beecham I, et al. Cytosponge-trefoil factor 3 versus usual care to identify Barrett's oesophagus in a primary care setting: a multicentre, pragmatic, randomised controlled trial. Lancet (London, England) 2020;396(10247):333–44.

[56] P, Dent J, Armstrong D, Bergman JJ, Gossner L, Hoshihara Y, et al. The development and validation of an endoscopic grading system for barrett's esophagus: the prague C & M criteria. Gastroenterol 2006;131(5):1392–9.

[68] Qumseya B, Sultan S, Bain P, Jamil L, Jacobson B, Anandasabapathy S, et al. ASGE guideline on screening and surveillance of Barrett's esophagus. Gastrointest Endosc 2019;90(3):335. 59.e2.

[83] Krishnamoorthi R, Singh S, Ragunathan K, Visrodia K, Wang KK, Katzka DA, et al. Factors associated with progression of barrett's esophagus: a systematic review and meta-analysis. Clin Gastroenterol Hepatol : The Official Clinical Practice Journal of the American Gastroenterological Association 2018;16(7):1046–55.e8.

[96] Codipilly DC, Chandar AK, Singh S, Wani S, Shaheen NJ, Inadomi JM, et al. The effect of endoscopic surveillance in patients with barrett's esophagus: a systematic review and meta-analysis. Gastroenterol 2018;154(8):2068–86. e5.

[119] Jankowski JAZ, de Caestecker J, Love SB, Reilly G, Watson P, Sanders S, et al. Esomeprazole and aspirin in Barrett's oesophagus (AspECT): a randomised factorial trial. Lancet (London, England) 2018;392(10145):400–8.

[144] Sharma P, Brill J, Canto M, DeMarco D, Fennerty B, Gupta N, et al. White Paper AGA: advanced Imaging in Barrett's Esophagus. Clinical gastroenterology and hepatology : the official clinical practice. Journal of the American Gastroenterological Association 2015;13(13):2209–18.

[150] Wang GQ, Abnet CC, Shen Q, Lewin KJ, Sun XD, Roth MJ, et al. Histological precursors of oesophageal squamous cell carcinoma: results from a 13 year prospective follow up study in a high risk population. Gut 2005;54(2):187–92.

[200] Gupta S, Li D, El Serag HB, Davitkov P, Altayar O, Sultan S, et al. AGA clinical practice guidelines on management of gastric intestinal metaplasia. Gastroenterol 2020;158(3):693–702.

[201] Banks M, Graham D, Jansen M, Gotoda T, Coda S, di Pietro M, et al. British society of gastroenterology guidelines on the diagnosis and management of patients at risk of gastric adenocarcinoma. Gut 2019;68(9):1545–75.

[233] Blair VR, McLeod M, Carneiro F, Coit DG, D'Addario JL, van Dieren JM, et al. Hereditary diffuse gastric cancer: updated clinical practice guidelines. Lancet Oncol 2020;21(8):e386–97.

3 Staging of oesophageal and gastric cancer

Richard P. Owen | Nicholas D. Maynard

INTRODUCTION

Survival after a diagnosis of gastric and oesophageal cancer is highly variable, even with curative treatment.[1] The need for accurate staging is no longer limited to identifying patients who may be cured and those for whom cure is not possible, but provides material for a more informed discussion about treatment options through stratification of predicted outcomes and measurement of factors that influence treatment decisions. Taken together, this information can therefore help inform patients' decisions regarding the treatment of their disease and manage the expectations of treatment outcomes. Increasing staging accuracy has resulted in a more complex staging process, with multiple possible investigations and results requiring a range of expertise to perform and interpret. In the context of a cancer diagnosis, these investigations should happen expediently, which has in part driven regional specialisation to higher volume centres and standardisation of reporting so that outcomes can be compared on a like-for-like basis nationally and internationally.

STAGING CLASSIFICATIONS

Patients should be staged according to the TNM (tumour–node–metastasis) staging system proposed by Pierre Denoix in 1946.[2] T represents the extent of the primary tumour, N the extent of regional lymph node involvement, and M the presence or absence of distant metastases. A single TNM staging classification was agreed between the American Joint Committee on Cancer (AJCC), the Japanese Joint Committee (JJC), and the International Union Against Cancer (UICC) in 1987,[3] and multiple subsequent editions have been agreed. Currently, the Royal College of Pathologists use the American Joint Committee on Cancer TNM eighth edition (TNM8) classification as the reporting standard for gastric and oesophageal carcinoma, supported by the Association of Upper Gastrointestinal Surgeons.[4] Accordingly, TNM8 is used throughout this chapter.

✅✅ The eighth and most recent edition of the classification of gastric and oesophageal cancer was published in 2016 and takes into account advances in staging, diagnosis, and treatment that occurred since the last edition in 2009.[5] The eighth edition of TNM is used in the UK as standard practice.[4]

The prefixes of the TNM system are important to understand, especially for oesophagogastric cancer in which patients have frequently undergone neoadjuvant treatment.

c: clinical
p: pathological
yc: post neoadjuvant (radiation or systemic) therapy – clinical
yp: post neoadjuvant (radiation or systemic) therapy – pathological
a: autopsy

All oesophagogastric cancer should be confirmed histologically. Then, findings on clinical examination, imaging, direct luminal inspection, or laparoscopic inspection can be assessed and a clinical TNM staging assigned, which is designated with a 'c' prefix and is used to determine suitability for particular treatment options. The 'p' prefix refers to all the information from the clinical classification combined with the information gained from histopathological analysis. Pathological grading is more accurate in predicting prognosis and is therefore considered when planning adjuvant treatment.[6] Discrepancy between cTNM and pTNM is common,[7,8] particularly in gastric cancer staging,[9] and can therefore help evaluate the accuracy of staging methodologies. The 'y' prefix relates to patients who have undergone neoadjuvant treatment, and therefore acknowledges that the previous staging classification may have changed. TNM classifications are grouped into disease stages, and once the stage is established it should remain consistent in the medical records to allow for the selection and assessment of therapeutic interventions, and later audit. Final pathological stage grouping also provides the most accurate assessment of prognosis. In cases of doubt, where two classifications are given for T or N, then the lowest category is chosen. In situations of single-organ synchronous tumours, the TNM classification is based on the most advanced tumour, with either the number of tumours or 'm' recorded in parenthesis after the T stage. The prefix 'r' can be added in cases of recurrent cancer. The recent HERO consensus recommendations support the use of the Royal College of Pathologists Guidelines as a minimum dataset and provide explicit guidance on sample preparation and assessment, which will help benchmark pathological staging after oesophagogastric resection.[10]

OESOPHAGEAL CANCER STAGING

As described earlier, adequate and accurate staging of oesophageal cancer is crucial in planning treatment and to avoid unnecessary surgery, considering the negative impact resectional surgery has on an individual's subsequent quality of life.[11] Clinical assessment is an important early step in assessment, since some patients may require nutritional support, clearly lack the physiological reserve for major surgery, or do not want radical treatment, and recognising this from the outset is kinder and allows a more efficient delivery of healthcare.

Currently in the UK, core staging investigations include endoscopy with biopsy, multidetector contrast-enhanced computed tomography (CT), endoscopic ultrasound (EUS) with or without fine-needle aspiration (FNA) of suspicious lymph nodes, and positron emission tomography combined with CT (PET/CT).[12] Laparoscopy is also commonly used in patients with infradiaphragmatic oesophagogastric tumours. Other staging investigations that may be used in selected patients, usually to investigate further findings identified in the core staging investigations, are magnetic resonance imaging (MRI), ultrasound (US) imaging with or without FNA, endoscopic mucosal resection (EMR) for T1 lesions, endobronchial US (EBUS), and laparoscopic US.

The T, N, and M criteria for oesophageal cancer are listed in Table 3.1. In cases where a category cannot be established this is denoted with an 'x', with the exception of the M stage, since this is a binary output. The categories are the same for adenocarcinoma and squamous cell carcinomas. The T, N, and M criteria are required to establish the clinical stage grouping, as detailed in Table 3.2. In addition to the T, N, and M stages, TNM8 pathological stage groupings also include assessment of oesophageal cancer grade and location, with the latter relevant only to squamous cell carcinoma.

T STAGE

TNM8 includes T1 subcategories T1a and T1b to reflect the increasing role of endoscopic resection in early cancer, and the prognostic importance of submucosal invasion. T2 is invasion into the muscularis propria, and T3 is invasion into the oesophageal adventitia. In T4 oesophageal cancers, TNM8 considers the azygos vein, pleura, diaphragm, pericardium, and peritoneum within the T4a subcategory. T4b structures are the major blood vessels, vertebra, adjacent organs, and airways.

N STAGE

Confident N staging requires examination of at least seven lymph nodes, but in recognition that increasing lymph node yields are associated with improved survival, the National Oesophago-Gastric Cancer Audit (NOGCA) recommends a yield of at least 15 nodes, which is helpfully consistent with the standards of lymphadenectomy in gastric cancer.[13] In cases where fewer than seven lymph nodes are examined and found to be clear of cancer the staging would still be reported as pN0, but the possibility of understaging should be considered in treatment planning. Regional lymph nodes are confined to those within the oesophageal drainage zones – paratracheal, subcarinal, pulmonary ligament, paraoesophageal, diaphragmatic, paracardial, left gastric, common hepatic, splenic, celiac, and cervical paraesophageal level VI/VII nodes. Lymph nodes in other distant anatomical locations, such as supraclavicular nodes, are considered as metastatic disease.

Table 3.1   TNM8 cancer staging categories for oesophageal cancer

Category	Criteria
T category	
TX	Tumour cannot be assessed
T0	No evidence of primary tumour
Tis	High-grade dysplasia, defined as malignant cells confined by the basement membrane
T1	Tumour invades the lamina propria, muscularis mucosae, or submucosa
T1a	Tumour invades the lamina propria or muscularis mucosae
T1b	Tumour invades the submucosa
T2	Tumour invades the muscularis propria
T3	Tumour invades the adventitia
T4	Tumour invades the adjacent structures
T4a	Tumour invades the pleura, pericardium, azygos vein, diaphragm, or peritoneum
T4b	Tumour invades other adjacent structures, such as the aorta, vertebral body, or trachea
N category	
NX	Regional lymph nodes cannot be assessed
N0	No regional lymph node metastasis
N1	Metastasis in 1–2 regional lymph nodes
N2	Metastasis in 3–6 regional lymph nodes
N3	Metastasis in 7 or more regional lymph nodes
M category	
M0	No distant metastasis
M1	Distant metastasis

M STAGE

M staging refers to the presence of distant disease, including disease in non-regional lymph nodes. In TNM8, inability to establish M stage is regarded as M0, rather than Mx as in earlier editions of TNM.

GRADE

Tumour grade is reported using the standardised WHO histological grading system and is subdivided into well differentiated (G1), moderately differentiated (G2), and poorly differentiated (G3)[14] (Table 3.3). Grade reporting is of particular importance in both early cancers, when planning perioperative treatment or anticipating the risk of recurrence after endoscopic treatment, and in advanced cancers, since G3 lesions or those with signet ring morphology have a particularly poor prognosis.[15] Consequently, if the lesion is deemed G3 or signet ring type from the original diagnostic biopsy this should be recorded,[16] since it may be difficult to assess later after neoadjuvant treatment.[17] Poor inter-observer reliability in the pathological reporting of tumour grade and dysplasia is well known,[18,19] with one study showing that TNM7 staging was altered in 21% of patients with T1 or T2 node-negative oesophageal cancer. Therefore, TNM8 only includes grade in the pTNM

Table 3.2 TNM8 clinical stage groupings for oesophageal cancer

Clinical stage group	cT	cN	cM
Squamous cell carcinoma			
0	Tis	N0	M0
I	T1	N0–1	M0
II	T2	N0–1	M0
	T3	N0	M0
III	T3	N1	M0
	T1–3	N2	M0
IVA	T4	N0–2	M0
	T1–4	N3	M0
IVB	T1–4	N0–3	M1
Adenocarcinoma			
0	Tis	N0	M0
I	T1	N0	M0
IIA	T1	N1	M0
IIB	T2	N0	M0
III	T2	N1	M0
	T3–4a	N0–1	M0
IVA	T1–4a	N2	M0
	T4b	N0–2	M0
	T1–4	N3	M0
IVB	T1–4	N0–3	M1

Table 3.3 TNM8 pathological grade of oesophageal cancer

Adenocarcinoma

GX	Differentiation cannot be assessed
G1	Well differentiated. > 95% of tumour is composed of well-formed glands
G2	Moderately differentiated. 50–95% of tumour shows gland formation
G3[†]	Poorly differentiated. Tumours composed of nests and sheets of cells, with <50% of tumours demonstrating glandular formation

Squamous cell carcinoma

GX	Differentiation cannot be assessed
G1	Well differentiated. Prominent keratinization with pearl formation and a minor component of nonkeratinizing basal-like cells. Tumour cells are arranged in sheets, and mitotic counts are low
G2	Moderately differentiated. Variable histologic features, ranging from parakeratotic to poorly keratinizing lesions. Generally, pearl formation is absent
G3[‡]	Poorly differentiated. Consists predominantly of basal-like cells forming large and small nests with frequent central necrosis. The nests consist of sheets or pavement-like arrangements of tumour cells, and are occasionally punctuated by small numbers of parakeratotic or keratinizing cells

[†]If further testing of "undifferentiated" cancers reveals a glandular component, categorise as adenocarcinoma G3.
[‡]If further testing of "undifferentiated" cancers reveals a squamous cell component, or if after further testing they remain undifferentiated, categorise as squamous cell carcinoma G3.

Box 3.1 TNM8 anatomical sites for location staging of oesophageal squamous cell carcinoma

Upper: Cervical oesophagus to lower border of azygos vein
Middle: Lower border of azygos vein to lower border of inferior pulmonary vein
Lower: Lower border of inferior pulmonary vein to stomach, including the oesophagogastric junction

rather than cTNM stage groupings, thus avoiding reliance on endoscopic sampling to establish grade.

LOCATION

According to TNM8 definitions, oesophageal cancers occur throughout the length of the oesophagus and the proximal 2 cm of the stomach. Proximal overlap of cancer into the pharynx is rarely of surgical importance since the primary treatment is usually chemoradiotherapy, but distal overlap of oesophageal cancer into the stomach can alter the surgical approach. In the case of oesophageal squamous cell carcinoma (OSCC) tumour location influences the stage, and TNM8 specifies the cancer epicentre as the reference point and uses common radiological landmarks to define anatomical subsites (Box 3.1),[20] whereas in adenocarcinoma most tumours are distal.

For surgical planning, further anatomical descriptions of tumour location, assessed by imaging and endoscopically, are often used in multidisciplinary team (MDT) discussions since these help to plan the surgical approach and suitability for radiotherapy. It is useful to include these anatomical definitions here, to recognise that they differ from the TNM8 anatomical subsite descriptions and avoid confusion when terms may be used interchangeably in MDT:

- Cervical oesophagus: lower border of the cricoid to thoracic inlet, marked at the suprasternal notch and approximately 18 cm from incisors.
- Upper thoracic oesophagus: thoracic inlet to tracheal bifurcation (24 cm from the incisors).
- Middle thoracic oesophagus: tracheal bifurcation to the halfway point between tracheal bifurcation and the oesophagogastric junction (32 cm from the incisors).
- Lower thoracic oesophagus: the halfway point between tracheal bifurcation and the oesophagogastric junction to the oesophagogastric junction (40 cm from the incisors).
- Oesophagogastric junction.

The Siewert-Stein classification is used for oesophagogastric junctional tumours, with the tumour epicentre defining the type, separating them into type I (1–5 cm above the oesophagogastric junction), type II (from 1 cm above the oesophagogastric junction to 2 cm below it), and type III (more than 2 cm below the oesophagogastric junction).[21] Since TNM8, type III oesophagogastric junction cancers are classified and staged as gastric cancers.

Table 3.4   TNM8 pathological stage groupings for oesophageal cancer

Pathological stage group	pT	pN	pM	pGrade	pLocation
Squamous cell carcinoma					
0	Tis	N0	M0	N/A	Any
IA	T1a	N0	M0	G1, X	Any
IB	T1b	N0	M0	G1, X	Any
	T1	N0	M0	G2–3	Any
	T2	N0	M0	G1	Any
IIA	T2	N0	M0	G2–3, X	Any
	T3	N0	M0	Any	Lower
	T3	N0	M0	G1	Upper/middle
IIB	T3	N0	M0	G2–3	Upper/middle
	T3	N0	M0	X	Any
	T3	N0	M0	Any	X
	T1	N1	M0	Any	Any
IIIA	T1	N2	M0	Any	Any
	T2	N1	M0	Any	Any
IIIB	T4a	N0–1	M0	Any	Any
	T3	N1	M0	Any	Any
	T2–3	N2	M0	Any	Any
IVA	T4a	N2	M0	Any	Any
	T4b	N0–2	M0	Any	Any
	T1–4	N3	M0	Any	Any
IVB	T1–4	N0–3	M1	Any	Any
Adenocarcinoma					
0	Tis	N0	M0	N/A	
IA	T1a	N0	M0	G1, X	
IB	T1a	N0	M0	G2	
	T1b	N0	M0	G1–2, X	
IC	T1	N0	M0	G3	
	T2	N0	M0	G1–2	
IIA	T2	N0	M0	G3, X	
IIB	T1	N1	M0	Any	
	T3	N0	M0	Any	
IIIA	T1	N2	M0	Any	
	T2	N1	M0	Any	
IIIB	T4a	N0–1	M0	Any	
	T3	N1	M0	Any	
	T2–3	N2	M0	Any	
IVA	T4a	N2	M0	Any	
	T4b	N0–2	M0	Any	
	T1–4	N3	M0	Any	
	T1–4	N0–3	M1	Any	

N/A, Not applicable; *X*, not defined.

The pathological stage groupings for oesophageal adeno-carcinoma (OAC) and OSCC are different to reflect that the prognosis of early OSCC is worse than in early OAC.[22,23] While data supporting survival differences for OSCC in different locations is mixed,[24,25] TNM7 has recognised tumour location as a prognostic factor and it remains in pathological stage groupings for TNM8 (Table 3.4). Arguably, the pure pTNM stage groups are losing relevance for oesophageal cancer due to the widespread use of neoadjuvant treatment with alternative prognostic factors such as tumour regression and complete pathological response becoming increasingly important.[26,27] This has led to a new stage grouping specific to post neoadjuvant patients in TNM8, with the same groupings for oesophageal squamous cell and adeno-carcinoma (Table 3.5).

✔✔ In 2 045 and 5 686 patients with OSCC and adeno-carcinoma, respectively, there was no residual cancer (ypT-0N0M0) in 25% of squamous cell carcinomas and 13% of ad-enocarcinomas treated with neoadjuvant therapy, prompting the need for specific post neoadjuvant stage groupings.[27]

TNM8 also includes numerous other requirements for staging oesophageal cancer, which may influence clinical decisions in borderline cases and help guide therapeutic options. A complete list of these requirements is included in Box 3.2.

Table 3.5   TNM8 post neoadjuvant therapy (ypTNM) stage groupings

ypStage group	ypT	ypN	ypM
I	T0–2	N0	M0
II	T3	N0	M0
IIIA	T0–2	N1	M0
IIIB	T4a	N0	M0
	T3	N1–2	M0
	T0–3	N2	M0
IVA	T4a	N1–2, X	M0
	T4b	N0–2	M0
	T1–4	N3	M0
IVB	T1–4	N0–3	M1

Box 3.2   TNM8 registry data collection variables for oesophageal cancer

Clinical staging modalities (endoscopy and biopsy, EUS, EUS/FNA, CT, PET/CT)
Tumour length
Depth of invasion
Number of nodes involved, clinical
Number of nodes involved, pathological
Location of nodal disease, clinical
Location of nodal disease, pathological
Sites of metastases, if applicable
Presence of skip lesions: T(m)
Perineural invasion
LVI (lymphatic, vascular, both)
Extranodal extension
Type of surgery
Chemotherapy
Chemoradiation therapy (for ypTNM)
Surgical margin (negative, microscopic, macroscopic)
HER2 status (positive or negative), adenocarcinoma only

CT, Computed tomography; *EUS*, endoscopic ultrasound; *FNA*, fine-needle aspiration; *HER2*, human epidermal growth factor receptor two; *LVI*, lymphovascular invasion; *PET*, positron emission tomography; *ypTNM*, post neoadjuvant (radiation or systemic) therapy – pathological tumour–node–metastasis staging.

GASTRIC CANCER STAGING

As for oesophageal cancer, accurate gastric cancer staging is important to avoid unnecessary surgery, since outcomes from palliative gastrectomy cannot justify resection in most cases.[28] International consensus on gastric cancer staging has been more challenging than in oesophageal cancer due to the different aetiology and anatomical distribution of gastric cancers in different parts of the world.[29,30] Unlike in oesophageal cancer, nearly all gastric cancers are adenocarcinomas and numerous histopathological classifications exist,[14,31–36] making globally unified subtyping difficult to apply. Consequently, there is no differentiation in the TNM staging groupings to recognise the clear variability in the biological behaviours of gastric cancers worldwide.[37] Ultimately, anticipation of limited availability of the immunohistochemical and genetic assays which would be required to biologically subtype gastric cancers have restricted their inclusion in TNM8. In general, distal gastric cancers have a lower mortality and are more common in Asian countries, whereas proximal gastric cancers are more common in the West and have poorer survival.[38–40] Whether very proximal lesions are staged as gastric or oesophageal cancers has evolved over the last iterations of TNM; with clinician's judgement used in TNM6,[41] all tumours with involvement of the oesophagogastric junction are staged as oesophageal in TNM7, to the current system in TNM8 where type III Siewert-Stein tumours (involving junction but tumour epicentre 2–5 cm below the oesophagogastric junction) are staged as gastric cancers. Note that gastric neuroendocrine tumours are also staged by TNM8. The TNM8 categories are shown in Table 3.6.

T STAGING

Similar to oesophageal cancer, TNM8 T staging now divides T1 disease into mucosal (T1a, tumour invades lamina propria or muscularis mucosae) and submucosal (T1b) to reflect increasing endoscopic treatment options for early gastric cancers. Within the earliest stage of in situ gastric carcinoma, high-grade dysplasia is now included in TNM8. T2 is invasion of the muscularis propria, T3 is invasion of the subserosa (with no invasion of the visceral peritoneum), T4a is invasion of the serosa, and T4b is invasion of adjacent structures.

N STAGING

N staging is an important prognostic feature in the radical treatment of gastric cancer. TNM8 defines the regional lymph node stations as paracardial and perigastric, along the greater and lesser curves (1–6), left gastric artery (7), common hepatic artery (8), coeliac trunk (9), splenic hilum (10), splenic artery (11), and the hepatoduodenal nodes (12). Other abdominal lymph node stations are classified as distant metastases (13–16, retropancreatic, mesenteric, and para-aortic). The required lymph node yield in gastric cancer is 15, despite no survival advantage seen in pN0 disease beyond 10 nodes, to acknowledge the potential for understaging and the survival benefits seen with yields of 30+ nodes for pN1–3 disease.[42] In support of higher lymph node yields, ratios of positive to negative lymph nodes have been shown as an independent prognostic factor, even where lymph node yields have been inadequate.[43,44]

M STAGING

M1 disease is classified as distant organ involvement, peritoneal metastases, positive peritoneal cytology, and omental tumour that is not a result of direct invasion from the primary tumour. Internationally, radical treatment of low-volume or isolated metastatic disease has given surprisingly good survival outcomes in some reports.[45–47] Few prospective trial data are available, but the Japanese phase III REGATTA trial showed no benefit from the addition of surgery to chemotherapy in patients with one non-curable factor (isolated liver, or peritoneal or para-aortic disease),[48] although whether this is applicable to current UK and European perioperative chemotherapeutic approaches is not clear. The potential for widening access to radical

Table 3.6   TNM8 cancer staging categories for gastric cancer

T category

TX	Primary tumour cannot be assessed
T0	No evidence of primary tumour
Tis	Carcinoma in situ: intraepithelial tumour without invasion of the lamina propria, high-grade dysplasia
T1	Tumour invades the lamina propria, muscularis mucosae, or submucosa
T1a	Tumour invades the lamina propria or muscularis mucosae
T1b	Tumour invades the submucosa
T2	Tumour invades the muscularis propria
T3	Tumour invades the subserosa
T4	Tumour perforates the serosa (visceral peritoneum) or invades the adjacent structures
T4a	Tumour perforates the serosa
T4b	Tumour invades the adjacent structures

N category

NX	Regional lymph nodes cannot be assessed
N0	No regional lymph node metastasis
N1	Metastasis in 1–2 regional lymph nodes
N2	Metastasis in 3–6 regional lymph nodes
N3a	Metastasis in 7–15 regional lymph nodes
N3b	Metastasis in 16 or more regional lymph nodes

M category

M0	No distant metastasis
M1	Distant metastasis

M1 includes positive peritoneal cytology, peritoneal seeding, and omental tumour not part of continuous extension.

Box 3.3   TNM8 registry data collection variables for gastric cancer

Tumour location
Serum CEA
Serum CA 19-9
Clinical staging modalities (endoscopy and biopsy, EUS, EUS/FNA, CT, PET/CT)
Tumour length
Depth of invasion
Number of suspicious malignant lymph nodes on baseline radiologic images
Number of suspicious malignant lymph nodes by EUS assessment
Location of suspicious nodes (clinical)
Location of suspicious nodes (pathological)
Number of tumour deposits
Lymphovascular invasion
Neural invasion
Extranodal extension
HER2 status (positive or negative)
MSI status
Surgical margin (negative, microscopic, macroscopic)
Sites of metastasis, if applicable
Type of surgery

CA19-9, carbohydrate antigen 19-9; *CEA*, carcinoembryonic antigen; *CT*, computed tomography; *EUS*, endoscopic ultrasound; *FNA*, fine-needle aspiration; *HER2*, human epidermal growth factor receptor two; *MSI*, microsatellite instability; *PET*, positron emission tomography.

treatment in a subset of M1 gastric cancer has meant further classifications of oligometastatic disease have been necessary, in particular for the further staging of peritoneal metastases. While several ways to quantify and site peritoneal cancer exist, in gastric cancer the Peritoneal Cancer Index is commonly used to set inclusion criteria for trials in cytoreductive surgery and intraperitoneal chemotherapy and has been shown to be prognostically important.[49–51] Another classification sometimes used is taken from the first English edition of the Japanese classification of gastric carcinoma, with peritoneal carcinomatosis graded as: P1, metastases to the adjacent but not to the distant peritoneum; P2, a few metastases to the distant peritoneum; and P3, numerous metastases to the distant peritoneum.[52] Several other ways to quantify peritoneal cancer exist, and in gastric cancer it is likely that more relevant and consistent ways of defining the extent of oligometastatic gastric cancer will be developed, especially if current trials, such as PERISCOPE II and RENAISSANCE, support radical treatments for these patients.[53,54]

While staging can be performed without specific assays, TNM8 does include a set of prognostic factors beyond the TNM category, including HER2 status. HER2-positive tumours are more commonly of the intestinal subtype, which is more prevalent in proximal or oesophagogastric junctional tumours, and geographically in the West, meaning these tumour types are more likely to be suitable for targeted therapies.[55] A full list of the TNM8 registry data collection variables for gastric cancer is in Box 3.3. As in oesophageal cancer, gastric cancer stage groupings have been devised for clinical staging, pathological staging, and post neoadjuvant treatment staging, to reflect better current international practices and provide more accurate prognostic detail (Table 3.7).

ENDOSCOPY

Fibre-optic endoscopy remains the most important investigation in the diagnosis of gastric and oesophageal cancers, and this is reflected in the UK's 2-week wait referral system for upper gastrointestinal red flag symptoms.[56] Diagnostic gastroscopy is a safe procedure, with a perforation risk of less than 0.05% and inpatient mortality risk of 0.008%, with cardiopulmonary complications as the most common cause of death.[57,58] In staging, endoscopy provides a wealth of information about the site and nature of the lesion, allowing for accurate surgical planning and direct tumour visualisation and biopsy. The sensitivity for the diagnosis of oesophagogastric cancer increases with multiple biopsies,[59,60] hence the current recommendation is for a minimum of six biopsies to be obtained from a suspected cancer along with photographic documentation of the lesion.[61] In cases where a tumour is impassable dilatation is not recommended, since perforation from dilatation will greatly worsen prognosis.

Table 3.7   TNM8 stage groupings for gastric cancer

Clinical staging

Stage 0	Tis	N0	M0
Stage I	T1–2	N0	M0
Stage IIA	T1–2	N1–3	M0
Stage IIB	T3–4a	N0	M0
Stage III	T3–4a	N1-3	M0
Stage IVA	T4b	N1-3	M0
Stage IVB	Any T	Any N	M1

Pathologic staging

Stage 0	Tis	N0	M0
Stage IA	T1	N0	M0
Stage IB	T1	N1	M0
	T2	N0	M0
Stage IIA	T1	N2	M0
	T2	N1	M0
	T3	N0	M0
Stage IIB	T1	N3a	M0
	T2	N2	M0
	T3	N1	M0
	T4a	N0	M0
Stage IIIA	T2	N3a	M0
	T3	N2	M0
	T4a	N1–2	M0
	T4b	N0	M0
Stage IIIB	T1-2	N3b	M0
	T3–4a	N3a	M0
	T4b	N1–2	M0
Stage IIIC	T3–4a	N3b	M0
	T4b	N3a–3b	M0
Stage IV	Any T	Any N	M1

Pathologic staging following neoadjuvant therapy

Stage I	T1–2	N0	M0
	T1	N1	M0
Stage II	T3–4a	N0	M0
	T2–3	N1	M0
	T1–2	N2	M0
	T1	N3	M0
Stage III	T4b	N0	M0
	T4a–4b	N1	M0
	T3, 4a, 4b	N2	M0
	T2, 3, 4a, 4b	N3	M0
Stage IV	Any T	Any N	M1

✔✔ Despite limited supporting data, the 2017 position statement and strong recommendation of the Association of Upper Gastrointestinal Surgeons and the British Society of Gastroenterology is that a minimum of six biopsies should be obtained from any suspected upper gastrointestinal malignancy.[61]

COMPUTED TOMOGRAPHY

Following diagnosis of oesophagogastric cancer, CT of the chest, abdomen, and pelvis provides the most cost-effective and efficient way to proceed with staging, since it can provide coarse local and distant staging information. To aid rapid staging, CT should be requested when there is a reasonable suspicion of cancer at endoscopy, ahead of confirmed histology.[61]

OESOPHAGEAL CANCER

CT can identify locally invasive lesions with high accuracy due to identifiable disruption of fat planes between the tumour and major structures, whereas in early T-stage cancer CT can only comment on the thickness of the oesophageal wall, and therefore accuracy is poor for early cancers (Fig. 3.1). Studies have quantified oesophageal wall thickness to assess T stage as follows: normal as < 5 mm, 'modified' T2 as 5–15 mm, T3 as > 15 mm with outer margin irregularity, and T4 as invasion of adjacent structures such as the trachea, aortic pericardium, or vertebral body.[62] In a small study of 41 patients, these oesophageal wall thickness

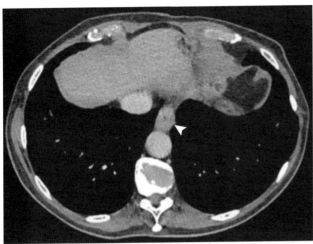
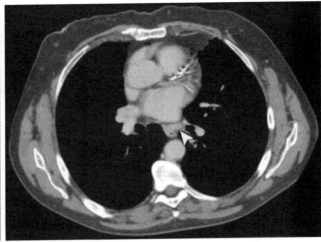

Figure 3.1 The left image shows a computed tomography (CT) image of a patient with a T3N0 type I junctional adenocarcinoma (tumour marked with the *white arrow*), and the right image shows a CT image of a patient with T3N2 lower oesophageal adenocarcinoma (enlarged lymph node inferior to left main bronchus marked with the *yellow arrow*, the primary tumour is not seen on this image).

cut-offs achieved accuracies of 75%, 79%, and 64%, in T1 or T2, T3, and T4 tumours, respectively, with an overall sensitivity of 60% and specificity of 69%.[63]

The accuracy of N staging from CT is also variable, since an arbitrary size cut-off of 10 mm is typically used as the sole deterministic factor in identifying nodal involvement. Using a size cut-off of 10 mm gives a poor sensitivity 50%, but a high specificity of 83%, with a higher specificity of 93% for abdominal lymph nodes.[64] More recently, logistic regression analysis has incorporated other CT-derived node parameters (node shape determined by the nodal axial ratio, and node heterogeneity determined by CT texture analysis) to achieve 87.5% sensitivity and 65.8% specificity.[65]

CT is the mainstay of identifying distant metastatic disease, however its sensitivity is limited, meaning further staging tests are usually required. A meta-analysis of 437 patients in seven studies showed the sensitivity and specificity for the diagnosis of distant metastases as 52% (95% CI 0.33–0.71) and 91% (95% CI 0.86–0.96), respectively.[64]

GASTRIC CANCER

In gastric cancer, CT is normally performed with intravenous contrast after drinking 750 mL of water or taking carbon dioxide-releasing granules to create negative intraluminal contrast and distension to highlight areas of wall thickening or projections into the gastric lumen. Some imaging protocols also recommend the administration of hyoscine butyl bromide to reduce movement artefacts by inducing gastric hypotonia. T-stage accuracy in gastric cancer is generally higher than in oesophageal cancer due to appreciation of a multi-layered wall corresponding to histological layers (Fig. 3.2). The overall accuracy of T staging by CT is 77%, but this has been shown to increase to 84% using volumetric scanning.[66] Similar volumetric CT protocols have also shown fairly good results in T1/T2 lesions with accuracies of 64.9% and 63.5% reported by two independent reviewers examining images in 148 patients with early gastric cancer.[67] The accuracy of CT to identify local organ invasion by gastric cancer has traditionally been poor, because inflammatory adhesions and local oedema can inhibit the ability of CT to discriminate true invasion. One study using CT identified

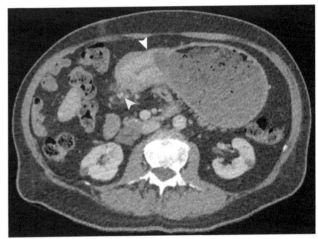

Figure 3.2 Axial computed tomography image of a patient with a T4aN1 obstructing pyloric adenocarcinoma (marked by the *white arrow*), fat stranding around the tumour, and small surrounding lymph nodes (marked by the *yellow arrow*).

pancreatic, hepatic, and colonic invasion with accuracies of 75%, 61%, and 78%, respectively, meaning CT is unreliable as the sole staging method to determine whether gastric cancer is resectable.[68] More advanced multiplanar reformation CT, now in common use in the UK, performed better, with pancreatic and transverse colonic or mesocolonic invasion identified by two reviewers with sensitivities of 82.6% and 87% and specificities of 98.4% and 100% in 149 T3 and T4 gastric cancers.[69]

CT staging of nodal status is variable, in part due to inconsistent and changing lymph node examination protocols in resected specimens, making a positive control difficult to standardise.[70] Typically a threshold of 6 mm is used for coeliac axis lymph nodes and 8 mm for perigastric lymph nodes is used, with lymph node shape, heterogeneous enhancement, central necrosis, and clustering of three or more lymph nodes all also described as features to determine lymph node involvement.[71] This lack of international consensus, changes in the nodal staging systems, and non-uniform evaluation of resected lymph nodes has made

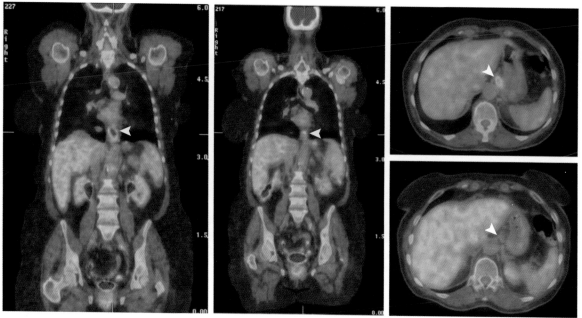

Figure 3.3   The coronal plane positron emission tomography/computed tomography (PET/CT) images on the left show an fluorodeoxyglucose (FDG) avid distal oesophageal adenocarcinoma before (left side) and after (right side) neoadjuvant chemotherapy. The tumour is marked with a *yellow arrow*. The axial PET/CT images on the right side show an FDG avid pericardial lymph node before (top) and after (bottom) neoadjuvant chemotherapy. The lymph node is marked with a *white arrow*.

it difficult to determine the accuracy of CT to correctly N-stage gastric cancer. One systematic review from 2009 found that the sensitivity for identifying N stage was 50–89.9% with a specificity of 62.5–91.9%.[72] These findings are consistent with more recent studies.[73]

Accurate recognition of distant metastases in gastric cancer by CT alone is appealing, since it is readily available, would reduce the need for invasive investigations, and help limit the expectations of offering radical therapy. A study of 350 patients with gastric cancer staged with CT showed 96.6% accuracy for the identification of distant metastases and an accuracy of 87.4% to identify resectable disease.[74] A previous systematic review has shown reduced sensitivity and specificity for hepatic and peritoneal metastases of 74% and 99%, and 33% and 99%, respectively.[75] Both of these studies highlight the well-recognised concerns of poor detection of peritoneal metastases by CT. Studies looking at this issue in isolation have not performed much better, with a sensitivity of 50.9% and specificity of 96.2% for the CT identification of peritoneal metastases, allowing for equivocal findings taken as positive identification.[76] More complex predictions of peritoneal metastases using CT radiomics, tumour size, presence of ascites, and Bohrmann classification are described and can improve the detection of metastatic disease, but are unlikely to replace further staging tests in patients who may be suitable for radical treatment.[77–80]

✔✔ Numerous small studies show that the accuracy of CT to correctly identify T, N, and M stages in oesophagogastric cancer is limited. The relative availability, safety, and affordability of CT means its use is recommended, but it should not be relied upon as a sole staging investigation in most patients planned for radical treatment.[12,81,82]

PET/CT

The Warburg effect observes that cancer cells generally produce energy by a high rate of glycolysis with the production of lactic acid, rather than the relatively low levels of glycolysis with subsequent oxidation of pyruvate in mitochondria seen in normal cells.[83] This high glycolysis mode of metabolism results in preferential uptake of glucose by cancer cells in fasted-state patients, and therefore increased glucose accumulation. The glucose analogue 2-deoxy-2-[18 F]-fluoro-D-glucose, abbreviated to FDG, is the most commonly used isotope in cancer imaging. In PET scanning, administered FDG is taken up from the blood preferentially by tumour cells through GLUT1 transport. Once FDG is in the tumour cells, it is phosphorylated by hexokinase to form FDG-6- phosphate, which is not easily metabolised further and hence provides signal for detection.[84] FDG uptake can be quantified within regions of interest and is most commonly measured using the maximum Standard Uptake Value (SUVmax). When the SUVmax in a region of interest exceeds the background physiological signal, it can be termed 'FDG avid', although confusingly the term 'FDG avidity' is used synonymously with SUVmax. Fig. 3.3 shows PET/CT images of two patients with oesophageal cancer.

OESOPHAGEAL CANCER

PET/CT is currently recommended to be used in all patients with oesophageal cancer suitable for radical therapy by the National Institute of Health and Care Excellence (NICE), the European Society for Medical Oncology (ESMO), and NOGCA.[12,13,81] Therefore, while the additive effect of multimodal investigations remains critical to the personalisation of staging of each patient's tumour, these guidelines highlight that PET/CT has become the single most important investigation in staging oesophageal cancer, and PET/CT scanning should be the cornerstone of any staging algorithm for oesophageal cancer.

✓✓ National and international guidelines recommend PET/CT for the staging of oesophageal cancer suitable for radical therapy.[12,81]

In local staging of the primary tumour, PET/CT is limited due to the unenhanced nature of the CT, lower resolution, and relatively large slices (usually 6 mm). Assessment of the liver is compromised for the same reasons. Much of the literature reports on older PET scanning alone, so accuracies are likely to be improved with combined scanning algorithms. In particular, combined contrast-enhanced CT and PET (PET/ceCT) could provide a more streamlined staging option in certain cases, with the potential for PET/ceCT to become the sole imaging requirement for staging most patients with oesophageal cancer.[85] Correct T staging was only reported in 42% of patients from PET scanning in a study of 75 patients.[86] Early cancers are also less likely to be detected by PET scan, presumably due to a low volume of metabolically active tumour cells, with FDG avidity in only 18% and 43% of T1a and T1b tumours, respectively, compared to 90% of T2 and 98% of T3 tumours in the same study.[87] The grading of the metabolic activity of a tumour with FDG avidity has been of prognostic interest, since it provides an objective metric that has been suggested to predict survival, although SUVmax is probably only relevant in the context of its change in response to neoadjuvant therapy, rather than the absolute value pre-treatment.[88]

For N staging, a study of 149 patients staged with PET scanning was 72% accurate and provided additional staging information to CT in 14.3% of patients.[87] A more recent meta-analysis of 10 studies shows a sensitivity and specificity of PET/CT for the detection of regional lymph node metastases of 57% (95% CI 43–70%) and 85% (95% CI 76–95%), respectively, which was a slight improvement over CT alone.[64] Fig. 3.4 shows the CT and PET/CT images of a patient with oesophageal cancer with a positive paratracheal lymph node. As in primary tumour assessment, PET/CT offers a prognostic advantage when nodal FDG avidity reduces in response to neoadjuvant therapy, as demonstrated in an observational study and a further validation study of 294 and 200 patients, respectively, which showed an association of nodal response with unresectable disease, early recurrence, and death[89,90] (also see Fig. 3.3, right-sided images).

The main benefit of PET/CT is the detection of distant metastases, as this will prevent patients from having radical treatment with no chance of cure and potentially high morbidity. Fig. 3.5 shows pelvic metastatic disease in a patient with oesophageal cancer. Two meta-analyses found similar sensitivities of 71% (95% CI 62–79%) and 67% (95% CI 58–76%) and specificities of 93% (95% CI 89–97%) and 97% (95% CI 90–100%) for the detection of distant metastases by PET scan,[64,91] which exceeded the performance of CT scanning. Whether the use of PET/CT changes management has been more debatable, with earlier studies showing mixed results, albeit with very different routine staging pathways prior to PET scan.[92,93] Two more recent studies investigating the impact of PET/CT in routine oesophageal cancer staging have found that additional staging detail was frequently added and clinically relevant changes were

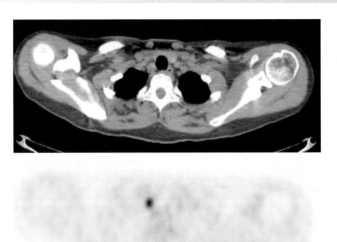
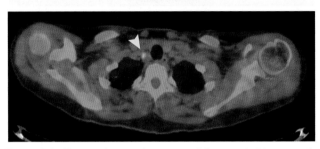

Figure 3.4 The top image shows an axial computed tomography (CT) image at T1 in a patient with mid-oesophageal squamous cell carcinoma. The positron emission tomography (PET) scan (middle image) at the same plane shows a focus of FDG uptake in the right paratracheal lymph nodes. The lowermost image shows PET and CT fusion, demonstrating the FDG avid lymph node *(yellow arrow)*.

made in 17% and 23% of treatment plans.[94,95] Since clinical management changes are common after PET/CT, and it is a non-invasive test, NICE guidelines support the use of PET/CT earlier in the staging process than EUS.[12]

PET/CT becomes of less value if the primary tumour is not FGD avid, since the sensitivity of detection of primary tumour, regional lymph node involvement, and distant metastases is reduced. In the case of very early tumours, the chance of both FDG avidity and distant metastases is low and therefore the utility of PET in T1 disease is debatable, but low FDG avidity has also been described in some more advanced mucinous or very poorly differentiated cancers, prompting some caution in the interpretation of PET/CT in these subgroups.[96] Despite this, studies of tumour heterogeneity and clonal evolution raise the potential for differential FDG uptake between the primary tumour and downstream metastatic sites, and an import driver of tumour evolution is neoadjuvant therapy.[97] Therefore our position is to support the use of PET/CT for primary assessment and for restaging, including in situations where FDG avidity was initially low.

GASTRIC CANCER

PET/CT is not well established in gastric cancer, with the FDG avidity rate in the primary tumour ranging from 75.2% to 80.6%, compared to oesophageal cancers with FDG avidity rates approaching 100% for T2 and above cancers.[98,99]

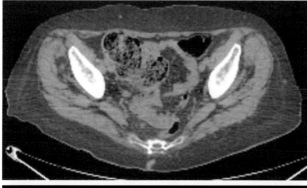
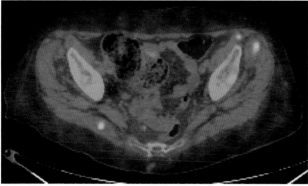

Figure 3.5 The top image shows an axial computed tomography (CT) scan at the iliac crests of a patient with oesophageal cancer. The lower image shows a positron emission tomography (PET)/CT image at the same level and demonstrates FDG avid areas in the muscle, bowel and bone, consistent with metastatic disease.

This inferior FDG uptake rate has been linked to cancer subtype, with non-intestinal growth-type tumours showing significantly lower FDG uptake than intestinal growth-type tumours.[96] Consequently, the ability of FDG/PET to identify regional lymph node involvement and distant metastases is reduced. One study of 279 patients showed that 4.7% of patients had metastatic disease not identified on other staging tests – and importantly, economic analysis of these data supported the use of PET/CT for staging of T2 and greater gastric cancer by reducing the requirement for further staging procedures.[99] Interestingly, this analysis did not show any difference in FDG avidity between Lauren tumour types, as had been previously described. Other studies have also recognised the enhanced ability of PET/CT to identify metastatic disease in gastric cancer over CT and staging laparoscopy, and highlighted a cost benefit to its use.[100,101]

The recent PLASTIC trial prospectively investigated PET/CT and staging laparoscopy together in 395 patients with T3 and greater gastric cancer, and found that PET/CT identified metastatic disease that was not identified at staging laparoscopy in only five patients and highlighted a delay in the diagnostic pathway when performing both tests. Additional clinically relevant findings were reported, however, in 22% of patients who underwent PET/CT.[102] A cost analysis has not yet been reported on these data.

The assessment of gastric cancer nodal stage by PET/CT is an area of some controversy, with reports that, in addition to the association between nodal stage and poorer prognosis,[103,104] FDG avid nodes are specifically related to worse outcomes.[105] Furthermore, it has also been shown that FDG

avid nodes are more commonly observed in patients with metastatic disease, thereby suggesting that more aggressive gastric cancer phenotypes might be identified by PET/CT before metastasis has occurred.[99]

✓ Considering the potential value of PET/CT in avoiding futile radical therapy, enhancing prognostic detail, and the financial benefit of avoiding further more invasive staging procedures, the authors support the use of PET/CT in all T2 and greater gastric cancers, while acknowledging that that this is not standard practice in most units and depends on the rapid availability of PET/CT.[99]

LAPAROSCOPY AND PERITONEAL CYTOLOGY

Staging laparoscopy is performed to detect low-volume abdominal metastatic disease, typically peritoneal, which is notoriously difficult to detect with other imaging modalities. For example, CT alone only diagnosed peritoneal metastases with a sensitivity of 52% of cases in oesophageal cancer and 33–90% in gastric cancer, meaning that without more accurate staging, patients might face neoadjuvant treatment with no prospect of curative resection.[64,74,75] While difficult to report objectively, staging laparoscopy also provides some degree of local tumour assessment and an opportunity to see how borderline fit patients can tolerate abdominal surgery, all of which may influence treatment planning.

In gastric cancer, a meta-analysis of five studies including 240 patients showed an overall sensitivity of 84.6% and a specificity of 100% for the diagnosis of peritoneal metastases.[106] A further systematic review and other small studies also confirm the high accuracy of staging laparoscopy, reporting sensitivities of 64.3–94% and specificities of 80–100% for the diagnosis of peritoneal metastases in gastric cancer.[107–109] M1 disease was detected in 16.7% and 31% in two studies of 222 and 657 patients with gastric cancer, respectively, thus highlighting the clinical impact staging laparoscopy has in gastric cancer.[110,111]

✓✓ NICE guidelines for oesophagogastric cancer recommend the use of staging laparoscopy for gastric cancer in situations where it might guide clinical management.[12]

Oesophageal cancer can have varying degrees of infradiaphragmatic oesophageal involvement, making the role of staging laparoscopy less clear. This has led to some heterogeneity in reports, in part due to the changing definitions of oesophagogastric junctional to gastric or oesophageal cancers. As in gastric cancer, accuracies for the identification of peritoneal metastases are high and have been reported to approach 100%,[112–115] with laparoscopic findings that would change the clinical course for patients seen in 10–38%, but these studies are of mostly oesophagogastric junctional cancers. Data for non-junctional oesophageal cancers is scarce, but one study of 511 patients showed that, although treatment decisions were changed in 20.2% of patients after staging laparoscopy, none of these were in patients with oesophageal cancer of the proximal two thirds.[116] Taken as one disease, staging laparoscopy in oesophagogastric cancer again identifies a high incidence of practice changing findings, with trends towards M1 identification being most frequent in gastric cancer, then oesophagogastric junctional cancer, and finally true oesophageal cancer.[116–121]

✔ Considering the very low risks associated with staging laparoscopy and the significant chance of identifying previously undiagnosed metastatic disease, its use is recommended in all patients with T2 or greater gastric or oesophagogastric junctional cancer with a significant infradiaphragmatic component.

The role of peritoneal cytology is less defined in the UK, with mixed utilisation of it as a staging investigation and variation in procedural protocols. In practice, the presence of tumour cells in peritoneal washings is not uncommon, even in otherwise localised cancer, and is associated with a poorer prognosis than in non-cytology-positive patients, as seen in a meta-analysis of 21 studies including 6 499 patients.[122] While TNM8 deems positive cytology as M1 disease and thus non-curable, a survival advantage has been shown in continuing treatment with curative intent, or using positive cytology as a selective feature for laparoscopic restaging, since conversion from positive to negative cytology after neoadjuvant treatment has shown a survival benefit from resection.[122–124] While it may be reasonable to consider radical treatment for patients in the latter situation, management of persistent cytology-positive patients with no macroscopic disease is more challenging and is likely to remain a controversial treatment decision. Accordingly, the issue of persistent cytology-positive gastric cancer is an area of active research, with the results of phase III trials exploring the role of cytoreductive surgery and intraperitoneal chemotherapy awaited following promising results from phase II trials.[54,125,126] Considering the outcome improvement seen with conversion of positive to negative cytology, whether there is a role for extended neoadjuvant therapy and serial cytological assessment has not been assessed. Overall, the role of peritoneal cytology for the staging of oesophagogastric cancer remains undefined in the UK and European guidelines, but is recommended in the Japanese gastric cancer guidelines along with staging laparoscopy, albeit as a weak recommendation.[127] A typical protocol for obtaining washings for peritoneal cytology includes aspiration of ascitic fluid if present, and if no ascites is present, 50–100 mL of normal saline is instilled into the subhepatic space, the left upper quadrant, and the pelvis, and then washings are aspirated.[128]

✔ Peritoneal cytology clearly adds prognostic detail and may create a future therapeutic opportunity as a part of staging T2 and greater gastric cancer, and is therefore recommended.[118,122] Accordingly, oesophagogastric cancer units need a consistent methodology for obtaining peritoneal cytology and a clear algorithm for the management of cytology-positive patients. Ideally, units performing routine peritoneal cytology will participate in research to help define a future national consensus.

ENDOSCOPIC ULTRASOUND AND MUCOSAL RESECTION

OESOPHAGEAL CANCER

In comparison to CT, EUS has been shown as superior in T and N stage determination in oesophageal cancer, with the exception of lymphadenopathy distant to the oesophagus.[127] A meta-analysis of 44 studies involving 2 880 patients

assessed the T and N staging performance of EUS in OSCC, finding an overall accuracy of 79% for T staging and 71% for N staging.[129]

Since EUS can visualise the layers of the oesophageal wall, it is of particular interest in staging of superficial oesophageal cancers (Fig. 3.6). In squamous cell carcinomas, EUS is shown to differentiate T1a from T1b squamous tumours accurately – in a subset of the meta-analysis above, EUS had a sensitivity of 84% (95% CI 80–88%) and a specificity of 91% (95% CI 88–94%) to diagnose T1a lesions, and a sensitivity of 83% (95% CI 80–86%) and specificity of 96% (95% CI 95–97%) to diagnose T1b lesions. However, studies looking more broadly at all oesophageal cancer subtypes have not achieved similar precision, with frequent over- or understaging, and therefore mucosal resection provides the most accurate T-stage assessment of superficial cancers.[130,131]

✔✔ EUS is currently the best imaging resource to stage T1 oesophageal cancer, but if T1 oesophageal cancer is suspected, EMR should be offered for accurate discrimination of T1a from T1b oesophageal cancers, with EUS used when the endoscopist cannot exclude advanced stage on the basis of endoscopic appearance of nodular lesions.[132]

To stage T4 OSCC, EUS also performed well with a sensitivity of 84% (95% CI 79–89%) and a specificity of 96% (95% CI 95–97%). Generalising these results to the UK population is difficult due to the differences in histological type and location of tumours. Smaller studies in Western countries have, however, produced similar results, and show superior performance of EUS over CT in the T and N staging of oesophageal cancer, although the performance of EUS to discriminate T1a from T1b adenocarcinoma remains limited[86,133,134] (Fig. 3.7).

Like most dynamic imaging studies, EUS is operator dependent and can be anatomically limited in cases where a tumour is impassable, or in oesophagogastric junction tumours, particularly type III Siewert-Stein, due to difficulties in obtaining images without artefact from oblique

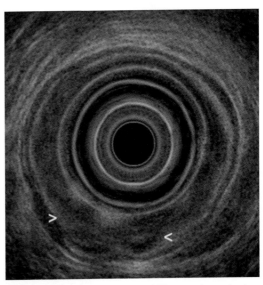

Figure 3.6 Endoscopic ultrasound of T1 oesophageal adenocarcinoma (*arrowheads*). (Courtesy Dr Ian Penman, Royal Infirmary of Edinburgh.)

probe orientation.[131] If a tumour is impassable by EUS, dilatation has been shown to be a safe way to enable intubation of the tumour to obtain the necessary access for assessment.[135] Published intubation failure rates are highly variable, but in more recent studies the frequent use of dilatation, and the selective use of finer US probes, has resulted in intubation failure rates as low as 2.9%.[136] Most impassable tumours have been shown to be squamous and staged as at least T3.[137] Endoscopic miniprobe is another technique used to negotiate malignant strictures impassable with standard EUS, but reductions in soundwave penetration make it frequently unsuitable for the staging of advanced oesophageal cancers.[138]

EUS lymph node imaging features suspicious for malignant involvement are a diameter greater than 10 mm, round shape, discrete borders, and a hypoechogenic pattern. Fig. 3.8 demonstrates EUS images of lymph nodes with suspicious features in two patients with oesophageal cancer. The most accurate assessment of local lymphadenopathy is achieved with FNA sampling of nodes guided by EUS,[139] although EUS/FNA of nodes outside of the resectable or radiotherapy field area is not always feasible. A large meta-analysis and systematic review of 76 studies including 9 310 patients showed that EUS/FNA increased the sensitivity of EUS alone from 84.7% (95% CI 82.9–86.4%) to 88% (95% CI 85.8–90.0%), and the specificity from 84.6% (95% CI 83.2–85.9%) to 96.4% (95% CI 95.3–97.4%).[140]

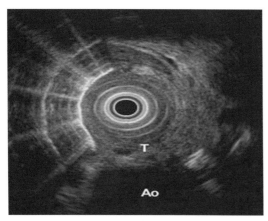

Figure 3.7   Endoscopic ultrasound of the oesophagus showing a T4 tumour *(T)* with extension into the aorta *(Ao)*. (Courtesy Dr Ian Penman, Royal Infirmary of Edinburgh.)

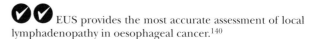 EUS provides the most accurate assessment of local lymphadenopathy in oesophageal cancer.[140]

The data available suggest that EUS, combined with FNA as required, provides the most accurate local staging of oesophageal cancer, especially in T1 disease, but whether EUS results in any change to clinical management is a more pertinent question in view of its invasive nature. A US study of 50 patients showed that clinical decision-making between surgeons was not significantly changed when EUS results were withheld.[141] A UK-based decision theory study of 501 patients showed that EUS only influenced clinical decisions in 0.4% of patients with T2–T4a oesophageal cancer, and this was less than the risks of the EUS itself.[94] In economic assessment, COGNATE, an eight-centre randomised trial of 223 patients, found that the addition of EUS to staging resulted in a significant improvement in quality-adjusted survival and a cost saving of £2 860 per patient; however, PET/CT was not a routine part of staging these patients.[142] A later systematic review has also found some potential for economic benefits from the addition of EUS but advises caution due to a lack of robust studies.[143]

Consequently, our practice follows the NICE recommendation to use EUS selectively in patients with early cancer (to determine suitability for mucosal resection as the first-line treatment, or whether neoadjuvant therapy may be beneficial where the T1b status is not certain), and in advanced tumours where a determination of airway or major vascular involvement cannot be confidently made with CT or PET/CT.[12]

EUS has little to add in the further staging of patients with CT and PET/CT staged T2–T4a oesophageal cancer, and its routine use in these patients is not recommended.[12,94]

GASTRIC CANCER

EUS is not regularly used in gastric cancer in the UK due to a tendency to understage tumour invasion and nodal status.[144] However, EUS does provide a more accurate assessment of T stage compared to CT for local disease staging, with obvious limitations in its role in identifying distant lymphadenopathy or metastases. In a 2015 Cochrane review of 7 747 patients from 66 studies, EUS was shown to achieve a sensitivity and specificity of 86% (95% CI 81–90%) and 90% (95% CI 87–93%), respectively, to discriminate T1/T2 from T3/T4 gastric cancer in a subset of 50 relevant studies

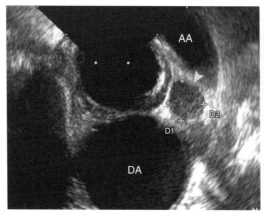
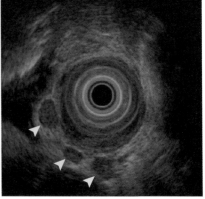

Figure 3.8 The left image shows an endoscopic ultrasound (EUS) image just below the arch of the aorta, demonstrating an enlarged lymph node *(yellow arrow)*. The right image shows an EUS image of a paraoesophageal lymphadenopathy with suspicious features of round shape, discrete borders, and hypoechogenicity, although all are <10 mm in size *(yellow arrows)*. *AA*, Ascending aorta; *DA*, descending aorta. *D1* and *D2* are measuring marks.

($n = 4\ 397$).[145] Subanalysis of 46 studies ($n = 2\ 742$) showed a sensitivity and specificity of 85% (95% CI 78–91%) and 90% (95% CI 85–93%), respectively, to discriminate T1 from T2 disease. A further subanalysis of 20 studies ($n = 3\ 321$) showed a sensitivity and specificity of 87% (95% CI 81–92%) and 75% (95% CI 62– 84%), respectively, to discriminate T1a from T1b disease. EUS has shown poorer performance in larger, ulcerated, or very proximal gastric cancers.[131]

The performance of EUS in N staging gastric cancer is poorer, with a meta-analysis of 44 studies including 3 573 patients showing that the sensitivity and specificity for the identification of metastatic lymph nodes were 83% (95% CI 79–87%) and 67% (95% CI 61–72%), respectively.[145] A more recent meta-analysis of 50 studies including 5 223 patients focusing on N staging in gastric cancer by EUS showed a sensitivity and specificity of 82% (95% CI 78–85%) and 68% (95% CI 63–73%), respectively.[146] While publication bias was not shown in either of these meta-analyses, attention is drawn to the wide heterogeneity, maybe partly consequent to the operator dependency of EUS.

EUS is not generally considered useful for the identification of distant metastases, especially considering that most patients would have previously undergone CT, but the identification of low-volume ascites by EUS is associated with poor clinical outcomes,[147] as might be expected.

✅ EUS can improve the accuracy of T and N staging in gastric cancer,[145] but this is unlikely to have a clinical impact on T2–T4a disease as staged by other modalities. Considering the invasive nature of EUS, its use should be reserved for situations where it might influence clinical decisions.[12]

An adequate EMR provides the most accurate approach to staging early oesophageal and gastric cancers since a formal histopathological assessment can be made of the mucosa and submucosa. The main value of EMR in this context is to identify T1a from T1b disease, to allow an informed MDT discussion regarding the next steps of treatment. Current NICE guidelines would support offering radical treatment to patients with T1b disease, and thus these patients should be formally staged to assess for nodal involvement or metastases.[12]

OTHER ULTRASOUND MODALITIES

Plain abdominal US is of limited diagnostic use in oesophageal cancer, as more sensitive imaging modalities would have been performed; however, US can occasionally be useful to identify, characterise, and sample distant lymphadenopathy. Most commonly, US is used to sample indeterminate cervical lymphadenopathy which, if confirmed as malignant, may render a patient unsuitable for curative therapy. A study of 567 patients demonstrated US/FNA as highly sensitive for the identification of cervical lymphadenopathy compared to CT alone (75% vs 25%), although the study included few true positive malignant nodes.[148] A study investigating the routine use of cervical US in 180 patients found that US gave no additional clinical information over CT and PET imaging.[149] The routine use of US appears to add little to modern staging practices.

For lesions in direct contact with the tracheo-bronchial tree and mediastinal lymphadenopathy, endobronchial US imaging can be used, especially where EUS cannot be performed for anatomical reasons. EBUS has been shown to provide some additional information to EUS in cases of suspected airway involvement, although data are too scant to quantify its role.[150] Similarly to EUS, it is doubtful that EBUS will change clinical management except in specific situations of suspected airway involvement that cannot be assessed by other less invasive means. There are little data to support its routine use, but a theoretical advantage of avoiding tumour seeding by FNA of mediastinal nodes has been described.[151]

Laparoscopic intraoperative US (LIOUS) can be used at the time of laparoscopy and can provide information on T, N, and M stage, as well as resectability. LIOUS has been shown to achieve significantly higher accuracy than CT alone in oesophagogastric cancer;[152] however, much of the benefit of LIOUS came from laparoscopy rather than US itself, and this, combined with improvements in other staging methods, has meant LIOUS is not widely used.[153]

MAGNETIC RESONANCE IMAGING

Generally MRI is used as a complementary staging modality for further characterisation of lesions identified by CT or PET/CT, typically in the liver, adrenal glands, or bone. For T staging primary oesophageal tumour staging, MRI was historically inferior to CT and EUS, with reported accuracies of 60% when compared to EUS (84%).[63] More recent data utilising different MRI imaging protocols suggest a similar performance to CT, with an overall T-staging accuracy of 81% and accuracy in assessing operability of between 75% and 87%.[154] For N staging conventional MRI performs poorly, with reported sensitivities of 25–62% and specificities of 67–88%.[155] Again, different MRI approaches have been shown to improve sensitivity and specificity to 81% and 98%, respectively.[156]

In gastric cancer, MRI provides T-stage accuracy comparable to CT, with a slight benefit in T1 cancers (50% vs 37.5%), but inferior to EUS.[157,158] In more advanced T stages, MRI accuracy did not differ significantly from CT. MRI performed poorly in N staging gastric cancer, with a systematic review identifying a median sensitivity of 68.8% and specificity of 75%, compared to CT which achieved 80% and 77.8%, respectively.[72] The superior soft tissue definition of MRI makes it more useful for locally invasive cancer in the neck and airways, especially when neck dissection is planned, but compared to CT, MRI is more expensive, less available, takes longer to perform, and can be easily affected by movement artefact, limiting its more general use in staging.

✅ MRI is mainly used as a complementary technique to further characterise lesions identified with other staging modalities. The use of MRI in more general staging is not currently supported.

RESTAGING

Restaging has become commonplace with the regular use of neoadjuvant chemotherapy (nCT) and chemoradiotherapy (nCRT) for radically treated oesophagogastric cancer in the UK. Restaging patients before surgery gives further prognostic information by not only measuring response to nCT/nCRT and helping guide further treatment, but also recognising patients whose disease has not responded and who may no longer be suitable for curative surgery. Recognition of complete pathological responders is also becoming increasingly important, since some patients may be more suitable for surveillance rather than resection. The SANO trial is investigating the safety of active surveillance of patients shown to have a complete pathological response to nCRT, as assessed through a two-part multimodal evaluation with gastroscopy and bite-on-bite biopsies 4–6 weeks after nCRT, then gastroscopy, bite-on-bite biopsy, PET/CT, EUS, and FNA of any suspicious nodes after a further 4–6 weeks.[159,160] Patients evaluated as having a complete response are then randomised to surgery or ongoing multimodal surveillance, which includes regular gastroscopy and bite-on-bite biopsies.

✔ While CT remains the most common way to restage oesophageal cancer after neoadjuvant therapy, current studies investigating the safety of surveillance after compete pathological response to chemoradiotherapy have meant that greater scrutiny of tumour response has been necessary, and CT alone is unlikely to be sufficient for restaging in the future.[159]

Any of the previously discussed staging modalities could potentially be used to restage a patient's oesophageal cancer, but PET/CT is increasingly being used as the first-line restaging modality. The use of PET/CT in this situation offers objective measures of tumour volume reduction and tumour metabolic activity, and remains the most sensitive test for new distant metastases and hence unresectable disease.[64] A study of 103 and 280 patients restaged with CT and PET/CT, respectively, showed PET/CT to significantly outperform CT in identifying patients who had unresectable disease, although 10.1% of unresectable patients were not identified by restaging with either modality.[161]

Beyond TNM staging, PET/CT has opened up further avenues for prognostication through measuring changes in FDG uptake in the primary tumour, and therefore metabolic activity, before and after nCT/nCRT. This metabolic response has been significantly associated with pathological response, albeit with a poor sensitivity.[162] Prior to these results, the MUNICON study had aimed to personalise nCT based on metabolic response, with patients only continuing on chemotherapy if they had demonstrated a metabolic response, with non-responders proceeding straight to resection after the first cycle of chemotherapy.[163] The results showed significantly better survival in the metabolic responders, but it is difficult to understand the relevance of these results in the context of the non-responder arm not receiving full nCT. MUNICON also reported no histological changes in non-responders, as had been previously commented upon,[162] implying that the mechanisms by which metabolic response associates with improved survival are biologically complex.

More recently, metabolic nodal response to nCT was described and has been shown, together with metabolic tumour response, to independently predict survival in patients after oesophagectomy.[89] Considering the poor results seen in patients with no response to nCT/nCRT, further opportunities for enhanced or emerging therapies are likely to develop and refinement of the definitions of

tumour and nodal metabolic response will be necessary.[164] For example, the phase II Alliance study personalised neoadjuvant treatment based on primary tumour PET response by switching the induction chemotherapy regimen, prior to completing nCRT and surgery, in patients who did not demonstrate metabolic response to one of two induction regimens, with promising results in patients who showed a metabolic response.[165]

✔✔ PET/CT offers important prognostic detail in patients when restaging after neoadjuvant treatment and is best able to detect incurable disease in this context.[161] Considering the well-known heterogeneity of oesophageal cancer and the observed clonal evolution changes resulting from neoadjuvant therapy, the authors recommend the use of PET/CT even in tumours which are initially of low FDG avidity.

CT scanning remains the most commonly used tool in restaging, but the ability of CT to predict nCT/nCRT pathological response is poor.[166] CT can identify patients no longer suitable for resection through identification of distant metastases, but PET/CT remains a more sensitive method for this, especially if the primary tumour is FDG avid. CT can identify volume reductions in primary tumours if these changes are substantial, but these do not correlate well with histological evidence of tumour regression.[167,168] Newer computational assessments of CT images have achieved more accurate predictions of tumour response, but this remains experimental.[169]

Clinical restaging mainly relates to change in dysphagia through treatment, with improvement of swallow taken as a sign of tumour response, suggesting disease progression or new metastases are less likely. Standardised dysphagia scores are used to assess swallow objectively to help identify changes. Several studies have not demonstrated a correlation between improvement in dysphagia following neoadjuvant therapy and pathological response or improved survival, suggesting dysphagia alone is not a good predictor of neoadjuvant response.[170–172]

The role of endoscopic reassessment after neoadjuvant therapy depends largely on the clinical objective. Routine restaging with endoscopy in a series of 100 patients suggested a complete pathological response in 30%; however, half of these patients had residual disease on histological assessment after oesophagectomy.[173] A meta-analysis of 23 studies of 1 281 patients showed that the sensitivity and specificity of endoscopic biopsy after nCRT for predicting complete pathological response were 34.5% (95% CI 26.0–44.1%) and 91.0% (95% CI 85.6–94.5%), respectively.[174] Since a central role of restaging is to establish that a patient continues to have resectable disease, endoscopy alone does not seem to be a practical investigation, with its use best suited to assessing patients who might be for surveillance rather than resection in cases of suspected complete pathological response, combined with other imaging modalities such as EUS and PET/CT.[175]

EUS offers the most accurate clinical T-staging modality of oesophageal cancer, and therefore its main use in restaging is for the assessment of complete pathological response.[159] Since EUS is more limited in assessing distant metastases, it has little role to play in restaging patients on a pathway to curative resection and poses additional risks from instrumenting the oesophagus. Oesophageal wall thickness reductions as assessed by EUS have been shown to correlate with tumour regression grade and overall survival.[176] A meta-analysis of 11 studies of 593 patients found a sensitivity and specificity of 96.4% (95% CI 91.7–98.5%) and 10.9% (95% CI 3.5–29.0%), respectively, for the identification of complete pathological response after nCRT.[174] For nodal response, a meta-analysis of 10 studies of 602 patients found a sensitivity and specificity of 62.0% (95% CI 46.0–75.7%) and 56.7% (95% CI 41.8–70.5%), respectively, for the identification of complete nodal response after nCRT.[174] Taken together, EUS therefore has a high false-negative rate for pathological response and only moderate accuracy in identifying ongoing lymph node involvement.

As in primary staging, MRI is not practical for the staging of distant metastases and is generally reserved for further characterisation of liver lesions, and may be used in selected patients to follow-up on liver lesions that were indeterminate before nCT/nCRT. In the assessment of primary tumours after nCRT, MRI was used to restage 51 patients, showing a high sensitivity but poor specificity of identifying response, meaning there was a likelihood to overstage and possibly overtreat patients if MRI was used in isolation.[177]

In gastric and oesophagogastric junctional cancers, repeat staging laparoscopy identified a new metastatic disease rate of 7.3% following neoadjuvant treatment, but since this does not change the treatment strategy from those in whom new metastases are identified at the time of resection, the benefits seem limited to resource and expectation management.[178] In contrast, conversion of positive to negative peritoneal cytology in patients with gastric cancer has shown a significant survival advantage, and this represents an exciting therapeutic niche.

MULTIDISCIPLINARY TEAM

The staging investigations described are complementary and must not be considered in isolation. The expertise needed to deliver and interpret the relevance of comprehensive staging of oesophagogastric cancer has increased with the numerous staging investigations discussed above. Not only does this require a wider range of experts, but evidence supports the role of this team working together to provide more complete and accurate staging,[179,180] resulting in improved outcomes after treatment.[181] In the UK, MDTs are generally arranged in two tiers – local MDTs involving an oncologist and radiologist, and a regional specialist oesophagogastric MDT, which should include an MDT coordinator, cancer nurse specialists, medical and clinical oncologists, surgeons, gastroenterologists, radiologists, histopathologists, specialist dieticians, and palliative care specialists.[12,182] Although most cases will go through the MDT staging process along a standard algorithmic pathway, some will not be straightforward and will require detailed multidisciplinary discussion to ensure appropriate staging is carried out, that the staging is interpreted correctly, and that the correct treatment decisions are made.

✔✔ Dutch guidelines recommend discussion of patients with upper GI malignancies in a specialist multidisciplinary tumour board. This is based on a prospective study of 252 patients which showed that the clinical plan changed in 34.5% of patients and the proposed treatment was changed from curative to palliative in 9.2% of patients.[180] Changes from palliative to curative treatment plans were rare.

SUMMARY

The approach to staging can be viewed from two perspectives – rigorous staging of all patients using all available methodologies, according to availability and expertise, to obtain the most accurate clinical staging possible in every patient, or a sequential approach which initially seeks to identify metastatic disease with CT, therefore identifying patients who are not suitable for radical treatment earlier in the staging process and reducing patient exposure to invasive and expensive tests and procedures. The authors' current staging practice uses gastroscopy and CT routinely, followed by PET/CT, for its higher sensitivity to detect M1 disease if the patient is fit for radical treatment and no metastatic disease is identified on CT. In tumours with an infradiaphragmatic component we use laparoscopy, considering the relatively poor sensitivity of CT and PET/CT to identify low-volume peritoneal metastases. We use other staging modalities in specific circumstances where a clinical decision may be altered by the result, such as EUS to stage cancers that could be managed endoscopically or without neoadjuvant chemotherapy. Box 3.4 summarises our staging approach, which we have unified for oesophageal and gastric cancer in view of the increasing evidence for PET/CT in both cancers.

Key points

- The eighth and most recent edition of the classification of gastric and oesophageal cancer takes into account advances in staging, diagnosis, and treatment that occurred since the last edition in 2009, and therefore should be used for staging all oesophagogastric cancers.
- After CT, PET/CT provides the most useful staging information in potentially curable oesophagogastric cancers and its use is recommended in both oesophageal and gastric cancer.
- The role of EUS in oesophageal cancer should be restricted to patients in whom a change in clinical management is likely. Specifically, this includes T1 and T4b cancers as staged by CT and PET/CT.
- Due to the potential for under- and overstaging, oesophageal cancers staged as T1 by EUS should be further staged with EMR.
- The use of staging laparoscopy and peritoneal cytology is recommended as a part of staging T2 and greater oesophagogastric cancer, since it adds prognostic detail and may enable future therapeutic opportunities.
- PET/CT should be the first-line restaging investigation for oesophageal cancer following neoadjuvant treatment as it is the most effective way to identify non-curable disease and adds prognostic detail.
- MRI and US can be used as adjuncts to staging in specific circumstances, but should not be routinely used for or replace the core staging investigations of CT and PET/CT for gastric and oesophageal cancer.
- The multiple complex staging modalities available mean MDT assessment is crucial to the interpretation and planning of additional investigations.

🌐 References available at http://ebooks.health.elsevier.com/

ACKNOWLEDGEMENT

This chapter in the sixth edition was written by Graeme Couper and we are grateful to him for those parts of the chapter which we have kept in this edition.

Box 3.4   Flowchart summarising the authors' staging process for oesophagogastric cancer

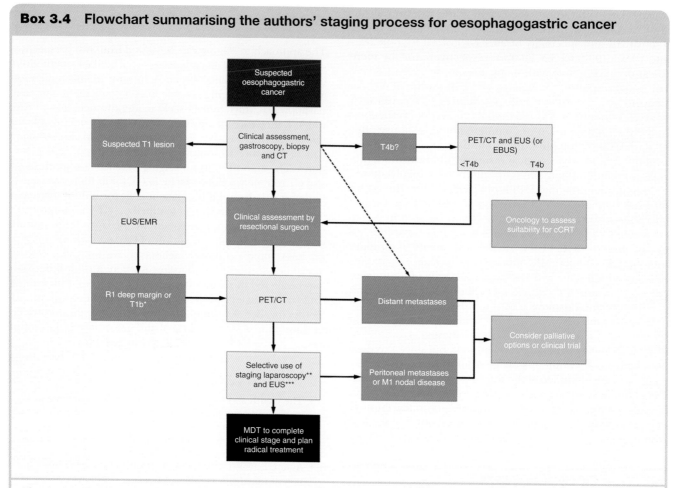

*Continued endoscopic surveillance of selected patients with low-risk T1b adenocarcinoma may be considered by MDT.

**Staging laparoscopy is reserved for patients with high suspicion of peritoneal disease due to bulky tumour, or tumours with an infradiaphragmatic component.

***EUS and nodal sampling reserved for patients with suspicious nodes that may affect resectability.

CT, computed tomography; *cCRT*, curative chemoradiotherapy; *EBUS*, endobronchial ultrasound; *EMR*, endoscopic mucosal resection; *EUS*, endoscopic ultrasound; *HER2*, human epidermal growth factor receptor two; *MDT*, multidisciplinary team; *PET*, positron emission tomography.

KEY REFERENCES

[4] Grabsch Heike I, Mapstone Nicholas P, Marco N. Dataset for histopathological reporting of oesophageal and gastric carcinoma [internet]. 2019. [cited 2021 Jun 12]. Available from: https://www.rcpath.org/profession/guidelines/cancer-datasets-and-tissue-pathways.html.

The current guidelines from the Royal College of Pathologists (developed on consultation with the BSG, AUGIS, the Association of Clinical Pathologists, and the British Division of the International Academy of Pathology), which detail the core data items required for the pathological reporting of oesophagogastric cancer, as well as guidance on non-core data items.

[5] Brierley J, Gospodarowicz MK, Wittekind C, editors. TNM classification of malignant tumours. 8th ed. Chichester, West Sussex, UK ; Hoboken, NJ: John Wiley & Sons, Inc; 2017.

The most recent TNM classification, which should be adopted by all centres to allow comparison of results.

[12] National Guideline Alliance (Great Britain), National Institute for Health and Care Excellence (Great Britain), Royal College of Obstetricians and Gynaecologists (Great Britain). Oesophagogastric cancer: assessment and management in adults [Internet]. 2018 [cited 2021 May 1]. Available from: https://www.ncbi.nlm.nih.gov/books/NBK481429/.

The most recent guideline from NICE detailing the recommendations for the assessment, staging, and management of oesophagogastric cancer in the UK.

[61] Beg S, Ragunath K, Wyman A, Banks M, Trudgill N, Pritchard DM, et al. Quality standards in upper gastrointestinal endoscopy: a position statement of the British Society of Gastroenterology (BSG) and Association of Upper Gastrointestinal Surgeons of Great Britain and Ireland (AUGIS). Gut 2017;66(11):1886–99

BSG document detailing the minimum quality standards expected in upper gastrointestinal endoscopy, including that malignant-looking lesions should be photo-documented and a minimum of six biopsies taken.

[81] Lordick F, Mariette C, Haustermans K, Obermannová R, Arnold D, ESMO Guidelines Committee. Oesophageal cancer: ESMO Clinical Practice Guidelines for diagnosis, treatment and follow-up. Ann Oncol 2016;27(Suppl. 5):v50–7.

[82] Smyth EC, Verheij M, Allum W, Cunningham D, Cervantes A, Arnold D, et al. Gastric cancer: ESMO Clinical Practice Guidelines for diagnosis, treatment and follow-up. Ann Oncol 2016;27(Suppl. 5):v38–49.

The current European guidelines for the management of oesophageal and gastric cancer, respectively.

[89] Findlay JM, Bradley KM, Maile EJ, Braden B, Maw J, Phillips-Hughes J, et al. Pragmatic staging of oesophageal cancer using decision theory involving selective endoscopic ultrasonography, PET and laparoscopy. Br J Surg 2015;102(12):1488–99.

A UK-based study concluding that the risk of EUS outweighed the benefit in patients with T2–T4a oesophageal cancer.

[132] Fitzgerald RC, di Pietro M, Ragunath K, Ang Y, Kang J-Y, Watson P, et al. British Society of Gastroenterology guidelines on the diagnosis and management of Barrett's oesophagus. Gut 2014;63(1):7–42.

These guidelines detail the diagnosis and management of Barrett's oesophagus, and include recommendations for PET/CT, EUS, and EMR for superficial oesophageal cancer.

[140] Puli S-R, Batapati Krishna Reddy J, Bechtold M-L, Ibdah J-A, Antillon D, Singh S, et al. Endoscopic ultrasound: it's accuracy in evaluating mediastinal lymphadenopathy? A meta-analysis and systematic review. World J Gastroenterol 2008 21;14(19):3028–37.

Meta-analysis of 2 558 patients with oesophageal cancer undergoing EUS reporting high sensitivity and accuracy rates for T and N stages.

[161] Findlay JM, Gillies RS, Franklin JM, Teoh EJ, Jones GE, di Carlo S, et al. Restaging oesophageal cancer after neoadjuvant therapy with (18)F-FDG PET-CT: identifying interval metastases and predicting incurable disease at surgery. Eur Radiol 2016;26(10):3519–33.

A UK-based study showing that restaging oesophageal cancer patients after neoadjuvant treatment with PET/CT is more sensitive than CT for detecting interval disease progression.

[180] van Hagen P, Spaander MCW, van der Gaast A, van Rij CM, Tilanus HW, van Lanschot JJB, et al. Impact of a multidisciplinary tumour board meeting for upper-GI malignancies on clinical decision making: a prospective cohort study. Int J Clin Oncol 2013;18(2):214–9.

A study demonstrating the impact of team compared to individual decision-making. This prospective study reported change in the management plan in 34.5% of cases from the treatment plan of the presenting physician.

4 Preoperative assessment and perioperative management in oesophageal and gastric surgery

Shiwei Han | James Helman | Donald E. Low

INTRODUCTION

Perioperative management strategies have been shown to be important in postoperative outcome following oesophageal and gastric surgery. The overriding principle of preoperative assessment is to identify comorbidities that may complicate the patient's operative intervention and perioperative recovery. Identification, recognition, and treatment of these comorbidities allow the patient to be optimised prior to undergoing surgery to reduce the incidence of perioperative mortality and postoperative complications.

Recently, the role of the multidisciplinary team (MDT) and of standardised perioperative/recovery pathways have become increasingly important. In this chapter, we will review principles of preoperative assessment and perioperative management in the context of oesophagogastric surgery and examine recent developments in this field.

PHYSIOLOGICAL STRESS DURING THE TREATMENT OF OESOPHAGOGASTRIC MALIGNANCY

The multimodal nature of the treatment of oesophagogastric malignancy imparts significant physiological stress and there are specific comorbidities that can affect a patient's tolerance to treatment. Clinical outcome following major surgery involves the interplay between patient characteristics (e.g. comorbidities), disease characteristics (e.g. tumour stage, grade, and cell type), choice of treatment modality (e.g. surgery, chemotherapy, radiotherapy, or a combination of several modalities), and postoperative recovery.[1] The results and interpretation of preoperative testing allows a prediction of patient tolerance and enables assignment of a treatment approach tailored to the individual patient.

DIAGNOSIS

The diagnosis of gastro-oesophageal malignancy is based on a good clinical history and examination, with the utilisation of appropriate further investigations.

✓ Clinical assessment undertaken at the primary care consultation must highlight important symptoms, including dysphagia and odynophagia, to trigger further investigation. Studies have shown that an under-appreciation of the importance of dysphagia in younger patients can lead to a delay in presentation and an advanced tumour stage, resulting in a poorer prognosis.[2]

Standard staging investigations for oesophagogastric malignancy (Box 4.1) typically include endoscopy, endoscopic ultrasound (EUS),[3] computed tomography (CT) and positron emission tomography (PET)[2] with or without staging laparoscopy (for oesophagogastric junctional, cardiac, or gastric tumours). Among the currently available staging modalities, EUS is considered the best for T stage and assessment of regional lymph nodes, whereas PET is most accurate for the detection of distant nodal and metastatic spread.[4] EUS has shown poor accuracy in distinguishing early-stage tumours limited to the mucosa (cT1a) from those extending into the submucosa (cT1b).[5] Therefore, endoscopic resection (ER), which is essential for the accurate staging of early-stage cancers, should be performed for early-stage tumours (sT1a and cT1b ≤ 2 cm) as it provides more accurate information on the depth of tumour invasion than EUS.[6] The addition of fine-needle aspiration (FNA) to EUS (EUS-FNA) has shown greater sensitivity and accuracy than either EUS alone or CT scan in the evaluation of cN staging, especially in assessing locoregional and celiac lymph nodes.[7] Apart from being increasingly useful in the initial staging of oesophageal cancer, 2-deoxy-2-[18 F]-fluoro-D-glucose positron emission tomography (FDG-PET) scanning has been identified as a potential tool for assessing the therapeutic response after neoadjuvant therapy and detection of recurrent malignancy.[8] However, FDG-PET is not able to distinguish a good from a complete pathologic response, which would potentially impact future therapeutic decisions.[8]

MULTIDISCIPLINARY TEAM EVALUATION

Patients referred for specialist oesophagogastric treatment are reviewed and discussed by the MDT. This consists of a lead clinician (often a surgeon or a medical specialist in oncology), medical and clinical oncologists, a radiologist (who may have an interest in interventional radiology), a

Box 4.1 Oesophagogastric cancer diagnostic and staging investigations

- Endoscopy
- Endoscopic ultrasound without fine-needle aspiration
- Computed tomography
- Positron emission tomography
- Staging laparoscopy

Box 4.2 Criteria for the diagnosis of malnutrition according to the ESPEN guidelines.

Definition of malnutrition

- Phenotypic criteria
- Weight loss (%): > 5% within past 6 months or > 10% beyond 6 months
- Low BMI (kg/m^2): < 20 if < 70 years or < 22 if > 70 years; Asia: < 18.5 if < 70 years or < 20 if > 70 years
- Reduced muscle mass: reduced by validated body composition measuring techniques
- Etiologic criteria
- Reduced food intake or assimilation: ≤ 50% of energy requirements >1 week, or any reduction for > 2 weeks, or any chronic gastrointestinal condition that adversely impacts food assimilation or absorption
- Inflammation: Acute disease/injury or chronic disease related

BMI, Body mass index; *FFMI*, fat-free mass index.
Fat-free mass can be measured objectively by bioelectrical bioimpedance analyses, dual-energy X-ray absorptiometry, computed tomography, ultrasound, or magnetic resonance imaging.

histopathologist, specialist nurses, and MDT coordinators. Other members of the MDT may include gastroenterologists, dieticians, palliative care nurses, intensivists, and anaesthetists. MDT discussion allows presentation of the radiological and histopathological findings in the context of patients' physical assessment, functional reserve, mental and nutritional status, and social support network.

The MDT has become the cornerstone of cancer treatment in order to provide an unbiased and evidence-based approach to the treatment of malignancy. Presentation to an MDT can produce important changes in management in up to 26% of patients.[9] The role of the cancer specialist nurse is critical in providing a means of communication with the patient and family in order to ascertain their expectations from treatment along with further information regarding social and support networks. In our centre this initial comprehensive interview takes place before travel to the speciality centre and is routinely recognised as valuable in-patient satisfaction surveys. This initial communication includes providing specific information regarding the make-up of the care team, required investigations, and potential treatment options. This also provides a contact person (key worker) within the clinical team for the patient and family.

✔ Centralisation of oesophagogastric cancer treatment has further improved the opportunities for informed multidisciplinary discussion through increasing specialisation and higher volume centres, resulting in improved clinical outcomes.[10] This has in turn led to increased recruitment to clinical trials, a process that has been further facilitated by the presence of clinical oncologists as part of the MDT discussion.

NEOADJUVANT THERAPY

MDT discussion allows for the formulation of a plan based on evidence-based principles including surgery with or without neoadjuvant therapies, given the premorbid status of the patient and characteristics of the tumour. Assessment of physiological issues is important because, although some patients may benefit from multimodality therapy, some will be considered inappropriate on the basis of physiologic health or frailty. Several studies have demonstrated a survival benefit in the use of neoadjuvant chemoradiotherapy prior to esophagectomy for the treatment of oesophageal cancer. Although this combination therapy has been shown to be effective, it may have a significant physiological impact on the patient. Timing of surgery around neoadjuvant chemoradiotherapy is also an important consideration, as in our institution we would recommend surgery 4–6 weeks following the cessation of neoadjuvant chemoradiotherapy; however, surgery within 4–10 weeks is generally considered to be appropriate.

NUTRITION

Nutritional assessment and optimisation are a cornerstone of good pre- and perioperative care in cancer surgery and should be a component of the MDT review.

Preoperative malnutrition and associated immunosuppression have been shown to be well correlated with septic complications and mortality following oesophageal cancer surgery.[11] The mechanism of malnutrition is often related to dysphagia, disease cachexia, or neoadjuvant chemotherapy. Criteria for the diagnosis of malnutrition have been updated by the European Society of Clinical Nutrition and Metabolism (ESPEN), focusing on building a global consensus around core diagnostic criteria for malnutrition in adults in clinical settings (Box 4.2). There was strong consensus that the key first step in the evaluation of nutritional status is malnutrition risk screening to identify "at risk" status by the use of a validated screening tool. As such, the Nutrition Risk Screening (NRS) and Subjective Global Assessment (GSA) are frequently used to define patients at risk for malnutrition and their assessment has been implemented in the German Society for Nutritional Medicine guidelines. The second step is the assessment for diagnosis and grading the severity of malnutrition. Preoperative nutrition therapy is proposed for severely malnourished patients defined by weight loss > 10% within 6 months, body mass index (BMI) < 18.5 kg/m^2 if < 70 years of age or < 20 kg/m^2 if ≥ 70 years of age, Subjective Global Assessment Grade C, serum albumin < 30 g/L (with no evidence of hepatic or renal dysfunction), or NRS > 3.[12–14] In these severely malnourished patients, surgery should be timed to allow improvement in nutrition status.

As many patients have to undergo neoadjuvant therapy first, this should be a window of opportunity to improve nutritional status and physical condition. Preoperative nutritional support, either by the enteral or parenteral route, was able to reduce postoperative complications and hospital stay in patients at high risk for malnutrition.[15]

The relative merits of enteral over parenteral methods of feeding in the malnourished patient have been the subject of debate for several years. The proposed benefits of enteral feeding include improved gut oxygenation, colonisation with gut flora serving to reduce septic complications, and a reduced cost compared to parenteral feeding.[16] There are several potential approaches to enteral feeding (Box 4.3).

Nasojejunal feeding is often poorly tolerated for long periods by patients, and thus is not routinely used at our institution. Thus, we advocate surgical placement of feeding jejunal tubes either by an open or a laparoscopic approach. We often combine this procedure with other procedures such as subcutaneous port placement or diagnostic laparoscopy.

At the time of surgery, many surgeons would advocate the routine placement of a feeding jejunostomy to ensure nutrition through the perioperative period and allow a more measured approach to reinstating oral nutrition. This can simplify discharge and avoid postoperative problems during the critical healing period, as in our patients jejunal tube feeding is initiated on postoperative day 1. It is important to emphasise that feeding jejunostomies can still be associated with complications in a proportion of cases,[17] which should be discussed with the patient prior to placement. In our own experience, we have found that placing a large 14 Fr feeding tube decreases problems with tube obstructions. In recent years the development of endoscopic stents has served as a well-tolerated treatment modality to bypass obstructing oesophageal lesions and allow oral enteral feeding, either for preoperative optimisation or as a palliative measure. However, despite these benefits, fully covered oesophageal self-expanding metal stents (SEMSs) are associated with an increased risk of migration (6–43.8%)[18] that may significantly impact upon the patient's nutritional status and surgical resection. In a recent multicentric study, SEMS placement as a bridge to surgery was associated with poor oncologic outcome and decreased 3-year survival when compared with propensity-matched controls.[19] Furthermore, many clinical oncologists are hesitant to use radiotherapy in a patient with an oesophageal metal stent. Thus, the future of stents as a nutritional bridge during neoadjuvant therapy remains inconclusive, with further studies required.

The role of the dietician or nutritionist in optimising perioperative nutrition is important in ensuring that the short- and long-term nutritional requirements of these patients are met. Current practice suggests that most centres employ a dedicated specialised gastrointestinal dietician who will nutritionally assess patients regularly in the postoperative period. Dietician-delivered intensive nutritional support has been shown to reduce severe postoperative complications after esophagectomy.[20]

PREOPERATIVE ASSESSMENT

In general terms, the most familiar and simple classification of preoperative physical status and risk is that of the American Society of Anesthesiologists (ASA)[8] (Table 4.1). The criteria for assigning ASA class include the presence of a systemic disease that affects activity or is a threat to life. The classification system alone does not predict the perioperative risks, but used with other factors (e.g. type of surgery, frailty, level of deconditioning), it can be helpful in predicting perioperative risks. A large-scale study including more than 2 million surgery cases showed that ASA has strong, independent associations with postoperative medical complications and mortality across procedures.[21] Another large-scale systemic review showed that ASA > 2 confers a 4.87-fold increase in postoperative pulmonary complications.[22] Several other clinical risk indices have been developed, including the Eastern Cooperative Oncology Group (ECOG) performance status and the Charlson comorbidity index. ECOG performance status allows assessment of the effect of oesophagogastric cancer on the daily living abilities of the patient. The Charlson comorbidity index predicts the 10-year mortality for a patient who may have a range of comorbid conditions such as heart disease, AIDS, or cancer (22 conditions in total). This index allows quantitative scoring of a patient's comorbidities and may provide a useful tool in the preoperative assessment. In 2013, the American College of Surgeons National Surgical Quality Improvement Program (ACS NSQIP) implemented a free online surgical risk calculator based on the evaluation of outcome data on 1.4 million patients. The individual surgical risk can be estimated based on the operative procedure and 20 parameters assessing patient characteristics, including certain comorbidities and the ASA score described earlier. The output includes risk estimation in different categories, for example development of pneumonia, cardiac complications, or renal failure. This tool might be useful and handy to assess and discuss procedure risk with the individual patient.[23] Despite the actual clinical value of risk assessment, scoring remains difficult.

Box 4.3   Approaches to enteral feeding

- **Jejunal feeds:** nasojejunal tube, surgical or interventional radiologically placed jejunal tubes
- **Stomach feeds:** percutaneous gastrostomy (PEG) – not advisable due to potential compromise of the gastric conduit
- **Endoscopic removable temporary stents:** self-expanding plastic or metal (SEMS) stents

---

Table 4.1   The American Society of Anesthesiologists' assessment of physical status

Grade	Definition
ASA 1	Normal healthy patient
ASA 2	Patient with mild systemic disease
ASA 3	Patient with a severe systemic disease that limits activity but is not incapacitating
ASA 4	Patient with incapacitating disease that is a constant threat to life
ASA 5	Moribund patient not expected to survive 24 hours with or without surgery
ASA 6	Declared brain-dead patient whose organs are being removed for donor purposes

ASA, American Society of Anesthesiologists.

Box 4.4   Cardiac preoperative investigations

- **History:** including functional capacity
- **ECG:** identifies electric conductional abnormalities
- **Stress testing:** exercise, pharmacological, echocardiography or radioisotope investigation and CPX

CPX, Cardiopulmonary exercise testing; *ECG*, electrocardiogram.

CARDIAC ASSESSMENT (BOX 4.4)

As described previously, oesophagectomy or gastrectomy places significant physiological stress upon the cardiovascular system. Up to 10% of patients undergoing oesophagectomy will have a cardiovascular-related complication.[24] Furthermore, with increasing oesophagogastric surgery being undertaken in the elderly population, accurate identification of patients at risk from cardiovascular complications (associated with ischaemia or dysrhythmia) can help guide treatment planning.

HISTORY

A thorough history and appropriate clinical examination will help identify major cardiovascular risk factors. Any pertinent findings will help guide further investigations that may be required, including a full cardiology assessment prior to undertaking major surgery.

FUNCTIONAL CAPACITY

Exercise capacity provides a useful measure of functional cardiorespiratory reserve. Poor exercise tolerance correlates with an increased risk of perioperative complications that are independent of age and other patient characteristics.[25] However, the ability to climb a flight of stairs does not preclude a patient from having underlying cardiorespiratory disease, and prior to undertaking surgery the majority of oesophagogastric surgeons and most anaesthetists would advocate the use of further cardiac investigation in all elderly patients or patients with multiple risk factors.

The 2014 American College of Cardiology/American Heart Association (ACC/AHA) guidelines on perioperative cardiovascular evaluation suggest a risk calculator-based assessment of the individual patient.[26] The ACS NSQIP risk calculator described above, the Gupta Perioperative Cardiac Risk calculator, or the Revised Cardiac Risk Index (RCRI) may be used. These risk assessment tools balance patient characteristics, comorbidities, and the surgical procedure to predict the risk of a major adverse cardiac event (MACE). MACEs include postoperative death or myocardial infarction. With the new guidelines, combined assessment of patient characteristics and surgery leads to a procedure being categorised as low risk when the risk for MACE is < 1% and elevated risk when the risk for MACE is ≥ 1%. The ACC/AHA guidelines suggest further cardiac work-up for patients with elevated risk and poor or unknown functional status[26] (Fig. 4.1).

INVESTIGATIONS (BOX 4.5)

Electrocardiogram

Electrocardiogram (ECG) is the most basic objective cardiac assessment, usually as part of any preoperative work-up prior to major surgery. It remains a useful baseline test to identify electric conductional abnormalities within the heart that may indicate further structural abnormalities that warrant further investigations. Patients with no prior history of cardiac disease but with an abnormal ECG represent a group that must undergo a higher level of investigation and are potentially amenable to intervention and risk reduction prior to surgery.

Cardiopulmonary exercise testing

The recommendation of the 2014 ACC/AHA guidelines on perioperative cardiovascular evaluation endorses cardiopulmonary exercise testing (CPX) for patients undergoing high-risk surgery in whom functional capacity is unknown.[26] A meta-analysis of studies assessing the discriminatory ability of CPX to predict increased morbidity and mortality after surgery suggested an anaerobic threshold of approximately 10 mL O_2/kg/min as the optimal discrimination point.[26]

Stress testing

Cardiac stress testing is a well-validated, non-invasive modality that has been shown to accurately predict patients at risk of cardiac complications following noncardiac surgery.[27] Preoperative, non-invasive stress testing has been recommended in the 2014 ACC/AHA guidelines on perioperative cardiovascular evaluation for patients with poor or unknown functional status (see Fig. 4.1).[26] Exercise-induced hypotension is a sign of possible ventricular impairment secondary to coronary artery disease and warrants further investigation with a coronary angiogram or myocardial perfusion imaging. Cardiac stress echocardiography and radioisotope investigation (to measure cardiac perfusion) are also used to provide a more detailed cardiac assessment. The identification of reduced left ventricular ejection fraction by the latter modalities has been significantly associated with the development of cardiac complications following major surgery.[28]

OPTIMISATION

Preoperative physical cardiopulmonary rehabilitation

Preoperative cardiopulmonary fitness has been shown to be well correlated with postoperative outcome following major surgery.[29] The use of intensive preoperative exercise has been shown to improve cardiopulmonary fitness prior to major surgery.[30] Although intensive preoperative exercise improves cardiopulmonary fitness, this short-term improvement has not been conclusively shown to correlate with postoperative outcome following major surgery and cancer resection.

Beta-blockade

The hypothesis is that adrenergic beta-blockade slows the heart rate and as a result improves ischaemic ventricular dysfunction. Patients on long-term beta-blockade exhibit adrenergic hypersensitivity if the therapy is withdrawn, and therefore beta-blockade should always be continued and the intravenous route should be utilised until oral intake can be resumed in this patient population. A systematic review for the 2014 ACC/AHA guidelines on perioperative cardiovascular evaluation included a meta-analysis on different randomised controlled trials (RCTs) assessing the outcome after

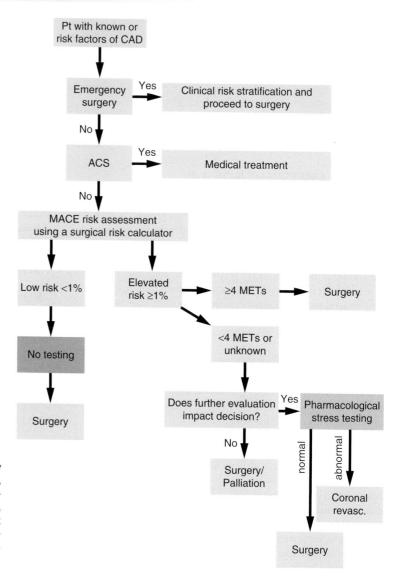

Figure 4.1 Preoperative cardiac assessment for coronary artery disease. MET refers to the activity level of a patient, with 1–3 METs being light activity (TV watching, slow walking) and 4–6 METs being moderate activity (bicycling). *ACS*, Acute coronary syndrome; *CAD*, coronary artery disease; *MACE*, major adverse cardiac event; *MET*, metabolic equivalent of task; *Pt*, patient. (Adapted and modified from 2014 ACC/AHA Perioperative Clinical Practice Guideline.)

Box 4.5 Preoperative pulmonary risk-reduction strategies

- Cessation of cigarette smoking for a minimum of 8 weeks
- Aggressively treat airflow obstruction in patients with COPD or asthma
- Optimise haemoglobin concentration either with iron supplementation or transfusion if absolutely necessary
- Treat any respiratory tract infection with antibiotics, having first cultured the sputum
- Begin patient education regarding adequate exercise and lung-expansion techniques with the assistance of a physiotherapist
- Encourage the patient to lose weight if obese

COPD, Chronic obstructive pulmonary disease.

---

besides a decrease in risk for a myocardial infarction, risk of stroke, death, hypotension, and bradycardia was increased with the treatment.[31] Therefore, no recommendation can be made concerning beta-blocker therapy. Early initiation and titration of beta-blockers prior to surgery might be considered in selected patients; however, no beta-blocker therapy should be initiated on the day of surgery.[26]

✓✓ The 2014 ACC/AHA focused update on perioperative beta-blockade for non-cardiac surgery[31] states that perioperative beta-blockade started within 1 day or less before non-cardiac surgery prevents nonfatal myocardial infarction but increases the risk of stroke, death, hypotension, and bradycardia. So far, there are insufficient data to recommend beta-blockade started 2 or more days prior to surgery without any reservations.

Other relevant cardiac medication

Statins. Current ACC/AHA guidelines on perioperative cardiovascular care recommend that patients continue statin treatment throughout the perioperative period. To date, the evidence regarding the cardioprotective effects of statins in

preoperative new-onset beta-blocker therapy in patients at risk, where beta-blocker therapy was initiated within 2 days prior to surgery. The main conclusion was that the pooled outcome of these RCTs is conflicting, basically showing that the perioperative period is low. For patients undergoing gastroesophageal surgery, statin therapy may be initiated if clinical risk factors exist.[26]

Anticoagulants. In performing oesophagogastric surgery on patients on anticoagulation, the major concern is when is it safe to perform surgery without increasing the risk of haemorrhage or increasing the risk of thromboembolism (e.g. venous, arterial) after discontinuing treatment.

Aspirin/clopidogrel

✓ Traditionally patients are advised to stop aspirin or clopidogrel 7–10 days prior to undergoing major surgery. However, in the case of patients who have had a bare-metal coronary stent placed within 6 weeks or a drug-eluted stent placed within 6 months of oesophagogastric surgery, the advice of the American College of Chest Physicians is to delay surgery if possible or to continue aspirin and clopidogrel through the perioperative period. For surgery beyond this time period, it is suggested that patients may continue aspirin and stop clopidogrel, as aspirin is believed to be associated with fewer bleeding complications when continued. The role of bridging with short-acting anticoagulants like heparin cannot be recommended at this point.

Warfarin. Patients on warfarin are typically told to stop therapy 4–5 days prior to undergoing major surgery, with the acquisition of an international normalised ratio (INR) assay on the day of surgery. Patients at high risk with mechanical heart valves, atrial fibrillation, or venous thromboembolism should have an anticoagulation bridging plan with heparin for the perioperative period[32] (Table 4.2). Thereby, therapeutic-dose low molecular weight heparin should be discontinued 24 hours before surgery and reassumed in a therapeutic dose 48–72 hours after surgery and with stable hemostasis. Therapeutic-dose intravenous unfractionated heparin, which is preferred in patients with chronic kidney failure, should be discontinued 4–6 hours before surgery and reassumed accordingly.[32] However, in low-risk patients, warfarin can be discontinued perioperatively and for moderate-risk patients, bridging has to be weighed up with bleeding risks (Table 4.3).

✓✓ In an RCT, Douketis et al. assigned 950 patients on warfarin for atrial fibrillation to non-bridging therapy and 934 patients to receive bridging therapy. Statistically, non-bridging was non-inferior to bridging anticoagulation when comparing the risk for arterial thromboembolism but superior in the context of risk reduction for major bleeding.[33]

In addition, patients who have recently sustained a venous thromboembolism may be considered for placement of temporary caval filters prior to radical surgery.

PULMONARY ASSESSMENT

Oesophageal surgery has significant effects on pulmonary physiology that may predispose to complications. The incidence of postoperative pulmonary complications following oesophagogastric surgery ranges from 16% to 30%, with an associated increase in operative mortality. Assessment of underlying pulmonary reserve is often recommended for identifying patients more likely to suffer from postoperative pulmonary problems and then instituting effective aggressive preventative strategies including regular chest physiotherapy, early mobilisation, and lung spirometry. For example, a patient with chronic obstructive pulmonary disease (COPD) and sputum retention should be identified as high risk preoperatively to allow the introduction of these preventative strategies early in the postoperative period; if not, this patient may require multiple therapeutic bronchoscopies in the postoperative period to treat mucus accumulation and lobar collapse. In an RCT, preoperative respiratory rehabilitation versus no preoperative rehabilitation was investigated in 60 patients undergoing esophagectomy. Yamana et al. reported significantly decreased complications and an especially decreased incidence of postoperative pneumonia in the preoperative rehabilitation group.[34]

HISTORY

A thorough history along with an appropriate examination will help identify pulmonary risk factors that will be important in the perioperative period. Risk factors for postoperative pulmonary complications include age, pathologic pulmonary function tests, performance status, increased serum creatinine, current cigarette use, and transthoracic resection.[35] Further pulmonary comorbidities that are important in the recovery following major surgery include COPD, asthma, pulmonary fibrosis, or any further restrictive lung disease and previous pulmonary emboli. In the medication history it is important to specifically ask about the use of oral bronchodilator therapy that may be administered as a nebuliser in the postoperative period. Furthermore, the use of oral steroids will need consideration for cover with intravenous hydrocortisone during the perioperative period.

INVESTIGATIONS

Pulse oxygen saturation

Assessment of pulse oxygen saturation (SpO_2) by oximetry can help stratify risk, particularly before high-risk surgeries.[36] Arterial blood gas (ABG) analysis is rarely needed as part of preoperative assessment. Based on clinical experience, indicators that an ABG analysis might be useful include a resting $SpO_2 < 93\%$, an abnormal serum bicarbonate, and severe abnormalities on pulmonary function tests (PFTs) (e.g. forced expiratory volume in 1 second [FEV_1] < 1 L). In general, patients with hypercapnia are identified based on established clinical risk factors, such as severe COPD or neuromuscular disease, rather than by routine ABGs. Several small case series have suggested a high risk of postoperative pulmonary complications among patients with a $PaCO_2 > 45$ mmHg, a finding usually seen only in patients with severe COPD, but the risk associated with this degree of $PaCO_2$ elevation is not necessarily prohibitive.[37]

Chest X-ray

Definitive evidence regarding which patients will benefit from a preoperative chest radiograph is lacking. On the other hand, it is reasonable to obtain a preoperative chest radiograph in patients with known cardiopulmonary disease and in those over 50 years of age undergoing high-risk

Table 4.2   Clinical care pathway at Virginia Mason Medical Center

Initial Contact	Initial Assessment/ Staging	Preoperative Arrangement/ Restaging	Surgery	
Phone interview Within 24 hours of referral: • PMH • Current symptoms • Assess dysphagia and weight loss • Current investigations • Travel arrangements Ensure previous notes, investigations, films, pathology are available Preparation of tailored patient schedule ≥ physiologic and staging investigations completed in 48 hours	**Consultations** • Medical oncology • Radiation oncology • Cardiology • Thoracic surgery • Gastroenterology **Investigations** • CT • PET/CT • EGD/US • Path review • PFT • Selective objective cardiac testing **Nutritional assessment** Thoracic tumour board Within 7 days of consult– communicate results the following day to patient and referring physician Initiate neoadjuvant therapy Appropriate patients with cT2–4, N1–4, Mx	**Restaging 2–4 weeks** Following neoadjuvant therapy: • CT • EGD/US • Tumour board **Surgical approach** Tailored according to: • Tumour/Barrett characteristics • Patient physiology • Previous surgery • Conduit availability	**Thoracic epidural placed preoperatively** • Bupivacaine 0.05% • Hydromorphone 10 μg/mL Single-dose second-generation cephalosporin Selective SQ heparin Minimise blood loss/ transfusion **No routine central venous catheter** Restrictive fluid administration intraoperatively Target < 4 L crystalloids Immediate extubation **On-table epidurogram** to verify correct epidural placement Immediate postoperative anaesthesia PCEA with pain service monitoring, no bolus **Admit to PPICU (step-down unit)**	**Medication** **Pain Control** **Positioning and Mobilisation** **Haemodynamics and Respiratory** **Imaging** **Drainage tube** **Nutrition** **Consult**
1. Description Surgery and Pathway	**2.** Description Surgery and Pathway	**3.** Description Surgery and Pathway	**Critical Measurable Goals**	

*Oral protocol: Ward nurse direct advancement of liquid oral intake from 15 cc/hour ≥ ⅔ cup/hour.

CD, Chest drain; *CT*, computed tomography; *CPAP*, continuous positive airway pressure; *CXR*, chest X-ray; *D/C*, discharge; D5/½NS, dextrose 5% and 1/2 concentration normal saline; *EGD*, gastroscopy; *F/U*, follow-up; *HOB*, head of the bed; *IV*, intravenous; *J-tube*, jejunostomy tube; *MAP*, middle arterial pressure; *NGT*, nasogastric tube; *NSAID*, non-steroidal anti-inflammatory drug; *PCA*, patient-controlled analgesia; *PCEA*, percutaneous epidural analgesia; *PET*, positron emission tomography; *PFT*, pulmonary function test; *PMH*, past medical history; *POD*, postoperative day; *PPI*, proton pump inhibitor; *PPICU*, post procedural intensive care unit; *PSY*, psychiatric consult; *PT*, physical therapy; *QoL*, quality of life; *RT*, respiratory therapy; *SQ*, subcutaneous; *UGI*, upper gastrointestinal contrast study; *US*, ultrasound.

POD 0	POD 1	POD 2–3	POD 4–5	POD 6–7
PPICU "step-down unit"	Surgical ward	Surgical ward	Surgical ward	Surgical ward / DC

• Antiemetic protocol
• Continue beta-blocker and ASA
• IV PPI – monitor gastric pH
	• Continue beta-blocker + ASA
	• Selective start routine medications down J-tube
	• IV PPI (esomeprazole)
		• Consider:
		  ○ Dulcolax suppository
		  ○ Lasix
		• Start oral crushed PPI when NGT removed
			• Consider erythromycin if delayed gastric emptying
			• Continue oral PPI
			• Transition all medications to J-tube
				• Oral PPI
				• All routine medications and analgesics given as liquid or crushed via a J-tube

• PCEA ± PCA
• Avoid bolus adjustment
• Consider:
  ○ IV acetaminophen
	• PCEA ± PCA
	• Consider ketorolac
		• PCEA ± PCA
		• Consider ketorolac
			• Transition from PCEA
			• J-tube scheduled oxycodone
			  ± NSAID
				• Provide prescriptions 24–48 hours prior to discharge

• Keep HOB > 45° • Compress stocking • Chair 4–6 hours postoperatively • 100 ft walk 12–14 hours postoperatively • Avoid CPAP • Maintain MAP > 70 mmHg Treat MAP < 70 mmHg • Decrease epidural rate/no bolus • Epinephrine drip • Infuse up to 2L crystalloid • Recovery room postoperative CXR	• Keep HOB > 45° • Compression stocking • 200 ft walk ×2 in PPICU • Transfer to ward • Maintain MAP > 70mmHG • Avoid CPAP	• Keep HOB >4 5° • Compression stocking • In chair 2–3 hours/day • 200 ft walks 6–8/day • Reinitialise CPAP if needed	• Keep HOB > 45° • Compress stocking • Chair 80% of day • Independent activity • Routine vital signs	• Keep HOB > 45° • Chair 80% of day • Independent activity • Discharge planning • Routine vital signs
• CD to 20 cm suction • NGT – low continuous wall suction • Foley catheter	• CXR (2 view) • D/C apical CD if no air leak and low output • CD water seal	• CXR (2 view) • Witnessed UGI POD 3-4 • May D/C 2nd CD (except Ivor Lewis) • F/U CXR in 4 hours • Ivor Lewis: CD until oral intake	• CXR (2 view) • D/C NGT when contrast study shows good gastric emptying (target day 3–4) • In IL D/C 2. CD when oral intake	• CXR (2 view) for clinical issues only
• IV fluid basal rate 70 cc/hour D5/½NS • MAP < 70 consider fluid bolus (max 2L)	• IV basal rate 50 cc/hour D5/½NS • J-tube 10 mL/hour and selective medications	• J-tube 30 cc/hour advance to goal • No oral intake • D/C IV fluids	• J-tube target rate and transition to nocturnal feed • Start oral protocol* when no gastric emptying delay on UGI • Dietary 1–2 days prior to D/C • Social work – PRN • ± Rehabilitation • Home healthcare services for J-tube	• Advance oral protocol • J-tube teaching for patient and family • Dietary: ○ Nutritional oral and J-tube protocol over next 4–6 weeks
• Pain service • PSY elderly patients • Selective RT • PT mobilisation	• Dietary			
Immediate Extubation **Maintain MAP >70 mmHg** **Mobilise Day of Surgery**	**Transfer to Ward** **Initiate Enteric Feeding** **Mobilise 2-4 Walks**	**J-Tube Feeding to Goal** **Assess Gastric Emptying** **Remove NG and Chest Drain**	**Independent Mobility** **Start Oral Intake**	**Discharge Day 6-7** **Routine post discharge goals** • Represent at MTB recommendations to referring and primary care MDs) • J-tube removed 4–12 weeks post discharge • QoL and patient satisfaction assessment • Commit to 3 years follow-up

Table 4.3   Risk stratification for perioperative thromboembolism

Risk Stratum	Indication for Anticoagulation Therapy with Vitamin K Antagonists		
	Mechanical Heart Valve	Atrial Fibrillation	VTE
High	• Any mitral valve prosthesis • Any caged ball or tilting disk aortic valve prosthesis • Recent (within 6 months) stroke or transient ischaemic attack	• CHADS$_2$ score of 5 or 6 • Recent (within 6 months) stroke or transient ischaemic attack • Rheumatic valvular heart disease	• Recent (within 3 months) VTE • Severe thrombophilia (e.g. deficiency of protein C, protein S or antithrombin; antiphospholipid antibodies; multiple abnormalities)
Moderate	• Bileaflet aortic valve prosthesis and one or more of following risk factors: atrial fibrillation, prior stroke or transient ischaemic attack, hypertension, diabetes, congestive heart failure, age > 75 years	• CHADS$_2$ score of 3 or 4	• VTE within the past 3–12 months • Non-severe thrombophilia (e.g. heterozygous factor V Leiden or prothrombin gene mutation) • Recurrent VTE • Active cancer (treated within 6 months or palliative)
Low	• Bileaflet aortic valve prosthesis without atrial fibrillation and no other risk factors for stroke	• CHADS$_2$ score of 0 to 2 (assuming no prior stroke or transient ischaemic attack)	• VTE > 12 months and no other risk factors

CHADS$_2$, Congestive heart failure, hypertension, age ≥ 75 years, diabetes mellitus, and stroke or transient ischaemic attack; each item adds one point to the total score. High risk may also be considered in patients with a prior thromboembolism during temporary interruption of VKA; *VTE*, venous thromboembolism.
Adapted from 9th ed: American College of Chest Physicians Evidence-Based Clinical Practice Guidelines.

surgical procedures such as oesophageal surgery. Chest radiographs add little to the clinical evaluation in identifying healthy patients at risk for perioperative complications. A meta-analysis of studies of routine preoperative chest radiographs demonstrated a low yield for abnormalities that actually change preoperative management. Of 14 390 preoperative radiographs, there were only 140 unexpected abnormalities and only 14 cases where the chest radiograph was abnormal and influenced management.[38] The prevalence of abnormal preoperative chest radiographs increases with age. In a review of studies, 21.1% of all preoperative chest radiographs were abnormal, but the prevalence of abnormal studies for patients under 50 years of age was only 4.9%. A preoperative chest X-ray (CXR) will elucidate obvious chest abnormalities. However, its greatest value resides as a reference comparison with postoperative films.

Pulmonary function testing

Preoperative PFT with spirometry in conjunction with clinical history and examination can be used to establish baseline lung function, evaluate dyspnoea, detect pulmonary disease, and evaluate operative risk. Low FEV_1 or forced vital capacity (FVC) has been shown to be well correlated with postoperative pulmonary complications.[39] Abnormal PFT results will allow identification of patients at risk of postoperative pulmonary complications and employment of preventative strategies in the perioperative period. However, routine pulmonary function testing can be time-consuming and expensive, and some surgeons would advocate a more measured approach, with PFTs being used in patients with pulmonary risk factors.

OPTIMISATION

As discussed previously, the benefits of preoperative exercise or rehabilitation have been shown to improve cardiopulmonary fitness and postoperative outcome following major cancer resection. Identification of patients at risk of pulmonary complications may provide a justification for altering the method of surgical resection. Patients with very poor pulmonary function who previously would have been deemed unfit to undergo resection may benefit from a minimally invasive approach. Aggressive chest physiotherapy and early mobilisation may also help to reduce the incidence of pulmonary complications associated with oesophagogastric surgery in this cohort. There are several preoperative pulmonary risk factors that may be optimised in patients with impaired lung spirometry who are undergoing upper gastrointestinal surgery (Box 4.5).

NEUROLOGICAL ASSESSMENT

HISTORY

Identification of patients with neurological risk factors is another crucial element of the preoperative global assessment. These risk factors include previous cerebrovascular accidents (CVAs), transient ischaemic attacks (TIAs), epilepsy, dementia or cognitive decline, and neuropsychiatric disorders. These factors can lead to severe neurological complications, including delirium that may significantly impact upon postoperative recovery. Furthermore, postoperative delirium was found to be associated with advanced age, benzodiazepine administration in the ICU, and surgical complications.[40] The reported incidence of postoperative delirium following major surgery is highly variable, ranging from 9% to 50%, and more common in the elderly population.[40,41] A report from our institution showed that delirium affects 9.2% of patients and is associated with increased length of hospital and ICU stay, increased costs, and increased pulmonary complications.[41]

INVESTIGATIONS

Several risk factors for postoperative delirium have been identified previously, including age, dementia, functional impairment, depression, psychotropic drug use, increased comorbidity (cardiac, pulmonary, renal, and neurological), laboratory abnormalities (electrolyte disturbance, anaemia, and low albumin), preoperative visual impairment, hearing impairment, alcohol use, institutional residence, and prior postoperative delirium. It is the accurate preoperative identification of these risk factors in vulnerable patients that will allow implementation of interventions to reduce delirium following major surgery.[42] The presence of pre-existing dementia or cognitive impairment has been shown in a previous study[43] to have the strongest correlation with postoperative delirium. The Mini-Mental State Examination (MMSE) provides a means of a quick assessment of a patient's cognitive state at admission that may allow prediction of patients vulnerable to postoperative delirium.[43]

✅ The National Institute for Health and Clinical Excellence (NICE) has published a guideline that outlines several preventative strategies against delirium.[44] It describes the use of a multi-intervention package including assessment and modification of key clinical factors that may precipitate delirium.

OPTIMISATION

The avoidance and treatment of postoperative delirium is a challenge, and thus prediction of vulnerable patients and employment of preventative strategies represent a more attractive option. A recent meta-analysis of 24 randomised trials assessed the efficacy of peri-operative interventions in decreasing the incidence of postoperative delirium.[45] The results endorsed perioperative geriatric consultations with multicomponent interventions and lighter anaesthesia as promising for reduction of postoperative delirium. Possible protection was further reported with prophylactic haloperidol, bright light therapy, and general as opposed to regional anaesthesia.[45]

RENAL ASSESSMENT

The presence of preoperative renal disease is a highly important factor that may impact the postoperative outcome. This is illustrated by several risk-scoring systems used to predict postoperative complications following major surgery, including renal disease as a variable, for example Possum, APACHE II, and Charlson scores. Due to improvements in perioperative care, patients with several medical comorbidities, including renal insufficiency that previously may have been refused surgical intervention, are now more likely to be considered for surgery. Thus, the assessment and optimisation of preoperative renal disease will gain increasing importance due to the changing demographics of the population undergoing oesophagogastric surgery.

HISTORY

Patients may or may not be aware of pre-existing renal disease. However, every elderly patient undergoing major surgery renal function should be assessed. Prior to the initiation of surgery, renal disease will influence many diagnostic and treatment modalities associated with oesophagogastric malignancy.

INVESTIGATIONS

All patients undergoing major oesophagogastric surgery will have basic laboratory blood tests that should include markers of renal function, i.e. serum urea, creatinine, and electrolytes. Together, these results will identify the presence or absence of underlying renal insufficiency and the impact of this upon serum biochemistry and electrolyte disturbance.

✅ In the presence of previously undiagnosed severe renal impairment, it would be prudent to investigate the aetiology to its conclusion with renal imaging, for example, ultrasound, MAG3 scan, or renal biopsy. This is especially important when a conservative approach to fluid utilisation is considered in the perioperative period (see 'Fluid management' section later).

OPTIMISATION

Previous studies have demonstrated that with good preoperative optimisation, patients with impaired renal function can undergo gastrectomy with similar results to patients with a normal creatinine clearance.[46] Patients with severe renal impairment requiring dialysis are considered inappropriate surgical candidates for major oesophagogastric resection. Active involvement and consultation with a nephrologist will help guide perioperative management strategies, including fluid and electrolyte management, in this complex cohort of patients.

ANAESTHETIC TECHNIQUE

Thus far, we have discussed a systems-based approach to preoperative assessment; in this next section we will move on to monitoring, assessment, and control of intraoperative factors that may adversely affect outcome following oesophagogastric surgery.

INTRAOPERATIVE MONITORING

During major surgery traditionally, invasive adjuncts have formed the mainstay of intraoperative monitoring. More recently, anaesthetists are moving away from these invasive monitoring mechanisms, instead attempting to safely monitor a patient during major surgery using as minimally invasive monitoring mechanisms as possible without compromising safety. The aim of intraoperative monitoring should be to safely monitor patients' vital systems whilst they undergo a general anaesthetic for major surgery that can impact and attenuate the body's normal homeostatic mechanisms. Inadequate perfusion of the end organs during major surgery not only increases the incidence of major complications – for example, CVAs, myocardial infarction, and renal failure – but also may result in anastomotic or graft ischaemia and resultant leakage.

THE CARDIOVASCULAR SYSTEM

Monitoring vital signs including heart rate and blood pressure can give clues as to a patient's intravascular volume, especially in challenging cases with significant blood loss. This monitoring can range from simple measures including a blood pressure cuff and an oxygen saturation finger probe, to central venous lines and arterial lines. The advantages of central lines include venous access away from the operating field to allow anaesthetists to administer intravenous solutions without disturbing the operating procedure. These lines also allow monitoring of the central venous pressure, which can be used to guide fluid administration during the intra- and immediate postoperative period. These lines are not without complications, including infection, pneumothorax during insertion, and venous thrombosis.

✔ We currently recommend the selective use of central lines in indicated cases with difficult venous access.

Arterial lines allow monitoring of the mean arterial pressure (MAP) to guide fluid administration during the intraoperative period. They also allow arterial blood to be sampled for blood gas analysis and to measure serum electrolytes, acid–base balance, and lactate, which all give vital clues as to the status of vital organs. The complications of arterial lines include infection and thrombosis. Arterial lines provide a useful intraoperative monitoring adjunct and we currently recommend their use in the majority of cases.

THE RENAL SYSTEM

From the measures described, ABG monitoring allows the measurement of serum electrolytes and lactate, both of which can indicate intraoperative renal impairment. The most common cause of renal impairment in a patient with no previous renal disease is renal hypoperfusion. Other causes include nephrotoxicity secondary to medication administered intraoperatively. Urinary catheterisation allows direct measurement of urinary output and an indirect measurement of renal function. This provides a less invasive approach to monitoring of renal function and is routinely used in all patients undergoing major oesophagogastric surgery.

ANAESTHETIC AGENTS

✔ The effect of the choice of anaesthetic agent upon inflammatory response and postoperative outcome following oesophagogastric surgery remains inconclusive.

Desflurane and sevoflurane have been shown to produce a reduced pulmonary inflammatory response and a decrease in the overall number of adverse events compared to propofol.[47] However, a more recent study suggested that sevoflurane caused a greater inflammatory response than propofol during thoracic surgery.[48] These studies are limited by heterogeneity in patient demographics and comorbidities, along with duration of surgery and one-lung ventilation. Thus, although volatile anaesthetics produce dose- and time-dependent effects upon the inflammatory and immune systems, the nature of these effects in the setting of oesophagogastric surgery requires further investigation.

AIRWAY MANAGEMENT

LUNG ISOLATION TECHNIQUES

Both gastric and oesophageal surgery can be performed in a patient intubated with a standard endotracheal tube. To allow intraoperative collapse of the right lung (during

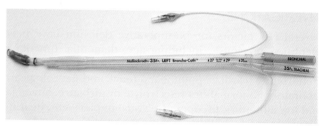

Figure 4.2 A left-sided double-lumen endobronchial tube.

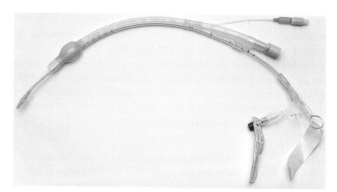

Figure 4.3 An endobronchial blocker.

a two-stage transthoracic oesophagectomy), a left-sided double-lumen endobronchial tube is most commonly used (Fig. 4.2). It is crucial to ensure correct placement of the tube and recognise inadvertent upper lobe occlusion. Usually, endobronchial tube position is confirmed through auscultation of the chest and fibre-optic bronchoscopy.

Single lung ventilation (SLV) is commonly used in oesophageal surgery to facilitate dissection by operating surgeons by increasing the space available within the thoracic cavity. However, SLV has been shown to result in an inflammatory response, with the time period of SLV and surgical manipulation increasing alveolar injury and leucocyte recruitment in the dependent lung. During re-expansion of the collapsed lung, alveolar recruitment and reperfusion lung injury provide an additional source of lung injury.[49] Protective strategies aimed at reducing intraoperative lung injury include using small tidal volumes and positive end-expiratory pressure (PEEP) during SLV, and this has been shown to reduce the inflammatory response following oesophagectomy, improve lung function, and result in early extubation.[50]

Endobronchial blockers (Fig. 4.3)

In some patients who are difficult to intubate in the presence of irregular dentition or limited temporomandibular joint movement, the use of a double-lumen endobronchial tube can be challenging due to its size. In this situation an endobronchial blocker passed fibre-optically through a single-lumen endotracheal tube may be beneficial to isolate the non-dependent lung. One important limitation to the routine use of endobronchial blockers is their tendency to migrate proximally or distally with mediastinal manipulation, resulting in sudden lung reinflation.

TIMING OF EXTUBATION

Immediate extubation following surgery has the advantage of giving the patient back control of their own respiratory system and allows them to begin their postoperative recovery immediately. In the past immediate extubation following major oesophagogastric surgery was not routinely considered. Furthermore, some patients with several respiratory comorbidities may require a measured approach to extubation. Patients with respiratory comorbidities are at greater risk from pulmonary complications and often require prolonged respiratory support.

✔ An operative approach that is individualised to patient and tumour characteristics, and based upon adhering to appropriate cancer principles with the minimising of blood loss and appropriate perioperative fluid administration, has allowed immediate extubation in up to 99.5% of cases following oesophagectomy.[51]

The benefits of early extubation have been clearly demonstrated, with reduced mortality and morbidity.[52] Early extubation has the additional benefit of reducing the requirement for postoperative ICU admission, instead allowing patients to be managed in a high-dependency setting, facilitating early mobilisation and reducing overall cost. Postoperative extubation must be predicated on the basis of good pain control and is a prerequisite for early mobilisation.

FLUID MANAGEMENT

Perioperative fluid management involves a careful balance between maintaining perfusion pressure and oxygen delivery to vital organs and the newly fashioned anastomosis, and the prevention of excessive fluid accumulation that may delay recovery of gastrointestinal function, impair wound or anastomotic healing, and increase cardiac and respiratory complications.[53] Patients undergoing major oesophagogastric surgery have several sources of loss of fluid, including bowel preparation, dehydration secondary to tumour dysphagia, blood loss, insensible and nasogastric losses, wound exudation, urinary output, and evaporative fluid losses from open abdominal and chest cavities.

Recent publications have suggested that a more restrictive "fluid as needed" approach to fluid management during major surgery may be beneficial, with improved gastrointestinal recovery time and reduced respiratory complications.[54]

✔✔ Two studies have demonstrated the benefits associated with perioperative fluid restriction, specifically in the setting of oesophagectomy.[55,56] Kita et al.[55] found that maintaining a central venous pressure of < 5 mmHg and an adequate urinary output with intraoperative fluids administered at 4–5 mL/kg per hour resulted in reduced postoperative respiratory complications following oesophagectomy. Neal et al.[56] demonstrated a reduction in oesophagectomy-related morbidity by using a standardised multimodal management plan that included thoracic epidural analgesia, early extubation, and avoidance of excessive intraoperative fluid administration.

Goal-directed fluid therapy includes minimising blood loss and maintaining haemodynamic stability, and this requires regular communication between surgeon and anaesthetic teams, i.e. during transhiatal dissection, where the blood pressure routinely decreases and anaesthetists typically respond by increasing fluid administration. In oesophagogastric surgery the monitoring of haemodynamic parameters is more challenging, as the most validated method remains transoesophageal Doppler, the use of which is not possible in the context of oesophagectomy.[57] Other monitoring measures to allow goal-directed fluid administration include arterial lines to monitor arterial pressure variation and the FloTrach/Vigileo system (Edwards Lifesciences, Irvina, CA) to predict intravascular hypovolaemia.[58] Clear evidence and the optimal method for monitoring in goal-directed fluid therapy are yet to be determined; however, this approach to intraoperative fluid administration would appear to be beneficial in theory.

POSTOPERATIVE ANALGESIA

With inadequate postoperative pain relief patients are less likely to mobilise, take part in respiratory exercises and comply with standard postoperative goals. Hence the importance of good postoperative analgesia in the implementation and effectiveness of multimodality clinical pathways cannot be overstated.

Thoracic epidural analgesia for oesophagectomy has been shown to be a highly effective method of postoperative pain relief.[59] Furthermore, the proven benefits of thoracic epidural analgesia following oesophagectomy include earlier recovery of bowel function, reduced pulmonary complications, and early extubation.[60] Further less well-validated benefits have been described, and these include reduced anastomotic leak and improved gastric conduit microcirculation.[61,62] However, aggressive epidural bolus dosing can reduce systolic arterial pressure and thus conduit perfusion. Measures to counteract this effect include changing the rate of epidural and avoidance of bolusing, avoidance of hypovolaemia, and the judicious use of vasopressor therapy.[63]

Epidural analgesia has been shown to be a highly effective method of reducing postoperative pain in gastrectomy.[64] Epidural analgesic therapies can vary between continuous infusions and patient-controlled analgesia (PCA). The advantages of the latter include subjective titration of the patient's pain and adequate treatment; however, usually a safety mechanism or lockout is in place to prevent the patient from overusing the PCA. Recent studies have suggested that a combined regimen of patient-controlled epidural analgesia during the day with a night-time infusion can help to reduce postoperative pain, and specifically pain associated with coughing, and provide a better sleep pattern.[65] The efficacy of epidurals in the immediate postoperative period can be optimised by the use of an "on theatre table" epidurography to verify accurate placement and optimal level of the epidural catheter before leaving the theatre.[38]

Other methods of effective postoperative analgesia following oesophagogastric surgery include intravenous PCA, which is often the next line in the analgesic ladder following epidural analgesia. The main disadvantage of PCA following major surgery is that it requires a well-orientated patient to be able to coordinate and administer their own pain relief. So, in some situations the patient may not be able to do this, resulting in inadequate analgesia and increased risk of postoperative complications.

Extrapleural intercostal nerve blockade is another method of effective pain control following thoracotomy. An indwelling catheter may be left in the extrapleural space, most commonly during the operation, to allow the continuous infusion of local anaesthetic to the thoracotomy region. Extrapleural intercostal nerve blockade has been shown to be as effective as thoracic epidural analgesia in controlling thoracotomy-related pain and allowing recovery of pulmonary function in an RCT.[66] Despite these benefits, extrapleural intercostal nerve blockade has yet to gain widespread acceptance, with thoracic epidural analgesia remaining the perceived gold standard for pain control following thoracotomy.

OESOPHAGOGASTRIC CLINICAL PATHWAYS

In February 2019, the Enhanced Recovery After Surgery (ERAS) Society, which had previously established ERAS guidelines for colorectal, gastric, bariatric, liver, and gynaecologic surgery, published the first guidelines for oesophagectomy, expanding standard recommendations to cover areas unique to oesophageal resection. These guidelines, developed by international experts, represent the most comprehensive infrastructure for directing the perioperative management of patients undergoing oesophagectomy.[67] These oesophagectomy-specific ERAS guidelines were developed to provide an evidence-based platform to be applied by the MDT caring for oesophagectomy patients. The implementation of a clinical pathway for oesophagogastric cancer requires the personal commitment of all members of the care team and will impact a patient's treatment at virtually every stage; these individuals and teams should be involved in formulating and adapting the clinical pathway.

- Key players in the implementation of clinical pathways include:
  - an oesophagogastric cancer nurse specialist;
  - oesophagogastric surgeons;
  - an anaesthetist;
  - recovery room staff;
  - pain service;
  - ICU and ward nursing;
  - physical therapy;
  - dieticians;
  - social service team;
  - surgical trainees.

One recent meta-analysis study (accepted by Disease of the Esophagus) demonstrated that the ERAS pathways reduced postoperative pulmonary complications and decreased hospital stay in oesophagectomy patients. These pathways should be reassessed and updated every 24–36 months to allow continued re-evaluation of goals by the entire team and to look for areas in which outcomes can be improved over time. It is important to understand that clinical pathways are not limited to the postoperative period, but instead a good pathway will begin at the time of initial consultation and support a patient's journey and goals until treatment has been completed.

PREOPERATIVE

In our institution this process begins at the time of initial telephone interview between the patient and the oesophagogastric nurse specialist within 24 hours of referral. This telephone interview will include a review of the patient's past medical history, their current symptoms (swallowing and weight loss), current investigations, travel arrangements (accommodation), and an initial description of the process of preoperative work-up, surgery, and postoperative recovery. This interaction allows specific planning to be made regarding what previous tests have been undertaken and what radiological examinations need to be obtained prior to the initial visit. In addition, specific plans are made to complete all staging and appropriate physiological tests within a specific time period (in our case, 48 hours) around the initial trip to the oesophagogastric unit. At the initial visit careful history, examination, and organisation of relevant clinical investigations as described previously in this chapter will provide an initial indication of physiological status. In particular, it is important to be able to adapt the surgical approach according to both tumour location and patient physiology; i.e. in patients with severe coronary artery disease, arrhythmias or cardiomyopathy we typically utilise a right thoracic approach so as to minimise cardiac manipulation during oesophageal mobilisation. Following physiological investigations and tumour staging, all patients should be presented at a multidisciplinary tumour board (see 'Multidisciplinary team evaluation' section) to allow an individually targeted goal-directed treatment plan to be formulated that considers both tumour and patient characteristics. A part of this MDT review will include reviewing suitability for enrolment in current clinical trials. The nutritional status of patients should also be discussed, with specific need for either a feeding jejunostomy or removable SEMS being included in the final recommendation (see 'Nutrition' section). At the MDT meeting, a plan is made regarding the timing of surgery in patients receiving neoadjuvant chemotherapy, but particularly chemoradiotherapy. Current recommendations indicate the optimum time for resection to be 4–6 weeks following completion of radiotherapy. Contact is maintained with the patient throughout neoadjuvant therapy by the oesophagogastric nurse specialist as well as post-treatment reassessments coordinated before surgery.

Restaging after chemoradiotherapy for locally advanced oesophageal cancer is a pivotal part of modern treatment individualisation. Restaging is critical for assessing the neoadjuvant treatment response of the primary tumour and regional lymph nodes, as well as detection of progressive disease including distant metastasis. The results of combined locoregional and distant restaging after neoadjuvant therapy stratifies oesophageal cancer patients into three groups: patients with 1) no evidence of residual locoregional disease nor distant spread, who might benefit from an active surveillance approach; 2) persistent locoregional disease with no evidence of distant spread, who require subsequent surgery; or 3) either persistent or no residual locoregional disease with evidence of distant spread, who should be offered systemic treatment, mostly with palliative intent.[68] At the time of publication no restaging approach has been identified that will reliably identify a concrete pathologic response to increase the utilisation described in group 1.

A multimodal locoregional restaging approach in our institution is usually taken within 2-4 weeks following neoadjuvant therapy. The approach currently includes contrast CT of the chest, abdomen, and pelvis, as well as upper endoscopy with ultrasound. The patient's restaging results will once again be reassessed by a multidisciplinary tumour board to confirm the following treatment plan.

INTRAOPERATIVE

Intraoperative aspects of the clinical pathway employed at our institution involve regular communication between the anaesthetic and operating teams. We routinely place a thoracic epidural in all of our patients undergoing oesophagectomy and liaise with the pain service to ensure their active involvement early in the postoperative period. During surgery we attempt to tailor the approach to minimise blood loss so as to reduce transfusion requirements. Over the past 6 years our median intraoperative blood loss has been 150 mL (interquartile range [IQR] 100–250 mL) during oesophagectomy, with a median operative time of 395 min (IQR 363–426 min). This has allowed us to adopt an increasingly conservative approach to intraoperative fluid utilisation (median 2700 mL [IQR 2300–4200 mL] for oesophagectomies over the past 2 years); as described previously, this reduces gastrointestinal recovery time and pulmonary complications. Immediate extubation postoperatively allows immediate introduction of the postoperative goal-directed pathway to allow enhanced recovery following oesophagogastric surgery.

POSTOPERATIVE

Postoperative care pathways allow the introduction of a targeted, goal-directed approach to postoperative recovery following major oesophagogastric surgery. They provide a template for all medical personnel interacting with these patients and can outline a goal-directed recovery for each patient. These pathways, once well established, can provide a framework for quality improvement and improving postoperative outcomes. With the implementation of enhanced recovery pathways, different groups showed that pulmonary complications, length of hospital stay, length of ICU stay, and total costs for oesophagectomy could be reduced.[69,70] A systematic review and pooled analysis of nine retrospective studies also found, in addition to the afore-mentioned parameters, anastomotic leakage rates to be reduced with enhanced recovery pathways.[71] Involvement of the entire healthcare team in the design and implementation of these pathways will help ensure all team members are committed to achieving specific recovery goals.

A simple schematic for a postoperative care pathway is shown in Table 4.3. It is imperative that patients should be provided with this pathway and dietary expectations prior to undergoing surgery, as this will help to guide their expectations regarding their postoperative recovery. The use of specific pathways will help patients, families, and their caregivers remain focused on a goal-orientated approach to recovery from major surgery. Through five revisions of our clinical care pathway over the past decade, we have seen our median length of hospital stay decrease from 10 to 8 days (median for the past 2 years).

Key points

- The principle of preoperative assessment is to identify comorbidities, and psychological and nutritional abnormalities that may complicate the patient's operative intervention and perioperative recovery.
- Several clinical risk indices have been utilised to assess operative risk, including ASA grade, Eastern Cooperative Oncology Group (ECOG) performance status, and the Charlson comorbidity index (CCI). Recently, the ACS NSQIP risk calculator has been introduced, enabling individual risk estimation in different categories.
- Poor exercise tolerance correlates with an increased risk of perioperative complications, which are independent of age and other patient characteristics. The use of intensive preoperative exercise has been shown to improve cardiopulmonary fitness prior to major surgery.
- Aggressive chest physiotherapy and early mobilisation may also help to reduce the incidence of pulmonary complications associated with oesophagogastric surgery in patients with respiratory risk factors.
- The ERAS Society guidelines on evidence-based infrastructure for management of oesophagectomy patients.
- The multidisciplinary team (MDT) has become the cornerstone of standardising and coordinating cancer treatment. It is the appropriate venue for making specific recommendations regarding the overall treatment approach and the requirement for nutritional supplementation.
- Surgical and anaesthetic techniques, methodology of intraoperative monitoring, minimising blood losses, and perioperative fluid management, as well as lung isolation techniques and intraoperative organ support, are all important perioperative factors that can influence clinical outcome following oesophagectomy or gastrectomy; producing basic platforms or pathways covering both surgery and anaesthesia perioperative standards will help coordinate intraoperative care.
- Immediate extubation following surgery has the advantage of allowing the immediate initiation of postoperative protocols involving pain control, physiotherapy, and early mobilisation.
- A more restrictive approach to fluid management during major surgery may be beneficial, with improved gastrointestinal recovery time and reduced respiratory complications. Goal-directed fluid therapy includes minimising blood loss and maintaining haemodynamic stability, and this requires regular communication between surgeon and anaesthetic teams.
- Thoracic epidural analgesia for oesophagectomy has been shown to be a highly effective method of postoperative pain relief. Furthermore, the proven benefits of thoracic epidural analgesia following oesophagectomy include earlier recovery of bowel function, reduced pulmonary complication, and early extubation.
- Postoperative care pathways allow the introduction of a targeted, goal-directed approach to postoperative recovery following major oesophagogastric surgery. They provide a template for all medical personnel interacting with these patients and can outline a goal-directed recovery for each patient.
- The implementation of a clinical pathway for oesophagogastric cancer requires the personal commitment of all members of the care team and will affect a patient's treatment at virtually every stage; these individuals and teams should be involved in formulating and adapting the clinical pathway.
- Due to the increasing complexity of the work-up of patients undergoing oesophagogastric cancer surgery, the involvement of a nurse specialist is important to ensure appropriate liaison with the patient and planning of every stage of treatment.

References available at http://ebooks.health.elsevier.com/

KEY REFERENCES

[31] Wijeysundera DN, Duncan D, Nkonde-Price C, Virani SS, Washam JB, Fleischmann KE, et al. Perioperative beta blockade in noncardiac surgery: a systematic review for the 2014 ACC/AHA guideline on perioperative cardiovascular evaluation and management of patients undergoing noncardiac surgery: a report of the American College of Cardiology/American Heart Association Task Force on Practice Guidelines. Circulation 2014;130(24):2246–64

This is a meta-analysis of 16 RCTs and one cohort study, comprising data on 12 382 patients and looking at postoperative outcomes related to preventive beta-blockade started before surgery. Of note, outcome data are analysed with and without the inclusion of the controversial DECREASE trials, which showed a decrease in overall mortality related to beta-blockade.

[33] Douketis JD, Spyropoulos AC, Kaatz S, Becker RC, Caprini JA, Dunn AS, et al. Perioperative bridging anticoagulation in patients with atrial fibrillation. N Engl J Med 2015;373(9):823–33

This is the first RCT comparing risk for arterial thromboembolism and risk for major bleeding among patients receiving bridging therapy and patients without bridging therapy. All patients included received warfarin treatment for atrial fibrillation.

[55] Kita T, Mammoto T, Kishi Y. Fluid management and postoperative respiratory disturbances in patients with transthoracic esophagectomy for carcinoma. J Clin Anesth 2002;14(4):252–6

This is the first trial to demonstrate significantly reduced length of hospital stay with reduced intraoperative fluid administration specifically in the setting of oesophagectomy.

[56] Neal JM, Wilcox RT, Allen HW, Low DE. Near-total esophagectomy: the influence of standardized multimodal management and intraoperative fluid restriction. Reg Anesth Pain Med 2003;28(4):328–34

This trial demonstrated a significantly reduced incidence of pulmonary complication and earlier extubation associated with intraoperative fluid restriction.

Surgery for cancer of the oesophagus

5

Peter J. Lamb

INTRODUCTION

Despite advances in surgical technique and perioperative care, oesophageal cancer remains one of the most challenging conditions confronting the surgeon. The principles of surgery are to achieve complete resection of the tumour and surrounding lymph nodes, and to perform a reconstruction with the optimal functional outcome and the minimum morbidity and mortality. This chapter discusses these principles, focusing on primary tumour resection, the rationale for lymphadenectomy, technical aspects of different surgical approaches including minimally invasive surgery, methods of reconstruction and anastomosis, management of postoperative complications, and outcomes of treatment.

In the UK, 70% of patients with oesophageal cancer have adenocarcinoma of the lower oesophagus or oesophagogastric junction. This chapter includes the surgical management of adenocarcinoma of the lower oesophagus and the cardia (Siewert type 1 and 2), which is frequently staged and treated as oesophageal cancer as well as squamous carcinoma. Subcardial adenocarcinoma (Siewert type 3) is covered elsewhere (Chapter 6).

Unfortunately, as a result of poor fitness and/or advanced disease, only 25–40% of patients with oesophageal cancer are suitable for potentially curative treatment. While radical treatment for adenocarcinoma of the oesophagus is multidisciplinary, surgery remains the primary mode of therapy. Outcome is strongly stage dependent; early tumours have excellent results with surgery alone (Chapter 7), but the majority who have transmural and/or node-positive tumours benefit from multimodality therapy, combining surgery with neoadjuvant chemotherapy, or chemoradiotherapy (Chapter 8). Surgery continues to have a key role in the primary treatment of squamous carcinoma, with outcomes similar to definitive chemoradiotherapy, and as a salvage procedure following failed oncological treatment. The multidisciplinary team must exercise judgement for each individual patient based on the site, histology, and stage of the tumour, and patient fitness and wishes.

SURGICAL PATHOLOGY

Tumour site and histology are both crucial factors; squamous cell carcinoma arising in the cervical and thoracic oesophagus and adenocarcinoma arising in the thoracic oesophagus and cardia differ in their mode of spread and response to therapeutic modalities. There is also variation in the pattern of lymph node spread and proximity to vital structures according to the precise tumour site.

SURGICAL ANATOMY

It is important that the anatomical divisions of the oesophagus are described to understand the surgical procedures adopted for tumours at each site (Fig. 5.1).

PATIENT SELECTION

A detailed preoperative assessment to accurately evaluate tumour stage and surgical risk is vital to a successful outcome (see Chapters 3 and 4). It is now established that enhanced recovery programmes and perioperative care pathways result in improved clinical outcomes and reduced length of stay, and are cost effective. Elements of such programmes include: preoperative assessment, planning and preparation before admission (prehabilitation), reducing the physical stress of the operation, using a structured, goal-oriented approach to recovery, and, above all, early mobilisation.

Patients and their families should be counselled in detail about treatment options, paying particular attention to the expectations, results, and limitations of surgery. It is crucial that a trained clinical nurse specialist in oesophagogastric cancer oversees the patient pathway. When UK surgeons and patients were questioned about the most important information to be included in such discussions there were notable differences, with surgeons rating short-term clinical outcomes (technical complications) most highly, while patients prioritised information related to long-term benefits of surgery. A consensus meeting developed the final core information set for surgery for oesophageal cancer[1] (Box 5.1).

PRINCIPLES OF OESOPHAGECTOMY

SURGICAL OBJECTIVES

Oesophagectomy should be undertaken only when a potentially curative R0 resection (complete removal of all macroscopic and microscopic cancer) is expected. Unlike some gastrointestinal tumours, including colorectal carcinoma, there is little evidence for resection in the presence of proven distant metastases.

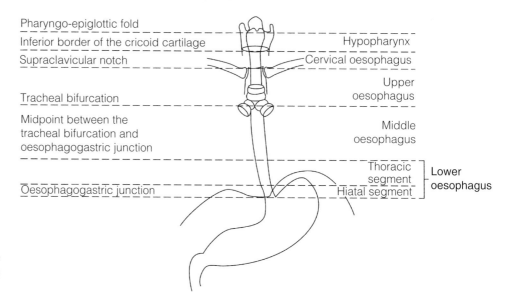

Pharyngo-epiglottic fold
Inferior border of the cricoid cartilage
Supraclavicular notch

Tracheal bifurcation

Midpoint between the tracheal bifurcation and oesophagogastric junction

Oesophagogastric junction

Hypopharynx
Cervical oesophagus
Upper oesophagus
Middle oesophagus
Thoracic segment
Hiatal segment
Lower oesophagus

Figure 5.1 Anatomical regions of the hypopharynx, oesophagus, and gastric cardia.

Box 5.1 Core information set for surgery for oesophageal cancer[1]

- In-hospital milestones to recovery
- Rates of open-and-close surgery
- In-hospital mortality
- Major complications (including re-operation)
- Milestones in recovery after discharge
- Longer term eating and drinking and overall quality of life
- Chances of survival

RESECTION OF PRIMARY TUMOUR

Accurate preoperative staging information is crucial to guide the optimal surgical approach and procedure. The majority of authors favour a subtotal oesophagectomy to take into account longitudinal spread in submucosal lymphatics for both squamous and adenocarcinoma. There is debate about the length of macroscopically normal oesophagus required to ensure a clear resection margin. In squamous carcinoma this relates primarily to the proximal margin, particularly if there is multifocal disease, which is common, or intramural lymphovascular spread, whereas in adenocarcinoma the distal gastric margin is usually the concern. A 10-cm resection margin is a goal to attain in both directions from the palpable edge of the tumour at surgery, *if this is possible*. In practice, this can often not be achieved but a minimum clearance of 5 cm should be targeted. When only a short proximal resection margin can be obtained through a thoracic exposure, a cervical phase with near total oesophagectomy must be considered. When there is concern at the time of surgery then a frozen section should be performed. Adenocarcinoma of the lower oesophagus commonly infiltrates the gastric cardia, fundus, and lesser curve. Extensive sleeve resection of the lesser curve and fundus with the formation of a tubular conduit is required to minimise the chance of a positive distal resection margin, particularly for Siewert type 2 tumours.

✓✓ Circumferential resection margin (CRM) is an independent prognostic factor for oesophageal cancer. A meta-analysis reported rates of CRM involvement of 45% according to the Royal College of Pathologists' (RCP) definition (tumour less than 1 mm from the resection margin) and 18% according to the College of American Pathologists' (CAP) definition (tumour at the resection margin). A positive CRM was associated with a worse prognosis regardless of histological subtype, T stage, or use of neoadjuvant therapy. Those positive according to CAP criteria had a worse overall survival.[2]

Radical en bloc resection techniques aim to produce a clear CRM. However, CRM can be influenced by a number of factors other than surgical technique, including case selection, type of neoadjuvant therapy, and histopathological assessment. The potential benefits of extended lymphadenectomy, discussed later, only pertain if the primary tumour has been completely excised (R0).

RESECTION OF LYMPH NODES

✓✓ There is no doubt that lymph node involvement and the number of lymph nodes involved are important independent prognostic variables for locoregional recurrence and survival. This was recognised by the RCP use the American Joint Committee on Cancer TNM seventh edition (TNM7), which subdivided the N stage according to the number of involved nodes (N1, 1–2; N2, 3–6; N3, ≥ 7). The Worldwide Esophageal Cancer Collaboration (WECC) has used pooled data from centres that have undertaken radical lymphadenectomy to report in detail the relationship between nodal involvement and survival.[3]

NODAL TIERS

Lymph node tiers for oesophageal cancer have been described according to lymphatic drainage of the oesophagus[4] (Fig. 5.2). However, there is confusion in the literature, with terms such as 'radical en bloc lymphadenectomy', 'extended lymphadenectomy', and 'two-field lymphadenectomy'

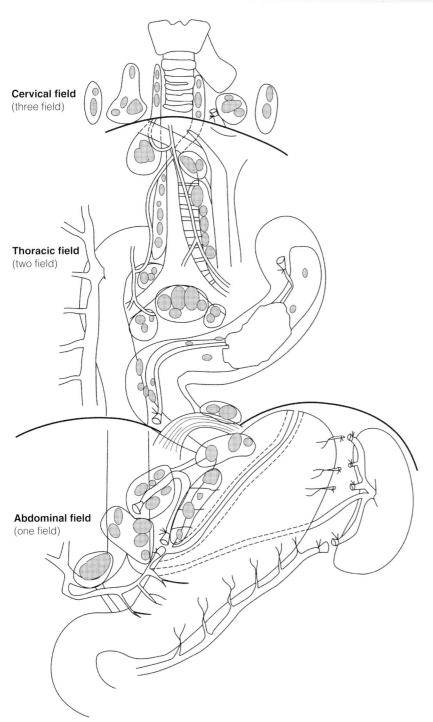

Cervical field
(three field)

Thoracic field
(two field)

Abdominal field
(one field)

Figure 5.2 Extent of resection and fields of lymph node dissection routinely carried out for cancer of the oesophagus.

used interchangeably to describe a variety of procedures. It has been proposed that the terminology used to describe the extent of lymphadenectomy should be standardised as follows.[5]

Radical lymphadenectomy

One-field lymphadenectomy describes an upper abdominal lymphadenectomy including removal of diaphragmatic, right and left paracardial, lesser curvature, left gastric, coeliac, common hepatic, and splenic artery nodes.

Two-field lymphadenectomy describes removal of the first field along with removal of the paraoesophageal nodes,

para-aortic nodes (together with the thoracic duct), and right and left pulmonary hilar, subcarinal, and right paratracheal nodes.

Three-field lymphadenectomy describes removal of the first and second fields along with a neck dissection clearing the brachiocephalic, deep lateral, and external cervical nodes, as well as right and left recurrent nerve lymphatic chains (deep anterior cervical nodes).

Non-radical lymphadenectomy

In this procedure only the nodes in direct proximity to the tumour, the oesophagus, and upper stomach are removed.

As for many solid-organ tumours, controversy persists as to the value of lymphadenectomy in oesophageal cancer. Some authors believe that lymph node metastases are simply markers of systemic disease, while others believe that cure can be obtained in many patients with positive nodes by a radical lymphadenectomy with clear resection margins.[6,7]

THE RATIONALE FOR LYMPHADENECTOMY

The arguments for radical lymphadenectomy are: optimal staging, improved locoregional control, and improved cure rates. Radical lymphadenectomy can also improve dissection of the primary tumour and increase R0 resection rates; for example, en bloc resection of the para-aortic nodes and thoracic duct requires a wider plane of dissection.

Optimal staging

Radical lymphadenectomy certainly allows more accurate pathological staging.[7,8] Current TNM staging relies not only on identifying positive lymph nodes, but also on how many are found. If an inadequate lymphadenectomy is undertaken, the phenomenon of stage migration means survival will tend to be poorer than that predicted by stage.

Locoregional tumour control

While oesophagectomy should not be undertaken without the potential for long-term survival, locoregional tumour control is an important benefit for those who are ultimately not cured. Radical lymphadenectomy has been associated with prolonged tumour-free survival, resulting from a combination of an increased R0 resection rate and the removal of involved nodes.[7,9,10] Locoregional recurrence can be further reduced by neoadjuvant therapy, whether chemotherapy or chemoradiotherapy, with an increase in R0 resection, and fewer positive nodes, associated with improved disease-free and overall survival in randomised trials.[11]

Improved cure rate

It is difficult to demonstrate that radical lymphadenectomy improves cure rates in a randomised controlled trial, and there are few in the literature.[12,13]

✔✔ There is an indication from a Dutch randomised trial[12,14] comparing radical transthoracic and less radical transhiatal resection that patients with a limited number of positive nodes (1–8) had significantly better survival following radical transthoracic oesophagectomy. Node-negative patients did well and those with a higher nodal burden did poorly irrespective of the radicality of surgery.

It has been shown by evaluating the sites of nodal involvement in patients who underwent neoadjuvant therapy and two-field oesophagectomy that long-term survival would have been compromised by limiting the extent of abdominal or mediastinal lymphadenectomy.[15] There is also a rationale for radical lymphadenectomy in patients believed to be node negative at staging, as 20% of these patients will ultimately be found to have lymph node metastases.[16] The role of radical lymphadenectomy in early-stage disease depends on the precise depth of invasion of the primary tumour, with the incidence of lymph node involvement rising sharply with submucosal invasion.

Further evidence in support of radical lymphadenectomy comes from the WECC, who reported on their multi-institution international database of over 4 600 resections in patients who had not had induction therapy.[6,17] Prognosis was highly dependent on the number of lymph nodes involved; patients with more than three nodes involved had a 50% likelihood of systemic disease and those with more than eight nodes involved had an almost 100% likelihood of systemic disease.[6] Importantly, survival depended not only on the number of nodes involved, but also on how many were removed at resection.[17] The number of lymph nodes removed was the third strongest predictor of survival after depth of invasion and number of nodes involved. This finding has been corroborated by the Surveillance, Epidemiology and End Results (SEER) database.[18] These international studies have recommended a respective lymph node yield of 23[17] and 30,[18] rather than the six nodes proposed for adequate staging in TNM7.

The role of a more extensive three-field dissection in oesophageal cancer is less clear. Five-year survival rates showed no significant difference between two-field and three-field dissection for lower third squamous carcinoma[8] and adenocarcinoma of the oesophagus. Selected patients with squamous and adenocarcinoma of the thoracic oesophagus might benefit from a formal three-field nodal dissection.[10] The potential benefit needs to be balanced against increased morbidity, particularly recurrent laryngeal nerve injury and pulmonary complications.

SUMMARY

There is little justification for oesophagectomy to be performed without an attempt to completely resect the primary tumour with an envelope of surrounding tissue. The majority of patients with oesophageal carcinoma have mediastinal lymph node metastases, and around three-quarters of patients with lower oesophageal tumours have involved upper abdominal lymph nodes. To perform a potentially curative resection for carcinoma in the middle and lower oesophagus, a dissection of upper abdominal and mediastinal lymph nodes is therefore logical. In practice, an infracarinal two-field lymphadenectomy is often performed for adenocarcinoma of the lower oesophagus and oesophagogastric junction.

✔ It is the author's opinion that a subtotal oesophagectomy with two-field lymphadenectomy is the operation of choice for patients with mid- and lower-third oesophageal cancer and type 1 and 2 tumours of the oesophagogastric junction.

RECONSTRUCTION OF THE OESOPHAGUS

ROUTE OF RECONSTRUCTION

POSTERIOR MEDIASTINAL

After oesophagectomy, the standard route of reconstruction is the posterior mediastinum. This provides the shortest distance between the abdomen and the apex of the thorax or the neck. Gastric or colonic substitutes are easily passed through the posterior mediastinum after completion of the oesophageal dissection in the thorax. The posterior mediastinal route is the preferred route of reconstruction in the primary surgical excision of oesophageal cancers.[19]

RETROSTERNAL (ANTERIOR MEDIASTINAL)

The potential space between the sternum and the anterior mediastinum is easily dissected by either blunt finger dissection or the use of a laparoscope through the abdominal and cervical incisions. The tip of an instrument is passed up to the neck in direct contact with the back of the sternum, taking care not to deviate from the midline. A laparoscopic sleeve can aid passage of the conduit from the abdomen to the neck in the retrosternal space. This route is most commonly used for reconstruction when there has been previous sepsis in the posterior mediastinum, such as following emergency treatment of gastric conduit necrosis. Its major disadvantage stems from the angulation of the oesophagus at the thoracic inlet, which can result in an unpleasant sensation on swallowing. When used for a colonic interposition, it is often necessary to resect the head of the clavicle and a small portion of manubrium to limit angulation and accommodate the graft.

PRESTERNAL

This is about 2 cm longer than the retrosternal route, which in turn is about 2 cm longer than the posterior mediastinal route. The only indication is when multiple previous reconstructions have compromised the other two routes.

ORGAN OF RECONSTRUCTION

RECONSTRUCTION WITH THE STOMACH

The stomach is the preferred conduit for reconstruction; it is easy to prepare, well vascularised, can be mobilised to the neck, requires a single anastomosis, and is durable in the long term.

There are important principles that must be observed in the preparation of the stomach as an oesophageal substitute:

1. **Right gastroepiploic arcade.** This is the main blood supply and is vital to the viability of the stomach when used as an oesophageal substitute. The gastrocolic omentum is opened and the entire course of the right gastroepiploic artery is carefully identified and preserved. Although the arcade is complete in the majority of patients, in some it is interrupted low on the greater curvature or is only in continuity through a small branch arching away from the stomach. It is important to recognise such variations at surgery, particularly in obese patients, and dissect well away from the stomach wall to avoid compromising the arcade (Fig. 5.3).
2. **Preservation of the intramural vascular arcade.** Extensive intramural anastomoses exist between the vascular arcades of the lesser and greater curvatures. This network must be preserved during resection of the lesser curvature and cardia of the stomach. The left gastric artery should be ligated at its origin as part of the en bloc resection. The right gastric artery contributes to the intramural network and should be preserved. The extent of resection of the lesser curvature is determined by a line connecting the highest point of the fundus (Fig. 5.4) and the lesser curvature at the junction of the right and left gastric arteries. This allows en bloc removal of the

RGEA/LGEA Anastomoses

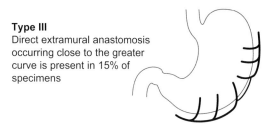

Type I
Continuous anastomosis between RGEA and the LGEA is present in 65% of specimens

Type II
No direct extramural anastomosis between the RGEA and LGEA is present in 15% of specimens

Type III
Direct extramural anastomosis occurring close to the greater curve is present in 15% of specimens

Type IV
Direct extramural anastomosis occurring away from the greater curve is present in 5% of specimens

Figure 5.3 Variations in vascular anatomy when mobilising the stomach as an oesophageal substitute. *RGEA/LGEA*, Right/left gastroepiploic artery.

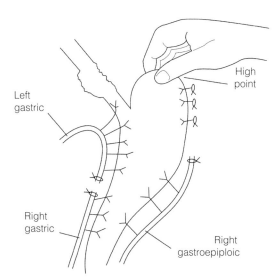

Figure 5.4 The high point of the stomach.

lesser curve lymph nodes, yet preserves the arterial network to the fundus. If the gastric tube is formed in the abdomen, care should be taken to angle the stapler along this line rather than at right angles to the lesser curve, to preserve this network. Care should also be taken to ligate the short gastric vessels away from the greater curvature of the stomach to preserve the extramural vascular network.

3. **Width of the gastric tube.** The author recommends adhering to the principles above and using a gastric tube of 5 cm width or greater to minimise the risk of ischaemia, as elegantly described by Akiyama et al.[20]

✓✓ A gastric tube should be used as a conduit rather than the whole stomach, as it provides a more durable functional outcome[21] and is also suitable for lower oesophageal cancers, when resection of the lesser curvature and cardia is required for oncological reasons.

4. **Gastric drainage.** The role of pyloroplasty or pyloromyotomy to prevent delayed emptying of the gastric conduit is a topic of debate.

✓✓ A systematic review identified a non-significant trend toward fewer postoperative complications with the use of pyloric drainage procedures.[22] As short-term complications of pyloroplasty are minimal, routine pyloroplasty is recommended to prevent early complications of gastric stasis and aspiration, as well as late emptying problems.

5. **Length of the gastric conduit.** Mobility of the gastric tube is important, as long-term function is better when the entire conduit lies with the thorax and on occasions the anastomosis may need to be high within the neck. The following steps should be considered to ensure adequate conduit length:

Kocher manoeuvre. The lateral aspect of the duodenum can be fully mobilised to the third part, and the peritoneum on the medial aspect divided to allow the 'C' of the duodenum to open and move caudally.

Excision of the lesser curve of the stomach. When the lesser curve of the stomach is short, an increase in length of the gastric conduit can be obtained by dividing the lesser curve between curved clamps. The gastric tube can then be stapled while held under gentle tension. If absolutely necessary, a tense right gastric artery can be sacrificed at the level of the pylorus, but this is rarely required.

Division of the right pillar of the diaphragm. This straightens and therefore shortens the route for the conduit.

RECONSTRUCTION WITH COLON

Indications for colonic reconstruction

The disadvantage of colonic transposition is that the function of the conduit deteriorates over time and it is less durable than the stomach in the long term. The main oncological indication for colonic interposition is tumours requiring extensive oesophageal and gastric resection. With current staging protocols, few such patients are candidates for resection. For extensive tumours of the oesophagogastric junction, an alternative and usually preferable approach is an extended total gastrectomy through a left thoracoabdominal incision using the jejunum to reconstruct. The number of patients who have had a previous gastric resection for peptic ulcer disease, precluding the use of stomach as the oesophageal substitute, is diminishing, and the choice of an oesophageal replacement in this situation lies between the colon and jejunum. The colon is also the preferred conduit after failed gastric interposition that has resulted in gastric necrosis.

Surgical technique

It is preferable to use the colon in an isoperistaltic fashion. The vascular pattern varies and careful selection of the correct vascular pedicle is important to ensure viability of the colon. Although the vascular supply determines the colonic segment for use in each case, the two preferred options are: 1) right colon based on the middle colic vessels; 2) transverse colon based on the ascending branch of the left colic vessels. Preoperative assessment with computed tomography (CT) angiography can be useful, particularly in patients with previous abdominal surgery, and careful intraoperative assessment of the vascular anatomy with temporary occlusion of the vessels before division is essential. Preoperative mechanical bowel preparation is routine.

The colon is mobilised and the mesentery inspected of its vascular supply. When right colon is being used, the right colic and ileo-colic vessels are temporarily occluded using vascular clamps. Once adequate perfusion of the conduit is assured, the occluded pedicles and the proximal ascending colon are divided. After anastomosis of the ascending colon to the oesophagus, the conduit is placed on sufficient stretch to prevent redundancy within the chest. The colon is then anchored in the straightened position with sutures to the hiatus, before the colo-jejunostomy or colo-gastrostomy is fashioned. Continuity of the large bowel is re-established, usually sacrificing the caecum to allow an ileo-colic anastomosis. An excellent technical description of the use of various segments of colon has been provided by DeMeester et al.[23] A useful refinement is resection of a short length of colon at either end of the graft, leaving redundant mesentery, to maximise blood supply to critical points of the graft.[24]

RECONSTRUCTION WITH THE JEJUNUM

The lower oesophagus and oesophagogastric junction can be replaced using a Roux-en-Y technique or by segmental interposition. A free graft of jejunum using a microvascular anastomosis can replace the upper oesophagus. It is sometimes possible to create a long loop of jejunum for replacement of the thoracic oesophagus, particularly when the proximal jejunum has adapted after previous gastric surgery.

A loop of jejunum is identified within the first 25 cm after the duodenojejunal flexure. Transillumination of the mesentery helps to identify the jejunal vascular tree precisely. It is important to appreciate that it is the free edge of the mesentery that will determine the length of the loop created rather than the length of the jejunum itself. The technique of microvascular free jejunal transfer for reconstruction of the upper oesophagus is well described elsewhere.[25] The indication for such a reconstruction is usually pharyngo-laryngectomy performed for carcinoma of the hypopharynx, postcricoid region, and cervical oesophagus. The operation is usually performed with a radical neck dissection as primary treatment or as salvage surgery following recurrence after radiotherapy.

SURGICAL APPROACHES TO OESOPHAGECTOMY

The primary purpose of any surgical approach is to allow optimal exposure to achieve complete resection of the oesophageal tumour and surrounding lymph nodes, and a reconstruction with minimum morbidity and mortality, and the best long-term quality of life. The choice of approach is dependent on tumour location, the extent of spread, and the fitness, age, and build of the patient. Traditionally oesophagectomy was performed by open surgery, but worldwide there has been increasing interest in totally minimally invasive oesophagectomy (MIO), hybrid surgery, and robot-assisted minimally invasive esophagectomy (RAMIE) during the last 10–15 years. UK practice for the surgical approach to oesophagectomy was published in the National Oesophago-Gastric Cancer Audit (NOGCA) Report 2012[26] (Box 5.2). The NOGCA Report 2018 demonstrated that there had not been a significant increase in the number of minimally invasive oesophagectomies in the UK in the 5-year period from 2012 to 2017.[27]

OPEN SURGICAL APPROACHES

TWO-PHASE SUBTOTAL OESOPHAGECTOMY

Two-phase subtotal oesophagectomy is accepted as the open approach of choice to the thoracic oesophagus.[26,27]

The first phase is abdominal mobilisation of the stomach through an upper midline or rooftop incision. The second phase is mediastinal dissection and oesophageal resection through a right thoracotomy. The stomach is delivered into the chest and an anastomosis fashioned at the thoracic inlet.

Abdominal phase

The procedure begins with a laparotomy to assess the primary tumour and exclude the presence of distant metastases. The stomach is mobilised on the right gastroepiploic and

Box 5.2 Surgical approach used for curative procedures for oesophageal cancer in the UK (n = 1 140)[26]

Two-phase subtotal oesophagectomy	77%	(49% open, 36% hybrid, 16% MIO)
Left thoracoabdominal oesophagectomy	15%	(97% open, 1% hybrid, 2% MIO)
Three-phase oesophagectomy	4%	(33% open, 12% hybrid, 55% MIO)
Transhiatal oesophagectomy	4%	(93% open, 0% hybrid, 7% MIO)

MIO, Minimally invasive oesophagectomy.

right gastric arcades, adhering to the principles outlined earlier. Preservation of a flap of omentum along the greater curve allows the formation of an omentoplasty around the anastomosis in the chest.

During hiatal dissection it is important to take an envelope of tissue around the tumour and to ensure adequate room for passage of the gastric conduit. For lower oesophageal and oesophagogastric junction tumours, it is routine to take a cuff of hiatal muscle and, anteriorly, all tissue posterior to the pericardium. The left and right pleura are entered and resected en bloc with the specimen. The lymphadenectomy begins at the origin of the right gastric artery, skeletonising the common hepatic artery, the root of the left gastric artery, and the splenic artery to the level of the posterior gastric artery. The omentum close to the transverse colon should be sutured to the abdominal wall to prevent postoperative diaphragmatic herniation.

The author recommends a feeding jejunostomy is routinely placed for postoperative nutrition, although some units do this selectively or use alternative feeding routes.

A systematic review of early nutrition after oesophagectomy demonstrated that a jejunostomy tube feeding was effective in meeting short-term nutritional requirements, but major tube-related complications occurred in 0–2.9%.[28]

Thoracic phase

The patient is placed in the left lateral decubitus position. The mediastinal phase is performed via a right posterolateral thoracotomy through the fourth or fifth intercostal space.

Division or resection of the arch of the azygos vein is required for exposure. The pleural incision is deepened along the line of the azygos vein to expose the descending aorta. The thoracic duct is identified and ligated with the tissue between aorta, oesophagus, and azygos, just above the level of the hiatus. The para-aortic lymph nodes and thoracic duct are mobilised en bloc, ligating aortic branches to the oesophagus. The anterior plane of dissection is along the pericardium, allowing the oesophagus to be slung. Dissection continues caudally to the right pulmonary hilum and the right bronchial, subcarinal, and left bronchial nodes are dissected en bloc. Diathermy and energy devices should be avoided in this region to prevent injury to the membranous parts of the tracheobronchial tree.

In high tumours, such as middle-third squamous lesions, a suprazygous dissection is performed.

The mediastinal pleura is incised along the course of the right vagus nerve towards the brachiocephalic and subclavian arteries. The right recurrent laryngeal nerve is preserved and the lymph node chain alongside it meticulously dissected. The pleura is incised along the border of the superior vena cava and the right paratracheal lymph nodes, located between the trachea and cava, are dissected. For tumours of the lower oesophagus and oesophagogastric junction the oesophagus is mobilised above the level of azygos but an infracarinal lymphadenectomy is routinely performed.

The stomach is delivered into the chest and the specimen removed after sleeve resection of the lesser curvature. The oesophagus is transected once sufficient gastric conduit length is confirmed. The oesophagogastric anastomosis is fashioned in the apex of the thorax. In addition to ensuring an adequate resection margin, it is important that the whole gastric conduit is within the thorax for a good functional outcome. If a lower anastomosis is fashioned, differences in abdominal and mediastinal pressure promote reflux and inhibit gastric emptying, resulting in troublesome long-term symptoms. Once the anastomosis and the gastrotomy line closure is completed, the omentum is passed posterior to the conduit and forms a 'wrap' around both the anastomosis and the staple line.

✔✔ A meta-analysis has demonstrated that omentoplasty to reinforce the anastomosis is a safe technique that reduces the incidence of anastomotic leak after oesophagectomy.[29]

LEFT THORACOABDOMINAL OESOPHAGECTOMY

The left thoracoabdominal approach provides excellent exposure of the hiatus and is appropriate for selected patients with tumours that have significant involvement of the cardia,[30] and for those requiring extended total gastrectomy. A good operative description is given by Sundaresan.[31] It is important to use a circumferential incision to divide the diaphragm rather than a radial incision that denervates the left diaphragm. The Japanese Clinical Oncology Group trial has shown that, for proximal gastric cancer, the left thoracoabdominal approach has a higher complication rate and no survival benefit compared to the alternative transhiatal approach to gastrectomy.[32]

THREE-PHASE OESOPHAGECTOMY

Exposing the oesophagus in the left neck provides good access for anastomosis. Although it does not allow resection of much more oesophagus than a two-phase approach, it should be considered for tumours of the upper middle third of the oesophagus when there is concern about involvement of the proximal margin. It does allow for a formal nodal dissection in the neck in patients with high nodal disease in the mediastinum. It was originally thought that leakage of a cervical anastomosis caused less morbidity than a thoracic leak. This is not always the case, and must be balanced against the potential increased risk of gastric tip necrosis and anastomotic stricture with a cervical anastomosis.

When a preoperative decision is made the first phase should mirror the thoracic dissection described in the preceding section, with mobilisation of the oesophagus to the root of the neck. The second phase of the operation is routine gastric mobilisation with the patient supine. This can be performed synchronously with a left-sided cervical dissection (third phase). The oesophagus is divided in the neck, and the oesophagus and stomach delivered on a tape to the abdomen, allowing the gastric tube to be formed with resection of the specimen. The gastric tube is then delivered to the neck behind a Foley catheter, or within a laparoscopic camera bag, for anastomosis. When an intraoperative decision is made to convert to a three-stage procedure, then the gastric tube is created during the thoracic phase and delivered into the neck during the cervical phase.

TRANSHIATAL OESOPHAGECTOMY

Controversy exists about the role of oesophagectomy without thoracotomy for oesophageal cancer. Proponents argue

that outcome is dependent on disease stage rather than operative technique. Opponents argue that there is improved survival for some undergoing oesophagectomy with two-field lymphadenectomy, which is not performed with a transhiatal approach. The rationale for lymphadenectomy has been discussed earlier in the chapter.

Orringer published a series of over 2 000 transhiatal resections that demonstrates an improvement in outcomes over 30 years with refinements of the technique.[33] A modified transhiatal technique, originally described by Pinotti, allows almost the entire procedure to be undertaken under direct vision, ensuring adequate local clearance and avoiding contact with the tumour.[34]

At present there are selected indications for transhiatal oesophagectomy, and thoracoscopic-assisted oesophagectomy is now an alternative in these cases:

1. To provide a gastric conduit for reconstruction in pharyngolaryngo-oesophagectomy (PLOG) for carcinoma of the hypopharynx and cervical oesophagus. In this situation oesophagectomy without thoracotomy can be safely performed. Radical neck dissection is carried out at the same time and reconstruction fashioned using the stomach through the posterior mediastinal route.
2. For resection of intraepithelial squamous carcinoma of the oesophagus. These tumours rarely disseminate via the lymph nodes. If the tumour is confined to the epithelial layer, resection by transhiatal oesophagectomy is appropriate (Chapter 7).
3. Patients with high-grade dysplasia and intramucosal adenocarcinoma in Barrett's oesophagus in whom endoscopic treatment is not an option (Chapter 7).

The debate will continue over which operative procedure is most appropriate for the treatment of lower-third oesophageal carcinoma. Few randomised studies have been performed and no clear survival advantage has emerged for a particular technique.

✔✔ A meta-analysis comparing transthoracic and transhiatal approaches did not demonstrate a significant difference in 5-year survival; however, it was subject to significant heterogeneity.[35] The strongest evidence for a survival advantage comes from the Dutch trial,[12,14] which included 220 patients with adenocarcinoma of the middle and lower oesophagus. More nodes were dissected with a radical transthoracic approach and significance was reached for an increased survival in this group for type 1 tumours, which continued with long-term follow-up. Patients with a low burden (1–8 nodes) of nodal disease appeared to benefit most from extended transthoracic oesophagectomy.

Pharyngolaryngo-oesophagectomy for carcinoma of the hypopharynx and cervical oesophagus

Resection of squamous cancer in this region requires resection of the larynx, lower pharynx, cervical trachea, thyroid gland, and the cervical oesophagus. It is often the primary treatment for patients who have received radical radiotherapy for other malignancies in the region, and salvage therapy following relapse after chemoradiotherapy. If the tumour is located in the hypopharynx only (postcricoid region), the thoracic oesophagus may be conserved and a free graft of je-junum transferred by microvascular anastomosis. If tumour has extended to the lower part of the cervical oesophagus, a total pharyngolaryngo-oesophagectomy and gastric trans-position, with pharyngogastric reconstruction, is required. The conduit can be provided by either a transhiatal or tho-racoscopic approach.

MINIMALLY INVASIVE OESOPHAGECTOMY TECHNIQUES

During recent decades, progress has been made in reduc-ing the morbidity of open surgery by the introduction of minimal access techniques across many surgical specialties. It is important that this is also explored for oesophagecto-my. Surgical access undoubtedly adds to the trauma of oe-sophagectomy, but it is unclear by how much, as whatever approach is taken the extensive dissection represents a ma-jor physiological challenge. For MIO techniques, it is vital that the core outcomes rated most highly by patients and specialists (see Box 5.1) are comparable with those from open surgery, including short-term morbidity and mortali-ty, and long-term oncological outcomes and quality of life. It follows that the same principles must be adhered to as for open surgery, in resection of the primary tumour and lymph nodes, preparation of the stomach as an oesophageal substitute, and anastomotic technique.

Evaluation of the outcomes of minimally invasive tech-niques is made more difficult by a number of different pro-cedures being labelled as MIO.

The term MIO should be reserved for operations involv-ing both thoracoscopic mobilisation of the oesophagus and laparoscopic mobilisation of the stomach. Hybrid procedures using minimally invasive techniques for only the abdominal or chest phase should be termed 'laparoscopically' or 'tho-racoscopically assisted oesophagectomy' (LAO and TAO, re-spectively).[36]

MINIMALLY INVASIVE OESOPHAGECTOMY (THREE-PHASE)

The first publications from Luketich et al.[37] describing total MIO with cervical anastomosis held out the potential of it being the approach of choice. However, the procedure was technically challenging and the learning curve was steep. For surgeons who did not routinely perform a cervical anasto-mosis for lower-third tumours, this operation added, in their view, unnecessary complexity and risk. Despite great inter-est, only a few centres published their early results,[38–43] and some highlighted concern of an increased conduit necrosis rate.[39] A multicentre feasibility study (Eastern Cooperative Oncology Group) comprising 106 patients in 16 institutions suggested short-term outcomes were acceptable when the technique was disseminated, but included only small num-bers from most centres.[44] After around 500 cases, Luketich changed his standard approach to a two-phase MIO with an intrathoracic anastomosis and reported a subsequent re-duction in mortality and recurrent laryngeal nerve injury.[45] Non-randomised comparative studies suggest three-phase MIO has similar outcomes to open surgery.[42,43]

Three-phase MIO has been compared with open surgery in a multicentre randomised controlled trial (TIME trial). The primary outcome of pulmonary infection was re-duced in the minimally invasive group, although in-hospital mortality was similar.[46] A criticism of the trial was an unusually high incidence of recurrent laryngeal nerve palsy in the open surgery group. A 3-year follow-up from the trial identified no differences in survival between MIO and open surgery.[47]

MINIMALLY INVASIVE OESOPHAGECTOMY (TWO-PHASE)

Luketich and colleagues changed their practice to a two-phase MIO with intrathoracic anastomosis.[45] This has be-come their preferred approach with a mortality rate of 0.9% for 520 cases, comparable with the best series of open oe-sophagectomy.[48] They caution a steep learning curve; many surgeons have found it technically difficult to replicate the two-field lymphadenectomy and intrathoracic anastomosis of open surgery. This is highlighted by the EsoBenchmark data from high-volume centres, which reported an intratho-racic anastomotic leak rate of 15.9% and up to 23.3% for end-to-side double-stapling techniques.[49] If technological advances can overcome these aspects, there is no doubt it will become an attractive technique for many units.

HYBRID PROCEDURES
Laparoscopically assisted oesophagectomy

The most frequently performed hybrid procedure in the UK (see Box 5.2) is a two-phase operation with a laparoscopic ab-dominal phase and an open thoracic phase. This approach allows extracorporeal gastric conduit formation, and allows familiar conditions to perform a mediastinal lymphadenecto-my and intrathoracic anastomosis. The benefit of laparoscop-ically assisted oesophagectomy over open surgery remains unclear given the conflicting results of two major trials.

The French multicentre MIRO trial randomised 207 patients and reported a significant reduction in major post-operative morbidity, including pulmonary complications, for laparoscopically assisted oesophagectomy (36%) compared to open oesophagectomy (64%), with a similar mortality.[50] There was no significant difference in 5-year overall survival (hybrid 59% vs open 47%). However, complications were a risk factor for poor long-term outcome, suggesting that hybrid surgery could be associated with improved oncological results.[51]

The UK multicentre ROMIO (Randomised Oe-sophagectomy: Minimally Invasive or Open) trial randomised over 500 patients and has identified no difference between groups in overall postoperative morbidity, pulmonary compli-cations, or recovery, including fatigue at 3 months following surgery.[52]

Thoracoscopically assisted oesophagectomy

This is a three-stage procedure comprising thoracoscop-ic oesophageal mobilisation followed by an open abdom-inal phase and a cervical anastomosis. The technique has been popularised by the Brisbane group and, by avoiding thoracotomy, aims to reduce chest complications and pain.

Thoracoscopic mobilisation in the prone position provides excellent visualisation and a relatively short single-lung ventilation time. Open gastric conduit formation, together with manual transfer of the conduit through the mediastinum to the neck, aims to minimise the risk of conduit ischaemia. Potential disadvantages are the need for a cervical phase and that it is not suitable for more advanced tumours of the oesophagogastric junction. Smithers et al. published a non-randomised comparison of this procedure with open oesophagectomy, finding it to be safe and comparable to the open approach with respect to postoperative recovery and cancer survival.[42] When they evaluated long-term health-related quality of life, the only difference was lower pain scores than the Ivor–Lewis group.[53]

ROBOTIC-ASSISTED MINIMALLY INVASIVE ESOPHAGECTOMY

The emergence of robotic technology has the potential to overcome some of the obstacles to widespread uptake of MIO; the learning curve and technical dexterity difficulties in reproducing the lymphadenectomy and intrathoracic anastomosis of open surgery.

✔✔ A randomised trial of 112 patients reported a reduction in surgery-related complications after three-phase RAMIE (59%) compared to three-phase open oesophagectomy (80%). Anastomotic leak rates were over 20% in both groups.[54]

At present, RAMIE is only carried out in a small number of centres. A large, single-centre propensity score–matched analysis reported that 350 patients undergoing two-phase RAMIE had equivalent short- and long-term outcomes to patients undergoing open oesophagectomy.[55] It is not clear how reproducible the results of RAMIE techniques will be if they are disseminated into wider practice, and the optimal technique for RAMIE needs to be determined before it can be considered the approach of choice for oesophagectomy.

✔ An international registry from specialist centres reported on 856 RAMIE cases with acceptable postoperative mortality (3%) and short-term oncological outcomes.[56] However, they identified variations in the use of robotic surgery during the thoracic and abdominal phases, anastomotic technique, and extent of lymphadenectomy. A high overall anastomotic leakage rate of over 20%, and up to 33% with a robotic hand-sewn intrathoracic anastomosis, was observed.

OVERVIEW OF MINIMALLY INVASIVE OESOPHAGECTOMY TECHNIQUES

Minimally invasive oesophagectomy techniques (MIOT) and RAMIE techniques have generated huge worldwide interest, and there has been an increase in the number of procedures performed. However, a series of hybrid and totally minimally invasive resections have been reviewed collectively showing no advantage, or a relatively small advantage of a minimally invasive approach.

Hospital Episode Statistics (HES) data in England[57] showed no difference in 30-day mortality (4.0% for MIOT, 4.3% for open) or 30-day postoperative morbidity (38% for MIOT, 39% for open). There was a slightly shorter length of stay for minimally invasive approaches. However, there was also a significantly higher re-intervention rate for MIOT, including a higher re-operation rate (8.8% vs 5.6%). MIO resections had twice the re-intervention rate of hybrid procedures.

✔✔ A meta-analysis has reported better global quality of life, physical function, fatigue, and pain 3 months after minimally invasive surgery compared with open surgery. However, no such differences remained at a longer follow-up of 6 and 12 months.[58] High-quality evidence is also lacking between MIO and hybrid procedures; a meta-analysis found that MIO was associated with lower morbidity, but a higher leakage rate and lower lymph node count, compared to hybrid procedures.[59]

The TIME and MIRO trials both identified potential benefits in early pulmonary complications, although these did not translate into improved mortality. This was also reflected in a recent meta-analysis of 32 315 patients undergoing open oesophagectomy, MIO, and RAMIE procedures.[60]

It is still not clear how reproducible the results of total MIO and RAMIE will be in wider clinical practice. The technical difficulty in replicating high-quality open surgery has led some centres to focus on optimising perioperative care pathways rather than surgical access. While we do not yet have robust evidence to recommend that MIO and RAMIE approaches should replace open oesophagectomy, they will certainly have an important role in the future.

ANASTOMOSIS TECHNIQUE

Meticulous technique is essential to minimise the risk of leakage after oesophagogastric anastomosis. Despite improvements in perioperative care, the recent Oesophago-Gastric Anastomosis Audit (OGAA) reported a mortality of around 11% for patients after an anastomotic leak.[61] The universal surgical principles relating to anastomosis apply – adequate blood supply, absence of tension, and accurate approximation of epithelial edges. The mobility and vascularity of the gastric conduit is of particular importance and is highlighted earlier in the chapter. The high point of the gastric tube is the logical site to fashion an anastomosis and is easily identified by applying traction to the conduit. The right gastroepiploic artery provides an adequate blood flow to maintain vascularity in this region of the fundus.

INTRATHORACIC OESOPHAGOGASTRIC ANASTOMOSIS

Circular stapled, linear stapled, and single- and two-layer hand-sewn anastomosis have been described, but no significant difference in leak rates has been demonstrated at open surgery. The technical difficulty, and learning curve, in replicating an intrathoracic anastomosis with MIO and RAMIE are reflected by relatively high reported leak rates.[49,56] The author recommends a circular stapled anastomosis for ease of repetition and training. A low-profile head is inserted into the proximal oesophageal stump, already prepared with stay sutures and a carefully placed purse-string suture. The anastomosis should be kept at least 3 cm from the gastric staple line to avoid angles of poorly perfused gastric wall. If there is redundant stomach, then more of the fundus can be excised with the specimen and the anastomosis placed on the high greater curve. This technique should provide intact 'doughnuts' of oesophageal and gastric tissue to confirm anastomotic integrity. The anastomosis can be covered with a cap of pleura and wrapped in transposed omentum. The rate of benign anastomotic stricture formation is reduced if a larger 28-mm–diameter stapler can be used.[62] The staple head can also be inserted transorally, allowing a double-staple technique similar to that in colorectal surgery. However, with this technique there is a real risk that cross-stapling will create angles of relative ischaemia.

CERVICAL OESOPHAGOGASTRIC ANASTOMOSIS

The OGAA confirmed that anastomotic leakage is more frequent in the neck than the chest, although the mortality rates do not differ between these sites.[61] Both hand-sewn and semi-mechanical side-to-side cervical anastomosis, with a linear stapled posterior wall and a hand-sewn anterior wall, have been described. Orringer[63] reported a reduction in the cervical anastomotic leak rate and long-term stricture rate with a semi-mechanical anastomosis. However, most were performed during transhiatal oesophagectomy for lower-third tumours, so that a sufficient length of cervical oesophagus could be left without compromising the resection margin. A semi-mechanical anastomosis is difficult if the purpose of the cervical phase is proximal clearance; in this situation, a high anastomosis using interrupted sutures to a short proximal oesophageal stump allows greater clearance.

POSTOPERATIVE MANAGEMENT

A detailed account of early postoperative care after oesophageal cancer surgery is described in Chapter 4, and the author recommends the use of clinical care pathways such as that from the Virginia Mason Medical Center (see Table 4.2. Pathways provide focus on the key components of good postoperative care – fluid balance, pain control, early mobilisation, clearance of sputum, and GI function, and early removal of chest drains once oral fluids have recommenced. It is the author's practice to routinely give patients early enteral nutrition via a feeding jejunostomy. There is no evidence that the routine use of contrast radiology to assess the oesophageal anastomosis is of value in patients who are asymptomatic in the postoperative phase.[64] The surgeon, a cancer nurse specialist, and a dietician should counsel patients prior to discharge from the hospital.

POSTOPERATIVE COMPLICATIONS

The postoperative complication rate of oesophagectomy is relatively high, in the region of 30–40%. The timely recognition and management of complications is a vital role of the specialist oesophagogastric cancer team and it is one of the key factors that determine not only in-hospital mortality rates, but also long-term quality of life and even oncological outcomes (Box 5.3). The concept of 'failure to rescue' patients with a major postoperative complication is

---

Box 5.3 Adverse outcomes directly linked to postoperative complications following oesophagectomy

- Increased postoperative mortality
- Increased length of hospital stay
- Increased hospital readmissions
- Early cancer recurrence
- Increased health resource utilisation
- Decreased quality of life
- Decreased long-term survival

Box 5.4 Esophagectomy Complications Consensus Group – summary of recommendations for reporting outcomes and quality measures[55]

1. Routinely record both 30-day and in-hospital mortality, and 90-day mortality
2. Comorbidity assessment – Routine recording of ASA, ECOG, and Charlson Comorbidity Index
3. Blood product utilisation – The number of units transfused, intraoperative and postoperative
4. Record the transfer of a patient to a higher level of postoperative care
5. Recording complication severity using the Clavien–Dindo classification
6. Record all readmissions to primary or secondary hospitals within 30 days of discharge, including timing and cause of readmission
7. Record the discharge location and discriminate between home and other medical facilities

ASA, American Society of Anesthesiologists; *ECOG*, Eastern Cooperative Oncology Group.

---

now recognised as a key marker for hospital quality of care. The marked differences in mortality between high- and low-volume centres are associated less with a difference in complication rate than they are with the ability to effectively rescue patients from a complication. Comparison between case series and analysis of the outcomes of randomised trials has been limited by a lack of standardisation, both in the definition of complications, and those reported.

The Esophagectomy Complications Consensus Group (ECCG) has now reported a standardised system for defining and reporting complications[65] (Box 5.4). The ECCG 2015–2018 outcomes reported a 30-day and 90-day mortality of 2.0% and 4.5%, respectively, with 22% of patients requiring an escalation in care during hospital admission.[66]

GENERAL COMPLICATIONS OF OESOPHAGECTOMY

These complications (see also Chapter 4) can be minimised by improved preoperative patient evaluation and adherence to perioperative care pathways. Respiratory complications constitute the largest proportion of this group. Pain is the major contributor to decreased ventilation and atelectasis, which leads to bronchopneumonia and respiratory failure. Major pulmonary complications occur in around 15–30% of cases following oesophagectomy.[50,66]

Major haemorrhage is uncommon and routine blood loss is less than 500 mL, with only around 10% of patients requiring transfusion.[66]

SPECIFIC COMPLICATIONS OF OESOPHAGECTOMY

ANASTOMOTIC LEAKAGE AND GASTRIC CONDUIT NECROSIS

Anastomotic leak is defined as a full-thickness defect involving the oesophagus, anastomosis, staple line, or conduit irrespective of presentation or the method of identification. A classification of anastomotic leak and gastric conduit necrosis is shown in Box 5.5.[65] Anastomotic leakage is influenced by a variety of factors, including cancer hypermetabolism, malnutrition, anastomotic blood supply, anastomotic tension, and surgical technique.

✔ Although anastomotic leak rates of around 5% should be targeted by specialist centres, recent multicentre studies have reported leak rates of 12–14%[61,66] and even higher for some series of MIO and RAMIE.[49,56]

While there is no role for a routine postoperative contrast swallow following oesophagectomy, patients with clinical suspicion of a leak or failure to progress should be actively investigated. The diagnostic test of choice is usually computed tomography (CT) with intravenous and oral contrast; this will demonstrate the presence of a leak or collection and other causes of deterioration, and can be performed in a ventilated patient. If clinical condition allows, a contrast swallow can provide further information about a confirmed leak and assess response to treatment. Diagnostic algorithms including C-reactive protein and pleural drain amylase have also been proposed.[67]

> **Box 5.5 Esophagectomy Complications Consensus Group – classification of anastomotic leak and gastric conduit necrosis following oesophagectomy[55]**
>
> **Anastomotic leak**
> - Type I: Local defect requiring no therapy or treated medically/with dietary modification
> - Type II: Local defect requiring interventional but not surgical therapy (e.g. interventional radiology drain, stent, or bedside opening of wound)
> - Type III: Local defect requiring surgical therapy
>
> **Conduit necrosis**
> - Type I: Focal conduit necrosis identified at endoscopy. Treatment – additional monitoring or non-surgical therapy
> - Type II: Focal conduit necrosis identified at endoscopy and not associated with free leakage. Treatment – surgical therapy not involving oesophageal diversion
> - Type III: Extensive conduit necrosis. Treatment – conduit resection with diversion

✔ Video endoscopy has a vital role,[68] both in assessing the extent of an anastomotic leak, and in particular identifying the presence of gastric necrosis (Box 5.5).

Early anastomotic disruption (within 48–72 hours) is rare and is usually the result of technical error. The patient should be re-explored for correction of the technical problem. Total gastric necrosis can, rarely, occur with catastrophic consequences. This must be diagnosed early by endoscopy, resuscitation given, and the patient immediately returned to theatre for the formation of a cervical oesophagostomy and closure of the viable component of the gastric remnant. At a later date, a retrosternal colonic interposition can be used to restore intestinal continuity.

✔ Late leaks usually manifest between the fifth and tenth postoperative days and are due to ischaemia of the tissues or tension on the anastomotic line. For leaks from the oesophagogastric anastomosis, an intensive non-operative approach is usually appropriate, with nasogastric decompression, radiological-guided chest, and mediastinal drainage, antibiotic and antifungals, and enteral nutrition via a jejunostomy (Fig. 5.5).[68] Operative intervention is required if the leak is not controlled and is usually limited to washout of the pleural cavity and drainage, with or without insertion of a T-tube.

There has been an increase in the use of oesophageal stents as treatment for anastomotic leak. The author does not recommend the routine use of stents as a primary treatment. They may prevent adequate drainage of sepsis, migrate, or even erode into surrounding structures, leading to haemorrhage and airways complications. A recent development in the management of anastomotic leak has been the use of endoscopic vacuum therapy. This is only suitable in certain situations but may have an improved fistula closure rate and mortality compared to oesophageal stenting.[69] Although anastomotic leakage is associated with an increased mortality, it is possible to rescue the vast majority of patients with the aggressive non-operative approach described (Fig. 5.5).[68]

CHYLOTHORAX

Damage to the thoracic duct during oesophagectomy can be minimised by formal identification during dissection and carefully ligating the duct low in the mediastinum between the oesophagus, azygos and aorta. An incidence of 2–3% during open resection is commonly reported and is more common with squamous cell carcinoma. High-volume chyle leaks, of over 1 L per day, are usually apparent during the first few days after surgery when jejunostomy feed is commenced. Early re-exploration is recommended for these leaks, as the damaged thoracic duct or side branch is usually easily identified, following a bolus of cream, at the time of re-exploration.[70] If left untreated the chyle leak results in malnutrition and significant immune suppression. Leaks of less than 500 mL/day often resolve with enteral feeding using medium-chain triglycerides. Persistent chyle leakage following re-exploration is a difficult management problem and is often due to abnormal lymph anatomy around the hiatus. Patients require total parenteral nutrition and can benefit from insertion of a pleuroperitoneal shunt, to allow reabsorption of chyle. There is also now a role for interventional radiology approaches to embolise or disrupt lymphatic flow.

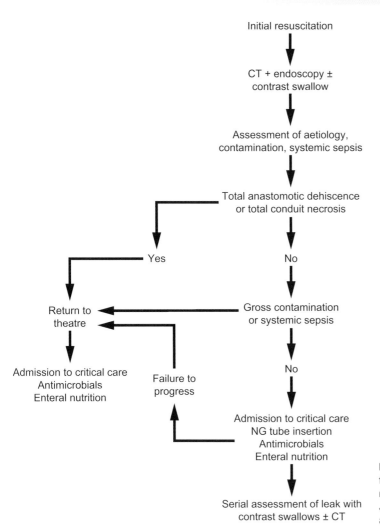

Initial resuscitation

↓

CT + endoscopy ±
contrast swallow

↓

Assessment of aetiology,
contamination, systemic sepsis

↓

Total anastomotic dehiscence
or total conduit necrosis

Yes   No

Return to theatre   ←   Gross contamination
                          or systemic sepsis

Admission to critical care   Failure to   No
Antimicrobials   progress
Enteral nutrition   Admission to critical care
                                             NG tube insertion
                                             Antimicrobials
                                             Enteral nutrition

Serial assessment of leak with
contrast swallows ± CT

Figure 5.5 Algorithm for the management of anastomotic leak following oesophagectomy. *CT*, Computed tomography; *NG*, nasogastric. (Modified with permission from Dent B, Griffin SM, Jones R, et al. Management and outcomes of anastomotic leaks after oesophagectomy. Br J Surg 2016;103(8):1033–8.)

RECURRENT LARYNGEAL PALSY

The incidence of recurrent laryngeal palsy is higher with cervical oesophagogastric anastomoses. If the palsy is transient but unilateral, the opposite cord will often compensate. If the palsy is permanent, Teflon injection of the cord or a formal thyroplasty can restore adequate voice volume and a satisfactory cough.

DIAPHRAGMATIC HERNIATION

The widened hiatus, through which the gastric conduit has passed, is a potential site of herniation in the early and late postoperative period. The transverse colon is usually the lead point, but other intra-abdominal contents including small bowel can be involved. It is important to recognise this complication on a postoperative chest radiograph as, once confirmed by a CT scan, urgent re-operation is indicated. The incidence is increased following laparoscopic gastric mobilisation and technical steps should be taken, as described earlier, to prevent this complication.

BENIGN ANASTOMOTIC STRICTURE

Strictures are relatively common following stapled intrathoracic anastomosis and usually respond to between one and three endoscopic dilatations.[62] Refractory strictures,

although rare, are more common following a cervical anastomosis.

LONG-TERM GASTROINTESTINAL SYMPTOMS

GASTRIC EMPTYING

Gastric emptying problems can be minimised by the routine use of a pyloroplasty or a pyloromyotomy, although some units selectively use pyloric dilatation or Botox injection as an alternative strategy. Emptying problems are less frequent when the anastomosis is in the apex of the thorax. Procedures that leave part of the stomach in the abdomen predispose to duodeno-gastro-oesophageal reflux. Prokinetic agents such as low-dose erythromycin can improve symptoms of gastric emptying.

DUODENO-GASTRO-OESOPHAGEAL REFLUX

Acid and alkaline reflux is common and although acid suppressants, prokinetic agents, and lifestyle advice can control it, it can be troublesome.

DUMPING SYNDROME

'Dumping' symptoms after oesophagogastric reconstruction are relatively common and often improve in the first year following surgery. They are usually adequately treated by the avoidance of high carbohydrate loads. It is becoming clear that there are complex changes in enteroendocrine function after oesophagectomy that are associated with reduced appetite, weight loss, and postprandial hypoglycaemia.[71]

DIARRHOEA

Complaints of altered gastrointestinal function are common after oesophagectomy and have been linked to dietary intake, altered gastric emptying, changes in enteroendocrine function, vagotomy, and impaired exocrine pancreatic function. Patients will often respond to specialist dietetic support and pancreatic enzyme supplements.[72]

OVERALL RESULTS OF SINGLE-MODALITY SURGICAL THERAPY

Survival for patients with oesophageal cancer is strongly related to the stage of disease. Patients with stage 1 disease can expect a 3-year survival of greater than 80%, emphasising the importance of early detection. Surgical resection alone is the treatment in fit patients with T1 tumours of the middle and lower thirds of the oesophagus that are not suitable for endoscopic therapy. In stage III disease, surgery alone produces relatively poor results, with a 5-year survival of only around 25% of cases, predominantly those with a low burden of lymph node disease. There is evidence that both neoadjuvant chemotherapy and chemoradiotherapy provide an additional benefit for patients[11] (see Chapter 8).

Overall survival following surgical resection for all stages of oesophageal tumour has improved over the past 25 years, with a reduction in postoperative mortality. The reasons for this are listed in Box 5.6. There is overwhelming evidence to confirm the influence of surgeon and unit case volume and specialisation on the outcome of site-specific cancer surgery.[73,74] Centralisation of oesophagogastric resection in specialist units in the UK has provided sufficient caseload to support strong multidisciplinary teams and allow publication of a robust national oesophagogastric cancer audit.[26,27]

The overall results of surgical therapy in oesophageal cancer should not only be analysed in terms of hospital mortality and patient survival. Assessment of quality of life (patient-related outcomes) as an outcome measure is essential and there is evidence relating it to overall survival.[75] The fact that it takes 9 months for quality of life to recover following surgery illustrates the scale of trauma that oesophagectomy produces. Very few new data have

become available on single-modality surgery for oesophageal cancer, as increasingly published results include patients having multimodality treatment.

SHORT-TERM OUTCOMES

Although individual units achieved considerably better results, a comprehensive review demonstrated a marked improvement in overall short-term outcomes during the latter part of the last century. The review by Jamieson et al.[76] confirmed that the average hospital mortality rate following oesophagectomy had continued to decrease, from 28% (1953–1978), to 13% (1980–1988), to 8.8% (1990–2000).

✅ Since the year 2000, case series from specialist centres have regularly reported in-hospital mortality rates of less than 5%,[7] including a huge series of over 20 000 esophagectomies from China,[77] and Low's series of 340 patients, with an in-hospital mortality of 0.3%.[48] Encouragingly, these results are now being replicated in multicentre randomised trials,[12] and large national audits.[27,78]

It is also apparent that, while there is a recognised learning curve for oesophagectomy, patient outcomes are not compromised by supervised trainee involvement in transthoracic oesophagectomy.[79] To allow *effective* comparison between different series, it is recommended that data should be routinely recorded for both 30-day and in-hospital mortality, and 90-day mortality.[65] It is also important that postoperative outcomes data accurately take into account the case mix, using techniques such as the validated adjustment model used in the UK national audit.[80]

LONG-TERM OUTCOMES

Trying to identify improvements in long-term outcome for adenocarcinoma over time from surgery alone is difficult because of the widespread use of neoadjuvant treatment for locally advanced disease. More recent 'surgery-alone' series reflect operations for early disease that would not allow fair comparison with the earlier publications. The continued reporting of results combining adenocarcinoma and squamous cell cancers has made interpretation more difficult; there is some evidence to suggest that adenocarcinomas tend to fare worse, although this may simply reflect a more advanced stage at presentation.

There does appear to have been some improvement in long-term outcome. In a review of the 1980s, Muller et al. found that 56% of all resected patients survived the first postoperative year, 34% the second, 25% the third, 21% the fourth, and 20% the fifth year after resection.[81] As discussed, the Dutch randomised trial reported a 5-year survival for adenocarcinoma of 34% and 36% after transhiatal and transthoracic resection, respectively.[14] A population-based study from Sweden evaluated survival with resection alone: the 5-year survival increased from 19.7% in 1987–1991 to 30.5% between 2001 and 2005.[82] However, not all studies have reported such good outcomes; patients in the surgery-alone arm of the OEO2 trial had a 5-year survival of only 17.6%.[83] In England and Wales between 2012 and 2018 the overall 5-year survival following oesophagectomy, including patients undergoing multimodality therapy, was 47.1%.[84]

Box 5.6 Reasons for improved results for oesophageal resection

- Earlier diagnosis
- Increase in specialist units
- Multidisciplinary team approach
- Better patient selection
- Use of neoadjuvant chemotherapy and chemoradiotherapy
- Improved perioperative management
- Enhanced recovery programmes

✅ The primary determinant of overall outcome is the stage of the tumour at diagnosis. WECC data included surgery-alone patients from several decades and produced separate survival curves for adenocarcinoma and squamous cancer. Five-year survival for adenocarcinoma was approximately 80% for TNM7 stages 0 and 1A, approximately 64% for stage 1B, 50% for 2A, 40% for 2B, and 25% for 3A.[85]

There is currently a focus on trying to develop more accurate predictive models at a patient level to help tailor treatment and follow-up. The AUGIS survival predictor, using 14 preoperative and postoperative variables, has been shown to provide greater accuracy than TNM staging alone.[84]

SUMMARY AND FUTURE RESEARCH

The main areas of progress in surgery for oesophageal cancer have been the introduction of a multidisciplinary approach in cancer centres, improved disease staging, the introduction of enhanced recovery pathways, the development of new surgical and endoscopic techniques for the management of early tumours including minimally invasive and robotic oesophagectomy, and the introduction of multimodality therapy for locally advanced disease. The future of oesophageal cancer surgery will be based on procedures tailored to the individual patient. Those with a low burden of lymph node disease will be targeted with increasingly effective multimodality regimens, including a radical en bloc oesophagectomy with two-field lymph node dissection. Neoadjuvant regimens will be tailored by genetic profiling to determine the best therapeutic strategy for each patient. Despite all this, significant improvements in long-term outcome for oesophageal cancer will only be achieved if increased focus is placed on earlier detection.

Key points

- Subtotal oesophagectomy should be carried out in patients with tumours of the middle and lower oesophagus to ensure clear resection margins.
- Two-phase oesophagectomy with two-field lymphadenectomy is recommended for lower oesophageal adenocarcinoma, particularly those with a low nodal burden.
- The stomach is the preferred conduit for oesophageal reconstruction.
- Minimally invasive oesophagectomy and robotic techniques have been shown to have comparable short- and long-term outcomes to open surgery in specialist centres.
- There is evidence to confirm the influence of surgeon and unit case volume on the outcome of oesophageal cancer surgery.
- The short- and long-term results of surgical resection for all stages of oesophageal tumour have improved over the past 20 years.
- Multimodality therapy including high-quality surgery should be considered for patients with >T1b N0 tumours.
- Outcome is strongly stage dependent – the focus must be on early detection.

ACKNOWLEDGEMENT

This chapter in the sixth edition was written with Professor Mike Griffin and I am grateful to him for those parts of the chapter which I have kept in this edition.

▶ RECOMMENDED VIDEOS

- Laparoscopic oesophagogastrectomy with colonic interposition – https://tinyurl.com/y8o8y5fz
- Transhiatal oesophagectomy – https://tinyurl.com/yd2hmy4k
- Minimally invasive oesophagectomy (three-phase) – https://tinyurl.com/ycabw4ll
- Minimally invasive oesophagectomy (two-phase) – https://tinyurl.com/y9fjahmj
- Intrathoracic oesophagogastric anastomosis – https://tinyurl.com/yce85w7y
- Robot-assisted Minimally Invasive Oesophagectomy – https://youtu.be/e6xpDBe915U

KEY REFERENCES

[2]. Evans R, Bundred JR, Kaur P, Hodson J, Griffiths EA. Meta-analysis of the influence of a positive circumferential resection margin in oesophageal cancer. BJS Open 2019;3(5):595–605. PMID: 31592511.

[3]. Rice TW, Rusch VW, Apperson-Hansen C, et al. Worldwide esophageal cancer collaboration. Dis Esophagus 2009;22:1–8. PMID: 19196264.

[12]. Hulscher JB, van Sandick JW, de Boer AG, Wijnhoven BPL, Tijssen JGP, Fockens P, et al. Extended transthoracic resection compared with limited transhiatal resection for adenocarcinoma of the esophagus. N Engl J Med 2002;347(21):1662–9. PMID: 12444180
  This important trial suggests that both techniques are safe but that there is lower morbidity in the transhiatal group and a trend to longer survival in the extended transthoracic group.

[14]. Omloo JM, Lagarde SM, Hulscher JB, Reitsma JB, Fockens P, van Dekken H, et al. Extended transthoracic resection compared with limited transhiatal resection for adenocarcinoma of the mid/distal esophagus: five-year survival of a randomized clinical trial. Ann Surg 2007;246:992–1000. PMID: 18043101.

[21]. Zhang W, Yu D, Peng J, Xu J, Wei Y. Gastric-tube versus whole-stomach esophagectomy for esophageal cancer: a systematic review and meta-analysis. PLoS One 2017;12(3):e0173416. PMID:28267808.

[22]. Arya S, Markar SR, Karthikesalingam A, Hanna GB. The impact of pyloric drainage on clinical outcome following esophagectomy: a systematic review. Dis Esophagus 2015;28(4):326–35. PMID: 24612489.

[28]. Weijs TJ, Berkelmans GHK, Nieuwenhuijzen GAP, Ruurda JP, van Hillegersberg R, Soeters PB, et al. Routes for early enteral nutrition after esophagectomy. A systematic review. Clin Nutr 2015;34(1):1–6. PMID: 25131601.

[29]. Wiggins T, Markar SR, Arya S, Hanna GB. Anastomotic reinforcement with omentoplasty following gastrointestinal anastomosis: a systematic review and meta-analysis. Surg Oncol 2015;24(3):181–6. PMID: 26116395.

[35]. Boshier PR, Anderson O, Hanna GB. Transthoracic versus transhiatal esophagectomy for the treatment of esophagogastric cancer: a meta-analysis. Ann Surg 2011;254(6):894–906. PMID: 21785341.

[46]. Biere SS, van Berge Henegouwen MI, Maas KW, Bonavina L, Rosman C, Garcia JR, et al. Minimally invasive versus open oesophagectomy for patients with oesophageal cancer: a multicentre, open-label, randomised controlled trial. Lancet 2012;379(9829):1887–92. PMID: 22552194.

[47]. Straatman J, van der Wielen N, Cuesta MA, Daams F, Garcia JR, Bonavina L, et al. Minimally invasive versus open esopha-

geal resection: three-year follow-up of the previously reported randomized controlled trial: the TIME Trial. Ann Surg 2017;266(2):232–6. PMID: 28187044.

[50]. Mariette C, Markar SR, Dabakuyo-Yonli TS, Meunier B, Pezet D, Collet D, et al. Hybrid minimally invasive esophagectomy for esophageal cancer. N Engl J Med 2019;380(2):152–62.

[51]. Nuytens F, Dabakuyo-Yonli TS, Meunier B, Gagniere J, Collet D, D'Journo XB, et al. Five-year survival outcomes of hybrid minimally invasive esophagectomy in esophageal cancer: results of the MIRO randomized clinical trial. JAMA Surg 2021:e207081. https://doi.org/10.1001/jamasurg.2020.7081.

[52]. Blazeby JM. The ROMIO Group. Minimally invasive or open oesophagectomy for localized oesophageal cancer. Results of the ROMIO phase 3 randomized controlled trial. J Clin Oncol 2021; 39(15)_suppl.

[54]. van der Sluis PC, van der Horst S, May AM, Schippers C, Brosens LAA, Joore HCA, et al. Robot-assisted minimally invasive thoracolaparoscopic esophagectomy versus open transthoracic esophagectomy for resectable esophageal cancer: a randomized controlled trial. Ann Surg 2019;269(4):621–30. PMID: 30308612.

[58]. Kauppila JH, Xie S, Johar A, Markar SR, Lagergren P. Meta-analysis of health-related quality of life after minimally invasive versus open oesophagectomy for oesophageal cancer. Br J Surg 2017;104(9):1131–40.

[59]. van Workum F, Klarenbeek BR, Baranov N, Rovers MM, Rosman C. Totally minimally invasive esophagectomy versus hybrid minimally invasive esophagectomy: systematic review and meta-analysis. Dis Esophagus 2020;3(8):doaa021. https://doi.org/10.1093/dote/doaa021.

[65]. Low DE, Alderson D, Cecconello I, Chang AC, Darling GE, D'Journo XB, et al. International Consensus on Standardization of Data Collection for Complications Associated With Esophagectomy: Esophagectomy Complications Consensus Group (ECCG). Ann Surg. 2015 Aug;262(2):286-94. https://doi.org/10.1097/SLA.0000000000001098. PMID: 25607756.

[66]. Kuppusamy MK, Low DE; International Esodata Study Group (IESG). Evaluation of International Contemporary Operative Outcomes and Management Trends Associated With Esophagectomy: A 4-Year Study of >6000 Patients Using ECCG Definitions and the Online Esodata Database. Ann Surg. 2022;275(3):515-525. https://doi.org/10.1097/SLA.0000000000004309. PMID: 33074888.

Surgery for cancer of the stomach

6

Takeshi Sano

INTRODUCTION

There seem to be two different worlds for surgeons who confront gastric cancer. In Japan and Korea, where nearly half of the tumours are T1, 'advanced gastric cancer' usually means non-early tumours that are still potentially curable by radical surgery. Surgeons have developed minimally invasive techniques for T1 tumours and perform meticulous extended dissection for 'advanced' cancers. In the rest of the world, where patients present with much more advanced disease, the chance of cure by surgery is limited and surgeons' best efforts are often not rewarded. Furthermore, the prevalence of a new disease called oesophageal adenocarcinoma has increased significantly in Western countries, almost overtaking distal gastric cancer, which is rapidly decreasing. Under the circumstances, surgeons in different parts of the world naturally have different strategies and standards to confront the disease. However, the ideal treatment for a patient with gastric cancer, wherever diagnosis is given, ought to be the same provided the disease is the same.

This chapter provides a Japanese perspective on surgery for gastric cancer from an international viewpoint, with the goal that surgeons in different circumstances are able to select the best available treatment to achieve a common goal.

MODES OF SPREAD AND AREAS OF POTENTIAL FAILURE AFTER GASTRIC CANCER SURGERY

Gastric cancer arises in the mucosa and seldom metastasises until it penetrates the muscularis mucosae. The submucosal layer has numerous lymphatic and venous capillaries through which cancer cells spread, first to the lymph nodes and subsequently to the liver. Once the tumour penetrates the serosa, peritoneal dissemination becomes common. The depth of tumour invasion (T-category) is an important prognostic factor itself and is closely correlated to all patterns of metastasis.

A rational approach to surgery for gastric cancer requires an understanding of the modes of spread of this cancer and how it recurs after surgery. This knowledge is essential to define the aims and limitations of radical surgery.

In addition, it should be noted that the patterns of failure after gastric cancer surgery have been variously reported using similar classifications but with different definitions. An example is shown in Table 6.1: hepatic and lymph node recurrences are categorised as distant and local failure, respectively, in the Dutch D1/D2 trial,[1,2] but as regional failure in the Intergroup 0116 study.[3]

METASTATIC PATHWAYS

LYMPHATIC SPREAD

Lymphatic spread is the most common mode of dissemination in gastric cancer and lymph node metastasis is histologically proven in 10% of T1 tumours, with the rate increasing as the invasion deepens, to up to 80% of T4a tumours.[4,5]

The lymphatic drainage system from the stomach has been well demonstrated in lymphography studies (Fig. 6.1). Unlike other parts of the digestive tract, the stomach has multidimensional mesenteries that contain dense lymphatic networks.[6] Cancer cells can flow out of the stomach through any of these routes via the nearby perigastric nodes to reach the nodes around the coeliac artery. They then enter the para-aortic nodes and finally flow into the thoracic duct and enter the systemic circulation, which can cause systemic metastasis. In particular, bone marrow carcinomatosis occurs most frequently in cases with extensive nodal disease.[7]

The stomach has the largest number of 'regional lymph nodes' of any organ in the human body. After a total gastrectomy with D2 lymphadenectomy, more than 40 lymph nodes can usually be collected with careful retrieval. Of the malignant tumours listed in the Union for International Cancer Control TNM (UICC/TNM) classification,[8] stomach cancer requires the largest number of nodes to be examined as a minimal requirement to allow a pN0 diagnosis (16 nodes) and also requires the largest number of positive nodes for the highest N category (pN3b, 16 or more positive nodes). Cancers in most other organs are staged as III or IV when a lymph node metastasis is pathologically confirmed, while pT1N1 and pT2N1 in gastric cancer are staged as IB and IIA, respectively. This suggests that lymphatic metastasis from gastric cancer may remain in the dense lymphatic filters for some time and that patients with nodal metastasis can still be cured by adequate dissection.

PERITONEAL SPREAD

Peritoneal metastasis is the most common type of failure after radical surgery for gastric cancer.[9] Once the tumour penetrates the serosal surface (T4a), cancer cells may scatter in the peritoneal space. They can be implanted in the gastric bed or any part of the peritoneal cavity and subsequently cause intestinal obstruction or ascites. Peritoneal metastasis

Table 6.1   Different definitions of patterns of failure in the Dutch and American trials on gastric cancer surgery

Pattern of failure	Dutch D1/D2 trial[1,2]	US Intergroup 0116[3]
Local	Gastric bed, anastomosis, regional lymph nodes	Gastric bed, anastomosis, residual stomach
Regional	Peritoneal carcinomatosa	Liver, lymph nodes, peritoneal carcinomatosa
Distant	Liver, lung, ovary, and other organs	Outside the peritoneal cavity

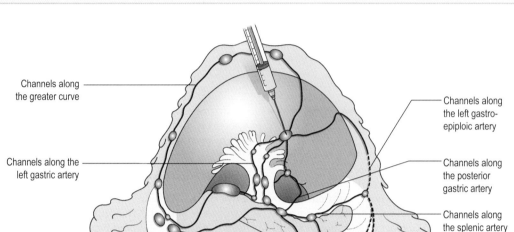

Channels along the greater curve

Channels along the left gastric artery

Channels along the superior mesenteric vein

Channels along the left gastro-epiploic artery

Channels along the posterior gastric artery

Channels along the splenic artery

Channels crossing the pancreatic surface

Figure 6.1   Lymphography of the stomach. (Courtesy of K. Maruyama.)

is much more common in diffuse-type cancers than the intestinal type[10] and later causes peritonitis carcinomatosa, a characteristic recurrent pattern of gastric cancer that is relatively uncommon in colorectal adenocarcinomas which are mostly of the intestinal type.

Peritoneal lavage cytology is a sensitive test for this type of metastasis. Almost all patients with positive cytology subsequently develop peritoneal recurrence even after macroscopically curative surgery. Since the UICC/TNM seventh edition (TNM7), positive cytology ('cy+') has been included in the definition of pM1 for gastric cancer classification.

In general, surgery has no curative role in treating this mode of spread. However, in some exceptional cases where a small number of peritoneal metastases exist in the upper abdomen but peritoneal cytology is negative, complete removal of these visible nodules may bring cure.

Peritoneal metastasis is refractory to systemic chemotherapy. Intraperitoneal chemotherapy with or without hyperthermia is being vigorously tested in various centres and some promising results have been reported,[11] but the evidence is not yet compelling.

HAEMATOGENOUS SPREAD

Liver metastasis is relatively uncommon at the time of diagnosis of gastric cancer, but is commonly seen as a part of systemic failure. In the 15-year follow-up report of the Dutch D1/D2 trial liver metastasis was found, either as the sole site or with other sites, in 102 of 319 deaths with recurrence.[12] Liver metastasis occurs predominantly in intestinal-type tumours. Unlike in colorectal cancer, liver metastasis from gastric cancer is usually multiple and associated with other modes of spread, including peritoneal and/or extensive lymph node metastasis. Resection is rarely indicated, but with careful patient selection and R0 resection, long-term survival can be expected.[13]

METASTASIS BY UNCERTAIN PATHWAY

Lung, bone, or other distant metastases are relatively rare at the time of diagnosis and appear as part of systemic dissemination at the terminal stage. These may be regarded as haematogenous spread, but as many such cases lack liver metastasis, the initial route of spread may be the lymphatic–caval system mentioned above rather than the venous portal–caval route.

Ovarian metastasis (Krukenberg tumour) may occur especially from diffuse-type tumours, including signet-ring cell carcinoma. It is not uncommon for patients to present with ovarian tumours, and histological proof of signet-ring cells in the resected ovary leads to the diagnosis of gastric cancer. Ovarian metastasis may occur as part of peritoneal spread but, considering the absence of peritoneal disease in some cases and the usual association with lymphatic involvement, it may be considered as a special form of lymphatic spread.

Retroperitoneal spread frequently occurs in advanced diffuse-type tumours. It causes urinary tract obstruction and/or 'frozen pelvis' symptoms. This is usually considered as part of peritoneal dissemination, but it may occur as a purely retroperitoneal disease without visible or cytological disease within the peritoneal cavity. Direct tumour extension from the gastric body to the retroperitoneal space through the inside of the mesogastrium around the celiac artery is a possible route of spread.

DIRECT EXTENSION

Gastric cancer penetrating the serosa sometimes extends to the adjacent organs or structures. When the operation is potentially curative, these may be excised en bloc with the stomach. It is of note that, in a considerable proportion of apparent T4b cases, pathological assessment shows only inflammatory adhesion without direct tumour invasion.[14]

Gastric cancer can extend intramurally to the oesophagus or duodenum, continuously or intermittently via submucosal lymph capillaries. Frozen section diagnosis is often needed for confirmation of clear margins.

INTRAOPERATIVE SPILLAGE

Surgery itself can be a cause of cancer spread, especially in terms of peritoneal dissemination. A T4a tumour penetrating the gastric serosa without visible or cytological peritoneal disease sometimes recurs in the peritoneal cavity after potentially curative surgery. There are two possible explanations for this: 1) cancer cells had already been implanted but the cytology test was not sensitive enough; 2) there were no free cancer cells before surgery, but operative manipulation caused cancer cell spillage from the tumour surface.

Even serosa-negative tumours can recur in the peritoneal cavity after surgery, and these cases are usually associated with lymph node metastasis. A possible explanation for this is that during lymph node dissection lymphatic channels were broken and cancer cells in the lymph nodes spilled out. This was proven in a unique study from Korea,[15] although it has not been confirmed whether these spilled cells can implant and grow.

Intraoperative spillages of cancer cells could be prevented by careful non-touch isolation techniques and/or the use of clips or vessel-sealing devices. However, the simplest means to prevent cancer cell implantation during surgery will be peritoneal wash with a large volume of saline before abdominal closure. A small-scale randomised study showed a significant survival benefit of extensive intraoperative peritoneal lavage (EIPL) in gastric cancer patients with positive cytology.[16] However, the effect was not expanded in another randomised controlled trial (RCT) in which EIPL after curative resection was tested.[17]

SUMMARY

Of the four patterns of spread of gastric cancer (lymphatic, peritoneal, haematogenous, and direct), lymphatic metastasis occurs at the earliest stage, which can lead to other types of metastases. Surgical control of this spread at an early phase of the disease may prevent subsequent systemic failure.

THE CONCEPT OF RADICAL GASTRIC CANCER SURGERY

Surgery plays an essential role in the curative treatment of gastric cancer. Although radical surgery has been attempted in many centres worldwide, it is Japanese surgeons who have been at the forefront of the practice of radical gastric resection and lymphadenectomy.

GASTRIC CANCER SURGERY IN JAPAN

The Japanese Classification of Gastric Carcinoma was established in 1962 and played a key role in the standardisation of surgery and pathology for gastric cancer in Japan. Detailed clinicopathological information, especially on lymph node metastasis, was prospectively collected from a large number of institutions and the optimal extent of lymphadenectomy was eagerly sought. The concept of 'lymph node groups' was established and the dissection of group 1 and 2 nodal stations was proposed as the standard radical surgery, which Japanese surgeons almost blindly accepted and followed.

This concept has never been tested in a randomised trial in Japan. As D2 gastrectomy is safely performed with good results in the country, Japanese surgeons think it unethical even to plan a trial in which half of the patients should undergo surgery that they consider inferior (D1).

The National Clinical Database (NCD) was launched in 2011 to collect nationwide data covering more than 95% of major surgeries in Japan. Detailed clinicopathological information including postoperative morbidity/mortality of about 50 000 gastrectomies per year has been collected, and a recent analysis of 71 307 total gastrectomies revealed hospital volume to have an impact on postoperative mortality, even in this high-incidence country.[18]

DEVELOPMENT OF GASTRIC CANCER SURGERY IN THE WEST

The Japanese documentation system and excellent treatment results have influenced the Western concept of radical surgery for gastric cancer. Some surgeons visited Japanese institutions to convince themselves of the feasibility and efficacy of the technique and have successfully reproduced the results in the West.[19] However, most non-specialist surgeons could not overcome their scepticism and were reluctant to practise this aggressive surgery on their patients. An important obstacle is the difficulty in directly comparing the results between Japan and the West due to the following two issues.

DIFFERENT STAGING SYSTEMS

The UICC and the American Joint Committee on Cancer (AJCC) unified their TNM staging system in their fourth edition in 1985. The N category in that edition was defined according to the anatomical location of the involved lymph nodes: metastasis in the perigastric nodes within 3cm of the primary tumour was staged as N1; metastasis in the other perigastric nodes and those along the named branches of the coeliac artery as N2. Although the Japanese definitions of nodal groups 1 and 2 were different, the basic concept of the two systems was similar in that the anatomical location of the involved lymph nodes determined the N category. Thus, the treatment results of tumours staged by the two different systems were able to be compared, neglecting minor differences.

In 1997 the UICC/AJCC adopted the numerical N category in the 5th edition, and the Japanese classification and the TNM classification became totally distinct systems. The Japanese results were able to be expressed using the new TNM system because the number of positive nodes in each case was also recorded, but the reverse was impossible because the anatomical data were no longer available in the West. Japanese surgeons and pathologists continued to use their system as the primary staging method, thus sticking to the surgical significance of lymph node anatomy, and they use the TNM system only when they write English papers. On the other hand, Western surgeons' interest in lymphadenectomy may have diminished because the N category was determined regardless of the extent of lymphadenectomy.

DIFFERENT DISEASE HYPOTHESES

A hypothesis that gastric cancer in the West may be a different disease to that in Japan prevails and prevents positive discussion to advance optimal treatment for gastric cancer patients on a global level. In the studies biologically analysing and comparing surgical specimens, evidence to support the hypothesis is scanty except for a recent study[20] demonstrating a difference in signatures of tumour immunity that might influence clinical results. The following are the currently discussed differences.

Proximal location

It has been repeatedly highlighted that Western gastric cancers are predominantly located in the proximal stomach while Japanese tumours are found mostly in the distal stomach. This might suggest that these are different diseases. However, this needs careful consideration.

Adenocarcinoma of the lower oesophagus and the oesophagogastric junction is one of the most rapidly increasing malignant tumours in the West, especially among White males.[21] This trend, together with the rapid decrease of distal gastric cancers, makes it plausible that Western gastric cancer arises mostly in the proximal stomach. However, lower oesophageal adenocarcinoma is a new, distinct disease with a different aetiology and contrasting patient backgrounds,[22] and therefore should be considered separately from 'classical' gastric cancer. In three large-scale Western surgical trials, the Dutch D1/D2,[1] the British MRC D1/D2,[23] and United States INT0116 studies,[3] the proportion of proximal third tumours was 10.3%, 30.5%, and 19.5%, respectively, and was not significantly different from that in the Japanese D2/D3 study (19.1%)[24] (Fig. 6.2). This suggests that, as far

as surgically targeted gastric cancers are concerned, tumour location is not largely different between the West and Japan. The apparent predominance of proximal tumours in the West may be a simple reflection of the mixture of different diseases, i.e. increasing oesophageal and decreasing gastric adenocarcinomas.

Patient factors

Western patients with gastric cancer are much more likely to be obese and more frequently have comorbidities, especially of cardiovascular diseases, than their Japanese counterparts. Although this does not mean that the disease is different, it certainly affects surgical process and outcomes. In particular, obesity hampers the completion of extended lymphadenectomy for gastric cancer, even in specialist Japanese centres. It has been shown to be an independent risk factor for postoperative morbidity.[25]

THE ROLE OF RADICAL SURGERY IN WESTERN PRACTICE

Due to decreased incidence and technically demanding therapeutic requirements, gastric cancer in the West is today considered as a disease that should be treated in specialist centres. Several studies have shown relationships between the hospital/surgeon's volume of gastric cancer treatment and operative mortality.[26] Given the accelerated 'proximal shift' of the disease and the increasing surgical risks in Western patients, the trend of centralisation will further progress.

✓ Although solid evidence of extended lymphadenectomy is yet to be established, D2 gastrectomy without splenectomy or pancreatectomy is officially recommended by the European Society of Medical Oncology.[27] National Comprehensive Cancer Network (NCCN) guidelines for gastric cancer in the USA also recommend D2 for potentially curable gastric cancer with the condition that experienced surgeons perform it in specialist cancer centres.[28] However, as the possible benefit of this extensive surgery could be easily offset by increased mortality, careful selection of patients is important even in specialist centres. There is an increasing move towards tailoring operations, taking not only the stage of the disease but also patient-related factors into account.

OUTCOMES AFTER RADICAL SURGERY FOR GASTRIC CANCER

The International Gastric Cancer Association (IGCA) launched a staging project and the survival data of more than 25 000 gastric cancer patients who underwent R0 gastrectomy in specialised centres around the world were collected and analysed (57 institutions in 17 countries).[29] The eligibility criteria included: adenocarcinoma in the stomach or of Siewert type 2 or 3; gastrectomy performed between 2000 and 2004; no lost to follow-up before the fifth postoperative year; no neoadjuvant therapy; and sufficient histological data. Table 6.2 shows the stage-specific 5-year survival rates of Japanese and Western patients in this project according to the eighth UICC TNM and, in addition, those of another dataset selected from the US National Cancer Database using similar criteria.[30] Even in this comparable setting in a project,

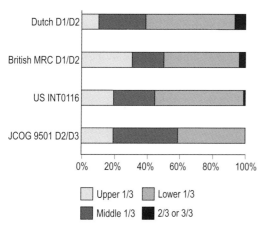

Figure 6.2 Proportion of the primary tumour location in prospective trials of gastric cancer surgery.

Table 6.2 Stage-specific 5-year survival rates after R0 gastrectomy according to the 8th edition of the TNM classification (International Gastric Cancer Association staging project[29] and USA National Cancer Database[30])

Pathological Stage	Japan		West*		Whole		USA NCDB	
	n	5-year SR (%)	n	5-year SR (%)	n	5-year SR (%)	n	5-year SR (%)
IA	5 394	93.8	463	86.0	10 606	93.6	1 501	81.0
IB	1 119	89.4	227	74.9	2 606	88.0	1 095	68.5
IIA	924	84.6	259	68.7	2 291	81.8	1 245	59.3
IIB	847	74.5	276	57.2	2 481	68.0	1 432	46.4
IIIA	956	60.3	376	42.0	3 044	54.2	2 310	30.5
IIIB	653	40.4	287	20.9	2 218	36.2	1 896	20.1
IIIC	389	21.1	167	16.2	1 350	17.9	1 067	8.3

*Data from 26 institutions from 9 countries in Europe and North and South America.
SR, Survival rate.

the Japanese 5-year survival rates were better than Western ones by about 15% at all pathological stages. The additional US data show further lower survival rates in the real world, probably due to stage migration caused by insufficient nodal staging. The reasons for this are multifactorial as mentioned above, but there may be some unknown essential tumour difference between the East and West.

SUMMARY

There are large differences between Japan and the West in incidence, staging system, tumour location, and patient factors. Consequently, the concept of radical surgery has developed separately in Japan and the West. Today in the West, gastric cancer is considered a disease to be treated by specialists, preferably with D2 lymphadenectomy without splenectomy.

PRINCIPLES OF RADICAL GASTRIC CANCER SURGERY

EXTENT OF GASTRIC RESECTION

The primary objective of gastric cancer surgery is to adequately excise the primary lesion with clear longitudinal and circumferential margins. Selection of gastrectomy depends on the tumour location and the mode of infiltration in the stomach wall. Preoperative diagnosis should focus on this and careful assessment of lateral tumour spread is indispensable.

RESECTION MARGINS

Proximal resection margin is the main determinant in selecting a total or distal gastrectomy. During surgery for T2 or deeper tumours, the resection line should be determined with a sufficient margin from the palpable edge of the tumour. A 5-cm margin has traditionally been recommended.[31] In some guidelines, 8 cm is recommended for diffuse-type tumours,[32] but this would necessitate most tumours of the gastric body requiring a total gastrectomy or oesophagogastrectomy.

According to Japanese treatment guidelines,[33] a 5-cm margin is recommended for tumours showing an infiltrative growth pattern with indistinct borders or diffuse-type histology, but 3 cm is usually sufficient for those showing an expansive growth pattern with grossly distinct borders, for which the histology is most frequently of the intestinal type.

For gastric cancers invading the oesophagus, a 5-cm margin is not necessarily required, but frozen section examination of the resection line is desirable to ensure an R0 resection.

In cT1 tumours, lateral mucosal extension should be preoperatively detected or excluded by stepwise biopsy, and placing clips on the negative border is helpful to accurately resect impalpable lesions.

TYPE OF GASTRECTOMY

Common types of gastrectomy for gastric cancer are as follows.

Total gastrectomy

This involves removal of the whole stomach including the cardia (oesophagogastric junction) and the pylorus. It is indicated for tumours arising at or invading the proximal stomach.

Distal (subtotal) gastrectomy

This involves removal of the stomach including the pylorus but preserving the cardia. Two-thirds or more of the stomach is usually removed for gastric cancer. It is indicated for middle or lower third tumours with sufficient resection margins mentioned earlier.

Proximal gastrectomy

This involves removal of the stomach including the cardia but preserving the pylorus. It is indicated for proximal tumours with or without oesophageal invasion, where more than half of the distal stomach can be preserved.

Other resections for T1 tumours

Some function-preserving gastrectomies such as pylorus-preserving gastrectomy (PPG) are applied to T1 tumours.

Total gastrectomy 'de principe' for distal cancers

Some European surgeons have argued that all cancers of the stomach, even those in the distal third, should be treated by total gastrectomy. This principle is based on the experience of frequent involvement of the proximal resection margin and consequent anastomotic local recurrence. Theoretically, total gastrectomy ensures more certain negative margins and sufficient lymphadenectomy. In addition, the possible occurrence of multicentric cancer in the gastric stump can be prevented. On the other hand, total gastrectomy is associated with a higher operative morbidity and mortality, increased risk of long-term nutritional problems, and impaired quality of life compared to distal gastrectomy.

✓✓ Randomised trials comparing total and distal gastrectomies in distal gastric cancer have failed to show a survival benefit for total gastrectomy.[34]

The policy of total gastrectomy 'de principe' should be abandoned for the following reasons:

1. Provided that the rules on safe margins of resection listed above are adhered to, a positive proximal resection margin is rare. If the margins are still positive, this usually indicates an aggressive and extensive malignancy, and resection line involvement will not be a major determinant of prognosis.
2. The lymph nodes that can be removed only by total gastrectomy, station numbers 2 (left cardia), 4sa (upper greater curve), 10 (splenic hilum), and 11d (distal splenic artery [SpA]), are seldom involved in distal gastric cancers. If they are involved, again this indicates an

aggressive malignancy and extended surgery would not alter the survival outcome.
3. The incidence of second primary cancer in the gastric stump is low. Long-term surveillance by endoscopy may detect a new lesion that can be removed by endoscopic submucosal dissection.

LYMPHADENECTOMY

Lymph node metastasis is the most common mode of spread in gastric cancer. Histological nodal metastasis has been proven in 80% of T4a/T4b tumours, and even T1 tumours have a 10% probability of lymph node metastasis (T1a 3%, T1b 18%).[4,5] Unlike hepatic and other distant metastases, lymph node metastasis from gastric cancer can be surgically removed for potential cure provided it is confined to the regional area. The optimal extent of lymphadenectomy, however, has been controversial.

LYMPH NODE GROUPS IN THE FORMER JAPANESE CLASSIFICATIONS

Japanese surgeons and pathologists have extensively investigated the distribution of lymph node metastasis. They recorded it using standardised anatomical station numbers (Fig. 6.3)[40] and then classified the stations into three groups, basically according to the incidence of metastasis (N groups 1–3). As the pattern of lymph node metastasis varies with the location of the primary tumour, N groups 1–3 were separately defined depending on the primary tumour location. These numbers of nodal groups were also used to express the grade of nodal disease (N1–3) and the extent of lymphadenectomy (D1–3); for example, cancer

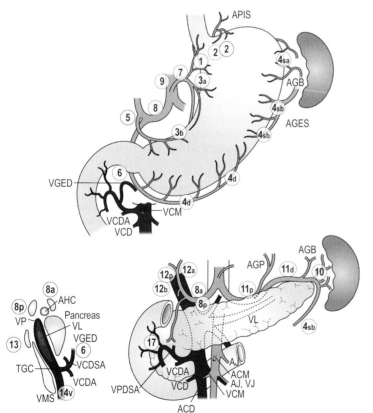

Figure 6.3 Station numbers of lymph nodes around the stomach. *ACM*, A. colica media; *AGB*, Aa. gastrica breves; *AGES*, A. gastroepiploica sinistra; *AHC*, A. hepatica communis; *AJ*, A. jejunalis; *APIS*, A. phrenic inferior sinistra; *TGC*, truncus gastrocolicus; *VCD*, V. colica dextra; *VCDA*, V. colica dextra accessoria; *VCM*: V. colica media; *VGED*, V. vastroepiploica dextra; *VJ*, V. jejunalis; *VL*, V. lienalis; *VMS*, V. mesenterica superior; *VP*, V. portae; *VPDSA*, V. pancreaticoduodenalis inferior anterior. (Modified from the Japanese Classification of Gastric Carcinoma, 3rd English ed.[40])

with metastasis to a node in the second group was designated as N2, and complete dissection of up to the second group nodes was defined as D2.

Since its first edition published in 1962, the Japanese Classification of Gastric Carcinoma (JCGC) has undergone periodic revisions, and in each subsequent edition the definitions of lymph node groups have been slightly modified. The Dutch and MRC D1/D2 trials were conducted using the N and D ('R' at that time) definitions of the 11th edition of the JCGC[35] (Table 6.3) while the Taipei D1/D3 trial[36] used the 12th edition,[37] in which the lymph nodes were grouped from N1 to N4. In the 13th edition,[38] the nodal grouping was completed, with four groups (N1–3 and 'M') in five categories of the primary tumour location; the Japanese D2/D3 trial[24] was reported using it. This definition was based on the 'dissection efficiency index' of each lymph node station,[39] calculated using the incidence of metastasis and survival data of a large number of patients.

Outside Japan, it is widely believed that Japanese N1 nodes are perigastric and N2 nodes are those along the coeliac artery and its branches. Although this expression roughly reflects the nodal groups, it is apparently incorrect in terms of the original concept of grouping based on the primary tumour location. The misunderstanding appears to be due to the over-complicated definitions of the JCGC. In the latest (14th) edition (3rd English edition[40]), the traditional nodal grouping system has been abandoned and the simplified 'D' has been defined according to the type of gastrectomy (Fig. 6.4).[33]

NEW DEFINITION OF LYMPHADENECTOMY

The new 'D' definitions in the Japanese Treatment Guidelines[33] are simple, practical, and mostly compatible with those in the 13th edition of JCGC, with only some exceptions. D1, D1+, and D2 (D3 is no longer included) are defined for the two major types of gastrectomy, total and distal, regardless of the tumour location. It should be noted that the lymph nodes along the left gastric artery (LGA; no. 7), which used to be classified as N2 for tumours in any location, are now included in the D1 category for any type of gastrectomy. This is based not only on the previously mentioned efficacy index analysis, but also on the view that surgery for gastric carcinoma should as a minimum include the division of the LGA at its origin.

✔ The JGCA recommends that non-early, potentially curable gastric cancer should be treated by D2 lymphadenectomy. D1 or D1+ should be considered as an option for T1 tumours. In a poor-risk patient or under circumstances where D2 cannot be safely performed, D1+ can be a substitute for D2.

Table 6.3 Lymph node groups used in the Dutch and MRC D1/D2 trials (Japanese classification, 11th edition)

	Location			
	AMC, MAC, MCA, CMA	A, AM	MA, M, MC	C, CM
Group 1 (N1)	1, 2, 3, 4, 5, 6	3, 4, 5, 6	3, 4, 5, 6, 1	1, 2, 3, 4 s
Group 2 (N2)	7, 8, 9, 10, 11	7, 8, 9, 1	2†, 7, 8, 9, 10†, 11	4d‡, 7, 8, 9, 10, 11, 5*, 6*
Group 3 (N3)	12, 13, 14, 110*, 111*	2*, 10*, 11, 12, 13, 14	12, 13, 14	12, 13, 14, 110*, 111*

*Resection or non-resection of these nodes does not affect the D number.
†These nodes should be excised if the primary tumour site is the MC. If the primary tumour site is MA or M, removal is optional.
‡In proximal gastrectomy, non-resection of these nodes does not affect the D number.
A, Lower third; M, middle third; C, upper third.

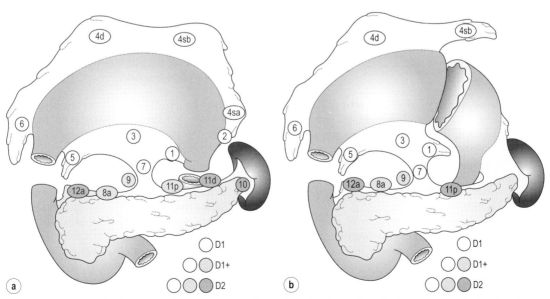

Figure 6.4 (a) Definitions of lymphadenectomy (D) in total gastrectomy. (b) Definitions of lymphadenectomy (D) in distal gastrectomy. (Modified from Japanese gastric cancer treatment guidelines 2010 (ver. 3).[33])

D2 LYMPHADENECTOMY – EVIDENCE

D2 lymphadenectomy is the gold standard for potentially curable advanced gastric cancer in Japan and Korea, while general surgeons in the West have been reluctant to adopt this radical approach.

In Japan, the benefits of D2 over less extensive dissections have never been tested in a randomised study. Instead, D2 was compared with more extensive surgery, D2 plus para-aortic nodal dissection (PAND), in a well-designed, multi-centre RCT.[24] This confirmed that D2 and D2 + PAND were performed with low operative mortality (0.8%) by specialist surgeons but failed to show a survival benefit of PAND. They have abandoned this super-extended lymphadenectomy as a means of prophylaxis, but they still will not consider that D2 might not be superior to D1. A single institutional RCT in Taipei showed a significant survival benefit of D2/3 over D1,[36] which is thus far the only RCT that showed superiority of extended lymphadenectomy for gastric cancer.

✔✔ In the West, where D0/D1 was the standard, D2 was tested as an experimental treatment in two large RCTs.[1,23] In both trials, D2 was associated with higher morbidity and mortality than D1, and no significant survival benefit of D2 was shown.

In these trials, total gastrectomy in the D2 arm was performed via pancreatosplenectomy, which caused high morbidity and mortality. Despite these negative results for D2, the Dutch group continued the follow-up of the patients for 15 years and finally published remarkable results.[12] They compared the recurrence of gastric cancer in both arms on the basis of autopsy findings and found a significantly lower rate of gastric cancer death in D2 than in D1 patients. They concluded the study by stating that D2 should be performed as a potentially curative surgery for gastric cancer.

✔ There are several non-randomised observational studies in Europe that suggest the benefits of extended lymphadenectomy, and today the guidelines officially recommend D2 lymphadenectomy for medically fit patients in specialised, high-volume centres with appropriate surgical expertise and postoperative care.[27]

NUMBER OF LYMPH NODES AND EXTENT OF LYMPHADENECTOMY

In the Western literature, the definition of extent of lymphadenectomy for gastric cancer is often ambiguous. The number of retrieved lymph nodes is sometimes used as a surrogate for 'D', e.g. extended lymphadenectomy means retrieval of 25 or more nodes.[41] This is a useful method to retrospectively assess the volume of lymphadenectomy in a gastrectomy where anatomical information of dissected lymph nodes is unavailable.

Generally, the more extensive the surgery is, the more lymph nodes are retrieved. However, the number of retrieved nodes in a gastrectomy specimen is influenced by other factors as well:

1. **Who picked up the nodes from which condition of the specimen for what goal.** More nodes are retrieved when a surgeon tries to pick up as many nodes as possible in a fresh specimen than when a pathologist picks up swollen nodes from a formalin-fixed specimen up to the minimal requirement number.
2. **Disease stage.** In advanced disease with multiple lymph node metastases, the nodes are hard and easily recognised, even if they are small.
3. **Patient factors.** In obese patients, the lymph nodes are not easily recognised.

✔ Thus, it should be kept in mind that the number of retrieved lymph nodes is a combination of surgery and pathological handling, and does not necessarily reflect the extent of lymphadenectomy. Surgeons should plan and perform lymphadenectomies according to anatomical extent rather than to fulfil an aim of removing 25 or more nodes.

BURSECTOMY

Bursectomy is the complete removal of the lesser sac (omental bursa) that comprises of the lesser/greater omenta, the anterior sheet of the transverse mesocolon, and the pancreatic sheath. It is performed in potentially curative gastrectomy for T4a tumours penetrating the serosa of the posterior gastric body with the aim of removing possible cancer seeding inside the bursa. However, in a large RCT conducted in Japan enrolling 1 204 patients comparing omentectomy and bursectomy, no survival benefit of bursectomy was shown in any subgroup of the tumour condition.[42] The procedure will soon become history.

SPLENECTOMY

Embryologically the spleen and the body of the pancreas arise in the dorsal mesentery of the foregut, sharing the vessels and lymphatics with the stomach, and in gastric cancer surgery these two may be removed together with the stomach as a total mesogastric excision.[6]

✔ On the other hand, all clinical studies have shown that splenectomy with or without distal pancreatectomy significantly increases operative morbidity and, in the West, mortality, without obvious survival benefit.[43] Today splenectomy for gastric cancer is avoided in most countries. However, this needs some consideration.

Proximal gastric cancer may metastasise to the splenic hilar nodes (no. 10) via the gastrosplenic ligament (no. 4sa), and/or the left gastroepiploic lymphatics (no. 4sb). The incidence of no. 10 metastasis increases up to 25–30% when the tumour invades the greater curvature of the upper gastric body.[39] These can be completely cleared by splenectomy, and up to 25% of patients with positive no. 10 nodes survive more than 5 years.[44] Total gastrectomy with splenectomy can be performed by specialist surgeons without increasing mortality.[24]

Although a number of observational studies have demonstrated a lack of survival benefit or even a negative prognostic effect of splenectomy,[43] these are all heavily biased, retrospective comparisons and cannot advocate for spleen preservation. Medium-sized RCTs conducted in Chile[45] ($n = 187$) and Korea[46] ($n = 207$) to compare total gastrectomy

(TG) and TG + splenectomy (TG + S) were both inconclusive. Then, a multicentre RCT was conducted in Japan,[47] in which 503 patients with proximal gastric cancer were randomised to receive TG or TG + S during a curative operation. TG + S showed higher operative morbidity (23.6%) than TG (16.7%), but similar mortality (0.4% vs 0.8%). After complete 5-year follow-up the survival curves almost overlapped, showing statistically significant non-inferiority of TG to TG + S in terms of survival. In this trial, tumours invading the greater curvature of the stomach were carefully excluded, and the incidence of histological metastasis in no. 10 nodes was very low (2.4%). They concluded that splenectomy should be avoided in TG for proximal gastric cancer that does not invade the greater curvature. The JGCA treatment guidelines have been revised, providing a new definition of D2 lymphadenectomy that does not include no. 10 nodes for TG.[33]

DISTAL PANCREATECTOMY

Distal pancreatectomy and splenectomy (DP + S) used to be part of D2 gastrectomy for proximal gastric cancer regardless of the presence or absence of pancreatic invasion of the tumour, and was actually performed in the Dutch and British D1/D2 trials.[1,23] The aim of the routine use of this aggressive procedure was complete dissection of the lymph nodes along the SpA (nos. 11p and 11d) and those in the splenic hilum (no. 10).

However, DP + S is associated with high operative morbidity including pancreatic leakage and abscess formation, even in specialist Japanese centres.[48] Since the technique of complete dissection of no. 11 nodes without pancreatectomy has been established,[49] DP + S is currently indicated only for tumours directly invading the pancreas.

It is of note that pathological assessment in apparent T4b cases shows that adhesion to the other organ is often inflammatory rather than neoplastic.[14] In order to avoid unnecessary DP + S in ambiguous cases, it may be worthwhile to surgically separate the adhesion without DP + S, paying special attention not to injure the pancreatic parenchyma.

EXTENDED RESECTIONS

The goal of surgery for potentially curable gastric cancer is to achieve R0 resection by standard gastrectomy with sufficient resection margin and adequate lymphadenectomy. Some tumours may exceed this range but still be resectable. In such cases, extended resection should be considered.

EN BLOC RESECTION OF INVOLVED ADJACENT ORGANS

Proximal gastric cancer may invade the distal pancreas, necessitating pancreatosplenectomy as discussed above. Middle to distal third gastric cancer may invade and penetrate the transverse mesocolon. When the invasion involves major colic vessels, then partial colectomy may be necessary for en bloc resection.

When a distal tumour invades the pancreatic head or extends to the duodenum for a long distance intramurally, a pancreaticoduodenectomy may enable en bloc tumour resection. However, this operation is rarely indicated as such tumours are frequently associated with other non-curative factors such as peritoneal disease. Although some case series from high-volume centres suggest a survival benefit in R0 resection, the selection criteria are difficult to define.[50]

Tumours penetrating the anterior wall of the stomach may invade the lateral segment of the liver and can usually be removed by partial liver excision without segmentectomy.

EXTENDED LYMPHADENECTOMY

The role of extended lymphadenectomy exceeding D2 is ambiguous. Prophylactic PAND did not improve the survival of standard D2 in a large-scale Japanese RCT[24] and has subsequently been abandoned in Japan.

On the other hand, in a series of phase II studies for bulky nodal disease or limited para-aortic nodal metastasis, neoadjuvant chemotherapy followed by gastrectomy with D2 + PAND showed excellent survival results.[51] PAND in combination with intensive chemotherapy may remain as a last means to enable R0 resection for a cure to such extensive nodal disease.

The retropancreatic lymph nodes (no. 13) are not regional nodes of gastric cancer and the prognosis of patients with positive no. 13 nodes is extremely poor. However, for distal tumours invading the duodenum no. 13 nodes are considered as regional nodes according to the TNM rules, and indeed some patients with a pyloric cancer invading the duodenum survive after dissection of positive no. 13 nodes.[52]

RESECTION OF LIVER METASTASES

Unlike for colorectal cancer, liver resection for gastric cancer is rarely indicated. In the literature, only some case series from high-volume Japanese centres suggest a possible survival benefit in selected cases.[53] In Koga et al.'s study,[53] for example, of 5 520 patients who underwent gastric cancer surgery during a 20-year period, 121 (2.2%) had synchronous liver metastases and 126 (2.3%) developed metachronous metastases, and only 42 patients underwent liver resection, of whom eight had survived more than 5 years at the time of analysis. A more recent pooled analysis of 256 patients undergoing R0 resection in five cancer centres in Japan showed a 31.1% 5-year survival rate.[54] Careful patient selection is mandatory: minimal serosal invasion of the primary tumour, less than three liver metastases, and 5 cm or smaller tumours may be the candidate.

LAPAROSCOPIC GASTRECTOMY

Laparoscopic gastrectomy gained a high popularity in Eastern Asia where early-stage, distal tumours suitable for this procedure prevailed. First, the safety and feasibility by experienced surgeons were tested in prospective studies for stage I disease, where the benefit of reduced operative bleeding and early recovery was confirmed. Then, large-scale RCTs were conducted, and non-inferiority in long-term survival to open distal gastrectomy was shown not only for stage I but also for stage II and III diseases.[55–58] It should be noted that these RCTs only included distal tumours deemed resectable with distal gastrectomy. TG has some technical issues, particularly for anastomosis, and still needs further technical development and expertise.

Laparoscopic distal gastrectomy has rapidly become standardised in the Japanese general practice, and according to the latest report of the NCD, it accounted for 52% of 33 177 distal gastrectomies performed for all stages of the disease in 2019.[59] In the West, experience of laparoscopic gastrectomy for cancer is still limited to highly specialised institutions and scientific evidence of its efficacy is weak. A recent review of the European literature showed that laparoscopic gastrectomy can be safely performed with similar oncological results to the open procedure.[60]

Various concerns have been expressed regarding laparoscopic gastrectomy for advanced disease[61]: intra-abdominal exploration of the disease extent may be insufficient; ideal movements of hard devices are hampered by large tumours; non-touch manoeuvre is difficult in diffuse tumours; resection line determination may be difficult without tactile sensation, and so on. Although laparoscopic surgery has many advantages for both patients and medical staff, the priority of cancer surgery is cure of the disease, which cannot be compensated by minimal invasiveness. Some experts are able to perform all kinds of complicated procedures such as an extended gastrectomy as mentioned earlier, but generalisation needs extensive training. In the meantime, open and laparoscopic gastrectomy should be appropriately selected according to patient risk and surgeon expertise.

SUMMARY

Radical surgery for gastric cancer comprises of gastric resection with adequate margins and systematic lymphadenectomy. TG 'de principe' should be abandoned. The Japanese Association has totally remodelled and simplified the definition of D2, which has potential to be the world standard. More extended surgery including combined resections of the involved organs shows no evidence of improving survival, but may become necessary for R0 resection on an individual case basis. Laparoscopic distal gastrectomy has been increasingly employed, especially for Stage I gastric cancer, but its application to TG or advanced disease should be carefully considered.

GASTRIC RESECTION WITH D2 LYMPHADENECTOMY TECHNIQUE

Below is a basic description of the open gastrectomy technique . Procedures specific to a laparoscopic approach are also covered.

INCISION

An upper midline incision is used for resection of non-cardia gastric cancer. For a bulky proximal tumour, especially in an obese patient, an inverted T-shaped or bilateral subcostal incision is useful.

For proximal gastric cancer invading the oesophagus, either a transhiatal (TH) or left thoracoabdominal (LTA) approach is selected. LTA provides excellent exposure of the paracardiac area and lower mediastinum but is associated with an increased morbidity. A Japanese randomised trial compared TH and LTA for Siewert type 2 and 3 gastric cancer invading the oesophagus within 3 cm and showed no survival improvement but increased morbidity in the LTA approach.[62]

INTRAOPERATIVE STAGING

The sensitivity and specificity of diagnostic imaging to stage gastric cancer is not sufficient to allow preoperative selection of optimal treatments. Surgical exploration or staging laparoscopy provides information on the T and M categories, especially on peritoneal metastasis. However, even by careful intraoperative palpation and inspection, lymph node metastasis cannot be accurately staged. Sentinel node diagnosis is not yet reliable due to the complicated lymphatic network around the stomach. Therefore, for radical gastrectomy, a systematic lymphadenectomy should always be considered unless the tumour is diagnosed as T1.

D2 LYMPHADENECTOMY PROCEDURE

DISTAL GASTRECTOMY

Kocherisation

Mobilisation of the duodenum facilitates a safe and smooth procedure for the subsequent infrapyloric lymphadenectomy in open gastrectomy. The assistant should hold the descending portion of the duodenum to stretch the parietal peritoneum. The peritoneum close to the duodenum should be incised and the incision extended along the duodenum. The assistant should then 'roll up' the duodenum and proceed to the back of the pancreatic head, staying close to the posterior pancreatic fascia, and mobilise the pancreatic head. The para-aortic area should be palpated and, if suspicious nodes exist, they should be sampled.

Omentectomy

Although omentectomy is not necessarily a part of D2 dissection, it is usually performed in open gastrectomy for T3/T4 tumours to remove possible tumour spread into the omenta. The omentum is removed from the right side of the transverse colon and the duodenum. It is then dissected along the transverse colon toward the lower pole of the spleen.

When omentectomy is omitted in D2 gastrectomy, the incision line of the omentum should be at least 3 cm away from the right gastroepiploic arcade so that the no. 4d lymph nodes along the arcade are completely dissected.

Division of left gastroepiploic vessels

At the lower splenic hilum and the pancreatic tail, the left gastroepiploic artery (LGEA) arises from the end of the SpA, sometimes as a branch of the lower polar SpA. The LGEA and the vein of the same name should be ligated and then cut. As the lymph nodes along the LGEA (no. 4sb) are rarely metastatic from distal gastric tumours, the dissection does not have to include the trunk of this artery. However, tumours in the gastric body, especially those located on the greater curvature, may metastasise to the splenic hilar nodes (no. 10) via no. 4sb. The LGEA should be dissected at the origin in these cases.

On the greater curve of the stomach, there is usually some avascular area between the first branch of the LGEA and the short gastric arteries, and this will be a landmark of the upper limit of dissection in distal gastrectomy.

Infrapyloric node dissection (no. 6)

In distal gastric cancers, a precise dissection of no. 6 lymph nodes is essential because they are most frequently involved, and the dissection of positive nodes can still bring a cure.

The (second) assistant should hold the transverse colon and gently stretch the mesocolon. The middle colic vein should be identified and pursued to the approach of the gastrocolic venous junction point (Fig. 6.5). Identify the accessory right colic vein (ARCV), right gastroepiploic vein (RGEV), gastrocolic trunk, and the anterior superior pancreatico-duodenal vein (ASPDV). The middle colic vein usually drains directly into the superior mesenteric vein (SMV).

The RGEV should be ligated and cut prior to its junction with the ASPDV. A small vein draining from the pancreas to the RGEV should be carefully cauterised. When no. 6 nodes are grossly metastatic, dissection of the nodes in front of the SMV (no. 14v) should be considered.

Then, the gastric antrum should be pulled up and the gastroduodenal artery (GDA) identified between the duodenum and the pancreas. The GDA is exposed distally as far as the origin of the right gastroepiploic artery (RGEA) (Fig. 6.6). The infrapyloric artery arises near the origin of the RGEA. The RGEA and the infrapyloric artery should be ligated and cut together or separately at their origin.

The GDA should be pursued proximally to its origin from the common hepatic artery (CHA). A large, flat lymph node (no. 8a) usually covers the CHA. The peritoneum covering this node at its right edge is opened and the surface of the CHA exposed. Using this procedure, no. 5 (suprapyloric) and no. 8a nodes are separated. A gauze is placed to the right of the no. 8a node, which will serve as a landmark of the correct layer in the subsequent suprapyloric dissection.

Suprapyloric nodes dissection (no. 5) and transection of the duodenum

The assistant pulls down the pylorus and the duodenum to stretch the suprapyloric area. The right gastric artery (RGA) and the superior duodenal arteries (SDAs) are identified and the serosa between them incised. The previously placed gauze is encountered, protecting the GDA and CHA.

The SDA arising from the GDA and/or the proper hepatic artery (PHA) is cut. The origin of the RGA and the right gastric vein that runs just close to the artery and drains into the portal vein is then exposed. The RGA and vein together are ligated and cut to dissect no. 5 nodes. The anterior peritoneum of the hepatoduodenal ligament is removed to expose the PHA for subsequent no. 12a dissection.

The duodenum is transected using a linear stapler and the staple line sutured with seromuscular stitches.

Exposure of the oesophageal hiatus

The assistant pulls down the stomach to stretch the lesser omentum. It is incised close to the liver and the incision extended toward the right cardia. The accessory left hepatic artery is sometimes encountered and can be dissected. If it is large and replaces the proper left hepatic artery then it should be preserved. In this case, the division of the LGA needs special attention, as described later.

At the upper end of the lesser omentum, the peritoneum covering the right diaphragmatic crus is excised to enter the oesophageal hiatus. The crus is exposed towards the coeliac artery, which will be helpful for later dissection around the coeliac axis.

Dissection of the upper border of the pancreas (nos. 8a, 9, 11p and 12a)

This is the core of D2 lymphadenectomy. The nerve tissue surrounding the major arteries in this area does not have to

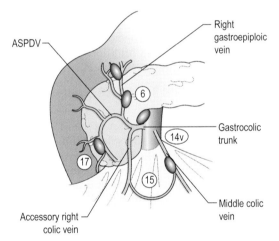

Figure 6.5 Infrapyloric veins and lymph nodes. *ASPDV,* Anterior superior pancreatico-duodenal vein.

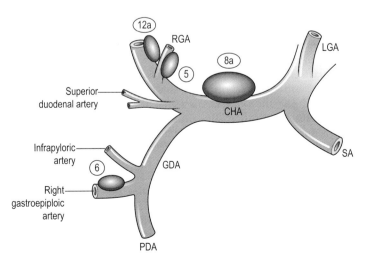

Figure 6.6 Branches of the common hepatic artery and lymph node numbers. *CHA,* Common hepatic artery; *GDA,* gastroduodenal artery; *LGA,* left gastric artery; *PDA,* pancreatico-duodenal artery; *RGA,* right gastric artery; *SA,* splenic artery.

be removed in lymphadenectomy for gastric cancer because the lymphatic tissue between the nerve and the arterial adventitia is sparse and the perineural infiltration at this level is very rare.

The assistant should gently pull down the pancreas and expose the field of dissection. The peritoneal covering is incised along the upper border of the pancreas and the vascular structures (CHA, SpA, left gastric vein [LGV], etc.) broadly identified. The lymphadenectomy should be started at the no. 8a nodes that have already been exposed. There are small vessels between no. 8a nodes and the pancreatic parenchyma that may require careful coagulation. The surface of the CHA should be exposed towards the coeliac axis until the root of the SpA appears. The LGV often drains to the splenic vein across the CHA and is ligated and cut.

A change of direction is then necessary and the CHA should be exposed towards the hepatoduodenal ligament. The lymph nodes are dissected along the PHA (no. 12a), exposing the left side of the portal vein.

The dissection then turns back towards the coeliac artery behind the CHA. The LGV draining to the portal vein is most frequently encountered at this point and it is ligated and cut. The lymph nodes on the right side of the coeliac artery are then dissected.

The bifurcation of the coeliac artery (to the CHA and SpA) is identified, and the anterior surface of the coeliac artery is exposed until the LGA appears, surrounded by thick nerve fibres. The LGA sometimes arises very close to the aorta. The LGA is ligated (usually double) and cut at the origin. The surface of the diaphragmatic crus exposed previously is encountered, and the dissection of no. 9 lymph nodes is completed by removing lymphatic tissue in this area.

The left side of the coeliac artery is not easy to expose because, unlike the right side that can be accessed directly from the free peritoneal surface, the left side is covered by complicated fusion of the retropancreatic fascia and the parietal peritoneum.

When the accessory left hepatic artery arising from the LGA is to be preserved, the LGA should not be ligated but dissected at the origin, which exposes its trunk longitudinally until the origin of the 'proper' LGAs (sometimes two) appear. These are ligated and dissected to leave the arterial arcade from the coeliac artery to the left liver exposed.

The SpA originating from the coeliac artery immediately passes behind the pancreas then reappears on the upper border of the pancreas and winds towards the spleen (Fig. 6.7). The left side of the coeliac artery and the proximal part of the SpA are dissected. In distal gastrectomy for distal tumours, dissection around the proximal 4–5 cm of the artery is sufficient. Note that there are lymphatic channels from the infrapyloric no. 6 area to the SpA nodes crossing the surface of the pancreas, and the no. 11p nodes often have metastases from pyloric tumours (Fig. 6.1).

Dissection of the upper lesser curvature nodes (nos. 1 and 3a)

The lymph nodes along the lesser curve (no. 3) are most frequently involved with tumours of the gastric body and therefore complete removal is essential. The assistant should pull down the stomach. The lesser omental surface is lifted and incised close to the gastric wall, and then peeled away towards the cardia. The anterior trunk of the vagal nerve is cut

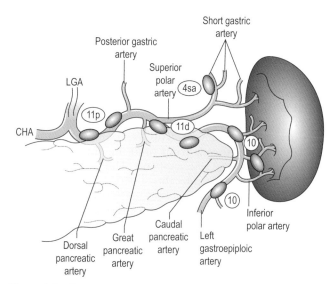

Figure 6.7 The splenic artery and its branches. *CHA*, Common hepatic artery; *LGA*, left gastric artery.

and the left cardia nodes (no. 1) dissected. The posterior vagal trunk is then cut and the stomach reflected. Complete nos. 1 and 3 dissections by removing the lymphatics on the posterior aspect of the cardia.

TOTAL GASTRECTOMY

Most aspects of D2 lymphadenectomy in TG are common to those in distal gastrectomy. Additional procedures are as follows.

DISSECTION OF THE UPPER GREATER CURVATURE NODES (NOS. 2 AND 4SA)

Following the division of the LGEA at its origin, the upper stomach is raised to inspect the splenic hilum from inside the lesser sac. The wall of the left bottom of the lesser sac is the dorsal gastric mesentery, which connects the upper greater curve of the stomach, the spleen, and the pancreatic body and tail. The gastrosplenic ligament is part of the dorsal mesentery.

The winding SpA and its terminal branches are broadly identified. The gastrosplenic ligament should be held and kept tense. The ligament is dissected close to the spleen, dividing the short gastric vessels towards the superior pole of the spleen. The peritoneal fusion at the back of the gastric fundus is then incised and the upper stomach mobilised from the abdominal wall.

The left paracardiac area has arterial supply from either the oesophagocardiac branch of the left subphrenic artery or the left cardiac branch of the LGA. Lymphatic flow from this area can directly reach the left para-aortic network.

Dissection along the distal SpA (no. 11d) and splenic hilum (no. 10)

Following the 11p dissection, the procedure is continued along the SpA towards the spleen. The winding SpA gives off several branches to both the pancreas and the stomach (Fig. 6.7). The great pancreatic artery, although not so large as its name suggests, is an important blood supply to the pancreatic tail. The caudal pancreatic artery arises near the splenic hilum and these pancreatic branches are preserved.

The remaining dorsal mesentery connects the posterior aspect of the upper stomach and the SpA and vein, and includes the posterior gastric artery and vein. This artery usually arises in the middle of the SpA and nourishes the dorsal part of the cardia. It should be ligated and cut at the root. Cancers in the upper stomach, especially those located on the posterior wall, frequently metastasise to the SpA nodes through the lymphatic channels in this mesentery.

The dissection is sometimes dangerous owing to kinking of the artery. Appropriate traction by the second assistant is particularly helpful.

SPLENECTOMY

Splenectomy is required when the tumour invades the tail of the pancreas and/or splenic hilum without other non-curative factors. It may also be indicated for complete dissection of no. 10 lymph nodes in tumours invading the greater curvature of the proximal stomach.

Mobilisation of the pancreas and spleen is started at the lower border of the pancreas. The bottom of the anterior sheet of the mesocolon is incised close to the pancreas. Several vessels arising from the pancreas to the anterior mesocolon (posterior epiploic arteries) should be cut.

The pancreatic body is lifted and entered behind the pancreas, leaving the retropancreatic fusion fascia to the retroperitoneal space. This is continued towards the spleen until the pancreatic tail is lifted. If the proper layer is entered, no vessels are encountered in this procedure.

The assistant should pull down the left kidney. The pancreatic tail is pulled up with the lower pole of the spleen. Then the parietal peritoneum behind the spleen can be visualised from its medial aspect. It is then incised and the spleen mobilised. This incision is continued towards the cardia, mobilising the whole dorsal mesentery from Gerota's fascia covering the kidney and left adrenal gland.

When the pancreas and spleen have been totally mobilised, the surgeon moves to the left side of the patient to continue the procedure.

The assistant should hold the reversed spleen. With the tail of the pancreas held in the left hand, the lymph nodes are dissected along the distal SpA. The SpA is double ligated and cut, then the vein, and the spleen is removed from the pancreas.

When the pancreas is also removed for tumour invasion, the SpA is ligated and dissected as close to the root as possible. Then the vein is ligated and cut close to the resection line, and the pancreas transected.

SUMMARY

✓ D2 lymphadenectomy is a systematic, standardised, technically demanding procedure that necessitates thorough knowledge of the anatomy of the major gastric arteries and veins.

RECONSTRUCTION AFTER GASTRIC RESECTION

A number of reconstruction methods have been proposed for gastrectomy. Each has advantages and disadvantages,

and should be selected according to surgical and oncological conditions in each patient. The following points should be considered in selection:

1. **Safety of surgery.** In gastrectomy for advanced tumours (curative or palliative) or for patients with high operative risk, any procedure after removal of the tumour should be simple and safe so as not to prolong the surgical time or increase the postoperative complications.
2. **Possible local recurrence.** In locally advanced tumours with wide serosal involvement and/or apparent nodal metastasis, gastric bed recurrence should be prepared for and a reconstruction with the least risk of obstruction should be selected.
3. **Long-term quality of life.** In gastrectomy with a high probability of cure, a reconstruction to maximise quality of life should be selected. Reflux of bile and alkaline duodenal juices into the oesophagus should be prevented. At the same time, long-term nutritional status should be considered.

RECONSTRUCTION AFTER DISTAL GASTRECTOMY (FIG. 6.8)

While Roux-en-Y (R-Y) and Billroth II (B-II) reconstructions are widely used, Billroth I gastroduodenostomy (B-I) is also frequently employed in Eastern Asia.

✓✓ Numerous RCTs and case series comparing these methods have been published with inconsistent results. A recent meta-analysis suggests that R-Y shows some clinical advantages over the other two methods.[63]

ROUX-EN-Y

INDICATIONS

Advantages of R-Y over B-I are the absence of duodenal juice reflux, safe anastomosis with a very low leak rate, and low risk of obstruction at gastric bed recurrence. Weak points include loss of easy endoscopic access to the duodenal papilla and possible nutritional problems due to non-physiological food passage, although no clear evidence has proven this. The R-Y procedure involves the jejunum and this may cause adhesive obstruction or an internal hernia in future. So-called 'Roux-en-Y syndrome', characterised by chronic abdominal pain and nausea that are aggravated by meals and associated with malnutrition, used to be reported mainly after ulcer surgery, but has not been observed as a serious problem recently.

R-Y reconstruction is applicable for most distal gastrectomies. The following are particularly good indications:

1. Tumours involving the gastric body for which the remnant stomach after resection is small;
2. Patients who suffer from reflux oesophagitis before surgery;
3. Patients with high operative risks for whom anastomotic leak must be prevented;
4. Locally advanced disease with high risk of gastric bed recurrence.

In special patients with biliary tract problems or duodenal pathological conditions that require endoscopic access or follow-up, B-I reconstruction might be considered.

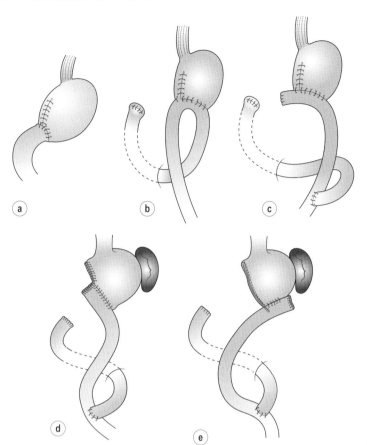

Figure 6.8 Reconstructions after distal gastrectomy. (a) Billroth I. (b) Billroth II isoperistaltic. (c) Roux-en-Y. (d) Roux-en-Y (hand-sewing). (e) Roux-en-Y (stapler).

PROCEDURE

The duodenum is transected using a linear-type stapler and many surgeons add covering seromuscular stitches. The jejunum 20–30 cm distal to the Treiz ligament is divided and the jejunal limb is pulled up either via the ante- or retrocolic route. In T4a/T4b tumours that have a significant risk of local recurrence involving the mesocolon, the antecolic route is preferred. Gastrojejunostomy is achieved either by stapler or hand-sewing; different anastomotic sites and jejunal directions are selected accordingly (Fig. 6.8d,e). The jejunojejunostomy is made 40 cm distal to the gastrojejunostomy. The mesentery holes are closed to prevent internal hernia.

When the retrocolic route is selected, the gastrojejunostomy site should be pulled down below the mesocolon and be fixed to it to prevent torsion or obstruction of the jejunal limb in the narrow space above the mesocolon.

BILLROTH I

INDICATIONS AND PROCEDURE
Advantages of B-I over R-Y are physiological food passage, simple anastomosis without jejunal manipulation, and preserved endoscopic access to the duodenal papilla. B-I is useful for distal tumours at an early stage for which a relatively large proximal stomach can be preserved and recurrence is not thought likely. Weak points of B-I are duodenal juice reflux, possible anastomotic leak and possible obstruction at recurrence. Thus, B-I should be avoided in cases with high operative risks, small remnant stomach, the preoperative presence of oesophageal reflux, or locally advanced disease.

Gastroduodenostomy is made either by hand-sewing or using a circular stapler. When the anastomotic tension is high, Kocher's mobilisation of the duodenum is useful to reduce it.

RECONSTRUCTION AFTER TOTAL GASTRECTOMY (FIG. 6.9)

R-Y is the standard reconstruction after TG. It is simple, safe, and gives relatively good functional results. Weak points are early satiety due to lack of reservoir and consequent long-term malnutrition. Careful dietetic surveillance and education is essential.

ROUX-EN-Y

INDICATIONS
There is virtually no contraindication for R-Y. In rare cases where endoscopic access to the duodenum needs to be maintained for biliary tract problems, a jejunoduodenostomy is added about 30–40 cm from thee oesophagojejunostomy (double-tract R-Y; Fig. 6.9b).

PROCEDURE
The jejunum is transected 20–30 cm from the Treiz ligament. Either the ante- or retrocolic route is selected according to the criteria mentioned in the section on distal gastrectomy. The retrocolic pathway provides the shortest route and the least tension on the limb mesentery, especially in obese patients with a large omental residue.

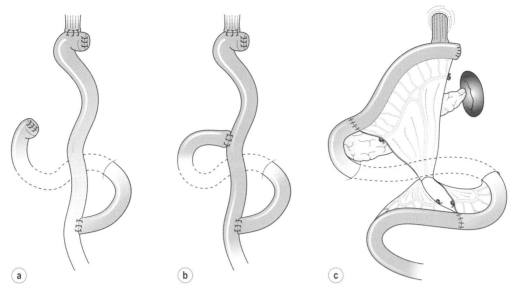

Figure 6.9 Reconstructions after total gastrectomy. (a) Roux-en-Y. (b) Double-tract Roux-en-Y. (c) Jejunal interposition.

Jejunal vessels are carefully prepared so that the mesentery tension is reduced, preserving the blood supply to the anastomotic site.

Oesophagojejunostomy is undertaken using a circular stapler. A 25-mm anvil is applicable in most cases. A larger size can be selected in patients with a large oesophagus and jejunum.

The jejuno-jejunostomy is performed 40–50 cm below the oesophageal anastomosis. A shorter limb may cause reflux and a longer one may be disadvantageous from a nutritional viewpoint. In the double-tract method, the jejuno-jejunostomy is made 20 cm distal to the jejunoduodenostomy.

In a laparoscopic procedure, oesophagojejunostomy has been an obstacle associated with frequent leakage and/or postoperative stenosis. A newly devised anastomotic method using the linear stapler is now widely used in totally intracorporeal oesophagojejunostomy, resulting in reduced complications.[64]

JEJUNAL INTERPOSITION

This method is employed to maintain the physiological food passage to the duodenum.

However, there is no solid evidence that this reconstruction has a long-term nutritional advantage over standard R-Y.

The length of the interposed jejunum can be shorter (20–30 cm) than the jejunal limb in R-Y, probably because the jejunal juice can flow down the natural route without reflux.

POUCH FORMATION

Various operations have been devised to increase the reservoir capacity of the jejunum, with inconsistent results – some patients eat remarkably well but others suffer from severe stasis or regurgitation.

Various types of jejunal pouch have been devised and tested in RCTs or prospective observation. The technique is expected to be standardised in the near future.

A recent meta-analysis of 17 RCTs and 8 observational studies comparing reconstruction with or without pouch after TG showed that pouch creation improves long-term functional and nutritional outcomes without greater perioperative morbidity.[65]

SUMMARY

There is no single best reconstruction method after gastrectomy. Priority should be given to safety for poor-risk patients and to function for those with a high possibility of cure. Roux-en-Y, following both distal and total gastrectomy, could be the first choice. Pouch formation appears to improve quality of life after TG and this procedure is expected to be standardised.

EARLY POSTOPERATIVE COMPLICATIONS

Two major complications after gastrectomy for cancer are anastomotic leak and pancreatic fistula. They cause abdominal abscess, peritonitis, sepsis, or massive haemorrhage. Complications are more common in TG and extended lymphadenectomy than in distal gastrectomy and limited lymphadenectomy, respectively. Most prospective studies have shown that splenectomy and distal pancreatectomy significantly increase postoperative morbidity and mortality. Close management by experienced surgeons, especially for pancreatic fistula, is essential to avoid mortality.

Use of prophylactic drains after gastrectomy is controversial and there is no evidence that drains decrease postoperative complications or death.[66] Distal gastrectomy without intraoperative problems usually needs no drains. However, in TG or extended D2 dissection along the upper border of the distal pancreas, a suction drain along the pancreas gives useful information on pancreatic fistula or early anastomotic leak.

ANASTOMOTIC LEAK

Most anastomotic leaks after gastrectomy occur at the oesophagojejunostomy. Possible causes are tissue ischaemia or tension on the anastomotic line and these should be avoided by careful preparation of the jejunal loop. Correct usage of the anastomotic circular stapler is also important. Covering stiches are usually unnecessary but should be used when the continuity of the 'doughnut' of the resected oesophagus or jejunum is incomplete. The anastomotic method using a linear stapler developed for laparoscopic gastrectomy is increasingly used also in open surgery.

Early anastomotic leak occurring within 72 hours could be life-threatening without proper management, and it may present as septic episodes or contaminated drain discharge. Contrast swallow (Gastrografin) should be done whenever a leak is suspected. Drainage is crucial to treat anastomotic leakage. When a prophylactic drain has been appropriately placed and the leak is minor without evidence of local diffusion, a conservative treatment with fasting and adequate nutrition will suffice. When there is no drain or septic signs are evident, some active intervention is strongly advised. Endoscopic vacuum therapy is effective in select cases,[67] but re-operation should not be delayed. Anastomotic failure can be repaired in some early cases, or at worst a drain can be placed close to the leak site. A feeding jejunostomy should be constructed.

The management of a delayed leak is controversial. Usually drains have already been removed and meals are started. The patient may have some difficulty in swallowing and, although the patient may be afebrile, blood tests suggest continuous inflammation. When a contrast study reveals only a minor leak, fasting and adequate nutrition will be sufficient. A naso-intestinal tube placed beyond the jejuno-jejunostomy may be useful for enteral feeding. If the patient is septic, a drain must be placed. Contrast-enhanced computed tomography will be helpful whether the intervention is achieved surgically or radiologically. Surgery at this point is technically difficult due to severe adhesions in the upper abdomen but should be carried out when the abdominal infection is diffuse.

DUODENAL STUMP LEAK

A properly stapled duodenal stump rarely leaks. However, stump leak occurs when the duodenal tissue is damaged or becomes ischaemic. There is no evidence that covering stiches reduce leak, but some surgeons use them. Duodenal stump leak may also occur when the intraduodenal pressure increases due to afferent limb obstruction or possibly unusually strong peristalsis.

A prophylactic drain that is placed near the stump gives good information. If its discharge contains bile, it is an indication for immediate re-operation. Re-closure of the stump is usually very difficult due to tissue inflammation. If there is a major defect, a Foley-type catheter can be placed in the duodenum with a plan to form a controlled fistula. When the leak is from a pinhole on the staple line, a suction drain is placed close to it and retrograde insertion of a duodenal decompression tube from the jejunum should be considered. Feeding jejunostomy is useful not only for nutrition, but also for returning the suctioned duodenal content to the intestine. With good duodenal decompression, enteral feeding does not have to be stopped or reduced.

PANCREATIC FISTULA

After D2 lymphadenectomy, pancreatic leak may occur even without pancreatectomy. It is more common when the pancreatic capsule has been removed as a part of bursectomy or the pancreas has been mobilised for splenectomy. Placement of a prophylactic suction drain along the upper border of the pancreas is recommended in these operations. Increased amylase content in the drain fluid on the first or second postoperative day is a useful marker to predict later development of pancreatic fistula, and the fluid containing high amylase usually takes on a dark red (wine) colour. Suction drainage is also useful to prevent diffusion of pancreatic fluid and localise the fistula.

When the tail of the pancreas is resected, pancreatic leak is more common and drain placement is strongly recommended. A suction tube should be placed close to the stump via the shortest percutaneous route.

It is controversial as to whether the use of somatostatin analogues prevents pancreatic fistula. RCTs for pancreatic surgery have shown inconsistent results, and meta-analyses have not supported a positive effect.[68] No RCT has been conducted on this subject in gastrectomy.

When pancreatic leak occurs, management should concentrate on prevention of infection and abscess control. Adequate drainage is essential and radiological intervention should be considered. Abscess drainage takes time and may require frequent adjustments of the drain tip. When the abscess is localised and surrounded by a solid wall, saline irrigation of the cavity will enhance healing.

HAEMORRHAGE

Haemorrhage within the first few hours of surgery should be treated by early re-laparotomy. It must be remembered that drains can occlude with blood clot and the clinical suspicion of bleeding in a haemodynamically unstable patient is a sufficient indication to operate.

Secondary haemorrhage caused by intra-abdominal infection following anastomotic leak and/or pancreatic fistula is truly life-threatening. A poorly drained abscess causes pseudoaneurysm of a major artery which can then cause massive haemorrhage. In the stage of pseudoaneurysm, a small amount of bleeding may precede massive haemorrhage, which must not be overlooked. Immediate radiological intervention may detect an unruptured pseudoaneurysm that can be embolised. Once massive bleeding occurs, immediate angiography again should first be considered because it not only provides the chance of embolisation, but can also identify the bleeding point. In immediate re-laparotomy, the bleeding artery is sometimes difficult to identify or reach due to severe adhesion and/or inflammation.

POSTSPLENECTOMY INFECTION

There is increasing evidence that splenectomy predisposes the patient to an increased risk of bacterial infection in both the early postoperative period and probably for the remainder of their life. Immediate prophylaxis with twice-daily oral penicillin is now recommended for patients of all ages. The patient should also be immunised with vaccines against pneumococci, meningococcus, and *Haemophilus influenzae*. If the splenectomy has been planned as part of a radical procedure, these vaccines are most effective if administered preoperatively. The patient should have an annual influenza vaccine and an updated pneumococcal vaccine roughly every 3 years.

LATE SEQUELAE AND COMPLICATIONS

SIDE-EFFECTS AND POSTPRANDIAL SEQUELAE

No gastrectomised patient can eat in the same way he or she used to eat, at least during the first few postoperative months. Good dietary advice is essential and patients should understand what their stomach used to do and how they can cope with their status without part or all of their stomach. The author usually explains this as follows: 'The stomach has three major functions: 1) it stores the food that has been swallowed; 2) it digests and dilutes it; and 3) it slowly pushes it out to the duodenum (taking many hours after a greasy meal). These functions help the small bowel to effectively absorb nutrients. When the stomach has been removed, it is necessary to change eating habits to help the small intestine work as before: chew well, take time before the next bite, and have frequent small meals.'

Patients should also be able to accept that their stomach will never come back, and that the lost stomach functions are compensated not by medicine but by an appropriate eating style. Additional specific advice from a dietician will help further.

EARLY DUMPING SYNDROME

Early dumping syndrome appears within 30 minutes after a meal, or even during a meal. The rapid filling of the proximal small intestine with hypertonic food leads to rapid movement of fluid from the extracellular fluid compartment into the gut and also triggers a complex neurohumoral response. This produces various gastrointestinal and cardiovascular symptoms such as palpitation, bloating, cramping, diarrhoea, and nausea, requiring some patients to lie down for an hour after each meal. Most patients with early dumping syndrome can be treated by appropriate dietary adaptation. In severe cases, however, quality of life is restricted and malnutrition can occur rapidly. Careful management involving an experienced dietician should be considered.

LATE DUMPING SYNDROME OR REACTIVE HYPOGLYCAEMIC ATTACKS

Late dumping syndrome appears 2–3 hours after a meal and is characterised by faintness, severe hunger, dizziness, and cold sweating, which are symptoms of hypoglycaemia. Rapid inflow of carbohydrate to the jejunum causes oxyhyperglycaemia, which induces hyperinsulinaemia followed by hypoglycaemia. Glucagon-like peptide-1 (GLP-1) secreted from the proximal jejunal mucosa is thought to play a role in this hypersecretion of insulin.

Dietary adaptation is again the main treatment for late dumping syndrome. Patients are advised to decrease the carbohydrate load in their main meals and to take small amounts of carbohydrate between main meals. Those with frequent attacks should carry dextrose tablets to eat at the first sign of symptoms.

In a large-scale investigation into dumping syndrome after gastrectomy (*n* = 1 153),[69] early dumping syndrome was more commonly experienced than late dumping syndrome (68% vs 38%) and the incidence varied according to the type of gastrectomy but not the postoperative period. Early and late dumping syndromes have different aetiologies and appear independently. During follow-up, a careful history should be taken and appropriate dietary advice should be given.

NUTRITIONAL PROBLEMS

Gastrectomy may cause deficits of specific nutrients. Of the three major nutrients, fat absorption particularly decreases because mixing with duodenal contents (bile acid, pancreatic lipase) and jejunal absorption become insufficient. Patients with fat malabsorption complain of steatorrhoea, which can be treated with pancreatic enzyme supplements.

VITAMIN B$_{12}$

Vitamin B$_{12}$ binds to intrinsic factor secreted by the parietal cells of the stomach and is absorbed in the ileum. After TG, patients absorb no vitamin B$_{12}$ and body stores are gradually depleted, resulting in megaloblastic anaemia, although this may take up to 24 months to become clinically apparent. All patients should receive 1 mg of hydroxocobalamin intramuscularly every 3 to 6 months for life after TG. Vitamin B$_{12}$ deficiency can develop even after distal gastrectomy, leaving a small atrophic remnant. Mean corpuscular volume should be monitored in the blood test for gastrectomy follow-up.

VITAMIN D

Absorption of fat-soluble vitamins (A, D, E, and K) may decrease in patients with fat malabsorption. Of these, vitamin D malabsorption is clinically important, particularly in postmenopausal women. Combined with decreased calcium absorption after gastrectomy, it leads to metabolic bone disorders from 2 years after surgery. It is recommended that postmenopausal women and all patients over 70 years of age take an oral calcium and vitamin D supplement for life after a TG.

IRON

Iron absorption occurs predominantly in the duodenum and upper jejunum. In the presence of gastric acid, ferric iron (Fe^{3+}) in foodstuffs is deoxidised to easily absorbable ferrous iron (Fe^{2+}). Iron absorption may be reduced after gastric resection due to decreased acid and rapid food passage in the intestine. Iron-deficiency anaemia is common, and an oral iron supplement is useful.

Key points

- Lymphatic spread is the most common mode of dissemination in gastric cancer.
- Among the four patterns of spread of gastric cancer (lymphatic, peritoneal, haematogenous, and direct), lymphatic metastasis occurs at the earliest stage and this can lead to other types of metastases. Surgical control of this spread at an early phase of the disease may prevent later systemic failure and patients can still be cured by adequate dissection.
- Peritoneal metastasis is the most common type of failure after radical surgery for gastric cancer. Peritoneal metastasis is much more common in diffuse-type cancers than the intestinal type.
- Surgery itself can be a cause of cancer spread, especially in terms of peritoneal dissemination. Even serosa-negative tumours can recur in the peritoneal cavity after surgery. These cases are usually associated with lymph node metastasis. Adherence to the principles of good surgical cancer practice reduces the risk of spread.
- There is an increasing move towards tailoring gastric cancer operations, taking not only the stage of the disease but also patient-related factors into account.
- According to the Japanese treatment guidelines, a 5-cm resection margin is recommended for tumours showing an infiltrative growth pattern with indistinct borders or diffuse-type histology, but 3 cm is usually sufficient for those showing an expansive growth pattern with grossly distinct borders, the histology of which is most frequently the intestinal type.
- Randomised trials comparing total and distal gastrectomy in distal gastric cancer failed to show any survival benefit for TG (known as TG 'de principe').
- The JGCA recommends that non-early, potentially curable gastric cancer should be treated by D2 lymphadenectomy. D1 or D1+ should be considered as an option for T1 tumours. In a poor-risk patient or under circumstances where D2 cannot be safely performed, D1+ can be a substitute for D2.
- Although solid evidence of extended lymphadenectomy is yet to be established, D2 gastrectomy without splenectomy or pancreatectomy has been officially recommended by the European Society of Medical Oncology in 2009.

- The number of lymph nodes retrieved is a combination of the surgery and pathological handling and does not necessarily reflect the extent of lymphadenectomy. Surgeons should plan and perform lymphadenectomy according to anatomical extent rather than to fulfil an aim of removing 25 or more nodes.
- All clinical studies have shown that splenectomy or distal pancreatectomy plus splenectomy (DP + S) significantly increases operative morbidity and, in the West, mortality, without obvious survival benefit.
- A large RCT showed no survival benefit of splenectomy for proximal gastric cancer that does not invade the greater curvature. Splenectomy should be considered only for tumours on the greater curvature having a high incidence of metastasis in the splenic hilum. In the new edition of the JGCA guidelines, station no. 10 has been removed from the D2 definition.
- DP + S is associated with high operative morbidity, including pancreatic leakage and abscess formation, even in specialist Japanese centres. It is currently indicated only for tumours directly invading the pancreas.
- The role of extended lymphadenectomy exceeding D2 is ambiguous. Prophylactic para-aortic nodal dissection did not improve the survival over standard D2 in a large-scale Japanese RCT and has now been abandoned in Japan.
- Several RCTs and case series comparing Billroth I, Billroth II, and Roux-en-Y (R-Y) reconstruction after distal gastrectomy have been published with inconsistent results. A recent meta-analysis suggests that R-Y shows some clinical advantages over the other two methods.
- R-Y is the standard reconstruction after TG. A recent meta-analysis of 13 RCTs comparing R-Y or jejunal interposition with and without pouch showed some clinical advantages of pouch reconstruction.
- Complications are more common in TG and extended lymphadenectomy than in distal gastrectomy and limited lymphadenectomy, respectively. Most prospective studies have shown that splenectomy and distal pancreatectomy significantly increase postoperative morbidity and mortality.

 References available at http://ebooks.health.elsevier.com/

KEY REFERENCES

[5] Gotoda T, Yanagisawa A, Sasako M, et al. Incidence of lymph node metastasis from early gastric cancer: estimation with a large number of cases at two large centers. Gastric Cancer 2000;3:219–25. PMID: 11984739

Detailed analysis of 5265 early gastric cancers that provided the grounds of expanded indications for endoscopic submucosal dissection.

[12] Songun I, Putter H, Kranenbarg EMK, et al. Surgical treatment of gastric cancer; 15-year follow-up results of the randomized nationwide Dutch D1D2 trial. Lancet Oncol 2010;11:439–49. PMID: 20409751

Long-term follow-up of an RCT finally showed significantly fewer gastric cancer deaths after D2 dissection.

[16] Kuramoto M, Shimada S, Ikeshima S, et al. Extensive intraoperative peritoneal lavage as a standard prophylactic strategy for peritoneal recurrence in patients with gastric carcinoma. Ann Surg 2009;250:242–6. PMID: 19638909

A small-scale RCT showed that extensive peritoneal lavage before closure reduced peritoneal recurrence.

[39] Sasako M, McCulloch P, Kinoshita T, et al. New method to evaluate the therapeutic value of lymph node dissection for gastric cancer. Br J Surg 1995;82:346–51. PMID: 7796005

A new concept to evaluate lymphadenectomy was proposed based on the incidence of metastasis and survival of patients with positive nodes.

[65] Syn NL, Wee I, Shabbir A, et al. Pouch versus n pouch following total gastrectomy: meta-analysis of randomized and non-randomized studies. Ann Surg 2019;269:1041–53. PMID: 31082900

A meta-analysis showed clinical benefits of pouch formation after total gastrectomy.

[69] Mine S, Sano T, Tsutsumi K, et al. Large-scale investigation into dumping syndrome after gastrectomy for gastric cancer. J Am Coll Surg 2010;211:628–36. PMID: 20829078

Direct questionnaire to 1153 gastrectomised patients with various postoperative periods revealed actual conditions of dumping syndrome.

Treatment of early oesophageal and gastric cancer

7

Maria J. Valkema | Arjun D. Koch | J. Jan B. van Lanschot | Sjoerd M. Lagarde

INTRODUCTION

DEFINITION OF EARLY OESOPHAGEAL AND EARLY GASTRIC CANCERS

✓ Early oesophageal cancers and early gastric cancers (EGCs) are defined as tumours limited to the mucosa or submucosa (T1 stage) and do, by definition, not invade the muscularis propria. This is irrespective of the presence of lymph node metastasis.[1]

This chapter deals with the management of early upper gastrointestinal neoplasms, which is described in two parts: early oesophageal cancer (part A) and EGC (part B).

A. EARLY OESOPHAGEAL CANCER

RISK AND DEVELOPMENT OF EARLY OESOPHAGEAL CANCER

Oesophageal cancer is the seventh most common cancer globally, with approximately 572 000 new cases and 509 000 deaths in 2018.[2] The two main histologic subtypes are squamous cell carcinoma and adenocarcinoma. Worldwide, squamous cell carcinoma is most prevalent. Squamous cell carcinoma can develop in any part of the oesophagus but is mostly located in the middle third and develops from the stratified squamous epithelium of the oesophagus. In high-income countries, major risk factors are heavy drinking and smoking. Risk factors for high-incidence countries in parts of Asia and Africa have not been clarified yet and are thought to include environmental and dietary factors, drinking very hot beverages, and genetic factors. Adenocarcinomas account for the majority of cases in Western countries and the incidence continues to increase, whereas the incidence of squamous cell carcinoma is expected to decrease.[3] Major risk factors for developing adenocarcinoma are obesity and gastro-oesophageal reflux disease (GORD), which are also risk factors for the development of metaplastic columnar epithelium (Barrett's oesophagus). Metaplasia, in Barrett's oesophagus or in the intestinal columnar mucosa in the stomach or gastro-oesophageal junction, may progress to increasing grades of dysplasia and eventually to invasive carcinoma. Rarely, adenocarcinomas occur in the proximal or mid oesophagus in the absence of Barrett's oesophagus, and are thought to develop from (sub)mucosal glands or ectopic columnar epithelium (especially the cervical inlet patch).[4]

CLASSIFICATION OF EARLY OESOPHAGEAL CANCER

Early oesophageal cancer is confined to the mucosa (T1a) or extends into the submucosa (T1b) and is considered eligible for local endoscopic removal (Fig. 7.1). Early carcinomas comprise a spectrum from very subtle carcinomas to deep submucosal tumours. While subtle carcinomas can be difficult to detect, deep submucosal carcinomas are easier to identify, but assessment of endoscopic resectability can sometimes be difficult. Detection and early assessment of oesophageal lesions are performed with endoscopy using white light and (virtual) chromoendoscopy such as narrow-band imaging (NBI). Endosonography can be performed on indication to determine lymph node status. Histopathologic evaluation from endoscopically resected specimens is considered as the optimal staging step to determine the indication for subsequent therapy.

ENDOSCOPIC APPEARANCE OF EARLY LESIONS

✓ Superficial neoplastic lesions in the gastrointestinal tract are classified by their endoscopic appearance according to the Paris classification[1] (Fig. 7.2). Superficial lesions are classified as protruding (Paris 0–I), elevated (0–IIa), depressed (0–IIc), or excavated and often ulcerated lesions (0–III).

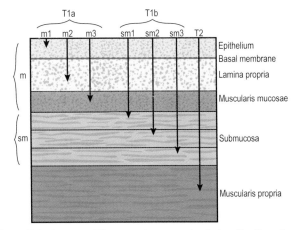

Figure 7.1 Layers of the oesophagus and subclassification of early oesophageal cancer related to the tumour invasion depth. *m*, Mucosa; *sm*, submucosa.

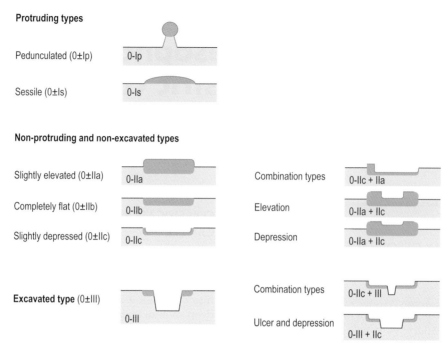

Figure 7.2 Paris classification: endoscopic appearance of superficial (type 0) neoplastic lesions. Type 0–I lesions are protruding, type 0–II lesions can be slightly elevated, flat and/or slightly depressed, and type 0–III lesions are excavated lesions (ulcers). The latter are distinguished from slightly depressed lesions by the amount of depression from the adjacent mucosa at a cut-off of 1.2 mm in the columnar epithelium and 0.5 mm in the squamous epithelium.

The Paris classification has been developed to unify the description of superficial lesions within the oesophagus, stomach, and colon.[1,5] The Japanese Society for Esophageal Diseases originally developed morphological criteria for cancers of the digestive tract and type 0 lesions were defined as endoscopically superficial cancers.

The Paris classification distinguishes three main subtypes within the type 0 category: protruding lesions (0–I), non-protruding non-excavated lesions (0–II), and excavated lesions (0–III) or 'ulcers' (see Fig. 7.2).[5] The protruding types protrude above the mucosal surface and may be pedunculated (0–Ip) or sessile (0–Is). Pedunculated polyps are narrow at the base, whereas sessile polyps have a width at the base equal to that of the top. Non-protruding lesions are classified as slightly elevated (0–IIa), flat (0–IIb), slightly depressed (0–IIc), or excavated (0–III). Depending on the depth of the depressed lesion relative to the adjacent mucosa, the lesion is classified as type 0–IIc or type 0–III. The cut-off is at 1.2 mm in the columnar epithelium of the oesophagus and in the stomach, and at 0.5 mm in the stratified epithelium of the oesophagus. Lesions that have both elevated and depressed components are classified into two groups: depressed lesions, in which most of the surface is depressed and there is elevation in a portion of the peripheral ring are classified as 0–IIc + IIa, while elevated lesions with a central depression encircled by the elevated ring at the periphery are called 0–IIa + IIc. The combined patterns of excavation and depression are called 0–III + IIc or 0–IIc + III, depending on the relative surface area of the ulcer and of the depressed area. The classification helps to predict the extent of invasion into the submucosal layer and thus the choice between endoscopic or surgical treatment, which is applicable to all neoplastic lesions throughout the gastrointestinal tract (Table 7.1). Type 0–I and 0–III are more at risk of submucosal invasion and thus not good candidates for endoscopic resection, in contrast to types 0–IIa, 0–IIb, and 0–IIc.[6]

Endoscopic staging before endoscopic resection does provide useful information on the prediction of invasion into the proper muscle layer. Lesions that are confined to the mucosa with or without the submucosa tend to move over the peristaltic waves, whereas peristaltic waves appear to curve around tumours that have invaded the proper muscle layer. The latter provides a strong argument against endoscopic resection. In most endoscopic resection techniques, submucosal injection of fluid is used to lift the early cancer from the proper muscle layer. This method has three major benefits: 1) it provides information on invasion depth and thus endoscopic resectability; 2) it facilitates endoscopic resection by increasing the visibility of and access to the submucosal resection plane; and 3) it provides a safety fluid cushion for resecting the superficial lesion without damaging the deeper layers when using snares, knives, or electrocautery.[7] The amount of lifting provides information on the invasion depth of the lesion. Mucosal or superficial submucosal lesions usually demonstrate complete lifting (m–sm1), whereas the lesions that infiltrate into the deeper submucosal layers often lift incompletely (sm2–sm3). A non-lifting sign most often represents invasion deeper than sm3.[7]

Other features that predict deeper invasion are the size of the lesion, poor tumour differentiation grade, and lymphovascular invasion (LVI). The histological features can be obtained through simple biopsy.

CHROMOENDOSCOPY

Chromoendoscopy is a technique that is used to highlight neoplastic changes in the mucosa that are less apparent

Table 7.1 Paris classification of type 0 superficial lesions[5]

Macroscopic Appearance	Paris Classification	Relative Frequency of Submucosal Invasion in Lesions in the Oesophagus	Relative Frequency of Submucosal Invasion in Gastric Lesions
Protruding	0–I	79%	57%
Pedunculated	0–Ip		
Sessile	0–Is		
	Non-protruding and non-excavated		
Slightly elevated	0–IIa	48%	29%
Completely flat	0–IIb	15%	20%
Slightly depressed	0–IIc	27%	40%
Elevated and depressed types	0–IIa + IIc		
	0–IIc + IIa		
	Excavated		
Ulcer	0–III	84%	–
Excavated and depressed types	0–IIc + III		
	0–III + IIc		

when white light is used. This is traditionally done by using dye spray to stain the mucosa during endoscopy.

Chromoendoscopy with Lugol's iodine solution is traditionally used to outline neoplastic areas in the squamous epithelium that can be recognised as Lugol-voiding lesions. The Japanese 2020 guideline advises to use iodine solution at a low concentration of ≤ 1% to prevent damage to the epithelium.[8] For Barrett's oesophagus, acetic acid can be used as stain, leaving dysplastic or cancerous areas more reddish than the surroundings. Virtual chromoendoscopy has become available as an alternative option for the use of stains. Examples are NBI, i-Scan, and Fujinon Intelligent Chromoendoscopy (FICE). These techniques employ a narrow-band optical filter using a spectrum corresponding with the absorption of haemoglobin to visualise the microvascular mucosal structure, which facilitates identification of abnormal microvessels.

For squamous cell carcinomas, a systematic review and meta-analysis reported similar diagnostic accuracy for Lugol chromoendoscopy and NBI to detect high-grade dysplasia or squamous cell carcinoma.[9]

In a per-patient analysis, the sensitivity and specificity of Lugol chromoendoscopy were 92% and 82%, respectively, and the sensitivity and specificity of NBI were both 88%. NBI is generally preferred since it has a shorter examination time and has no side-effects.[9] In patients with many multiform Lugol-voiding lesions, however, NBI has a higher chance of misdiagnosis of squamous cell carcinoma than with Lugol chromoendoscopy, as was reported in one randomised non-inferiority trial.[10]

ENDOSONOGRAPHY

Routine staging with endoscopic ultrasonography (EUS) for early lesions is not recommended, since EUS is not sufficiently accurate to distinguish T1a from T1b or T1 from T2. A meta-analysis assessing the diagnostic accuracy of EUS to differentiate T1a from T1b adenocarcinomas and squamous cell carcinomas reported a large degree of heterogeneity due to the site of the lesion, the histology, the frequency of the ultrasound probe, the method of use (radial versus linear or both), and the experience of the operator. For T1a staging the pooled sensitivity was 85% and pooled specificity was 87%. The pooled sensitivity and specificity for T1b staging were both 86%.[11]

In a setting of patients with Barrett's oesophagus who were referred for high-grade dysplasia or adenocarcinoma, a meta-analysis showed that performance of T staging with EUS to identify ≥ T1sm1 was suboptimal, with a sensitivity of 56%, specificity of 89%, positive predictive value of 63% and negative predictive value of 85%.[12] In a subsequent meta-analysis of the same research group, EUS was found to over-stage 9% of patients with Barrett's oesophagus and suspected early carcinoma and to under-stage another 9%.[13] Over-staging of pT1a carcinomas has been reported to occur in 20–40%, as reported in two cohort studies including squamous cell carcinoma patients.[14,15] In recent patient series including two prospective cohort studies, cT2-staged tumours by EUS have been reported to be overstaged in 30–40%.[16–18] To prevent over-staging and consequent overtreatment in cT2-staged lesions by EUS, endoscopic reassessment by an expert interventional endoscopist is recommended for cT2N0 adenocarcinomas.[16]

Endoscopic resection of defined mucosal abnormalities offers the most sensitive method of obtaining a T stage for early oesophageal neoplasia and should be considered before defining the overall treatment of the patient.

EUS with fine-needle aspiration (FNA) is advised to detect lymph node metastases when submucosal disease is suspected or when pT1b is histopathologically confirmed after staging endoscopic resection.[6,19,20] EUS outperforms positron emission tomography (PET) and computed tomography (CT) for clinical T staging and has similar accuracy compared to PET and CT for clinical N staging.[21] EUS has a pooled sensitivity for detecting N+ of 71% (95% confidence interval (CI) 49–87%) and a pooled specificity of 94% (95% CI 89–97%) in patients with high-grade dysplasia or adenocarcinoma in Barrett's oesophagus.[12] Patients with invasive submucosal or T2 disease being considered for oesophagectomy should undergo complete staging with EUS and diagnostic CT and PET-CT.[6]

Table 7.2   The revised Vienna classification of gastrointestinal epithelial neoplasia[22]

Category	Diagnosis	Clinical Management
1	Negative for neoplasia	Optional follow-up
2	Indefinite for neoplasia	Endoscopic follow-up
3	Mucosal low-grade neoplasia (low-grade adenoma/dysplasia)	Endoscopic resection or follow-up
4	Mucosal high-grade neoplasia	Endoscopic or local surgical resection
4.1	High-grade adenoma/dysplasia	
4.2	Non-invasive carcinoma (carcinoma in situ)	
4.3	Suspicious for invasive carcinoma	
4.4	Intramucosal carcinoma	
5	Submucosal invasion by carcinoma	Surgical resection

Table 7.3   Risk of lymph node involvement per histologic type related to invasion depth in the oesophagus[24–28,30,31,34]

Squamous cell carcinoma	m1	m2	m3	sm1 ≤ 200 µm	sm2/3
LN risk	0%	0–5.6%	9%	23%	29–48%
Adenocarcinoma	m1	m2	m3	sm1 ≤ 500 µm	sm2/3
LN risk	0%	0–2%	0–3%	0–9%	0–38%

REVISED VIENNA CLASSIFICATION

Large discrepancies between Western and Japanese pathologists in the diagnostic criteria for adenoma, dysplasia, and carcinoma in the gastrointestinal tract have led to considerable problems in the comparison between Western and Japanese data. This led to a consensus meeting in 1998 in Vienna, ultimately resulting in the Vienna classification of gastrointestinal epithelial neoplasia and the revised Vienna classification in 2002.[22] This classification allows not only for a more universal nomenclature of gastrointestinal epithelial neoplasia, but also corresponds more properly with clinical management. The revised Vienna classification is shown in Table 7.2. Histology from biopsies and resection specimens are nowadays classified according to the revised Vienna classification.

ENDOSCOPIC TREATMENT VERSUS SURGERY

The decision for endoscopic treatment or surgery depends on the extent of the disease, the risk of the individual patient to develop lymph node metastases, and the operative risk of the individual patient. In early cancers, endoscopic treatment is considered the therapy of choice for patients in whom the risk of lymph node metastases is below the mortality risk of oesophagectomy, taking patient preferences and patient performance status into consideration.

RISK OF NODAL INVOLVEMENT

For adenocarcinoma and squamous cell carcinoma, differences exist in the risk of developing nodal metastases (Table 7.3). The risk of lymph node metastases increases with the depth of tumour invasion in the oesophagus. T1a carcinoma is intramucosal carcinoma and can be subclassified according to the level of invasion into the epithelium (m1), the lamina propria (m2), or the muscularis mucosae (m3) (see Fig. 7.1). For assessment of the extent of submucosal invasion in T1b carcinomas, a pragmatic approach is to divide

the submucosa into three layers of equivalent thickness: superficial (sm1), middle (sm2), and deep (sm3). However, after endoscopic resection, the submucosal divisions cannot be obtained from the resected specimen since the full submucosa is not available for examination. The depth of tumour invasion is obtained by measuring from the lower limit of the muscularis mucosae in microns (µm). Pathologists should be aware of the finding of a duplication of the muscularis mucosae in Barrett's oesophagus to avoid overestimation of the invasion depth.[4] The cut-off between sm1 and sm2/3 is defined at 200 µm for squamous neoplasia and at 500 µm in Barrett's neoplasia.[6] Most international guidelines advise oesophagectomy at an invasion depth more than m3 in squamous carcinoma and more than m3 or sm1 in adenocarcinoma.

Specimens of endoscopic resection should be assessed according to standardised protocols, reporting on adverse prognostic features that could change patient management, including the depth of invasion, tumour size, tumour differentiation grade, margin status and presence of LVI.[23]

RISK OF LYMPH NODE METASTASES IN T1A

Many studies have been conducted to estimate the risk of lymph node metastases related to the extent of tumour invasion depth. It is likely that the rates of risk of lymph node involvement as reported based on surgical series have been subject to overestimation.[24] In these time periods, the estimation of exact tumour invasion in surgical specimens did not change patient management. Also, histopathologic analysis of surgical specimens is usually performed at slices of 5 mm, whereas endoscopically resected specimens are assessed at 2-mm intervals. As a consequence, reported estimates of lymph node metastases in surgical series might actually correspond to more deeply invading tumours and thus the true risk of lymph node metastases may be lower.

High-grade dysplasia or tumours not infiltrating deeper than the epithelium (m1) in Barrett's oesophagus or in the squamous epithelium have not been associated with the development of nodal disease.[25,26] The occurrence of lymph node metastases with m2 squamous cell carcinoma or adenocarcinoma is rare,[25,26] but has been reported up to 5.6% in a large, single-centre surgical series.[27] With squamous cell carcinoma invading up to m3, the node-positive rate has been reported to be 8.8% in a meta-analysis.[26] For mucosal adenocarcinomas the overall rate of lymph node metastases ranges between 0% and 3%.[24,25,28,29]

✓ Patients with high-grade dysplasia (in squamous epithelium or Barrett's oesophagus) and patients with intramucosal (T1a) adenocarcinoma have a low risk of lymph node involvement and are suitable for endoscopic ablative therapies as definitive treatment. Also, patients with squamous cell carcinoma not exceeding the epithelium (m1) or lamina propria (m2) are unlikely to develop lymph node metastases and are suitable for endoscopic therapy.

RISK OF LYMPH NODE METASTASES IN T1B

The risk of lymph node metastases in early oesophageal cancer increases with the depth of tumour invasion (Table 7.3) but is also dependent on the presence of additional risk factors. Several studies highlight the reasons for the difference in recommendations based on the presence of (histopathological) features when it comes to management of the disease.[28,30–34]

A recent meta-analysis evaluated 20 Asian studies including 3 983 patients who underwent surgery for early squamous cell carcinoma. The positive lymph node rate was 23% for tumours in sm1, 29% for sm2, and 48% for sm3.[26] Risk factors for lymph node metastases were tumour size > 20 mm, Paris type 0–I and 0–III tumours, poor tumour differentiation, deeper submucosal invasion depth, and LVI. Age, sex, and tumour location were not statistically significant risk factors for the development of lymph node metastases. The association between LVI and lymph node metastases was also reported in a meta-analysis including 4 749 patients with squamous cell carcinoma or adenocarcinoma from 23 studies in the USA, Europe, and Asia from 2000 to 2018 (odds ratio for lymph node metastases of 5.72 for patients with LVI compared to patients without LVI).[35]

In a large retrospective cohort study of 1 283 patients with T1a or T1b adenocarcinomas, a scoring system for the presence of lymph node metastases was developed based on tumour invasion depth, tumour size, and LVI. A subgroup of T1a adenocarcinomas could be defined with a high risk (> 15%) of nodal metastases, occurring in approximately 5% of the T1a tumours. Also a subgroup of T1b adenocarcinomas with low risk (< 5%) of nodal metastases could be defined, occurring in approximately 10% of the T1b tumours.[28] In another internally validated prediction model for T1b adenocarcinomas, the risk to develop lymph node metastases was associated with the presence of LVI, every 500-µm increase in invasion depth and every 10-mm increase in tumour size. Depending on the combination of these factors, lymph node risks ranged between 5.9% and 70%.[36]

Several series that included patients who underwent endoscopic resection have reported lower lymph node metastasis risks for submucosal adenocarcinoma than previously reported in surgical series.[37] In low-risk T1b sm1 adenocarcinomas,

defined as tumours with R0 resection margins after endoscopic resection, with well or moderate tumour differentiation and without LVI, the risk for lymph node metastases was less than 2%,[30,34] whereas high-risk sm1 disease is seen with a rate of 9% lymph node metastasis.[30] In T1b sm2–3 adenocarcinomas, the overall rate of lymph node metastasis is 0–22% for sm2 and 0–36% for sm3.[24,31] In subgroups of low-risk sm2 and low-risk sm3, the positive lymph node rates were 0–8% and 25–29%, respectively. In subgroups of high-risk sm2 and high-risk sm3, the lymph node rates were 28–36% and 37–38%, respectively.[31] In these patients the risk of lymph node metastases clearly exceeded the mortality rate of oesophagectomy, which is estimated to be 1.7–3%.[30,31]

For patients with an T1bN0M0 adenocarcinoma, strict follow-up after endoscopic resection might be a feasible option. In these patients, surgery might be safely postponed until lymph node metastases have been detected during follow-up examinations. This strategy has been investigated in a multicentre, multinational prospective study and the results are pending at the time of writing (PREFER study, NCT03222635).

✓ Step-up therapy with surgery and/or chemoradiotherapy is recommended for patients with a high risk for lymph node metastases with one or more of the following risk factors: poor tumour differentiation, LVI, positive vertical resection margins, or an invasion depth > m3 for squamous cell carcinoma and > m3 or sm1 for adenocarcinoma (Table 7.4).[6,8]

ENDOSCOPIC RESECTION

There are two commonly used methods to remove gastrointestinal neoplastic lesions. The first is endoscopic mucosal resection (EMR) and is based on the principle of creating a 'pseudopolyp' with the use of suction. This 'polyp' can be resected with a snare instrument. The second method is endoscopic submucosal dissection (ESD), in which the mucosa can be carefully dissected with the use of an endoscopic knife. EMR or ESD allow for thorough histopathologic assessment of the resected early cancer with the possibility of avoiding subsequent surgery when the removed lesion is found to be within accepted criteria.

ENDOSCOPIC MUCOSAL RESECTION

The principle of EMR is the removal of a mucosal lesion by resecting it from its deeper layers using a snare instrument (Fig. 7.3). This method does not allow for lesions larger than 2 cm to be removed en bloc.[38] Larger lesions can be removed by EMR, but only in a piecemeal fashion. This technique is fundamentally different from ESD, where the submucosal layer is carefully dissected in a stepwise manner. Using EMR, early neoplasia is often lifted from the proper muscle layer before resection by using different solutions of saline or viscous fluids for submucosal injection.[39–41] The lesions can then be sucked into a cap that is placed at the tip of the endoscope with a snare preloaded into the rim of the cap. After sucking the lesion into the cap, the snare is pulled. The content of the snare is then resected using a high-frequency current. An alternative resection method that is frequently used is the so-called 'band-and-cut' method (video reference: https://youtu.be/WltDtB-fKCUk). A lesion is sucked into a modified multiband ligator,

Table 7.4 Recommendations for management of early oesophageal cancer after initial endoscopic therapy with curative intent according to the ESGE 2015 Guideline[6]

	Fulfils Criteria	Recommendation
Squamous cell carcinoma	sm2 or >200 μm invasion, and/or Lymphovascular invasion, and/or R1 (vertical margins), and/or poor tumour differentiation	Consider chemoradiotherapy and/or surgery
	m1–m2, and en bloc R0, and no lymphovascular invasion	No further definitive treatment necessary
	m3–sm1 (≤200 μm), and en bloc R0, and good tumour differentiation, and no lymphovascular invasion	Curative in majority of cases. Discuss necessity of further treatment in multidisciplinary team
	R1 (horizontal margin), and absence of high-risk criteria	Consider endoscopic surveillance or re-treatment
Adenocarcinoma	>500 μm invasion, and/or lymphovascular invasion, and/or R1 (vertical margins), and/or poor tumour differentiation	Consider chemoradiotherapy and/or surgery
	m1–m3 in Barrett's oesophagus and en bloc R0	Perform subsequent ablative therapy of the residual Barrett's mucosa
	sm1 (≤500 μm), and en bloc R0, and good–moderate tumour differentiation, and no lymphovascular invasion	Curative in majority of cases. Discuss necessity of further treatment in multidisciplinary team. If no chemoradiotherapy and/or surgery is performed, perform ablative therapy of the residual Barrett's mucosa
	R1 (horizontal margin) or piecemeal resection, and absence of high-risk criteria	Endoscopic surveillance or re-treatment preferred over surgery

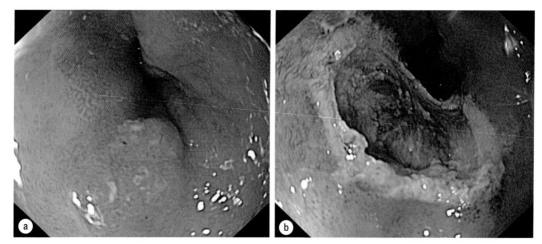

Figure 7.3 Intramucosal carcinoma in a segment of Barrett's epithelium (a) pre-endoscopic mucosal resection and (b) post-endoscopic mucosal resection.

and by ligating the mucosa bearing the lesion, a pseudopolyp is created that can be resected using a snare. This multiple-band mucosectomy allows for larger segments of neoplasia to be completely resected.[42] This method is mostly used in early Barrett's-related cancer but is also applicable in the cardia and antrum of the stomach or the rectum.

ENDOSCOPIC SUBMUCOSAL DISSECTION

ESD was originally developed in Japan for the local treatment of superficial EGC limited to the mucosal layer or with minimal invasion into the submucosal layer. The main goal of submucosal dissection is to retrieve the lesion en bloc for histopathological staging and to minimise the risk of local recurrence. ESD is performed in several steps (Fig. 7.4). First, the lesion is delineated by placing circumferential dots using electrocautery around the lesion, with a few millimetres of free margin. The lesion is then lifted from the proper muscle layer by submucosal injection in the same fashion as in EMR.[39–41] The solutions used are stained with either indigo carmine or methylene blue. This dye will colour the submucosal layer and facilitate recognition of the separate layers and blood vessels. After lifting the lesion, a full circumferential

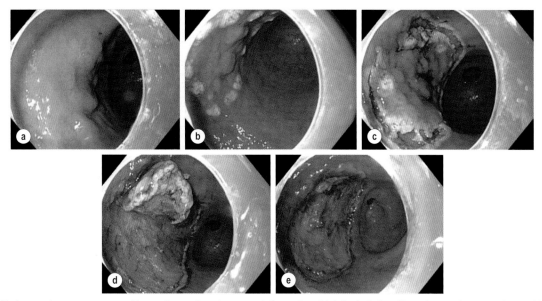

Figure 7.4 Early gastric cancer removed by endoscopic submucosal dissection. (a) A Paris 0–IIc + IIa early gastric cancer located in the antrum. (b–e) Markings are placed around the lesion (b) and after submucosal lifting and circumferential incision (c), the lesion is stepwise dissected (d) and finally fully removed (e). Histopathological assessment demonstrated a well-differentiated adenocarcinoma confined to the mucosal layer with a maximum extent into the muscularis mucosae and tumour-free resection margins.

incision of the mucosal layer is made, placing the markers just inside the circumferential cut. From this point onwards the submucosal layer is carefully dissected from the muscle layer, often with additional submucosal injections. Different approaches have been described using a tunnelled approach underneath the lesion in order to leave the lesion in its anatomical position until the final stage of the resection. This allows for better orientation and overview in the narrow lumen of the oesophagus. After markers have been placed, a distal incision is created first, followed by a proximal incision, and a submucosal tunnel dissection is performed towards the distal incision (video reference: https://youtu.be/OIM3iJ33LR0). The lateral circumference of the lesion is then used as a tether to keep the lesion in place and is cut in the final stage after complete submucosal dissection.

Different speciality knives have been developed for ESD. A breakthrough in ESD was the development of the insulated tip (IT) knife in 1996.[38] An insulated small ceramic sphere is mounted on the top of a high-frequency needle knife, allowing for safe and easy incision and separation of the mucosal and submucosal layers. Subsequently, the design of the original IT knife has been further adapted, leading, for example, to the IT-2 knife, the hook knife, the flex knife, the triangular tip (TT) knife, and the hybrid knife.[43] This hybrid technique combines electrocautery with a distance-dependent water-jet application, allowing for easier, faster, and safer submucosal lifting and cutting in ESD without having to change instruments.[44,45]

ESD is recognised as a challenging procedure reserved for centres with experience in the technique. ESD needs more operator skills, has a much longer learning curve, takes more time, and is more expensive than EMR. Common difficulties for ESD in the oesophagus include working within the tubular structure of the oesophagus and the delineation of neoplastic lesions, the circular cutting, and the stepwise and partial lifting of the lesion in an area with movement from the heartbeat and breathing. Over the last few years, more and more experience has been obtained with ESD in American and European

countries. Results regarding the (oncological) safety of ESD have been reported to comply with quality benchmarks.[46]

EMR VERSUS ESD

For early squamous cell cancer of the oesophagus, the local recurrence rate after endoscopic therapy ranges between 9% and 23% for piecemeal resections.[6] Achieving en bloc resection is therefore important, and they are preferably accomplished with ESD. Since some clinically sm1-staged lesions are overstaged, ESD may be attempted as an initial treatment.[8] EMR may be considered in lesions < 10 mm according to European guidelines.[6]

In early cancer in Barrett's epithelium the aim is complete resection of the lesion, for which EMR is the first treatment option in Western countries, whereas in Japan ESD is always primarily performed. Lesions up to 15 mm can be removed en bloc with EMR. ESD may be considered for larger lesions or lesions suspected of submucosal disease, for example macroscopically depressed lesions or when a non-lifting sign is present.

✔ The Japanese and European Society of Gastrointestinal Endoscopy (ESGE) guidelines recommend ESD as a first option for superficial oesophageal squamous cell cancer to achieve en bloc resection.[6,8] EMR can be considered for squamous cell carcinomas < 10 mm, when an en bloc resection is expected to be achieved.[6]

✔ For mucosal lesions in Barrett's oesophagus, EMR is the preferred choice in Western countries. ESD can be considered for lesions > 15 mm, poorly lifting lesions, and for lesions at risk of submucosal invasion.[6] In Japan, ESD is the preferred technique for superficial adenocarcinomas.[8]

OUTCOMES AFTER EMR AND ESD

A meta-analysis of 16 Asian and Western studies reported an en bloc rate of 97% and an R0 rate of 92% for patients who underwent ESD for squamous cell carcinoma (52% of patients had a tumour invasion depth at m1–2, 43% at m3–sm1, and 4.7% at ≥ sm2).[47] The R0 rate decreased to 78% in lesions with submucosal invasion. The overall local recurrence rate was 1.8% at a minimum of 3 years of follow-up.

For superficial adenocarcinoma, a systematic review reported that ESD achieved higher en bloc resections than EMR (96% versus 50%, respectively) and higher R0 rates (82% versus 40%, respectively).[8] At a mean follow-up of 2.8 years for patients treated with ESD and 4.2 years for patients treated with EMR, the local recurrence rates of adenocarcinomas were 2.5% with ESD and 12% with EMR.[8] However, local recurrences can usually be treated with redo EMR with good outcomes and comparable tumour-related survival.[48]

COMPLICATIONS AFTER EMR AND ESD

Strictures after EMR and ESD mainly occur in the narrower parts of the gastrointestinal tract such as the oesophagus, gastric cardia, and pyloric region. Stricture formation is seen more frequently with circumferential resections or large size perimeters and is induced through ulcer scar healing. These strictures are relatively easy to treat with balloon dilatation, with the exception of strictures after circumferential ESD, which can prove quite difficult to treat because of severe scar fibrosis. In the Japanese guidelines, ESD for whole-circumferential lesions is only recommended when the longitudinal length is ≤ 50 mm.[8] Apart from stricture formation, post-procedural bleeding occurs with ESD and EMR in approximately 0.9–3%, and perforation rates are seen in approximately 1.5% with ESD and 0.4% with EMR.[8,47] Most of these complications can be treated endoscopically or conservatively.

MUCOSAL ABLATION

In the remaining untreated segment of Barrett's oesophagus, recurrence of metachronous neoplastic lesions is seen in 11–30% of patients within 3 years after endoscopic treatment of the primary neoplasm.[48-50] Western guidelines recommend subsequent ablation of the Barrett's oesophagus after curative endoscopic treatment for high-grade dysplasia or adenocarcinoma. Radiofrequency ablation (RFA) is the first-choice ablation technique.[19,20,51] The role of mucosal ablation in the squamous epithelium is less evident and is therefore not recommended.

RFA can be performed with a balloon-based radiofrequency device that ablates the mucosa of the tubular oesophagus to the submucosa (circumferential ablation). With a focal RFA catheter, limited mucosal areas can be treated (video reference: https://youtu.be/d_O_nN5zu4w). Focal RFA is often used to eradicate the residual Barrett's mucosa after initial (circumferential) ablation, which usually requires multiple procedures. The most common complication after RFA is an oesophageal stricture, which occurs in approximately 5% of patients and is associated with a longer length of ablated mucosa and previous EMR.[52,53] Common symptoms after RFA are chest pain and odynophagia, which usually resolve after a week. Complete eradication of dysplasia or intramucosal carcinoma is seen in 84–95% of patients.[52-55] Long-term data of a prospective database of nine Dutch Barrett Expert Centres have shown that after successful endoscopic resection and RFA, the annual incidence of recurrence of high-grade dysplasia or adenocarcinoma was 0.8%.[55] Three-monthly follow-up visits within the first year after treatment were not associated with improved outcomes. Yearly surveillance is therefore recommended after successful eradication of the neoplastic lesion.

Other ablation techniques include argon plasma coagulation (APC) and cryotherapy, which are not as frequently used since RFA has become the mainstay technique. APC therapy eradicates the mucosa to a variable depth and usually multiple procedures are required. A randomised trial on the use of APC in patients with high-grade dysplasia or mucosal carcinoma in Barrett's epithelium has shown that APC decreases recurrences in comparison to patients who underwent surveillance, with a recurrence rate for neoplasia of 3.0% versus 37%, respectively.[56] A systematic review and meta-analysis of 405 patients with a median follow-up of 22 months reported a comparable efficacy of cryotherapy compared to RFA. The complete eradication rate of dysplasia was 85%. Oesophageal strictures occurred in 7% and post-procedural pain in 3%. Recurrences of high-grade dysplasia were seen in 18%.[57]

Omission of subsequent ablation therapy after endoscopic resection has been suggested for selected patients. A retrospective cohort study analysed 94 patients who underwent endoscopic surveillance after endoscopic resection for low-grade dysplasia, high-grade dysplasia, or low-risk adenocarcinoma and refused ablation because of comorbidity or old age. In 18% of patients progression was seen to high-grade dysplasia or adenocarcinoma, but all cases were amenable to curative endoscopic treatment.[58]

After curative endoscopic treatment for early squamous cell carcinoma, a regular follow-up protocol with high-resolution endoscopy, (virtual) chromoendoscopy, and targeted biopsies of suspect areas should be performed.

✔ To detect occurrence of metachronous oesophageal cancer, surveillance is recommended after endoscopic treatment for squamous cell carcinoma or adenocarcinoma at least once a year according to the Japanese guideline.[8] The ESGE guideline recommends surveillance with endoscopy at 3–6 months after endoscopic resection of squamous cell carcinoma followed by annual surveillance.

✔ In Western countries RFA is recommended after endoscopic resection for early neoplasia in Barrett's oesophagus. When complete eradication is achieved, yearly surveillance is recommended.[55] More frequent follow-up visits in the first year are not associated with improved outcomes.

SURGICAL RESECTION

OESOPHAGECTOMY

Oesophagectomy with extensive lymphadenectomy is considered as the definite treatment for patients with a non-curative endoscopic resection and/or high-risk criteria for lymph node metastases. Oesophagectomy should be considered based on patients' preference, taking into account the willingness to commit to endoscopic surveillance after endoscopic therapy (followed by subsequent endoscopic therapy if needed), and is considered for patients with the presence of multifocal disease, long-segment neoplasia, or impaired oesophageal function such as achalasia or dysphagia.[59]

The advantage of complete removal of the primary tumour and lymph nodes provided by surgery must be weighed against the potential mortality and morbidity of the procedure and the loss in long-term quality of life. Five-year overall survival of patients undergoing oesophagectomy and lymphadenectomy after non-curative endoscopic resection of cT1 adenocarcinoma or squamous cell carcinoma ranged from 83% to 100%, as reported in several retrospective studies.[60] The operative mortality for oesophagectomy in high-volume centres is 1–3%, which is better compared to low-volume hospitals.[20,61]

Oesophagectomy does have a long-lasting effect on the quality of life of patients. Two-thirds of patients who are disease free at least 1 year after oesophagectomy experience symptoms related to the surgery.[62] Most prevalent long-lasting symptoms include a feeling of early fullness after eating (79%), reduced energy or activity tolerance (73%), tiredness (71%), heartburn (71%), and bloating (60%). Based on another large patient cohort from a prospective trial, fatigue and decreased physical functioning do not seem to restore to pre-treatment levels at more than 6 years postoperatively, regardless of whether patients underwent neoadjuvant treatment or not.[63]

LIMITED RESECTIONS

Because of the associated high morbidity, mortality, and postoperative decreased quality of life, alternatives to a traditional oesophagectomy with lymphadenectomy have been explored. For limited surgical procedures to be successful, a degree of predictability of the lymph node drainage is required. For pT1 tumours, in one study patients with adenocarcinoma had the majority of positive nodes below the tracheal bifurcation, locally associated with the primary cancer in all but 2% of patients.[64] For squamous cell carcinoma the nodal site was less predictable, with the positive nodes widely distributed in the chest and upper abdomen.

For early adenocarcinoma, technical variations for resection of the diseased segment have been attempted. Two variations which have been described for patients with Barrett's high-grade dysplasia and intramucosal carcinoma are a limited resection of the oesophagogastric junction[65] and vagal-sparing oesophagectomy.[66,67] These patients carry a minimal risk for occurrence of lymph node metastases and lymphadenectomy can be omitted. The resection of the oesophagogastric junction with jejunal interposition (Merendino operation) is performed using a transabdominal approach, with splitting of the oesophageal hiatus to access the lower oesophagus. The dissection can be carried out through the diaphragmatic hiatus to the level of the tracheal bifurcation, incorporating a lower mediastinal and upper abdominal lymphadenectomy with or without preservation of the vagal innervation of the distal stomach. Following resection of the distal oesophagus, cardia, and proximal stomach, gastrointestinal continuity is restored by means of interposition of an isoperistaltic, pedicled jejunal loop to prevent postoperative reflux (Fig. 7.5).[65] The outcome of over 80 procedures for early Barrett's cancer was reported to be similar in terms of long-term survival compared with a radical oesophagectomy. The advantages were lower peri- and postoperative morbidity and a good postoperative quality of life. The procedure has been reported to be technically challenging to achieve good long-term functional results.[65]

A vagal-sparing oesophagectomy has been described for resection in patients with high-grade dysplasia and intramucosal adenocarcinoma of the lower oesophagus.[66,67] A gastric tube or colon pull-up is used for reconstruction. Fewer postoperative complications have been reported in comparison with transhiatal or en bloc resections (35% versus 56% and 76%, respectively).[66] Although there was a reduction in postvagotomy symptoms such as diarrhoea and dumping, these were not abolished.

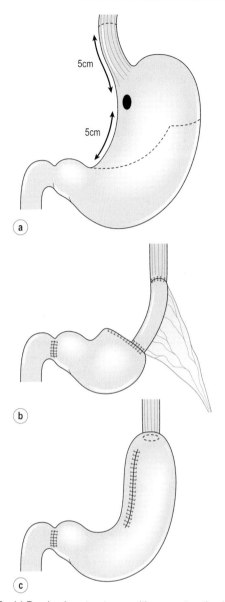

Figure 7.5 (a) Proximal gastrectomy, with reconstruction by (b) jejunal interposition or (c) gastric tube.

The transhiatal approach for oesophagectomy has been reported to reduce respiratory complications compared with transthoracic oesophagectomy with extended en bloc lymphadenectomy.[68] Although suitable for adenocarcinoma, the transhiatal approach does not address the issue of unpredictable lymphatic drainage of distally located squamous cell carcinoma. A systematic lymphadenectomy should therefore be performed with the benefits of a cervical and upper mediastinal lymphadenectomy being weighed against the added morbidity in this group.[64,69]

Minimally invasive oesophagectomy aims to reduce the trauma of the abdominal and/or thoracic incisions. A randomised controlled trial (RCT) comparing an double open approach to a combined thoracoscopic oesophageal mobilisation and a laparoscopic approach for gastric mobilisation reported a significant reduction in respiratory complications from the minimally invasive approach.[70] This was also the case in a comparative study examining open surgery with a hybrid approach consisting of a laparoscopic abdominal gastric mobilisation and an open thoracotomy.[71] There does not appear to be any detrimental oncological impact to using the minimally invasive approaches, compared with an open resection for invasive cancer, with a meta-analysis, including studies from the East and the West, reporting no difference in 1- to 5-year cancer survival.[72]

✅ Resection offers the most definitive treatment aimed at cure for early oesophageal neoplasia, taking away the need for long-term endoscopic surveillance. However, surgery has the potential for mortality and unpredictable effects on short- and long-term quality of life.

SENTINEL NODE BIOPSY

In breast cancer and melanoma surgery, sentinel lymph node biopsy (SLNB) has proven to be a valuable tool in lymph node mapping, with a sensitivity of more than 95%. When SLNB is negative in these tumours, lymphadenectomy can safely be omitted. The clinical application of SLNB in early oesophageal cancer is still considered experimental. SLNB in oesophageal cancer has a 17% higher detection rate for T1–T2 tumours (95%) compared with T3–T4 staged tumours, as was reported in a meta-analysis. For all T stages, the sensitivity was higher for adenocarcinomas.[73]

A pilot study has evaluated the feasibility of thoracolaparoscopic lymphadenectomy without oesophagectomy after endoscopic resection in patients with cT1N0M0 adenocarcinoma.[74] In this study, five patients first underwent lymph node dissection, followed by oesophagectomy in the same session. A median of 30 lymph nodes were removed per patient, but a median of 6 lymph nodes, most smaller than 5 mm, were found in the oesophagectomy specimen and thus had been retained during the lymph node dissection. In one patient discolouration of the oesophagus during two-field lymph node dissection occurred. Vascularisation during the procedure might have been compromised, which indicates a possible risk of lymph node dissection without oesophagectomy. A similar phenomenon has also been observed in a case series of patients with locally advanced oesophageal cancer.[75] In these patients the mobilised oesophagus was left in situ even when distant disease was detected at a relatively late phase of the procedure. Fatal adverse events occurred in one-third of patients. On the other hand, in more than half of the patients, leaving the mobilised oesophagus in situ was not accompanied by serious complications.

In a second phase of the pilot study, the feasibility of sentinel node navigation surgery (SNNS) was evaluated in five patients with cT1N0M0 adenocarcinoma who had undergone radical endoscopic resection and had an indication for subsequent surgery.[74] Prior to surgery, patients underwent SPECT/CT with the tracer technetium-99m. During surgery, the sentinel nodes (SNs) were identified using a gamma probe. Following removal of the SNs, lymphadenectomy was performed. In all patients at least one sentinel lymph node could be resected and none of the resected SNs contained micrometastases. In future, SNNS might become an option for patients who have a high risk of lymph node metastases after endoscopic resection of early adenocarcinoma of the oesophagus, but the effectiveness of this approach currently remains a topic of research.

ENDOSCOPIC TREATMENT VERSUS SURGERY IN PATIENTS WITH EARLY SQUAMOUS CELL CARCINOMA

Only retrospective studies have been conducted reporting outcomes of endoscopic resection in comparison to oesophagectomy. A systematic review and meta-analysis of retrospective studies between 2010 and 2019, most from East Asian countries and a few from Europe, reported comparable long-term outcomes for treatment with ESD or surgery for patients with squamous cell carcinomas up to T1-sm2.[47] The R0 rate was higher in patients treated with oesophagectomy (97%) compared to patients who underwent ESD (90%). The 5-year overall survival rate was comparable between the two treatments: 86% for ESD and 82% with oesophagectomy, as well as 5-year disease-specific survival (ESD: 98%, oesophagectomy: 94%). Metachronous recurrences were more often seen with ESD (7.4% versus 0% with oesophagectomy). ESD was associated with fewer post-procedural complications, most of which could be managed immediately, and with a shorter hospital stay.

ENDOSCOPIC TREATMENT VERSUS SURGERY IN PATIENTS WITH EARLY ADENOCARCINOMA

A Cochrane review has been conducted on this topic but no RCTs were identified that compared endoscopic treatment versus surgery for early neoplasia in Barrett's oesophagus.[76] The review described multiple retrospective studies but concluded that high-quality evidence could not be provided. The risk of selection bias was considerable, since in these time periods endoscopic therapy has been mostly offered to patients who were unfit for surgery. Also the use of RFA had not yet been adopted as part of standard treatment in most of the studies.

Some evidence may be provided from matched cohort studies. One comparative retrospective matched cohort study reported treatment outcomes for patients with mucosal adenocarcinoma treated with endoscopic treatment followed by APC ($n = 76$) versus treatment with surgery ($n = 38$). The recurrence rate was 6.6% in the endoscopic resection cohort and 0% in the surgery group after a median follow-up of 4 years. Endoscopic treatment was possible for the patients with a recurrence after endoscopic resection and a complete remission rate of 98.7% could be achieved. A complete remission rate of 100% was observed in the surgery group. The mortality rate and major complication rate was 0% after endoscopic resection, whereas after surgery major complications were seen in 32% and the 90-day mortality was 2.6%.[77]

A recently published population-based study reported outcomes for patients who underwent endoscopic resection or oesophagectomy for T1a or T1b small-sized (≤ 2 cm) oesophageal cancer after propensity score matching.[78] The propensity score-matched groups included 217 patients in each group; 89% of whom were patients with adenocarcinomas. Among patients with T1a carcinomas, overall survival was not different (78% with endoscopic therapy and 80% with surgery). For patients with T1b carcinomas, overall survival was better in the oesophagectomy group (79%) than in the endoscopic therapy group (45%). However, data on differences in patient comorbidities were not available and the survival difference may be (partly) attributed to selection bias.

ALTERNATIVES TO OESOPHAGECTOMY

ADDITIONAL CHEMORADIOTHERAPY AFTER ENDOSCOPIC RESECTION

Several small and retrospective studies, most including patients with squamous cell carcinomas, have investigated the possibility of chemoradiotherapy after non-curative endoscopic resection or en bloc resection with high-risk criteria for lymph node metastases. Overall survival ranged between 67% and 100% after a median follow-up of 2–5 years, and grade 3–4 serious adverse events were seen up to 25%.[79]

The Japanese prospective single-arm JCOG0508 trial investigated the efficacy and safety of selective adjuvant chemoradiotherapy after endoscopic resection with ESD or EMR in 83 patients with pT1b (sm1–2) tumours or pT1a tumours with LVI.[80] Chemoradiotherapy comprised 41.1 Gy in 23 fractions delivered to the locoregional lymph nodes combined with 5-fluorouracil (5-FU) on days 1–4 and 29–32, and cisplatin on days 1 and 29. In the group that received selective adjuvant therapy, 3-year overall survival was 91% (90% CI 84–95%). Since the survival rate was equivalent to treatment with surgery and no severe adverse events were reported, the authors concluded that adjuvant chemoradiotherapy after endoscopic resection for selected patients is a suitable, less invasive, alternative treatment option to oesophagectomy.

Another RCT has been initiated in China comparing oesophagectomy with definitive chemoradiotherapy consisting of cisplatin, 5-FU, and 60.2 Gy radiotherapy in patients with cN0-pT1b squamous cell carcinoma after ESD.[81] The trial is expected to be completed in 2027.

DEFINITIVE CHEMORADIOTHERAPY AS A PRIMARY TREATMENT OPTION

Definitive chemoradiotherapy can be considered when patients are unfit for resection or refuse an operation. A Japanese prospective non-inferiority trial has been conducted to compare oesophagectomy with chemoradiotherapy in patients with cT1bN0M0 squamous cell carcinoma (JCOG0502 trial).[82] Few patients accepted randomisation and therefore the majority of patients were included in the preference arms for either surgery or definitive chemoradiotherapy consisting of cisplatin, 5-FU, and 60 Gy radiotherapy given concurrently. In these study arms, 3-year overall survival was 94.7% for the 209 patients undergoing surgery and 93.1% for the 159 patients undergoing definitive chemoradiotherapy. The 5-year overall survival rate was 86.5% and 85.5%, respectively. The authors concluded that definite chemoradiotherapy showed a trend towards non-inferiority and should be considered as a treatment option for this patient group.

In several case series, definitive chemoradiotherapy as a primary treatment for cT1N0M0 squamous cell carcinoma has been reported to achieve a clinically complete response in approximately 90%, but local recurrences are common.[83–87] For those patients salvage may be possible with salvage surgery or salvage endoscopic resection. Salvage endoscopic resection after definitive chemoradiotherapy for patients with squamous and adenocarcinomas (cT1–3 and any N stage) has been reported to be technically feasible by European and American gastroenterologists.[88]

The data relating to the use of radiotherapy (without chemotherapy) for early adenocarcinoma of the oesophagus are not clear. This modality is an option of patients not suitable for surgery but who are considered suitable candidates for a definitive therapy. This is particularly the case if patients are considered high risk for residual primary disease or localised lymph node metastases.

ROLE OF A MULTIDISCIPLINARY TEAM

Because of the evidence for multimodality therapy in patients with locally advanced oesophageal cancer, management decisions are now typically made in a multidisciplinary setting, including the surgical oncologist, radiation oncologist, and medical oncologist. It is clear that for early oesophageal cancer the management discussions should also include an interventional endoscopist, allowing all the alternatives for therapy to be considered in the same multidisciplinary, collaborative environment. For endoscopic therapies, the better neoplasia eradication figures and procedural outcomes will probably be optimal in centres that have a specific interest in this problem with specialist interventional endoscopists who have strict follow-up endoscopy protocols in a multidisciplinary environment.

B. EARLY GASTRIC CANCER

RISK AND DEVELOPMENT OF EARLY GASTRIC CANCER

In the Western world the incidence of gastric cancer has steadily declined over many decades, yet worldwide it remains one of the most common malignancies. Most gastric cancers arise as a result of lifelong colonisation with *Helicobacter pylori*, which induces chronic active gastritis. An abundance of research over the past 20 years has yielded endoscopic and non-invasive methods to recognise not only this infection but also the various stages of the cascade leading from chronic gastritis via atrophic gastritis, intestinal metaplasia, and dysplasia to early and advanced gastric cancer. Cohort studies have revealed that the cancer risk increases with each step of the cascade.[89] Gastric cancer and thus EGC has a higher incidence in Japan and Korea. This part of the chapter deals with the management of EGC.

CLASSIFICATION OF EARLY GASTRIC CANCER

EGC usually arises in a mucosa that has undergone atrophic and metaplastic changes. These are recognisable with modern high-definition endoscopic equipment, in particular when combined with additional image-enhancement techniques, such as NBI. Against this background, most EGCs amenable for endoscopic resection can be recognised by experienced endoscopists.[90] Complete staging and classification of EGCs are usually done in three steps. The first step is a pre-interventional endoscopy. The endoscopic appearance and diameter of the tumour is determined, combined with histopathological sampling. The value of endosonography is limited.[91] The second step is the actual endoscopic resection, where the most valuable information is gathered from the submucosal lifting properties of the lesion. The third step is the final histopathological staging of the resected lesion. The resection of the lesion can be seen as a staging step with a potentially curative intent.

ENDOSCOPIC APPEARANCE

Experienced endoscopists performing EMRs or ESDs are trained to recognise and delineate early neoplasia, which includes assessment of invasion depth and thus the endoscopic resectability of the lesion.

Similarly to the oesophagus, early gastric superficial lesions are classified according to the Paris classification (Table 7.1 and see Fig. 7.2). Endoscopic staging before resection does provide useful information on the prediction of lymph node metastases. For instance, truly protruding lesions in the stomach demonstrate a 57% relative frequency of submucosal invasion, whereas non-protruding, non-excavated lesions demonstrate submucosal invasion in frequencies between 20% and 40%. In excavated lesions, often the proper muscle layer is already involved. Although the exact percentage of involvement of the muscle layer is not reported in the literature, this number comes close to 100% and the Paris 0–III excavated types of lesions are usually not resectable by endoscopic means. Also, lesions that do not show movement with peristalsis and/or have a non-lifting sign, as described previously in this chapter, are contraindicated for endoscopic resection. Other characteristics that predict submucosal or deeper invasion in the stomach are larger tumour size (> 30 mm), presence of discolouration (remarkable redness), and ulceration.[90] Additionally, tumour differentiation grade can be assessed through simple biopsy.

✔ Traditionally only well to moderately differentiated tumours up to 20 mm were amendable for endoscopic resection; however, a large Japanese study showed that these traditional indication guidelines were too strict.[92] A cut-off of ≤ 30 mm is now defined as amenable for endoscopic resection.[93]

The aforementioned Japanese retrospective cohort study assessed the occurrence of lymph node metastases in 5 265 patients who had undergone gastrectomy with lymph node dissection for EGC.[92] All specimens were reassessed for macroscopic appearance, size, ulceration, invasion depth and extent of submucosal invasion, differentiation grade, and lymphovascular involvement. The results are summarised in Table 7.5 and define the groups of patients who can be treated with EMR and ESD.[92,94]

Because undifferentiated tumours carry a high risk of lymph node metastases, these tumours have not been indicated for endoscopic resection (Table 7.5). Recently, the Japanese prospective JCOG1009/1010 trial has investigated whether undifferentiated cT1a EGCs, ≤ 2 cm and no LVI or ulceration might be amenable to endoscopic resection.[95]

In 275 patients meeting these criteria, curative ESD, requiring no additional treatment, was achieved in 71%. In this group no recurrences were seen during follow-up. Patients with non-curative ESD underwent additional gastrectomy. In the cohort of 275 patients 5-year overall survival was 99%. These criteria have not yet been included in the current guidelines, but are already considered as extended criteria for ESD in the fifth edition of the Japanese guidelines for gastric cancer.[96]

ENDOSONOGRAPHY

The role of endosonography remains debatable in EGCs. Endosonography lacks sufficient diagnostic accuracy in discriminating T1 from T2 lesions. The combined results of two large studies show a diagnostic accuracy for T3 and T4 tumours of 88–100%, with 64–85% accuracy for T2 lesions and 75–82% accuracy for T1 tumours.[97,98] T1 lesions are often overstaged, probably because of submucosal fibrosis, connective tissue hyperplasia, or ulceration. Diagnostic accuracy can be improved using mini-probes; however, complete assessment of larger lesions is difficult and bears the risk of underestimating the deepest invasion when parts of the lesion are missed and subsequently not assessed.[99] A German study assessing infiltration depth in early neoplasia of the oesophagus[91] demonstrated a similar diagnostic accuracy of 83.4% and 79.6% using either high-resolution endoscopy or endosonography, respectively. The authors believe the same applies for early neoplasia in the stomach. The accuracy in submucosal tumours is only around 50%.[91] For these reasons, many endoscopists rely on endoscopic assessment alone followed by histopathological assessment of the endoscopically resected specimen.

✔ Conventional endoscopic assessment of depth of infiltration in EGC has a similar accuracy compared to endosonography. For this reason, most experienced interventional endoscopists rely on endoscopic assessment and do not routinely perform endosonography before proceeding to EMR or ESD.

Hence, the resection of the lesion can be seen as a staging step with potentially curative intent and gives all the information necessary for accurate staging and further treatment planning when the lesion has progressed beyond the accepted criteria for endoscopic resection (differentiation, size, tumour depth, radicality, LVI).

Table 7.5 Criteria for endoscopic mucosal resection and endoscopic submucosal dissection for early gastric cancer, according to the proposed guidelines

Depth	Mucosal Cancer				Submucosal Cancer	
	No ulcer		Ulcer		sm1	sm2
Differentiation	≤20 mm	>20 mm	≤30 mm	>30 mm	≤30 mm	Any size
Good/moderate	EMR	ESD	ESD	S	ESD	S
Poor/undifferentiated	CS	S	S	S	S	S

CS, Consider surgery; EMR, suitable for endoscopic mucosal resection; ESD, suitable for endoscopic submucosal dissection; S, surgery; sm1, superficial submucosal layer; sm2, middle submucosal layer.

ENDOSCOPIC RESECTION

Endoscopic removal of EGC can be performed using EMR or ESD. These techniques have been previously described in this chapter. In Fig. 7.4 an example of a Paris 0–IIa + IIc lesion is shown, which is subsequently removed by ESD.

Factors related to technical difficulty with ESD for EGC have been addressed in a post hoc analysis of the JCOG0607 trial.[100] 'Difficult cases' were defined as ESD procedures taking longer than 120 minutes, occurrence of piecemeal resection, or perforation. Factors associated with technical difficulty were non-ulcerated tumours larger than 3 cm in size, location in the upper or middle part of the stomach, and age of the patient 60 years or younger.

ENDOSCOPIC TREATMENT VERSUS SURGERY

There are three observational studies describing EMR versus surgery, and five studies describing ESD versus surgery. All studies were from Asian countries. There are no large randomised trials. The quality of the data is therefore poor, but studies do not show statistically significant differences in survival nor in locoregional recurrences.

COMPLETE RESECTIONS

The aim of both EMR and ESD is to strive for complete resection of the neoplastic lesion.[101] In theory, using the ESD technique, lesions of all sizes can be removed. However, attempts at curative resection are limited by a number of anatomical factors that relate to the primary lesion. These factors are related to the relative frequencies of lymph node metastases, as described earlier in this chapter.

Larger lesions, poorer differentiation, or deeper penetration in the submucosal layer are associated with a rapidly increasing incidence of lymph node metastases. Routinely, after endoscopic resection, the resected specimens are stretched and pinned on cork or paraffin and sent for pathological assessment. This final staging step by the pathologist should provide the necessary information on 1) quantitative criteria (lateral margins, deeper margins, maximum extent of submucosal invasion) and 2) qualitative criteria (differentiation grade, lymphovascular involvement), which correspond with the risk of lymph node metastases.[92] This ultimate information is pivotal for further management. It mandates additional surgery or allows for a surveillance policy.

Because of an approximately 14% risk of metachronous gastric cancer over a 5-year period[102] and possible remnant neoplastic tissue, surveillance is usually carried out after endoscopic resection at 6-month intervals during the first year, followed by annual surveillance thereafter. Early detection of metachronous neoplasia can be treated by repeated endoscopic resection.

COMPLICATIONS OF ENDOSCOPIC RESECTIONS

Endoscopic treatment is now accepted worldwide for early gastrointestinal neoplasia as it replaces the need for major surgery associated with considerable morbidity and mortality. Endoscopic treatment is also superior in terms of postprocedural functional results. The obvious example is the avoidance of gastrectomy by endoscopic resection of an early neoplastic lesion. However, these novel endoscopic techniques also come with a risk of complications, ranging from bleeding and perforation to post-treatment strictures and, potentially, leading to considerable morbidity and even mortality. Most bleeding complications occur during the procedures and can be dealt with instantly. Superficial bleeding vessels are identified and treated either by using coagulation, adrenaline injections, or clips. Delayed bleeding also occurs and might necessitate subsequent re-intervention. A large prospective study found no risk factors for bleeding besides the presence of a gastric malignancy itself.[103] In expert hands, perforations occur during EMR and ESD in about 0.2% and 1–4% of cases, respectively. In Europe higher incidences of perforations after ESD are found (up to 20%).[104] This clearly demonstrates a difference in expertise in some Western referral centres compared to Japanese and Korean expert centres. This is mostly due to a much lower incidence of EGCs in the Western world, resulting in an insufficient exposure to this type of pathology and resection techniques. A panel of European experts has attempted to set standards regarding quality criteria for ESD in European countries.[105] Perforations can lead to pneumoperitoneum and in severe cases to generalised peritonitis. Usually, perforations are recognised immediately during the procedure and endoscopic management is possible and frequently adequate.[106] Closure with clips is a safe treatment option together with nasogastric drainage and fasting.[107] Advanced closure methods such as over-the-scope clips (OTSCs) have been introduced for closure of perforations. The OTSC device is a promising tool that can potentially close defects up to approximately 2 cm in size.[108]

ENDOSCOPIC MUCOSAL RESECTION VERSUS ENDOSCOPIC SUBMUCOSAL DISSECTION

In a recent meta-analysis, the data of 10 retrospective studies were pooled.[109] Some 4 328 lesions, 1 916 in the ESD and 2 412 in the EMR group, were pooled and analysed. The mean intervention time was longer for ESD than for EMR and the en bloc and histologically complete resection rates were significantly higher in the ESD group. As a consequence of its higher radicality rate, ESD provided lower recurrence rates. However, the perforation rate was significantly higher after ESD. Bleeding incidences did not differ between the two techniques.

✔ The 2015 ESGE guideline recommends ESD as a first treatment option for all EGCs with an exception only for small (< 10 mm) Paris 0–IIa lesions. In these small lesions an EMR could be considered.[6]

SURGICAL RESECTION

When local endoscopic procedures are not possible (too large) or other risk factors (submucosal invasion (sm1) > 500 μm, LVI, undifferentiated histology, large tumour size, and a tumour-involved vertical margin) for lymph node dissemination are present, surgery is recommended. The type of gastrectomy and extent of lymphadenectomy for EGC depend on the location of the tumour. In general, a total gastrectomy is performed for tumours in the middle and upper third of the stomach and a distal gastrectomy for tumours in the distal third. Operations can be performed via laparotomy or laparoscopy. Although cases with intra-abdominal adhesions after ESD have been described, a recent study with more than 1 700 patients showed no effect on short-term surgical outcomes during and after an additional laparoscopic gastrectomy.[110]

Before EMR and ESD were developed, the low recurrence rates and high 5-year survival rates of EGC have led to the development of less invasive gastric surgery, since formal gastric resection with lymphadenectomy is associated with significant morbidity and mortality. In Japan and Korea proximal gastrectomy for EGC in the upper third of the stomach and pylorus-preserving gastrectomy (PPG) for EGC in the middle portion of the stomach are well-accepted procedures. Segmental or local gastric resections with or without lymphadenectomy have been described for gastric tumours, but still have to be considered experimental. With increased experience with EMR and ESD, these procedures will hardly be necessary (hence a formal gastrectomy and lymphadenectomy should be performed only for high-risk lesions). However, when EMR/ESD is not available or technically not feasible, these procedures might be considered.

PROXIMAL GASTRECTOMY

Total gastrectomy with D1 or D2 lymphadenectomy is still the standard treatment for tumours in the upper third of the stomach. This type of resection is associated with the postgastrectomy syndrome, including dumping, epigastric pain, diarrhoea, hypoglycaemia, malnutrition, and anaemia. As nodal metastases in the distal gastric lymph nodes (stations 5 and 6) are rare in EGC of the proximal stomach, fewer extensive resections have been proposed. Proximal gastrectomy (see Fig. 7.5a) was developed as an alternative to total gastrectomy in order to reduce the long-term postoperative problems without compromising the oncological outcome. In proximal gastrectomy the proximal half of the stomach is resected, including a D1 or D1 + lymphadenectomy.[111] Several techniques for surgical reconstruction after proximal gastrectomy have been described, including reconstruction by jejunal interposition (to prevent severe gastro-oesophageal reflux and a gastric tube (see Fig. 7.5b,c), but the optimal method remains controversial. As could be expected due to the relatively high incidence of EGC in the East, most studies on proximal gastrectomy are from Japan and Korea,[112–114] while data from Western countries are scarce.[115] These studies have shown that proximal gastrectomy for upper EGC is a safe procedure with comparable 5-year survival rates. However, conflicting data have been reported on the long-term complications and quality of life. Some studies showed an improved clinical outcome after proximal gastrectomy with oesophagogastrostomy or jejunal interposition, while others report a markedly higher complication rate including anastomotic stenosis and reflux oesophagitis. Therefore, further evaluation on this type of gastric resection for proximal EGC is needed. As yet, randomised data are not available and it is unlikely that these studies will be performed with further development of ESD and EMR techniques.

PYLORUS-PRESERVING GASTRECTOMY

PPG is a function-preserving procedure initially described for the treatment of peptic ulcer disease[116] (Fig. 7.6). For patients with EGC, favourable functional results have been reported with PPG compared to conventional distal gastrectomy. In contrast to conventional distal or total gastrectomy, the suprapyloric (second-tier) lymph nodes are not resected in PPG. In

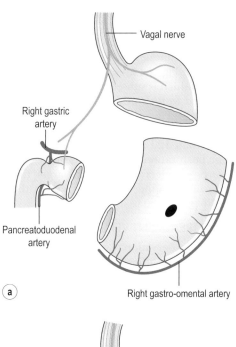

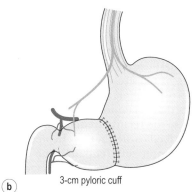

Figure 7.6 Pylorus-preserving gastrectomy, preserving the right gastric artery and the pyloric branch of the vagal nerve (a) and retaining a 3-cm pyloric cuff (b).

EGC this is probably justified, as 80–90% of EGCs are negative for lymph node metastases and the vast majority of positive lymph nodes are located in the first-tier lymph nodes only. Retrospective data of a Japanese database of 3 646 T1 tumours located in the middle third of the stomach showed only 0.2% metastases to the pyloric lymph nodes.[117] PPG is feasible for early tumours in the middle third of the stomach with the distal border at least 4 cm proximal to the pylorus. In PPG a distal gastrectomy is performed with preservation of the pylorus and both the right gastric artery and the pyloric branch of the vagal nerve, followed by a stomach-to-stomach anastomosis.[116] As a result, it is assumed that the pyloric function remains intact, preventing gastrointestinal symptoms such as dumping syndrome, epigastric fullness, reflux oesophagitis, bile regurgitation, and cholelithiasis.[118] There is one small, randomised trial comparing 81 patients with EGC.[118] They underwent either PPG or conventional gastrectomy, and there were no differences in early results. The incidence of early dumping syndrome was lower in PPG (8%) than in the conventional gastrectomy group (33%). Other late results including the incidence of gallstones were not different between the two groups.

High 5-year survival rates up to 98% have been reported after PPG with modified D2 lymph node dissection in patients with clinically diagnosed mucosal or submucosal gastric cancer (cT1) without lymph node metastases (cN0).[119] Similar to studies on proximal gastrectomy, most data on PPG are derived from studies done in Japan and Korea. An ongoing Korean multicentre RCT (KLASS-04), which compares laparoscopic PPG with laparoscopy-assisted distal gastrectomy for EGC in the middle-third of the stomach, may provide more clear evidence about the advantages and oncologic safety of PPG. In Western countries PPG is still considered investigational.

LOCAL (OR WEDGE) SEGMENTAL RESECTION

Local or wedge resection involves removal of only the tumour including the nearby lymph nodes and primary closure of the stomach (Fig. 7.7). In a segmental resection a limited segment between the lesser and the greater curvature of the stomach is resected, including the nearby lymph nodes, and a formal gastro-gastrostomy is performed (Fig. 7.8). Local and segmental gastric resections for (early) gastric cancer have the obvious potential advantage of a better functional postoperative outcome because digestive and reservoir functions of the stomach are mostly preserved. Several small studies show superior results on nutritional status and the incidence of dumping and reflux oesophagitis after local or segmental resection compared to a total or distal gastrectomy.[120–123] These procedures can be safely performed in EGC with favourable features that cannot be resected by EMR or ESD for technical reasons. As mentioned previously, the likelihood of lymph node metastases in these patients is very low and local or segmental resection with a limited lymphadenectomy seems justified. For EGC with unfavourable features local or segmental resection with only limited lymphadenectomy is still investigational. In these patients the risk of lymph node metastases and local recurrence is relatively high and no clear evidence exists that similar recurrence and survival rates can be achieved compared to standard gastric resections.

MINIMALLY INVASIVE SURGERY

Over the past decade there has been a notable trend towards laparoscopic or laparoscopically assisted surgery for EGC, especially in Japan and Korea. Minimally invasive surgery is regarded as an alternative to conventional open surgery in gastric cancer.[124] Several large Japanese and Korean RCTs on laparoscopic versus open surgery have been conducted.[124,125]

✔✔A meta-analysis including 3 411 patients showed that laparoscopy-assisted gastrectomy was significantly associated with fewer complications, less intraoperative blood loss, and shorter hospital stay. Long-term survival was similar to open surgery.[124]

A meta-analysis of randomised trials compared long-term surgical outcomes and complications of laparoscopy-assisted distal gastrectomy (374 patients) with open distal gastrectomy (ODG) (358 patients) for the treatment of EGC.[125] It was shown that laparoscopic resections lowered the rate of long- and short-term complications and promoted earlier recovery, with comparable oncological outcomes to ODG. The indication of laparoscopic gastrectomy has been extended to locally advanced gastric cancer. However, the oncological

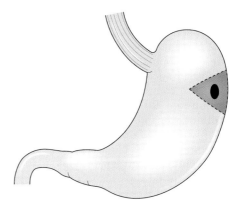

Figure 7.7 Local or wedge gastric resection.

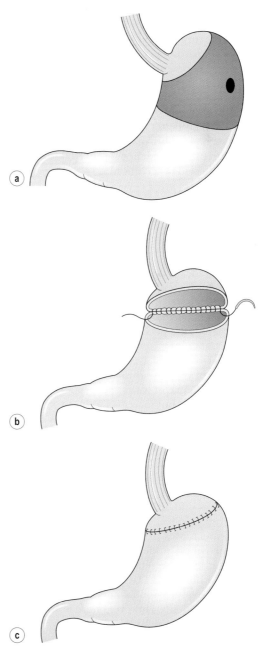

Figure 7.8 Segmental gastric resection. The tumour is removed by a limited segment resection between the lesser and greater curvature (a). A gastro-gastrostomy is then performed (b-c).

safety has long been debated. Recently, results of the randomised controlled LOGICA trial have been published.[126] The LOGICA trial compared laparoscopic and open gastrectomy in a Western population, with the majority of included patients having advanced carcinomas. Length of hospital stay, postoperative complications, in-hospital mortality, 30-day readmission rate, R0 resection rate, lymph node yield, 1-year overall survival, and quality of life were not different between laparoscopic and open gastrectomy. In the laparoscopic gastrectomy arm less blood loss and a longer operating time was seen. Although laparoscopic gastrectomy was not demonstrated to be superior to open gastrectomy, for experienced centres in Western countries laparoscopic gastrectomy can be considered as an alternative option.

Furthermore, with the accumulation of surgical experience and development of instruments, several advanced techniques, such as function-preserving surgery, SNNS, natural orifice surgery (NOTES), robot-assisted surgery, reduced port laparoscopic gastrectomy, and laparoscopic and endoscopic cooperative surgery (LECS) have also been explored and applied to gastric cancer patients. All these techniques could modify the extent of surgery in future and further reduce the risk of perioperative complications and generate potentially better results in quality of life. Although recent studies have confirmed the feasibility and safety of each procedure, more evidence is required for further popularisation of these new techniques.

LYMPHADENECTOMY

In gastric cancer, lymph node status is one of the crucial prognostic factors.[127] The type of resection and the extent of lymphadenectomy are largely based on the likelihood of lymph node metastases to first- and second-tier lymph nodes. However, in parallel with many other tumours it is still debatable whether (extended) lymphadenectomy in gastric cancer really leads to improved survival. The discussion is mainly focused on the adequacy of a limited D1 lymphadenectomy versus the necessity of extended D2 or even D3 lymphadenectomy.

The optimal extent of lymph node dissection remains controversial, not only in advanced gastric cancer but also in EGC. The incidence of lymph node metastases for mucosal EGC is only 2–4% but increases to up to 45% in mucosal tumours with unfavourable features such as depressed or ulcerated lesions, tumours larger than 30 mm in size, and tumours with undifferentiated histological type or with lymphovascular involvement.[92] Most patients with mucosal EGC can be safely treated by EMR or ESD without lymphadenectomy (Table 7.5). However, in submucosal EGC lymph node metastases are found in approximately 20%, with a wide range from 10% to 64%. In addition, approximately 5% of lymph node metastases from submucosal EGC are located in second-tier lymph nodes (mainly nodal stations 7, 8a, and 9).[92] Because of the relatively high risk of lymph node metastases in submucosal EGC and mucosal EGC with unfavourable features, a lymphadenectomy is generally performed in these patients. However, there is no consensus on the required extent of the lymphadenectomy. The Japanese Gastric Cancer Association (JGCA) recommends D2 lymphadenectomy for patients with EGC and clinically positive node(s) (cN+), but this guideline lacks clear evidence.[96] For patients without suspicion of positive lymph nodes (cN0),

currently no evidence exists that D2 dissection can improve survival rates in EGC. Considering the fact that in EGC the rate of lymph node metastases is relatively low and, when positive, these nodes are generally confined to the first-tier lymph nodes, D2 resection can probably be omitted in EGC.

✔ In Europe and the USA D1 resection is advocated for submucosal EGC and mucosal EGC with unfavourable features. The JGCA recommends a D1/D+ resection for all EGCs that are clinically node negative and do not meet the criteria for EMR or ESD.[96]

It is likely that with increasingly applied function-preserving (and minimally invasive) procedures, there will be a shift towards more limited (regional) lymphadenectomy. Ultimately a personalised approach based on patient and tumour characteristics will decide which type of lymphadenectomy might be performed. Sentinel node navigation might be helpful for this.

SENTINEL NODE BIOPSY

SN biopsy offers a targeted approach to lymphadenectomy. Obviously, gastric cancer patients with suspicious or proven lymph node metastases are not eligible for SLNB and a routine D2 lymphadenectomy is deployed. Also, in patients with advanced tumours (T3 and more), SLNB seems inappropriate. These patients already have a high probability of having first- or second-tier lymph node metastases. Moreover, in advanced tumours original lymphatic drainage routes might be obstructed or altered, resulting in a lower accuracy of the SLNB. In EGC the incidence of lymph node metastases is relatively low, i.e. approximately 3% for mucosal and 20% for submucosal tumours. Consequently, when D1 or D2 lymphadenectomy is performed for these tumours as part of standard surgical treatment, in the majority of patients no lymph node metastases are found. In these patients a less extensive resection without lymphadenectomy would probably have resulted in the same excellent disease-free survival rates but without the inherent surgical morbidity and mortality.

SLNB in EGC has been a focus for research in the past 10 years and many different techniques and protocols have been employed. In most study protocols a double-tracer method is preferred using a radioactive colloid, e.g. technetium-99 m, in combination with a dye agent such as isosulfan blue, patent blue violet, or indocyanine green. The day before surgery the radioactive colloid is injected endoscopically in four quadrants into the submucosal layer at or in the vicinity of the primary lesion. The dye agent is injected intraoperatively in the same manner. By this means the SN can be located by both a gamma probe for detection of a radioactive SN and by visualisation of a blue- or green-coloured SN.

Originally SN detection and accuracy rates were disappointing. Therefore clinical application of SN mapping in patients with EGC has been controversial for years. However, a recent meta-analysis and a prospective multicentre trial of SN mapping for EGC have shown acceptable SN detection rates and accuracy of lymph node status. In the recently published prospective study from the Japan Clinical Oncology Group, 400 patients with previously untreated cT1 or cT2 gastric adenocarcinomas smaller than 4 cm in diameter underwent SN mapping using a standardised dual tracer endoscopic injection technique. The SN detection rate was 97.5% (387 of 397). Of 57 patients with lymph node metastases by conventional haematoxylin and eosin staining, 93% (53 of 57) had positive SNs and the accuracy of nodal evaluation for metastases was 99% (383 of 387). Only four false-negative SN biopsies were observed.[128] The same study group has initiated a prospective multicentre non-randomised phase III study to evaluate long-term outcomes after tailored surgery using SN navigation for EGC. In this study patients with cT1N0 gastric cancer have been included. Depending on intraoperative SN status, either limited or distal or total gastrectomy with SN basin dissection (for negative SN) or standard gastrectomy with D2 LN dissection (for positive SN) is performed.[129]

✔ A prospective study in 397 patients has shown that the endoscopic dual tracer method for SN biopsy was safe and effective when applied to superficial, relatively small gastric adenocarcinomas.[128]

A meta-analysis showed that the pooled detection rate is 97%.[130] In studies conducted in Japan and studies published after 2012, cT1 stage and performing SLN biopsy ≥ 15 minutes after dye injection were related to a higher identification rate. Although recent studies have confirmed the feasibility and safety of the SN procedure, more evidence is required for further popularisation of the SN technique, especially in Europe and the USA, where early cancers are rare.

FUTURE DEVELOPMENTS

- Artificial intelligence (AI) systems are increasingly being investigated to assist real-time (early) detection, delineation, and prediction of the invasion depth of gastrointestinal neoplasms. These systems are trained for a specific task using many endoscopy images and videos, preferably high quality. Careful validation to assess diagnostic accuracy and clinical utility is awaited before these algorithms can be incorporated in daily clinical practise.
- The PREFER study (NCT03222635) investigated the possibility of a surveillance protocol after endoscopic resection for patients with T1bN0M0 adenocarcinoma. When a local recurrence is detected, the patient is offered subsequent endoscopic or non-endoscopic treatment.
- The Ad-ESD trial (NCT04135664) compared oesophagectomy with dCRT for cN0-pT1b oesophageal squamous cell carcinoma treated with ESD.[81]
- The KLASS-04 RCT (NCT02595086) compared laparoscopic PPG with laparoscopy-assisted distal gastrectomy for EGC in the middle-third of the stomach, and may provide more clear evidence about the advantages and oncologic safety of PPG.
- The applicability of SNNS in clinical practice for EGC is being evaluated in a prospective phase III study (UMIN000014401).

Key points

Early oesophageal cancer

- The macroscopic appearance of early oesophageal lesions is classified according to the Paris classification. The classification is relevant for predicting the extent of tumour invasion depth.
- Oesophageal mucosal cancer has a very low risk of lymph node metastases but it is slightly higher for squamous cell carcinoma compared with adenocarcinoma.
- Endoscopic resection with EMR or ESD provides the best method for T staging of early oesophageal cancer.
- For localised mucosal adenocarcinoma without additional high-risk criteria, endoscopic therapy is the gold standard.
- In Western countries, definitive endoscopic therapy for early adenocarcinoma in Barrett's mucosa consists of complete EMR of the mucosal cancer and ablation of the residual intestinal metaplasia.
- RFA provides the most efficient, durable ablation outcomes for intestinal metaplasia with associated low morbidity from the procedure.
- Endoscopic resection for localised intramucosal squamous cell carcinoma is an acceptable therapy as long as complete resection is possible. The role of ablative therapies is unclear.
- Oesophagectomy for early oesophageal cancer is reserved for fit patients with submucosal extension of the cancer and/or high-risk criteria for lymph node metastases and/or extensive mucosal neoplasia not suitable for endoscopic ablation.
- Radiotherapy typically with concurrent chemotherapy is an option for patients with early oesophageal squamous cell carcinoma but its role in the treatment of early adenocarcinoma is not clear. It remains an option for unfit patients not suitable for endoscopic therapy or surgery.

Early gastric cancer

- EGC is defined as a tumour that is limited to the mucosa or submucosa (T1); it is relatively rare in the Western world.
- EGCs are classified endoscopically according to the Paris classification.
- If technically possible, EGC can be removed by endoscopic resection and sent for pathology, where it is staged according to the revised Vienna classification. Endoscopic resection can be seen as a staging step with potentially curative intent.
- The 2015 ESGE guideline recommends ESD as a first treatment option for all EGCs.
- D1 resection is advocated for submucosal EGCs and mucosal EGCs that are clinically node negative and do not meet the criteria for EMR or ESD.
- Based on a RCT conducted in a Western population, laparoscopy-assisted gastrectomy is not associated with a shorter hospital stay compared to open gastrectomy. In addition, postoperative complications, in-hospital mortality, and 1-year overall survival are not different between laparoscopic gastrectomy and open gastrectomy.

🌐 References available at http://ebooks.health.elsevier.com/

ACKNOWLEDGEMENT

This chapter in the sixth edition was written by Mark Smithers and Iain Thomson, and we are grateful to them for those parts of the chapter which we have kept in this edition.

KEY REFERENCES FOR EARLY OESOPHAGEAL CANCER

[9] Morita FH, Bernardo WM, Ide E, et al. Narrow band imaging versus Lugol chromoendoscopy to diagnose squamous cell carcinoma of the esophagus: a systematic review and meta-analysis. BMC cancer 2017;17(1):54.

Systematic review and meta-analysis on NBI, including one RCT, assessing the diagnostic accuracy of narrow-band imaging compared with Lugol's iodine for identifying high-grade dysplasia and/or invasive squamous cell carcinoma in the oesophagus. Twelve studies were included in the meta-analysis showing that there was a statistically significant difference only for specificity, with NBI being superior to Lugol chromoendoscopy.

[11] Thosani N, Singh H, Kapadia A, et al. Diagnostic accuracy of EUS in differentiating mucosal versus submucosal invasion of superficial esophageal cancers: a systematic review and meta-analysis. Gastrointest Endosc 2012;75(2):242–53. PMID: 22115605.

Meta-analysis of 11 studies comprising 656 patients assessing the role of EUS in patients with HGD, early adenocarcinoma, or nodules in HGD. The aim was to assess whether the EUS would change management.

[12] Qumseya BJ, Brown J, Abraham M, et al. Diagnostic performance of EUS in predicting advanced cancer among patients with Barrett's esophagus and high-grade dysplasia/early adenocarcinoma: systematic review and meta-analysis. Gastrointest Endosc 2015;81(4):865–74. PMID: 25442088.

Systematic review and meta-analysis of 19 studies comprising 1019 patients to assess the accuracy of EUS in patients with high-grade dysplasia or mucosal and submucosal adenocarcinoma.

[13] Qumseya BJ, Bartel MJ, Gendy S, Bain P, Qumseya A, Wolfsen H. High rate of over-staging of Barrett's neoplasia with endoscopic ultrasound: Systemic review and meta-analysis. Dig Liver Dis 2018;50(5):438–45.

Systematic review and meta-analysis of 11 studies determined that EUS overstaged lesions in 9% and also understaged in 9% among patients with Barrett's oesophagus.

[26] Xu W, Liu XB, Li SB, Yang ZH, Tong Q. Prediction of lymph node metastasis in superficial esophageal squamous cell carcinoma in Asia: a systematic review and meta-analysis. Dis Esophagus 2020;33(12).

A systematic review and meta-analysis pooled 20 studies comprising 3983 patients to assess the incidence of lymph node metastases in patients with superficial squamous cell carcinoma. Tumour size, endoscopic appearance, differentiation grade, tumour invasion depth, and lymphovascular involvement were risk factors for lymph node metastases.

[35] Yang J, Lu Z, Li L, et al. Relationship of lymphovascular invasion with lymph node metastasis and prognosis in superficial esophageal carcinoma: systematic review and meta-analysis. BMC cancer 2020;20(1):176.

The association between lymphovascular invasion and lymph node metastases was investigated in a systematic review and meta-analysis of 23 studies in patients with adenocarcinoma or squamous cell carcinoma, indicating that lymphovascular invasion is strongly correlated with lymph node metastases.

[37] Sgourakis G, Gockel I, Lang H. Endoscopic and surgical resection of T1a/T1b esophageal neoplasms: a systematic review. World J Gastroenterol 2013;19(9):1424–37. PMID: 23539431.

Systematic review of endoscopic and surgical resection of T1a and T1b oesophageal neoplasms from 1997 to 2011. This includes 80 studies and 4241 patients with information on procedures and outcomes for both histologic variants.

[47] Yeh JH, Huang RY, Lee CT, et al. Long-term outcomes of endoscopic submucosal dissection and comparison to surgery for superficial esophageal squamous cancer: a systematic review and meta-analysis. Ther Adv Gastroenterol 2020;13:1756284820964316.

A systematic review and meta-analysis addressed long-term outcomes of ESD for early oesophageal squamous cell cancer, including five studies comparing ESD with oesophagectomy. Overall, disease-specific, and recurrence-free survivals were comparable between ESD and oesophagectomy.

[53] Orman ES, Li N, Shaheen NJ, et al. Efficacy and durability of radiofrequency ablation for Barrett's esophagus: systematic review and meta-analysis. Clin Gastroenterol Hepatol 2013;11(10):1245–55. PMID: 23644385.

Systematic review and meta-analysis of studies reported from 2008 to 2012, including one RCT, assessing the efficacy (18 studies, 3802 patients) and durability (6 studies, 540 patients) of RFA of Barrett's oesophagus for neoplasia and associated metaplasia.

[52] Chadwick G, Groene O, Markar SR, Hoare J, Cromwell D, Hanna GB. Systematic review comparing radiofrequency ablation and complete endoscopic resection in treating dysplastic Barrett's esophagus: a critical assessment of histologic outcomes and adverse events. Gastrointest Endosc 2014;79(5):718–31.e713.

EMR and RFA were compared in a systematic review of 22 studies, showing a low rate of adverse events with RFA compared with EMR.

[57] Tariq R, Enslin S, Hayat M, Kaul V. Efficacy of cryotherapy as a primary endoscopic ablation modality for dysplastic Barrett's esophagus and early esophageal neoplasia: a systematic review and meta-analysis. Cancer Control 2020;27(1):1073274820976668.

This systematic review and meta-analysis of 14 studies including 405 patients showed a complete eradication rate of dysplasia in Barrett's oesophagus of 85%, which was even 91% among high-quality studies. Adverse events were seen in 12% of patients.

KEY REFERENCES FOR EARLY GASTRIC CANCER

[1] The Paris endoscopic classification of superficial neoplastic lesions: esophagus, stomach, and colon: november 30 to december 1, 2002. Gastrointest Endosc 2003;58:S3–43. PMID: 14652541.

[6] Pimentel-Nunes P, Dinas-Ribeiro M, Ponchon T, et al. Endoscopic submucosal dissection: European society of gastrointestinal endoscopy (ESGE) guideline. Endoscopy 2015;47(9):829–54. PMID: 26317585.

Meta-analyses of 4329 lesions, 1916 in the ESD and 2412 in the EMR group, were pooled and analysed. The en bloc and histological complete resection rates were significantly higher in the ESD group; ESD provided a lower recurrence rate. However, the perforation rate was significantly higher after ESD; bleeding incidences did not differ between the two techniques. The results of the included studies led to the ESGE guideline.

[7] Kato H, Haga S, Endo S, et al. Lifting of lesions during endoscopic mucosal resection (EMR) of early colorectal cancer: implications for the assessment of resectability. Endoscopy 2001;33:568–73. PMID: 11473326.

Gotoda T, Yanagisawa A, Sasako M, et al. Incidence of lymph node metastasis from early gastric cancer: estimation with a large number of cases at two large centers. Gastric Cancer 2000;3:219–25. PMID: 11984739.

Based on the histopathological assessment of 5265 gastrectomy specimens with formal lymph node dissections, it has been demonstrated that differentiated EGCs less than 30mm in size and undifferentiated lesions without ulceration and less than 20mm in size have a negligible risk of lymph node metastases.

[22] Dixon MF. Gastrointestinal epithelial neoplasia: Vienna revisited. Gut 2002;51:130–1. PMID: 12077106.

[49] May A, Gunter E, Roth F, et al. Accuracy of staging in early oesophageal cancer using high resolution endoscopy and high resolution endosonography; a comparative, prospective, and blinded trial. Gut 2004;53:634–40. PMID: 15082579.

Conventional endoscopic assessment of depth of infiltration in EGC has a similar accuracy compared to endosonography. For this reason, most highly experienced interventional endoscopists rely on endoscopic assessment and do not routinely perform endosonography before proceeding to EMR or ESD.

[95] Takizawa K, Ono H, Hasuike N, et al. A nonrandomized, single-arm confirmatory trial of expanded endoscopic submucosal dissection indication for undifferentiated early gastric cancer: Japan Clinical Oncology Group study (JCOG1009/1010). Gastric Cancer 2021;24(2):479–91.

A prospective, non-randomised trial that included 346 patients with endoscopically diagnosed cT1aN0M0 EGCs, ≤2cm, without ulceration and undifferentiated adenocarcinoma. Patients underwent ESD and additional gastrectomy when resection was non-curative. En bloc resection was achieved in 99%, curative resection was achieved in 71%, and 5-year overall survival was 99% (95% CI 97.1–99.8).

[109] Facciorusso A, Antonino M, Di Maso M, et al. Endoscopic submucosal dissection vs endoscopic mucosal resection for early gastric cancer: a meta-analysis. World J Gastrointest Endosc 2014;6(11):555–63. PMID: 25400870.

[124] Zeng YK, Yang ZL, Peng JS, et al. Laparoscopy-assisted versus open distal gastrectomy for early gastric cancer: evidence from randomized and nonrandomized clinical trials. Ann Surg 2012;256(1):39–52. PMID: 22664559.

This meta-analysis included 3411 patients and showed that laparoscopy-assisted gastrectomy was significantly associated with fewer complications, less intraoperative blood loss, and shorter hospital stay. Long-term survival was similar.

[128] Kitagawa Y, Takeuchi H, Takagi Y, et al. Sentinel node mapping for gastric cancer: a prospective multicenter trial in Japan. J Clin Oncol 2013;31(29):3704–10. PMID: 24019550.

This prospective study in 397 patients showed that the endoscopic dual tracer method for SN biopsy was confirmed as safe and effective when applied to superficial, relatively small gastric adeno carcinomas.

8 Radiotherapy and chemotherapy in treatment of oesophageal and gastric cancer

Stephen Falk

INTRODUCTION

Cancers of the upper gastrointestinal (GI) tract represent a challenge for the practising oncologist. The majority of patients who present with either locally advanced or metastatic disease are typically of poor functional status and unsuitable for aggressive therapies. Notwithstanding, there are exciting developments, in systemic therapy in particular, with the development of immunotherapy yielding genuine survival advantages for patients in all stages of the disease. The ability to shape radiation beams in four dimensions and thus provide a more conformal or uniform treatment throughout the tumour volume is impacting on the routine treatment of upper GI tumours. Unresolved controversy remains around both sequence and optimal modalities of therapy for potentially curable oesophageal cancer.

Oncology is moving towards a more personalised biomarker-driven therapeutic approach. Factors that determine treatment choice can be broadly divided into factors relating to the patient and those relating to their disease. The former include age, performance status, comorbidities/physiological fitness, and treatment preference. Disease factors include macroscopic features such as the location of disease in the oesophagus and stomach and/or local invasion of mediastinal structures, and microscopic features such as histological type and biological characteristics. The strategic direction of research is to individualise therapy by biomarker discovery to predict response to specific therapies.

The identification of improved activity when chemotherapy and radiotherapy are given synchronously has led to chemoradiotherapy (CRT) becoming the primary organ-preserving approach in anal, cervix, and certain head and neck cancers, with surgery being reserved for salvage.[1] There is now good evidence that primary CRT has a significant role in oesophageal cancer treatment, either integrated into trimodality therapy or as sole curative modality.

Oncological therapies may be considered as:

1. potentially curative as sole modality;
2. adjuvant or additive therapy: additional treatment given before (neoadjuvant) or after (adjuvant) potentially curative local therapy, in an attempt to improve long-term outcome;
3. palliative – to prolong quantity and quality of life.

For potentially curative surgical therapy the objective is a resected tumour with no residual macroscopic disease and clear histological margins (R0), in the absence of metastatic disease. Similarly, non-surgical therapies should be seen in the context of their primary objective, categorised as previously outlined, with clarity regarding the number of patients needed to treat for any individual to benefit and also the, often understated, treatment-related morbidity and mortality risk. Thus, care needs to be taken in assessing how therapies combine in particular with surgery to deliver their primary objective, including altering patterns of relapse and improving survival, or providing a viable alternative to surgery, yet mindful that the mortality rates of preoperative therapy for oesophageal cancer are now similar to surgery.

OESOPHAGEAL CANCER

POTENTIALLY CURATIVE TREATMENT

Traditionally, chemotherapy and/or radiotherapy have followed local surgical therapy. Increasingly, in all GI tract cancers, preoperative oncological therapy is preferred.

Theoretical and generic issues of preoperative versus postoperative therapy treatment include:

Advantages
- a more easily defined and measurable target volume;
- determine response to treatment with cancer in situ;
- improved tumour oxygenation at the time of treatment;
- the potential to improve resectability and reduce the impact of tumour cell spillage at surgery;
- improved chance of an R0 resection and reduction in the risk of local recurrence;
- improved chance of treating micrometastatic disease;
- better tolerance of treatment prior to major surgery;
- improved swallowing and therefore nutrition prior to surgery;
- sparing those patients that progress early with metastatic disease major surgery.

Disadvantages
- overtreatment of some patients that do not need, or gain no benefit from, the treatment;
- reduced physiological reserve prior to major surgery, increasing risk of perioperative morbidity and mortality;
- may allow disease progression prior to definitive treatment.

PREOPERATIVE RADIOTHERAPY ALONE

There have been six randomised controlled trials (RCTs) of preoperative radiotherapy. Three trials were restricted to squamous cell carcinoma (SCC). A Cochrane group quantitative meta-analysis of preoperative radiotherapy using data from 1147 patients in five randomised trials has been performed. With a median follow-up of 9 years, in a group of patients with mostly SCC, the hazard ratio (HR) of 0.89 (95% CI 0.78–1.01) suggests an overall reduction in the risk of death of 11% and an absolute survival benefit of 3% at 2 years and 4% at 5 years. This result is not statistically significant (*P* = 0.062).[2] Preoperative radiotherapy as sole modality is not considered a standard of care.

POSTOPERATIVE RADIOTHERAPY

Given the morbidity of oesophagectomy, patients are often unfit for postoperative therapy to be given within a reasonable timeframe. Furthermore, attempts at radiation therapy are compromised by the need to irradiate the gastric pull-up.

The available literature largely considers patients with SCC alone. Six randomized trials and 13 retrospective studies that included a total of 8 198 patients were included in a meta-analysis of postoperative radiotherapy (PORT) in patients with resected SCC of the oesophagus.[3] The authors noted that PORT provided significant survival benefit compared with surgery alone in retrospective studies but not in RCTs. The randomised trials were deemed of low quality. The conclusion was that there was an improvement in disease-free survival and decreased risk of locoregional recurrence with PORT.

The meta-analysis observed that several of the studies included did not report resection status. In particular whilst longitudinal resection margin involvement in most series would be considered an incomplete resection in others circumferential resection margin involvement is variably reported as such.

To complicate matters, the definition of an R1 resection has changed in international staging manuals. Previously any distance from the resection margin was considered R0 but there is now consensus that R1 resection, and consequent worse prognosis as initially shown in rectal cancer, encompasses any disease within 1 mm of any resection margin.[4]

Postoperative radiotherapy is therefore not established in completely resected oesophageal cancer. There have been no contemporaneous RCTs addressing the role of PORT where there is an R1 resection, where the risk of locoregional failure is clearly higher than with surgery alone.

In the absence of randomised evidence, the knowledge that radiotherapy has a demonstrated role in reducing the risk of locoregional recurrence in surgically treated oesophageal cancer probably justifies considering patients with longitudinal resection margin and/or circumferential resection margin involvement for postoperative CRT on an individual patient basis. Pragmatically, common practice is to target patients where the risk of systemic disease relapse is lower, i.e. those with no, or a lower ratio of, involved lymph nodes. Such a selective policy was shown to have some benefit in an audit of two high-volume tertiary UK referral centres. This showed that postoperative CRT improved overall survival (median survival: 16 months [no postoperative CRT] vs 24 [postoperative CRT] months; HR = 0.46; 95% CI 0.24–0.89; *P* = 0.021) and relapse-free survival (median survival: 12 [no postoperative CRT] months vs 17 [postoperative CRT] months; HR = 0.5; 95% CI 0.27–0.92; *P* = 0.026) in the R1 subgroup.[5]

✔ The role of postoperative chemoradiotherapy following neoadjuvant chemotherapy remains uncertain. Highly selected patients with R1 resection and low or no lymph node burden may reasonably be offered therapy.

WHAT IS THE OPTIMAL PREOPERATIVE TREATMENT FOR OPERABLE OESOPHAGEAL CANCER?

This continues to be the subject of much expert debate, limited evidence base and thus widespread international variation in practice

PREOPERATIVE CHEMOTHERAPY

Preoperative chemotherapy (NCT) in both squamous cell and adenocarcinoma appears to achieve consistently good clinical response rates, as judged by symptom improvement, ranging from 47% to 61%. The mainstay of therapy is a platinum, e.g. cisplatin or oxaliplatin, with a fluoropyrimidine, e.g. 5FU infusion or oral capecitabine. These combinations seem to be active in both squamous[6] and adenocarcinoma,[7] although the benefit of adding a third drug such as an anthracycline, e.g. epirubicin, or taxane in SCC in particular, is less certain and therefore these are often omitted.

Randomised trials of pre- and perioperative chemotherapy

✔✔ The American Intergroup Trial (INT 0113) produced data on 440 randomised patients with a median follow-up of 46.5 months.[8] Adenocarcinoma (54%) was the predominant histology. The chemotherapy limb was given three preoperative courses (cisplatin and 5 days of infusional 5FU) and in stable or responding patients, two postoperative courses. There was no difference in survival.

Overall, 83% of patients received the intended three preoperative cycles of chemotherapy. The study, however, only managed a low operation rate of 80% in the chemotherapy arm, possibly reflecting a more prolonged chemotherapy regimen, leading to more toxicity. Any factor that precludes resection, resulting from chemotherapy, such as excess toxicity or delay in surgery in non-responding patients, clearly could counter any potential gains in responding patients. Further, only 32% of patients received both postoperative chemotherapy cycles. This theme of low postoperative chemotherapy rates is consistent through all perioperative studies and favours a complete preoperative rather than perioperative strategy. There was no difference in treatment-related mortality between the two arms (6% surgery [S] vs 7% chemotherapy [C] + surgery [S]; *P* = 0.33). On an intent-to-treat basis there was no difference in median survival (16.1 months C + S vs 14.9 months S), and 1-, 2- and 3-year (23% C + S vs 26% S) survivals.

✔✔ The Medical Research Council (MRC) OE02 study firmly established the role of neoadjuvant chemotherapy (NCT) at least in the UK.[9] A total of 802 patients were randomised to receive two courses of cisplatin and a 4-day infusion of 5FU followed by surgery (CS) after 3–5 weeks or immediate surgery alone (S) and showed a significant survival advantage for patients receiving preoperative chemotherapy. Two-year survival increased from 34% to 43% and 5-year survival from 17% to 23% (*P* = 0.004; hazard ratio 0.79, CI 0.67–0.93).

Whilst 66% of patients had adenocarcinoma, there was no evidence that the effect of chemotherapy varied with histology. The overall operation rate was similar in both, but there was a significant difference in the microscopic complete resection rate (60% CS vs 53% S; $P < 0.0001$). The postoperative mortality was equivalent in both arms at 10%.

The UK 'MAGIC' trial initially randomised patients with gastric cancer alone but late in its course was expanded to include tumours of the oesophagogastric junction. In 503 patients, three cycles of epirubicin/cisplatin and 5-fluorouracil (ECF) both before and after surgery increased 5-year survival from 23% with surgery alone, to 36%. In the MAGIC trial only ~ 55% received any postoperative chemotherapy.[10]

✓✓ The OE05 trial was designed to assess whether increased NCT (four cycles of ECX: epirubicin/cisplatin and capecitabine) resulted in a survival benefit compared to two cycles of cisplatin and 5FU (CF) building on the results of OE02,[11] but in adenocarcinoma alone. Although downstaging was greater in the ECX arm the overall survival at 3 years was the same.

The OE05 trial[11] is an important contribution; it is the largest reported randomised trial in localized oesophageal cancer and it included quality assurance of all components of modern staging and therapy, including EUS. Sixty-one percent of cases underwent PET-CT scanning. The study thus reflects the current UK model of care with centralised services serving populations of at least 1 million.

In the study, 87% of patients in the CF arm and 91% of patients in the ECX arm underwent surgery ($P = 0.043$). Postoperative mortality was the same in both arms. Downstaging was greater in the ECX arm: Mandard TRG 1-3, CF 15% vs ECX 32% ($P < 0.001$) and associated with better progression-free survival. Eight patients died receiving chemotherapy in the ECX arm as opposed to one in the CF arm, but overall survival was the same with 3-year survival: CF 39% (35–44%); ECX 42% (37–46%).

In summary, two cycles of cisplatin with fluoropyrimidine remains a standard of care for thoracic oesophageal cancer preoperative therapy alone given the absence of a survival benefit with intensified chemotherapy and an increased death rate on treatment.

- Meta-analysis of 15 RCTs involving 3 343 patients concluded that the 5-year overall survival (OS) rate was 27·9% with preoperative chemotherapy and 19·7% with surgery alone (RR 1·42, 95% CI 1·18–1·71, $P < 0·01$; high quality.[12] Adenocarcinoma patients who received NCT showed significantly better OS (HR 0·83; 95% CI 0·72–0·96, $P = 0·012$) and 5-year OS rate (RR 1·56, 95% CI 1·04–2·34, $P = 0·030$) than those who underwent surgery alone. In contrast there was no clear advantage for use of NCT for SCC histology.

POSTOPERATIVE CHEMOTHERAPY ALONE

Patients undergoing major resections for oesophageal carcinoma often have a prolonged postoperative phase. The start of chemotherapy is thus often significantly delayed due to poor performance status, and patients commonly choose not to continue. This is reflected in poor chemotherapy completion rates in studies that adopted a perioperative or 'sandwich' approach, e.g. Intergroup 0113 and MAGIC. A strategy that relied solely on postoperative treatment could have significant problems. As a consequence, there are few useful trials that address the question of adjuvant postoperative chemotherapy alone.

The literature is largely confined to patients with SCC. One meta-analysis of three randomized controlled trials and six retrospective studies comprised a total of 1 684 cases. Postoperative chemotherapy could improve OS (HR 0.78, 95% CI 0.66–0.91; $P = 0.002$) and disease-free survival (DFS) (HR 0.72, 95% CI 0.6–0.86; $P < 0.001$).[13]

CAN POSTOPERATIVE CHEMOTHERAPY BE WITHHELD WHEN NEOADJUVANT THERAPY HAS BEEN GIVEN?

There is no randomised data available. The UK MAGIC study was designed to give both preoperative and postoperative treatment. In practice only a minority of patients received postoperative treatment. Some believe that postoperative chemotherapy should be offered to patients with a heavy tumour burden after neoadjuvant therapy to try to improve what is likely to be poor outcome, while others believe that postoperative chemotherapy should only be administered to patients with a good response to neoadjuvant therapy. This author favours the latter approach given that the observed pathology reflects the responsiveness or otherwise to systemic chemotherapy.

PREOPERATIVE CHEMORADIOTHERAPY

Radiotherapy is commonly combined with chemotherapy for a number of theoretical reasons and is an attractive preoperative strategy. First, early administration of systemic therapy could deal with occult micrometastases that would lead to overt systemic metastases, and second, the optimum time to treat micrometastases is probably when their volume is minimal, supporting the application of chemotherapy as early as possible. Third, hypoxic cells exist in solid tumours in regions of poor vascularity and are likely to be more resistant to conventional radiotherapy treatment as sole therapy. These cells, however, may be more sensitive to the combined effects of cytotoxic agents and radiotherapy. Finally, certain chemotherapy drugs, such as 5-fluorouracil, cisplatin, gemcitabine and paclitaxel are known to be 'radiosensitisers', which result in normal and malignant tissues becoming more sensitive to ionising radiation.

Several strategies that combine systemic chemotherapy with radiation (as definitive locoregional treatment) have been explored:

- concurrent chemoradiation, in which chemotherapy and radiation are delivered synchronously in order to maximise radiosensitisation;
- neoadjuvant (pre-emptive) chemotherapy, in which chemotherapy is administered first, usually followed by assessment of response and implementation of definitive therapy;
- adjuvant therapy, in which systemic treatment is administered after completion of locoregional therapy in an attempt to control micrometastatic disease;
- combination of concurrent chemoradiation with either neoadjuvant or adjuvant chemotherapy.

There is good evidence that pathological complete response (pCR) rates are significantly higher with CRT than with radiotherapy or chemotherapy given alone. pCR and R0 resections are possible surrogate proxies of benefit to patients and do seem to translate into a survival benefit, which remains the gold standard assessment. A review of the MAGIC pathology data[14] showed on univariate analysis, high Mandard TRG (3,4, or 5) and lymph node metastases were negatively related to survival, but on multivariate analysis, only lymph node status was independently predictive of OS (HR = 3.36; 95% CI 1.70–6.63; $P < 0.001$).

Both radiotherapy and chemotherapy rely on achieving an acceptable balance between increased response rates in the tumour on one hand and normal tissue morbidity coupled with patient tolerance on the other. Whilst many side-effects of chemotherapy occur relatively early in presentation, e.g. hair loss, emesis, and myelosuppression, radiotherapy side-effects can present late, from 6 months to years after treatment. If radical surgery is added in combined modality therapy then the potential for higher levels of morbidity and mortality becomes significant.

Non-randomised studies of CRT have appeared in the literature since the late 1980s (reviewed by Geh et al.).[15] Pooled data from these studies is notable for the heterogeneity of approach, in terms of scheduling of chemotherapy and radiotherapy, and eligibility criteria. Geh et al. showed that, of 2 704 patients (squamous 68% and adenocarcinoma 32%), 79% were operated on with a pCR rate of 24% of those treated and 32% of those resected. The controversy and delay in implementing what is clearly an active therapeutic approach has revolved around the associated increased morbidity and postoperative mortality. Reported CRT-related deaths in the non-randomised series ranged from 0–15% (mean 3%). Postoperative deaths ranged from 0% to 29% (mean 9%). Adult respiratory distress syndrome, anastomotic leak and breakdown, pneumonia and sepsis were the commonest causes of death following oesophageal resection. Treatment-related deaths ranged from 3–25% (mean 9%) of all patients treated. It seems clear that the risk of chemotherapy-related toxicity, particularly myelosuppression, rises with the number of drugs used and the radiation dose-intensity of the CRT regimen. An increased risk of tracheobronchial fistula has also been reported. However, most of these reported series did not use contemporaneous radiotherapy planning and treatment techniques that allow greater precision and sparing of organs and tissues to within normal tissue tolerance.

Using modern radiotherapy techniques and fractionation, the randomised phase III CROSS study comparing surgery alone to preoperative CRT demonstrated a doubling of overall survival (OS) in favour of the preoperative arm (OS 49.4 months vs 24 months, HR 0.67), a pCR rate of 29% and no increase in surgical mortality (3.8% [S] vs 3.4% [CRT-S]). The 'CROSS' trial.[16] has been practice-changing.

In the 'CROSS' trial, 363 patients with operable oesophageal or oesophagogastric junction tumours were randomised to surgery alone or to a preoperative CRT regimen (NCRT) of weekly carboplatin (AUC2) and paclitaxel (50 mg/m²) concurrent with radiotherapy (41.4 Gy in 23 fractions). Of the 175 patients assigned to the CRT arm, 163 completed protocol treatment and the study reported a low incidence of grade 3/4 CRT toxicity (haematological,

6.8%; non-haematological, 16%). The R0 resection rates in the surgery and CRT + surgery arms were 67% and 92.3%, respectively ($P = 0.002$). The results of this study, would suggest that where preoperative CRT is delivered safely, there is a significant improvement in outcome compared to surgery alone.

The study also gives clues as to future directions. CRT delivered a major reduction in R1 resections that translated into a reduction in local failure from 20.5–7%. However, its effect on haematogenous spread remains limited (35.4–28.5%). Distant disease control clearly remains suboptimal with this approach.

Meta-analysis of 21 RCTs involving 3 138 patients were included in a comparison of NCRT with surgery.[12] Compared with surgery alone, NCRT was associated with increased OS (HR 0.74, 95% CI 0.66–0.82, $P < 0.01$; high quality), 5-year OS (RR 1.51, 95% CI 1.28–1.78, $P < 0.01$; (high quality) and R0 resection rate (RR 1.16, 95% CI 1.07–1.25, PP < 0.01; moderate quality). Improvement in outcome was seen in both adenocarcinoma and SCC histology

Repeated meta-analysis of randomised trials has shown that neoadjuvant chemoradiotherapy increases R0 resection rates, reduces locoregional recurrence and improves survival compared with surgery alone.[12]

WHICH PREOPERATIVE STRATEGY: NEOADJUVANT CHEMORADIOTHERAPY OR CHEMOTHERAPY?

To date there have been eight reported randomised phase III trials that include the comparison of NCRT with NCT. The largest trial to date, however, includes fewer than 240 patients. Not surprisingly therefore these studies have been underpowered to answer the question individually but have been subject to a number of meta-analyses the most recent published in 2020.[12] Compared with NCT, NCRT was associated with increased OS (HR 0.78, 95% CI 0.62–0.99, $P = 0.04$; high quality), 5-year OS rate (RR 1.48, 95% CI 1.06–2.07, $P = 0.02$; moderate quality), R0 resection rate (RR 1.13, 95% CI 1.07–1.20, $P < 0.01$; high quality), and pCR (RR 3.74, 95% CI 2.03.6.88, $P < 0.01$; moderate quality). The 30-day postoperative or in-hospital mortality rate was 7.7% with NCT and surgery versus 8.0% with surgery alone.

Among the SCC patients, meta-analysis provided high-quality evidence of a strikingly improved OS associated with NCRT compared with surgery alone, not observed with the use of NCT. In contrast, in patients with oesophageal adenocarcinoma there was longer OS following NCRT than following NCT, and the HR of NCRT versus surgery alone (HR 0.73, 95% CI 0.62–0.86; high quality) was better than that of NCT versus surgery alone (0.83, 0.72–0.96; moderate quality). The current data is moving towards NCRT.

Whether current trials will finally answer this question is a moot point. The current international study neo-AEGIS trial initially aimed to recruit 594 patients randomised between the 'CROSS' CRT regimen and perioperative chemotherapy and was initially powered to show a 10% improvement in 3-year survival. Due to poor accrual it has reduced its sample size to 540 and is now a non-inferiority design.

Earlier identification of non-responding patients to chemotherapy (e.g. by PET-CT scanning) could allow a change in neoadjuvant therapy direction to reduce the R1 resection rate, the number of involved lymph nodes and possibly translate into improved outcomes.

The good outcomes from surgery alone in stage I disease make neoadjuvant therapy difficult to justify. Given the frequent upstaging of clinical stage II disease when resected fit and young patients will often be offered preoperative therapy.

FUTURE DIRECTION

There is rightly a clear separation in current and future trials for adenocarcinoma and squamous carcinoma. The majority of adenocarcinoma patients will present with stage III disease (at least T3 with lymph node metastases). There are two issues to consider:

1. *Local control.*

Tumours frequently threaten the CRM, although a clear plane for surgical excision does not exist as it does for other anatomical sites such as the rectum. Disease present at or within 1 mm of the circumferential margin (R1) occurs in around one-third of cases and is a poor prognostic factor. Preoperative CRT has become a standard management strategy in rectal cancer for patients who have a threatened CRM on preoperative staging. MRI scanning revolutionised the identification of patients with rectal cancer at risk of a positive margin[17] and preoperative CRT is mandatory for cases where MRI predicts a positive margin. Such a paradigm shift is required for oesophageal cancer. Currently there is no agreed staging tool that accurately predicts R1 resection.

2. *Systemic control*

Whatever improvements in locoregional treatments are proposed, the strategy being addressed with new trials for stage III adenocarcinoma is systemic relapse, in other words overall survival. In particular larger RCTs using immunotherapy in addition to chemotherapy will become available, combination chemo-immunotherapy having demonstrated benefit in incurable disease as will be described later.

The provisional results of CheckMate 577 have been made available.[18] 794 patients, 70% of whom had adenocarcinoma, who had received NCRT and had residual pathological disease were randomised 2 to 1 to receive 1 year of nivolumab or placebo. The primary endpoint was disease-free survival, which was 11 months in the placebo group and 22.4 months in the investigational arm (HR.0.69 (0.56–0.86; $P = 0.0003$)). Whilst mature survival results remain not available this study potentially raises a step change in outcome.

Hopefully the addition of immunotherapy to NCT will improve systemic treatment for the disease. At the same time these studies will re-ignite the long-standing debate of the role of radiotherapy in the preoperative management of operable oesophageal cancer.

PATIENT SELECTION

With the introduction of targeted therapies biomarker-driven trials with new biological agents added to standard chemotherapy or selective CRT are likely to be the next step, with advance knowledge from their use in the advanced and metastatic disease setting.

Genetic profiling of pathology will become increasingly important. Grading of CRT response has been described by Mandard et al.[19] In this paper the significant predictor of disease-free survival after multivariate analysis was the tumour regression grade. Five grades of response ranging from no identifiable tumour to complete absence of regression potentially allow a more formalised approach to be adopted (Box 8.1). This system is, however, a subjective assessment. Without central quality control or an automated measuring system this is only one potential step.

- Preoperative chemotherapy remains a standard of care in the UK for adenocarcinoma of the thoracic oesophagus. The current neo-AEGIS trial directly compares perioperative chemotherapy (MAGIC) and neoadjuvant chemoradiotherapy (CROSS). Meta-analysis of the available data however suggests that there is high-quality evidence for a survival benefit of NCRT surpassing NCT over surgery alone in patients with oesophageal carcinoma of both histological types

DEFINITIVE RADIOTHERAPY AND CHEMORADIOTHERAPY

Surgery as a local treatment modality with neoadjuvant treatment for stage III disease, particularly adenocarcinoma, remains the gold standard against which new approaches to potentially curative treatment must be compared. It is also clear that there are consistently 35% long-term survivors in series of definitive non-surgical treatment of any histology. With an ageing population and the not inconsiderable risks of surgery, non-surgical treatment is a valid option for many patients. In particular the UK AUGIS database is starting to demonstrate very poor outcomes for surgically treated patients over the age of 80.

DEFINITIVE SINGLE AGENT RADIOTHERAPY

✅ With an increasingly elderly population it is not uncommon to be faced with patients who have localised disease on staging, particularly squamous cancers, but who clearly are not candidates for an operation and who, because of comorbidity, may not tolerate the chemotherapy component of a CRT treatment. There still is a role for radical radiotherapy alone.

Classical figures quoted for survival from radical radiotherapy come from Earlam and Cunha-Melo.[20] Mean survival figures of 8 489 patients at 1, 2 and 5 years were 18%, 8% and 6%, respectively. Modern radiotherapy in more selected patients can produce impressive survival results. In a series of 101 patients treated at the Christie Hospital in Manchester

---

Box 8.1 Mandard scoring

- TRG1 No residual cancer
- TRG2 Rare residual cancer cells
- TRG3 Fibrosis outgrowing residual cancer
- TRG4 Residual cancer outgrowing fibrosis
- TRG5 Absence of regressive change

between 1985 and 1994, 3- and 5-year survival figures of 27% and 21%, respectively, were recorded.[21] There was a slightly better survival for adenocarcinoma, but not reaching statistical significance. The majority of tumours (96/101) were of 5 cm or less in length. Importantly, the only significant prognostic factor was the use of diagnostic CT, introduced during the latter part of the study. This was used to plan the radiotherapy and led to an increase in field sizes.

DEFINITIVE CHEMORADIOTHERAPY

The adoption of CRT stems from high response rates but at the cost of increased toxicity. There are four randomised trials comparing radiotherapy alone with CRT. Three of these use low doses or low intensity of chemotherapy.

The biggest series with a major impact on treatment patterns has been the RTOG 85-01, Herskovic study.[22] A total of 123 patients were randomised to receive either radiotherapy alone to a dose of 64 Gy or two courses of cisplatin and infusional 5FU concurrent with 50 Gy of radiotherapy. Two more courses of chemotherapy were scheduled after the completion of the radiotherapy. A summary of the results of the randomised patients is shown in Table 8.1 and demonstrates the significant advantage of combined therapy, with survival increasing from 0– 30%.

A Cochrane collaboration meta-analysis indicated that the addition of chemotherapy to radiotherapy improved both local control and survival.[23] Thirteen randomised trials were included in the analysis. There were eight concomitant and five sequential radiotherapy and chemotherapy (RTCT) studies. Concomitant RTCT provided significant overall reduction in mortality at 1 and 2 years of 7% (95% CI 1–15%). The mortality in the control arm was 62% and 83% respectively. The local recurrence rate for the control arms was around 68%. The combined RTCT approach provided a reduction in local recurrence rate of 12% (95% CI 3–22%). There was, however, a significant increase of severe and life-threatening toxicities.

The high local failure rate of 45% in the Herskovic trial led to the Intergroup study 00123 (Minsky) that compared a regimen similar to the Herskovic regimen (modified with narrower radiotherapy fields, radiotherapy using 1.8 Gy/fraction and an alteration in the chemotherapy schedule to reduce anticipated toxicity), to the same schedule but with a higher dose of radiotherapy (64.8 Gy in 36 fractions).[24] In total, 236 patients, once again predominantly with SCC, were randomised in this study. The trial had to be closed prematurely due to an excess of treatment-related deaths in the experimental arm (11 vs 2), although the majority of these occurred before the higher radiation dose section of the treatment protocol had been received. Although this trial did not show better disease control with higher doses of radiotherapy (56% failure at 2 years compared to 52% in the standard arm) it did confirm the outcome of previous studies, of approximately 30% survival at 3 years with definitive chemoradiotherapy.

Another approach to improve local control was to use brachytherapy to intensify the radiotherapy dose to the tumour. Study RTOG 92-07 used the 50-Gy external beam and chemotherapy protocol from the Herskovic protocol and added an intraluminal brachytherapy boost with one of two methods of delivery, high-dose rate or low-dose rate.[25] Six

Table 8.1 Summary of results of the RTOG 85-01 study of Al-Sarraf et al. (1997)[28]

	RT	RT + CT	P value
Median survival (mth)	9.3	14.1	
Overall survival (%):			
1-year	34	52	
2-year	10	36	
5-year	0	30	0.0001
Rate distant metastases (%)	37	21	0.0017
Two-year local recurrence rate (%)	59	45	0.0125
Overall disease free (%)	11	36	< 0.001

CT, Chemotherapy; *RT*, radiotherapy.

of the 35 patients developed an oesophageal fistula and this toxicity was deemed unacceptable.

Following successful CRT or radiotherapy alone there is a significant rate of benign stricture formation. Inevitably such issues are worse when there is complete dysphagia prior to treatment. This ranges from 12–25% in more modern studies. However, good swallowing function can be maintained in the majority of patients. Even in those with a benign stricture, a full or soft diet can be maintained by dilatations in 71% of cases.[26] The higher pCR rates seen with CRT, the improved local control rates and altered patterns of failure in the literature have all contributed to CRT being adopted as a standard of care. The successful management of CRT-treated patients requires the same multidisciplinary nursing and dietetic support as for surgical patients.

FUTURE DIRECTIONS IN DEFINITIVE CHEMORADIATION

The next steps are further attempts at intensifying radiation dose, utilising techniques that allow the shape of radiotherapy fields to be individually tailored to the irregular-shaped target disease to achieve smaller radiation volumes and thus reduced normal tissue toxicity. This can be associated with greater tumour accuracy with breath-hold techniques to reduce documented tumour movement during treatment, which can be up to 3 cm superior and inferior with 3D and 4D CT planning techniques. Secondly, there needs to be optimisation of systemic therapy. What can reliably be achieved in routine practice was shown in the UK SCOPE 1 trial.[27] This study examined the addition of Cetuximab on survival. This proved a negative trial, but better than expected 2-year survival overall is attributed to an on-trial radiotherapy trials quality assurance (RTTQA). This consisted of all principal investigators' first plans, 10% of all subsequent plans, and trial-specific planning assessment forms for each patient submitted for central review that outlined and assessed the 3D dose distribution before treatment. Despite the fact that most patients had stage III disease, 38% of patients were older than 70 years, and 15% of patients had comorbidities that precluded surgery, the 2-year overall survival in all patients was 49%, and was 56% in those receiving CRT only.

The ability to predict which patients will respond to chemotherapy or CRT would allow greater certainty in a primary non-surgical approach. The current SCOPE2 trial schedules a PET scan after two cycles of treatment to prospectively evaluate whether changing or intensifying treatment in PET non-responders may confer benefit. Molecular markers predicting response to chemotherapy remain investigational, as does the integration of immunotherapies with radiation.

Local recurrence rates of 40–75% are recognised following definitive CRT. Indeed it is generally recognised that local failure is more common after chemoradiation than with surgery. The role of salvage oesophagectomy is controversial. An audit of 308 patients undergoing salvage oesophagectomy in 30 European centres showed 8.4% in-hospital mortality. There was a 43.3% 3-year disease-free survival rate and this appears a valid option for selected patients who justify endoscopic surveillance following therapy.[28]

Clearly, as patients continue to relapse with both metastatic and locoregional disease, systemic and local components of this treatment strategy need to be improved and intensified. Systemic treatments should either have independent activity in oesophageal cancer or have synergistic effects with radiotherapy in the form of radiosensitisation, or overcoming mechanisms of radioresistance. However, newer therapies need to be carefully integrated so as not to compromise the dose intensity of standard chemoradiotherapy.

PRIMARY DEFINITIVE CHEMORADIOTHERAPY OR SURGERY?

In practical terms, these are very different treatments. CRT is given as an outpatient over 4.5 weeks, delivering 23 fractions (approximately 2 min/day) of radiotherapy, concurrently with chemotherapy. This may be preceded by neoadjuvant chemotherapy. There is a 40–50% rate of World Health Organisation Grade 3–4 (serious or life-threatening) acute toxicities, predominantly haematological, as a result of the chemotherapy; this is largely manageable, but there is a mortality of less than 2%. Overall, greater than 90% of patients complete planned treatment. In the longer term, there may be a greater risk of post-therapy stricture requiring dilatation or a stent after CRT.

Ideally, decision-making regarding optimal therapy would be based on a randomised trial; however, a recent feasibility RCT of surgical versus non-surgical treatment for SCC of the oesophagus revealed such a study was not feasible in the UK alone because of the low number of incident eligible patients[29] This trial of very different approaches was enriched with integrated qualitative research involving audio-recorded recruitment appointments and interviews with patients to inform recruitment training for staff.

Definitive CRT treatments now report good survival figures,[27] rivalling those of surgery, stage for stage, particularly for SCC. Many squamous cancers are in the mid and upper oesophagus and their pattern of lymph node spread is less predictable. These areas can be safely treated with CRT with increasing sophistication of treatment delivery techniques. Further surgery in the upper oesophagus is particularly complex and mutilating where laryngectomy is required.

In squamous carcinoma of the oesophagus there is some evidence that a policy of primary CRT with surgery as salvage may be the direction for the future.[27,28] The evidence around equipoise in the treatment of patients with oesophageal adenocarcinoma is less robust. Tumours primarily of the lower oesophagus or oesophagogastric junction could be candidates for CRT but target volumes are more difficult and CRT is currently reserved where a surgical approach is either excluded by age, performance status, or comorbidity and, increasingly, patient choice.

There are two trials that address the additional value of surgery after CRT in squamous cell carcinoma and would give some support to a selective approach to its use.[30,31] These trials also suggest planned surgery is not routinely necessary following definitive CRT. Surgical results are worse in the elderly population with more comorbidities and CRT is a viable option.

In a French study (FFCD 9102), SCC patients were assessed after induction CRT using 5FU and cisplatin.[30] If they had achieved an objective response they were randomised (295 of 455 patients) to carry on with CRT or go to surgery. There was no significant difference between the 2-year survival rates for patients who had surgery (33.6%) and those who had CRT alone (39.8%). There were more early deaths in the surgery arm but CRT required more dilatations and stents.

In a German trial, 177 patients with T3 or T4 SCC were randomised to receive CRT + surgery or CRT alone.[31] The response rate to CRT was the same for both arms. There was a strong trend towards improved local tumour control in the arm with surgery. In responding patients the 3-year survival (45% and 44% respectively) was equivalent in both arms, whereas in non-responding patients the rates were 18% and 11%, respectively. The 3-year survival rate improved to 35% in non-responding patients undergoing complete tumour resection, implying that a subgroup of non-responding patients may benefit from surgery as an elective salvage procedure. Longer-term results confirm no clear survival difference between a surgical versus CRT approach.

Patient choice should play a vital part of decision-making and may be assisted by examining patient-reported outcomes. Quality of life is dependent upon the effects of treatment and the state of disease control. A prospective study evaluated the quality of life of patients surviving at least 3 years after surgery.[32] Although most aspects of quality of life returned to baseline, patients reported residual problems with reflux, dyspnoea and diarrhoea even 3 years after surgery. There are even fewer data regarding quality of life after CRT. A non-randomised study comparing CRT with treatment including surgery showed that quality of life was diminished after CRT, but the deterioration was less dramatic than following oesophagectomy.[33] Some 132 patients began treatment, 51 had CRT and 81 a combination treatment including surgery. Patients selected for chemoradiotherapy were older, more likely to have squamous cell cancer, and reported poorer health-related quality of life (HRQL) than those selected for surgery. At the worst

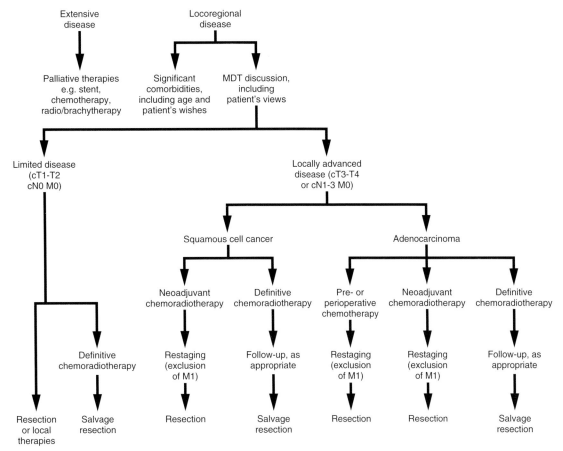

Figure 8.1 Algorithm for the management of oesophageal cancer.

expected time point after treatment, both groups reported multiple symptoms and poor function, but surgery was associated with a greater reduction in HRQL from baseline than CRT. Recovery of HRQL was achieved within 6 months after CRT, but complete recovery had not occurred 6 months after surgery.

Similarly, in the French study (FFCD 9102) of CRT, with or without surgery, quality of life was worse after surgery but not different between the treatment arms at 2 years.[30]

Fig. 8.1 summarises a suggested treatment algorithm for localised carcinoma of the oesophagus.

SMALL CELL OESOPHAGEAL CANCER

Small cell oesophageal cancer is a rare entity, accounting for around 2.5% of primary oesophageal cancers and is associated with a poor prognosis due to a high rate of metastatic disease. To complicate matters, at least 70% of patients have mixed histology, i.e. including at least a focus of squamous or more commonly adenocarcinoma. The literature is made up of small retrospective series from major institutions. The disease tends to have male preponderance and occurs in the mid and lower oesophagus. The median survival of untreated metastatic patients is less than 3 months. Treatment

is dependent on a separation between limited disease and extensive disease.

✔ The treatment of patients with extensive small cell carcinoma is palliative chemotherapy based on etoposide- and platinum-containing regimens if the performance status allows. Response rates to treatment are high and there is definite improvement in overall survival, but outcomes are universally poor, with median survivals of 8–11 months.

Due to the very high rate of systemic relapse, limited stage disease requires primary treatment with chemotherapy, again based on etoposide- and platinum-containing regimes. There is a role for consolidation treatment to enhance local control and to prevent local symptomatic progression. There are surgical series with good local control rates, but the majority of series concentrate on radiotherapy (doses up to 50 Gy) or chemoradiotherapy, avoiding the mortality risk and morbidity of surgery.[34,35] Local control rates with surgery are high but overall prognosis poor, with survival dictated by metastatic disease and median survivals in the range of 15–24 months. Oesophageal small cell carcinoma has low rates of brain metastases and prophylactic cranial irradiation is thus not required, unlike for a lung primary.

GASTRIC CANCER

POTENTIALLY CURATIVE TREATMENT

Non-surgical approaches are not considered curative for patients with gastric cancer as a sole modality but are used in a multimodal approach. Surgery provides high rates of cure in the early stages; however, less than 25% of patients present with early stage disease. The survival of the remaining patients with potentially curable, non-metastatic disease falls below 50%, and below 20% when the tumour invades through the muscularis propria and involves regional lymph nodes. These patients are candidates for multimodal therapy.

One controversial issue is where does the stomach begin for treatment purposes. In the TNM staging manual, tumours arising at the oesophagogastric junction (OGJ) or in the cardia of the stomach (within 5 cm of the OGJ) that extend into the OGJ are staged and treated as oesophageal rather than stomach cancers. However, tumours that arise beyond 5 cm of the OGJ, or are within 5 cm of the OGJ but without extension to the junction are classified and treated as gastric cancers. The relative limited tolerance of gastric mucosa has traditionally limited radiation protocols to treat 2 cm of macroscopically involved gastric mucosa only.

POSTOPERATIVE CHEMOTHERAPY

The goal of systemic therapy for gastric cancer is to reduce the late patterns of failure following successful surgical resection. The pattern of spread includes nodal, transcoelomic, and haematogenous. Chemotherapy, either systemic or intraperitoneal, has thus been used to try to reduce the incidence of widespread recurrence. Despite encouraging results for chemotherapy in advanced disease, proof of a benefit for adjuvant postoperative chemotherapy has been elusive in Caucasian populations.

Adjuvant chemotherapy (CT) has been widely explored in Western and Asian countries since the 1960s. Many of the regimens in the older studies have low response rates (10–30%) in advanced disease, compared with the higher expected response of more modern regimens such as ECF. Although adjuvant CT is not used routinely in the West, it represents standard practice in the East, following the reporting of two large RCTs in Asian patients. In the CLASSIC trial[36] 1 035 patients with stage II to stage IIIB gastric cancer were randomly assigned to eight 21-day cycles of capecitabine plus oxaliplatin after D2 gastrectomy or surgery alone. There was improved overall survival with chemotherapy (78% vs 69%, HR for death = 0.66%, 95% CI 0.51–0.85). However, only 67% of the patients assigned to chemotherapy received all eight cycles of chemotherapy as planned, and adverse events (most commonly neutropenia, nausea, vomiting, thrombocytopenia, and anorexia) led to chemotherapy dose modifications in 90% of patients.

The ACTS-GC trial[37] randomised 1 059 patients with stage II or III gastric cancer following D2 gastrectomy to observation or S-1, an oral fluoropyrimidine containing tegafur, gimeracil, and oteracil, for 1 year after surgery. There is a persistent survival benefit of S-1 from 61–71% (HR = 0.669 [0.54–0.828]). S-1 appears well tolerated with < 5% of patients reporting grade 3 or higher toxicities. S-1, however, is not widely available in Western countries and indeed whether it is well tolerated and efficacious in Caucasian populations is unknown.

A Cochrane review[38] identified 34 studies and 7 824 patients. Post-surgical chemotherapy showed an improvement in OS (HR 0.85; 95% CI 0.80–0.90) and an improvement in DFS (HR 0.79; 95% CI 0.72–0.87). The conclusion was that post-surgical chemotherapy should be used routinely for resectable gastric cancer where possible.

PRE- AND PERIOPERATIVE CHEMOTHERAPY

The MAGIC study[10] of perioperative ECF has already been described, and included 74% stomach, 14% oesophageal and 12% junctional cancers. The majority of resections were at least D1, with 40% having a D2. The proportion deemed to have had a potentially curative resection was 10% higher with chemotherapy (79% vs 69%). There was an improvement in overall survival (hazard ratio of 0.75, P = 0.009), with 5-year survival rates of 36% for chemotherapy and surgery versus 23% for surgery alone. Progression-free survival was also significantly prolonged.

Two European RCTs have evaluated NCT versus surgery alone. The ACCORD-07/FFCD 9703 trial,[39] which closed early because of poor accrual, randomised 224 patients to surgery alone versus two to three cycles of preoperative cisplatin and 5FU CT. This study included predominantly patients with oesophagogastric junction (OGJ) adenocarcinoma, with gastric primaries allowed later in the study and comprising 25% of the patients enrolled. At a median follow-up of 5.7 years, preoperative CT improved the R0 resection rate from 74 – 84% (P = 0.004), as well as increasing 5-year OS from 24% to 38% (P = 0.02).

The EORTC 4 0954 trial,[40] which also closed early because of poor accrual, randomised 144 patients (of a planned 360) to surgery alone versus two cycles of preoperative cisplatin and 5FU. Although this trial allowed the inclusion of type I and II OGJ tumours, 47.2% of patients had primary tumours in the middle and lower third of the stomach. At a median follow-up of 4.4 years, despite an improvement in R0 resection rate from 66.7–81.9%, there was no difference in overall survival between the two arms.

The phase III 716 patient FLOT4-AIO trial enrolled patients with locally advanced, resectable gastric or gastro-oesophageal junction adenocarcinoma and demonstrated that compared with fluorouracil or capecitabine plus cisplatin and epirubicin, a combination consisting of fluorouracil, leucovorin, oxaliplatin, and docetaxel (FLOT) improved OS, (hazard ratio [HR] 0·77; 95% confidence interval [CI; 0·63–0·94]; median OS, 50 months [38·33 to not reached] vs 35 months [27·35–46·26]). There was no significant difference in treatment-related adverse events among resectable gastroesophageal junction or gastric adenocarcinoma[41]

- FLOT is now standard of care for perioperative chemotherapy for operable gastric cancer[41]

POSTOPERATIVE CHEMORADIOTHERAPY

Radiotherapy has not been and is not routinely used in the management of stomach cancer in the UK. However, local recurrence can be a significant problem. The stomach and nodal areas are close to many crucial normal tissues with dose-limiting susceptibility to toxicity, such as kidney, spinal cord and small bowel.

In the British Stomach Cancer Group trial,[42] postoperative radiotherapy was one of the arms of the study. The other arms were FAM (5FU, doxorubicin and methotrexate) chemotherapy and a control surgery-only group. There was no difference in survival but the local recurrence rate was significantly better (54% surgery vs 32% with radiotherapy; $P < 0.01$).

✓✓ The American Intergroup INT 0116 (SWOG 9008) study (commonly referred to as the Macdonald study) reported that postoperative CRT shows a significant benefit to survival following gastric resection and has become standard of care in the USA.[43]

The regimen consists of 5FU–leucovorin (folinic acid) given in the first and last weeks of radiotherapy (45 Gy) and two 5-day courses of 5FU–leucovorin given monthly. With over 10 year follow up, the CRT arm maintains a survival advantage ()HR = 1.32 (95% CI, 1.10 to 1.60; $P = 0.0046$)). However, a significant proportion of the patients (54%) had only a D0 resection and the survival in the surgery-alone arm was relatively poor (41% 3-year survival). It is possible that the CRT was making up for less than adequate surgery, since survival outcomes in the combined modality arm of the Macdonald study are equivalent to European surgical-only studies where D1 and/or D2 dissection has been performed.

This seems to be the conclusion that can be drawn from the CRITICS trial,[44] which randomised 788 patients who had D1 or better lymphadenectomy with at least 15 nodes in the resection specimen to either perioperative chemotherapy or preoperative chemotherapy and postoperative chemoradiotherapy. Forty-seven percent of patients completed all protocol treatment in the chemotherapy-alone arm and 52% in the CRT arm. Five-year survival was identical at 40.8% in both groups. Similarly, the ARTIST trial[45] randomly assigned only patients who underwent a D2 resection for pathologically staged IB to IV (M0) gastric cancer to adjuvant chemotherapy of six cycles of capecitabine and cisplatin (XP) or two cycles of XP before and after concurrent capecitabine and radiotherapy (XPRT). With a median of 7 years of follow-up, there was no significant difference in DFS or overall survival. Because results suggest a significant DFS effect of chemoradiotherapy in subsets of patients however, the ARTIST 2 trial evaluating adjuvant chemotherapy and chemoradiotherapy in patients with node-positive, D2-resected GC is under way.

✓✓ A meta-analysis[46] of six trials comprising 1171 patients (excluding the CRITICS trial) concluded that while chemoradiotherapy was associated with significantly higher rates of 5-year DFS (odds ratio [OR] 1.56, 95% CI 1.09–2.24) and significantly lower rates of locoregional recurrence (OR 0.46, 95% CI 0.32–0.67), there was only a trend toward a survival benefit for CRT that was not statistically significant (OR for overall survival 1.32, 95% CI 0.92–1.99). Postoperative radiotherapy is not required when resection is complete

Practice varies around the world and in Asia postoperative chemotherapy is used whilst in Europe perioperative chemotherapy regimes are favoured. Why such wide international variation? There are frequently observed differences in outcomes between continents, with reported survival rates consistently higher in Asian studies. It is not clear whether a more radical extent of surgery can solely be responsible for this. Numerous hypotheses have been suggested to explain this observation. The first relates to the issue of stage migration, where a more extensive nodal dissection leading to more accurate prognostic stratification and upstaging in a proportion of patients may falsely suggest a treatment benefit. Other factors include inherent biological differences in the disease between the two populations, as well as differing tolerance and sensitivity to chemotherapeutic agents. None has clear supporting evidence.

✓✓ It is currently reasonable to adopt a standard approach using perioperative chemotherapy alone for gastric cancer other than early-stage disease.

INTRAPERITONEAL CHEMOTHERAPY

Peritoneal metastases (PMs) are detected in up to 30% of patients with advanced gastric cancer and are associated with a dismal prognosis, which makes the early use of intraperitoneal chemotherapy attractive. The primary advantage of heated intra-peritoneal chemotherapy (HIPEC) is the ability to target the tumour burden with up to 20-times higher concentrations of drug measured in the intraperitoneal compartment compared to plasma drug level. Studies to date have been performed primarily in Asia, limiting the interpretation of their results for Western populations. Two areas are of interest:

- HIPEC in patients at high risk of developing peritoneal recurrence based on preoperative assessments treated with "prophylactic intent"
  Meta-analysis[47] restricted to patients with serosal involvement and no distant or peritoneal metastases, in 1 062 patients showed the total relative risk of recurrence with this technique was 0.73 (95% CI 0.64–0.83, $P < 0.00001$). In particular, HIPEC showed a lower peritoneal recurrence rate compared to the control group (RR = 0.45, 95% CI 0.28–0.72, $P = 0.001$).
- HIPEC in the treatment of patients with evidence of gastric cancer peritoneal carcinomatosis (GCPC)
  Meta-analysis demonstrated a significant improvement in median OS with the addition of HIPEC to cytoreductive surgery (CRS) for GC (HIPEC+CRS vs. CRS, median OS 11.1 vs. 7.1 months, $P < 0.001$).[48] Multiple individual studies have suggested that patients with low volume PM and complete cytoreduction are most likely to benefit from HIPEC+CRS.

However, high procedure-related morbidity and mortality associated with the CRS–HIPEC approach continues to generate debate on its merits and has limited its applicability, particularly in Western populations which remain poorly studied.

FUTURE DIRECTIONS

Given the low compliance with postoperative therapies (40–60%) and downstaging advantages of treatment given before surgery, optimising and intensifying the neoadjuvant approach is being adopted in current clinical trials. Strategies include the addition of immunotherapy to chemotherapy as described for oesophageal cancer but also the addition of preoperative chemoradiation.

CRITICS2[49] randomises patients between:

- four cycles of docetaxel+oxaliplatin+capecitabine (DOC);
- two cycles of DOC followed by chemoradiotherapy (45Gy in combination with weekly paclitaxel and carboplatin); or
- chemoradiotherapy.

TOPGEAR is a randomised phase III trial comparing perioperative ECF chemotherapy with an experimental arm therapy of preoperative chemoradiation plus perioperative ECF chemotherapy.[50]

The addition of monoclonal antibodies such as bevacuzimab has not yielded anticipated benefits. The 1 000-patient UK ST03 MAGIC 2 study failed to demonstrate any survival benefit for the addition of bevacizumab to perioperative chemotherapy. Indeed, it showed that preoperative bevacizumab administration could be associated with an increased risk of postoperative anastomotic leak, specifically in those patients who undergo oesophagogastrectomy.[51]

The relative merits of standard therapies and novel biomarkers will drive improvements in outcome. Future studies should stratify by response to neoadjuvant therapy when deciding upon the administration of an additional adjuvant treatment.

PALLIATIVE SYSTEMIC THERAPY

The goals of palliative systemic therapies in patients with advanced upper GI cancer are to palliate symptoms, including malignant dysphagia, improve quality of life, and prolong survival. The benefits of treatment are largely confined to patients of good performance status (WHO 0 or 1) (Table 8.2).

Many patients are elderly, have comorbidities, and are unfit for treatment. A careful discussion of the possible benefits, risks, and limitations of therapy is mandatory for informed consent.

SQUAMOUS CARCINOMA OF THE OESOPHAGUS

A Cochrane meta-analysis identified four studies comparing chemotherapy or targeted therapy against best supportive care. Median OS was 8.0 months in the chemotherapy or targeted therapy arm versus 6.5 months in the BSC arm. HR 0.76 (95% CI 0.65–0.90).[52] The meta-analysis also indicated improved quality of life in the chemotherapy treated patients. A combination of platinum- and fluoropyrimidine-containing combination regimen such as cisplatin or oxaliplatin with intravenous 5FU or oral capecitabine is considered a standard of care. Good response rates (as defined by > 50% shrinkage of tumour volume) of the order of 35% can be achieved with cisplatin and 4- or 5-day 5FU infusion.[53] Response duration is variable and can range from 3 to 6 months. Consideration is often given to consolidation radiotherapy after successful chemotherapy to improve local control where recurrent growth may produce symptoms

Table 8.2   WHO performance scale

Grade	Explanation of activity
0	Fully active, able to carry on all pre-disease performance without restriction
1	Restricted in physically strenuous activity but ambulatory and able to carry out work of a light or sedentary nature, e.g. light housework, office work
2	Ambulatory and capable of all self-care but unable to carry out any work activities. Up and about more than 50% of waking hours
3	Capable of only limited self-care, confined to bed or chair more than 50% of waking hours
4	Completely disabled. Cannot carry on any self-care. Totally confined to bed or chair
5	Dead

for patients with a better performance status and expectation of life. Such therapy is unlikely to prolong survival but prolong the 'swallowing well' interval. Other agents such as paclitaxel are clearly active as single agents but have yet to demonstrate clear superiority in combination regimens. Some results are promising, with response rates nearer 50%.[54]

The programmed death 1 protein (PD-1) is a key immune checkpoint receptor that is expressed by activated T cells. Tumours use the PD-1 pathway to evade immune surveillance. PD-1 binds to its ligands PD1-L1 (B7-H1) and PD1-L2 (B7-DC), which are expressed on tumour cells, thereby causing immunosuppression and preventing the immune system from rejecting the tumour. Reported trials however are inconsistent in using this potential biomarker for eligibility purposes.

The first randomised trial that established the use of immunotherapy in oesophagogastric cancer was ATTRACTION 3[55] in patients who had failed initial chemotherapy for squamous cell carcinoma of the oesophagus. Overall survival was significantly improved in the nivolumab group compared with clinician's choice of second-line chemotherapy group (median 10·9 months, 95% CI 9·2–13·3 vs 8·4 months, 7·2–9·9; HR for death 0·77, 95% CI 0·62–0·96; P = 0·019). Survival benefit occurred regardless of tumour PD-L1 expression. There was an overall significant on-treatment improvement in quality of life for patients given nivolumab compared with those given chemotherapy and a subsequent decreased risk of deterioration in quality of life compared with patients treated with chemotherapy.

KEYNOTE 590[56] randomised 749 patients with locally advanced or metastatic adenocarcinoma or oesophageal squamous carcinoma to chemotherapy with or without Pembrolizumab. The results in squamous cell carcinoma patients were reported recently showing an improvement in the combination from 9.8 to 12.6 months (HR 0.72 (0.6–0.88)). A higher PDL-1 or immune score (CPS) score was associated with more benefit.

Immunotherapy typically has drug costs of £6–7000 per month and is thus unaffordable in many healthcare systems. Current trials are investigating the role of immunotherapy with chemotherapy in first-line treatment

✓✓ In patients with elevated CPS score and squamous histology immunotherapy in addition to chemotherapy is a newly established standard of care[56]

ADENOCARCINOMA OF THE OESOPHAGUS AND STOMACH

A number of controlled trials and meta-analyses have provided evidence for survival benefit of palliative systemic chemotherapy for patients with advanced gastric cancer compared with supportive care. In a meta-analysis of three trials comparing chemotherapy with best supportive care, there was a significant benefit in overall survival in favour of chemotherapy (HR 0.37, 95% CI 0.24–0.55), which translated into an improvement in median survival from 4.3 to 11 months.[57] Several cytotoxic agents are active against oesophagogastric cancer, including fluoropyrimidines, platinum agents (cisplatin and oxaliplatin), taxanes (paclitaxel, docetaxel), and irinotecan. Despite a large number of well-powered randomised trials, there is no clear winner and thus no international consensus as to the best regimen for initial or first-line chemotherapy for advanced oesophagogastric cancer. Tumour testing is mandated for HER2 status, MMR, and PDL1 or CPS score to identify subgroups where selective therapies may be appropriate

SINGLE-AGENT OR ATTENUATED THERAPY

Meta-analysis showed that combination chemotherapy improves survival compared to single–agent 5–FU and is standard of care.[57] The HR for death was 0.84 (95% CI 0.79–0.89) in favour of combination chemotherapy, but this translates into a mere 1-month survival advantage. The price of this benefit is increased toxicity as a result of combination chemotherapy certainly when administered at full dose. A recent UK clinical trial (GO2) addressed the issue of attenuation of doublet chemotherapy for patients unsuitable for full dose chemotherapy due to age or frailty. The lowest dose tested was non-inferior in terms of progression free survival (PFS) and produced less toxicity and better overall treatment utility.[58]

- There are early randomised clinical trials of palliative chemotherapy versus best supportive care that clearly show improved survival (8–12 months chemotherapy vs 3–5 months best supportive care).[57]
- The UK GO2 trial suggests that in elderly and/or frail patients chemotherapy doses can be reduced without any detriment in terms of quality of life or effectiveness of treatment[58]

COMBINATION REGIMENS

- Generally agreed standard of care is two chemotherapy drugs – fluoropyrimidine and a platinum agent.[59]

In one randomised comparison with FAMTX (5FU, doxorubicin and methotrexate), a total of 274 patients with adenocarcinoma or undifferentiated carcinoma of the oesophagus, oesophagogastric junction or stomach were treated. ECF was associated with a superior response rate (45% vs 21%) and median survival (8.9 months vs 5.7 months).[60] ECF has evolved over the years. Firstly, the requirement of three drugs rather than two, in particular the addition of epirubicin to this regimen. An individual patient data meta-analysis of the GASTRIC group concluded that there was no role for epirubicin in combination with a fluoropyrimidine and a platinum agent which is now generally agreed standard of care.[59] In addition it is very difficult to add further novel agents in particular immunotherapy into epirubicin containing regimens.

Secondly, cisplatin infusion requires hydration and prolonged infusion over 8 hours and can cause significant tinnitus, neuropathy, emesis, and a predictable decline in renal function. Oxaliplatin can be administered over 2 hours, does not require hydration but can cause both acute and chronic neuropathy. Thirdly, can protracted venous infusion of 5FU, with the inconvenience of the pumps and associated complications such as thrombosis, be eliminated by the use of modern oral fluoropyrimidines such as capecitabine? To answer these latter two questions the UK REAL2 trial[61] compared four different chemotherapy regimens in 1002 patients with advanced gastric cancer: ECF, EC plus the oral fluoropyrimidine capecitabine, and epirubicin plus oxaliplatin and either infusional FU (EOF) or capecitabine (EOX) The study was sufficiently powered to demonstrate non-inferiority.

✓✓ The REAL2 results demonstrated that oxaliplatin can be substituted for cisplatin with less renal toxicity and neutropenia and that oral capecitabine is a valid substitution for intravenous 5FU.[61] Although a secondary endpoint, there was a significant improvement in median survival for the EOX (epirubicin–oxaliplatin–capecitabine) regimen compared to the ECF regimen (11.2 months vs 9.9 months). There was no significant difference in response rates between regimens and a response rate of 40.7% in the ECF arm.

REAL2 also showed the incidence of thrombotic complications was reduced in the oxaliplatin arm compared to the cisplatin arm. Oxaliplatin-treated patients had significantly less grade 3–4 neutropenia, hair loss, and renal dysfunction, but they had significantly more peripheral neuropathy and diarrhoea.

OX, omitting the epirubicin, is now generally preferred over ECF as first-line therapy.

Importantly, there is a group of patients with locally advanced irresectable disease who may be downstaged sufficiently to undergo potentially curative surgery.

Other options include docetaxel-containing regimens. Docetaxel plus cisplatin and 5FU (the DCF or TCF regimen) was compared with cisplatin and FU alone in a multinational TAX-325 trial[62] that enrolled 457 patients. The group receiving docetaxel did significantly better in terms of response rates (37% vs 25%), and 2-year survival (18% vs 9%). Rates of any serious grade 3 or 4 toxicity during therapy were high in both groups (81% and 75%, respectively). DCF showed significant improvement compared with cisplatin/FU in measures of clinical benefit, including time to definitive worsening of performance status (median 6.1 months vs 4.8 months) and in the duration of preserved quality of life.

MONOCLONAL ANTIBODIES

A paradigm-changing study in this disease was the demonstration that trastuzamab (Herceptin) was as active in gastric cancer as breast cancer. Trastuzumab, a monoclonal antibody against human epidermal growth factor receptor 2 (HER2; also known as ERBB2), was investigated in combination with chemotherapy for first-line treatment of HER2-positive advanced gastric or oesophagogastric junction cancer. The ToGA trial was an international phase III study undertaken in 594 patients, randomised to capecitabine or fluorouracil plus cisplatin plus or minus trastuzumab.[63] Median overall survival was 13.8 months (95% CI 12–16; 16.0 months in those who would be considered HER2-positive (HER2 3 + or HER2 2 + and FISH +) in those assigned to trastuzumab plus chemotherapy compared with 11.1 months (95% CI 10–13) in those assigned to chemotherapy alone (HR 0.74; $P = 0. 0046$). There were no significant differences in toxicities, including cardiac, between the two groups. The proportion of HER2-positive tumours ranges from approximately 10–30% of all gastric cancers, being higher in oesophagogastric junctional cancers, Caucasian patients, and intestinal type pathology.

✔✔ Trastuzumab in combination with chemotherapy can be considered as a new standard option for patients with HER2-positive advanced gastric or oesophagogastric junction cancer.[63]

As yet, other antibodies have not been shown to have additional benefit to chemotherapy in the first-line setting. For example, bevacizumab, widely used in other cancers (e.g. colon and brain cancer), is a monoclonal antibody that binds to soluble VEGF and prevents binding to VEGFR. A survival benefit for adding bevacizumab to capecitabine plus cisplatin could not be shown in the global 774 patient, phase III AVAGAST trial.[64] There was no significant survival benefit (median 12.1 months vs 10.1 months, HR 0.87, 95% CI 0.73–1.03).

Similarly, several studies have explored the addition of the anti-EGFR monoclonal antibodies to standard chemotherapy regimens for first-line treatment. Benefit was not confirmed in the UK 553 patient REAL3 phase III randomised trial[65] comparing chemotherapy with and without the anti-EGFR agent panitumamab. In advanced colorectal cancer, the benefit of these agents is limited to patients whose tumours lack mutated RAS genes. An important point is that none of the trials performed in gastric cancer selected patients based upon biomarkers. However the RAS mutation rate in gastric cancer (6–10%) is much lower than colorectal cancer (45%).

Agents such as ramicuramab discussed later have failed to establish themselves as first-line therapy with a randomised trial showing no benefit in terms of overall survival with addition to standard chemotherapy[66]

IMMUNOTHERAPY WITH CHEMOTHERAPY

This is the major area of interest and clinical trial activity in advanced oesophageal and gastric cancer. Numerous large phase III trials have either completed or reported their early results. The outcome of reported trials is not entirely consistent for first-line treatments. The 763 patient KEYNOTE 062 showed no survival advantage for pembrolizumab or pembrolizumab plus chemotherapy when compared with chemotherapy in patients with programmed cell death ligand 1 (PD-L1) combined positive score (CPS) of 1 or greater, which makes up about half of all cases. Pembrolizumab was however non-inferior to chemotherapy, with fewer adverse events observed.[67]

CHECKMATE649 is the largest global randomised study ever undertaken in advanced gastric cancer. 1 581 patients were randomly assigned to one of three regimens: nivolumab at 260 mg every 3 weeks or 240 mg every 2 weeks plus chemotherapy; chemotherapy alone; or nivolumab plus ipilimumab (the latter date has not as yet been presented). 955/1581 patients randomised had a CPS score > 5. Median overall survival was 14.4 months with nivolumab plus chemotherapy vs 11.1 months for chemotherapy in the PD-L1 CPS ≥ 5 population (HR = 0.71; $P < 0.0001$). The differences were also statistically significant for the PD-L1 CPS ≥ 1 population (HR = 0.77; $P = 0.0001$) and for all randomly assigned patients, 13.8 vs 11.6 months (HR = 0.80; $P = 0.0002$).[68]

In contrast, ATTRACTION-4 contained only Asian patients with no survival advantage for immunotherapy treated patients. Median survival in the Asian study was over 17 months in both arms of the trial and post-progression therapy was given to more than 66% of patients, while in CHECKMATE649, only 39% of progressing patients received further treatment, indicating the disparity between the use of second and further lines of treatment in Western and Asian countries. Also, a higher proportion (27%) of control arm patients in ATTRACTION-4 received post-trial immunotherapy.[69]

It should be noted that these reports are currently preliminary data which raise important questions about optimal biomarker selection in particular mutational burden. These relevant issues regarding optimal patient selection may need to be addressed before adopting this treatment as a standard of care, even in healthcare systems that can afford such therapies

✔✔ The largest global randomised study ever undertaken in advanced gastric cancer (CHECKMATE649) suggests a modest survival benefit for the addition of immunotherapy to chemotherapy. Optimal patient selection by way of biomarker remains controversial.[68]

SECOND-LINE AND SUBSEQUENT TREATMENTS

In general, clinical trials assessing the efficacy of second-line therapy regimens after failure of first-line treatment have shown that response rates are lower than in previously untreated patients, and toxicity rates tend to be higher, related to declining performance status. Quality of life and minimisation of side-effects are key considerations when determining therapeutic approach. The COUGAR-02 UK trial[70] was a phase III randomised controlled trial, testing whether the addition of docetaxel to active symptom control would affect survival and quality of life. Median survival showed a modest, yet statistically significant, improvement in favour of the treatment arm (5.2 months vs 3.6 months, HR = 0.67) and adverse events were found to be generally manageable. Importantly, patients receiving docetaxel also showed improvement in terms of pain, nausea and vomiting, and disease-specific quality of life measures including dysphagia and abdominal pain. In this study, patients were of excellent functional status (100% WHO 0–2; 83% WHO 0–1), mandating that it is essential that the patient's overall health status is considered before commencing second-line therapies.

The German AIO trial, despite its poor accrual, also showed a statistically significant improvement in survival favouring irinotecan over best supportive care (BSC) from 2.4 months to 4.0 months, as well as a marked improvement in tumour-related symptoms (50% vs 7%). Again, patients were of excellent performance status at randomisation.[71]

The global TAGS trial randomised 507 patients with heavily pretreated metastatic cancer to either receive oral trifluridine/tipiracil or placebo. This oral drug is well tolerated in general which makes it an attractive proposition and achieved a 2.1 month improvement in survival from 3.6 to 5.7 months HR = 0.069 (0.56–0.85 P = 0.00003).[72]

Two landmark trials have shown that ramucirumab, a monoclonal antibody inhibiting VEGFR-2, is a valuable addition to therapeutic options. In the phase III REGARD trial, 355 patients with previously treated disease were randomly assigned to BSC plus either ramucirumab or placebo. Overall survival increased from 3.8 months to 5.2 months (HR 0.78, 95% CI 0.60–0.998). The most common adverse event in ramucirumab-treated patients was hypertension (16% vs 8% in the placebo group). Arterial thromboembolism is also noted in the treatment group. Ramucirumab was not associated with increased bleeding, venous thromboembolism, perforation, fistula formation, or proteinuria previously associated with other VEGF inhibitors such as bevacizumab.[73]

The phase III RAINBOW trial[74] compared weekly paclitaxel plus ramucirumab or placebo in 665 patients who had disease progression on or within 4 months after first-line combination therapy. Median overall survival was significantly better with ramucirumab (9.6 months vs 7.4 months, HR 0.807, 95% CI 0.678–0.962).

Genomes of tumours that are deficient in DNA mismatch repair (dMMR) have high microsatellite instability (MSI-H) and harbour hundreds to thousands of somatic mutations that encode potential neoantigens. Such tumours are therefore likely to be immunogenic, triggering upregulation of immune checkpoint proteins. This group of patients, in all diseases, is highly sensitive to immunotherapy with for example Pembrolizumab, which can achieve responses in 30–50% of patients with prolonged survival often in excess of 2 years in pretreated patients and is a standard of care[75]

ATTRACTION 2 randomised 493 patients after failure of two or more chemotherapy regimens to receive Nivolumab immunotherapy or placebo. Irrespective of PD-L1 expression the overall survival rates were 5.32 months in the experimental arm versus 4.14 months with placebo. Nivolumab is now approved the use in some countries in heavily pretreated disease.[76]

- The high cost of novel agents, in particular immunotherapy, precludes their use in many countries and limits their adoption into practice. Immunotherapy is proving to be of increasing interest but requires identification of appropriate biomarkers for patient selection. Where feasible, weekly paclitaxel plus ramucirumab is preferred standard second-line therapy.[74] If not, either single-agent irinotecan or docetaxel are appropriate single-agent chemotherapeutic choices.[70,71]

BEYOND CURRENT STANDARD THERAPIES AND FUTURE DIRECTIONS

The goal is appropriately targeted therapy. Patients for trials need to be selected by biomarker overexpression so that the population can be specifically enriched with the selected target. Failure to appropriately select patients is unlikely to demonstrate the potential efficacy of the targeted agent. Experience in other tumours subtypes suggest that the proportion of patients suitable for such therapy may be relatively modest. Two areas exemplify the field and demonstrate the need for and the utility of appropriate markers.

Neurotrophic tyrosine receptor kinase (NTRK)-1, NTRK2, or NTRK3 encode TRK gene fusion proteins which are implicated in oncogenesis of many solid tumours. Extremely rare in oesophagogastric cancer targeted therapies are available including Larotrectinib. Trials that established this use of agent were not disease-specific but for patients harbouring a NTRK gene fusion. Only one oesophageal cancer patient has been identified to date. The UK has funded all end-stage patients to receive such gene testing. For those rare patients with the gene fusion, typically sarcomas and saliva gland tumours and some paediatric cancers, the response rate was 75% with more than half ongoing for more than 12 months.[77]

The Cancer Esophagus Gefitinib trial demonstrated improved progression-free survival with the epidermal growth factor receptor (EGFR) tyrosine kinase inhibitor gefitinib relative to placebo in patients with advanced oesophageal cancer who had disease progression after chemotherapy. Rapid and durable responses were observed in a minority of patients. A pre-specified, blinded molecular analysis was conducted to compare efficacy of gefitinib with that of placebo according to EGFR copy number gain (CNG) and EGFR, KRAS, BRAF, and PIK3CA mutation status. In EGFR fluorescence in situ hybridization (FISH)-positive tumours (20.2%), overall survival was improved with gefitinib compared with placebo (HR for death, 0.59; 95% CI, 0.35 to 1.00; P = 0.05). In EGFR FISH-negative tumours, there was no difference in overall survival with gefitinib compared with placebo (HR for death, 0.90; 95% CI, 0.69 to 1.18; P = 0.46). There was no difference in overall survival for gefitinib versus placebo for patients with EGFR, KRAS, BRAF, and PIK3CA mutations, or for any mutation versus none, exemplifying the need for appropriate biomarkers.[78]

FUTURE STRATEGIES

Successful strategies to achieve the best outcomes for patients, require assessment, staging, and treatment to be closely coordinated and integrated in a multidisciplinary setting. Patient selection should become increasingly individually tailored by patient specific biomarkers rather than by histology and crude stage. The drive towards genomic sequencing and biomarker discovery with the routine use of PET to pick up early metastatic disease, help radiotherapy planning, and assist in early prediction of non-responders, seems likely to become a key decision-making tool.

Radiotherapy has an increasing role and has undergone rapid technological developments through improved imaging, both in terms of primary tumour localisation and treatment verification. Intensity-modulated treatment uses computer algorithms to optimise the delivery of radiation and spare normal tissue injury. More accurate radiotherapy techniques will allow safe dose escalation in cancers in the upper third of the oesophagus, where there is close proximity of the target volume to the spinal cord.

Systemic therapy is moving towards an era of personalised oncology. More than a decade of clinical experience with biologically targeted cancer agents has both shown their potential and exposed the inadequacies of historical pathology-based classification systems as a basis for treatment selection. Studies have repeatedly shown the huge variation in biological behaviour of patients who have been managed within classically defined disease entities. It is now generally acknowledged that improved biological profiling of individual patients is needed in order to better link patients with appropriate targeted therapies. This is where treatments are selected based on the characteristics of the individual tumour. Many patients will never benefit from current chemotherapy and biological therapies, including monoclonal antibodies, and biomarkers are needed to select those that will benefit the most from what may be relatively toxic and/or expensive treatment. We have seen the first of these in the form of HER2-positive oesophagogastric cancer, which predicts the benefit of the addition of trastuzumab to combination chemotherapy.[63] This will aid the process of new high-quality research trials aiming to develop new treatment strategies.

✔ As chemoradiotherapy emerges as an alternative to radical surgery, particularly in squamous carcinoma, accurately predicting and defining those patients who will achieve good remission prospectively is important, as is the identification of patients who require salvage surgery. New molecular markers may be important tools for the future.

Ultimately, a greater improved understanding of the epidemiology of these diseases will be necessary to allow the identification of disease at a far earlier stage. The current presentation with predominantly nodal and advanced stage disease is likely to limit the improvements that are possible with existing treatments.

The need for continued randomised trials is important. Major centres with high quality assurance and good research support can recruit sufficient patients to answer major questions that are important to improve the outcome for these diseases.

Key points

- Chemotherapy and radiotherapy have a major role, integrated with surgery, in the potentially curative treatment of oesophageal and gastric cancer. Surgery alone is now indicated only for early-stage disease.
- One standard treatment strategies for locally advanced adenocarcinoma of oesophagus and junctional tumours is six cycles of perioperative chemotherapy (MAGIC study).
- There is good evidence that pCR rates are significantly higher with chemoradiotherapy (CRT) than with radiotherapy or chemotherapy given alone. CRT achieves enhanced local therapy coupled with a systemic benefit.
- The CROSS trial using modern radiotherapy techniques and fractionation was an internationally practice-changing randomised phase III study comparing surgery alone to preoperative CRT. The study showed a doubling of overall survival (OS) in favour of the preoperative arm (OS 49.4 vs 24 months, HR 0.67).
- A meta-analysis of both chemotherapy and CRT concluded that there was strong evidence for a survival benefit of neoadjuvant chemoradiotherapy or chemotherapy over surgery alone in patients with oesophageal carcinoma. A clear advantage of neoadjuvant CRT over neoadjuvant chemotherapy has not been finally established.
- Current trials address the issue of the addition of immunotherapy to chemotherapy in perioperative trials
- The role of postoperative CRT following neoadjuvant chemotherapy remains uncertain. Highly selected patients with R1 resection and low or no lymph node burden may reasonably be offered therapy.
- Definitive CRT does provide an alternative to surgery in localised oesophageal cancer.
- In squamous cell carcinoma there is good evidence that a policy of primary CRT is a sustainable strategy (with or without surgical salvage), with equivalent results to surgery.
- The overall local control rate for definitive CRT is 70% in upper-third squamous cancers, for which it is presently the treatment of choice.
- The ability to predict which patients will respond to chemotherapy or CRT would allow greater certainty in a primary non-surgical approach.
- Better outcomes in gastric cancer can be achieved for all but early-stage tumours with the addition of perioperative chemotherapy to surgery (MAGIC).
- The American Intergroup postoperative CRT study reported a significant benefit to survival following gastric resection. However, this advantage is lost when further studies were performed where appropriate radical surgery is undertaken.
- Chemotherapy and radiotherapy have a major role in the palliative treatment of oesophageal and gastric cancer.
- Combinations of a platinum drug and fluoropyrimidine such as oral capecitabine have significant activity against advanced oesophagogastric cancer.
- The aim is to develop more targeted therapies. For the 10–30% of tumours that strongly overexpress HER2 the addition of trastuzumab improves survival from 11.1 months to 16 months.
- Ramucirumab, a monoclonal antibody inhibiting VEGFR-2, is a valuable addition to therapeutic options and is currently used in late stages of therapy.
- The programmed death 1 protein (PD-L1) is a key immune checkpoint receptor that is expressed by activated T cells. Major trials are now reporting small advantages in outcome in all stages of oesophageal and gastric cancer when administered in addition to chemotherapy.
- Immunotherapy will now need to develop biomarkers and other tools to identify those patients most likely to benefit from these costly treatments.

 References available at http://ebooks.health.elsevier.com/

KEY REFERENCES

[5] Teoh S, Virdee P, Mason J, et al. Role of adjuvant radiotherapy following neo-adjuvant chemotherapy (NACT) and surgery in oesophageal cancer – a multi-centre retrospective cohort study. Ann Oncol 2016;27(Suppl 2):ii117.

[8] Kelsen DP, Ginsberg R, Pajak TF, et al. Chemotherapy followed by surgery compared with surgery alone for localized esophageal cancer. N Engl J Med 1998;339:1979–84. PMID: 9869669.

This randomised trial of 440 patients compared chemotherapy (three cycles preoperative CF ± two cycles postoperative) plus surgery with surgery alone and found no difference in survival or pattern of metastatic disease.

[9] Allum WH, Stenning SP, Bancewicz J, et al. Long-term results of a randomized trial of surgery with or without preoperative chemotherapy in esophageal cancer. J Clin Oncol 2009;27:5062–7. PMID: 19770374.

The OE02 study demonstrated improved 2-year and 5-year survival and established preoperative chemotherapy (two cycles CF) as standard treatment in the UK.

[10] Cunningham D, Allum WH, Stenning SP, et al. Perioperative chemotherapy versus surgery alone for resectable gastroesophageal cancer. N Engl J Med 2006;355:11–20. PMID: 16822992.

The MAGIC study demonstrated improved 5-year survival for the perioperative chemotherapy limb (three cycles preoperative ECF + three cycles postoperative ECF) compared to surgery alone (36% vs 23%).

[11] Alderson D, Langley RE, Nankivell MG, et al. Neoadjuvant chemotherapy for resectable oesophageal and junctional adenocarcinoma: results from the UK Medical Research Council randomised OE05 trial (ISRCTN 01852072). ASCO Annu Meet 2015 2015;33:4002. Available from: http://meetinglibrary.asco.org/content/149773-156.

The OE05 trial compared four cycles of preoperative ECX with two cycles of CF chemotherapy and demonstrated that although downstaging was greater at 3 years with ECX, overall survival was the same.

[12] Clinical evidence for association of neoadjuvant chemotherapy or chemoradiotherapy with efficacy and safety in patients with resectable esophageal carcinoma (NewEC study). J eclinm 2020:100422.

This meta-analysis concluded that there was a 21% increase in survival at 3 years with preoperative chemotherapy. It also demonstrated that neoadjuvant chemoradiotherapy increases R0 resection rates, reduces locoregional recurrence and improves survival compared with surgery alone.

[16] van Hagen P, Hulshof MCCM, JJB L, et al. Preoperative chemoradiotherapy for esophageal or junctional cancer. N Engl J Med 2012;366:2074–84. PMID: 22646630.

The CROSS trial compared surgery alone to preoperative CRT using modern radiotherapy techniques and demonstrated a doubling of overall survival (OS) in favour of the preoperative arm.

[22] Al-Sarraf M, Martz K, Herskovic A, et al. Progress report of combined chemoradiotherapy versus radiotherapy alone in patients with esophageal cancer: an Intergroup study. J Clin Oncol 1997;15:277–84. PMID: 8996153.

This randomised trial compared definitive radiotherapy with chemoradiotherapy and demonstrated a significant advantage of combined therapy with survival increasing from 0 to 30%.

[27] Crosby T, Hurt CN, Falk S, et al. Chemoradiotherapy with or without cetuximab in patients with oesophageal cancer (SCOPE1): a multicentre, phase 2/3 randomised trial. Lancet Oncol 2013;14:627–37. PMID: 23623280.

[28] Markar S, Gronnier C, Duhamel A, et al. Salvage surgery after chemoradiotherapy in the management of esophageal cancer: is it a viable therapeutic option?. J Clin Oncol 2015;33:3866–73. PMID: 26195702.

[31] Stahl M, Wilke H, Lehmann N, et al. Long-term results of a phase III study investigating chemoradiation with and without surgery in locally advanced squamous cell carcinoma (LA-SCC) of the esophagus. J Clin Oncol 2008;26(Suppl):4530. abstr

These two trials give some support to a selective approach to using surgery after CRT in SCC.

[43] Smalley SR, Benedetti JK, Haller DG, et al. Updated analysis of SWOG-directed intergroup study 0116: a phase III trial of adjuvant radiochemotherapy versus observation after curative gastric cancer resection. J Clin Oncol 2012;30:2327–33.

This trial reported improved survival for CRT after surgery for gastric cancer but has been criticised for a lack of standardisation of surgery.

[46] Dai Q, Jiang L, Lin RJ, et al. Adjuvant chemoradiotherapy versus chemotherapy for gastric cancer: a meta-analysis of randomized controlled trials. J Surg Oncol 2015;111:277–84. PMID: 25273525.

This meta-analysis of six trials did not resolve the issue of whether chemoradiotherapy or chemotherapy was optimal in multimodal therapy for gastric cancer.

[57] Wagner AD, Syn NL, Moehler M, et al. Chemotherapy for advanced gastric cancer. Cochrane database Syst Rev 2017;8(8):CD004064.

This systematic review demonstrated a clear survival benefit for palliative chemotherapy over supportive care for advanced gastric cancer.

[59] Webb A, Cunningham D, Scarffe JH, et al. Randomized trial comparing epirubicin, cisplatin and fluorouracil versus fluorouracil, doxorubicin, and methotrexate in advanced esophagogastric cancer. J Clin Oncol 1997;15:261–7. PMID: 8996151.

[60] The GASTRIC. (Global advanced/adjuvant stomach tumor research international collaboration) group. Role of chemotherapy for advanced/recurrent gastric cancer: an individual-patient-data meta-analysis. Eur J Cancer 2013;49(7):1565–77.

Generally agreed standard of care is two chemotherapy drugs – fluoropyrimidine and a platinum agent.

[63] Bang Y-J, Van Cutsem E, Feyereislova A, et al. Trastuzumab in combination with chemotherapy versus chemotherapy alone for treatment of HER2-positive advanced gastric or gastro-oesophageal junction cancer (ToGA): a phase 3, open-label, randomised controlled trial. Lancet 2010;376:687–97. PMID: 20728210.

The ToGA trial randomised 594 patients and demonstrated improved overall survival for HER2-positive patients assigned to trastuzumab plus chemotherapy compared to chemotherapy alone.

[68] Moehler M, Shitara K, Garrido M, et al. LBA6_PR Nivolumab (nivo) plus chemotherapy (chemo) versus chemo as first-line (1L) treatment for advanced gastric cancer/gastroesophageal junction cancer (GC/GEJC)/esophageal adenocarcinoma (EAC): first results of the CheckMate 649 study. Ann Oncol 2020;31:S1191. https://doi.org/10.1016/j.annonc.2020.08.2296.

CHECKMATE 649 which is the largest global randomised study ever undertaken in advanced gastric cancer shows a survival advantage for the addition of immunotherapy to chemotherapy in advanced disease.

[70] Ford HER, Marshall A, Bridgewater JA, et al. Docetaxel versus active symptom control for refractory oesophagogastric adenocarcinoma (COUGAR-02): an open-label, phase 3 randomised controlled trial. Lancet Oncol 2014;15:78–86. PMID: 24332238.

COUGAR-02 shows a genuine but small survival advantage for 2nd line palliative chemotherapy over best supportive care.

9 Palliative treatments of carcinoma of the oesophagus and stomach

Natalie S. Blencowe | Ben E. Byrne

Despite improvements in the detection and treatment of oesophageal and gastric cancer, the outlook for most patients is poor. Patients may present late with advanced disease and despite some having localised disease, their general health and frailty precludes radical treatment. In these situations, effective palliative therapy is required, with the aim of improving quality of life. Each year in England and Wales about 60% of new patients with oesophageal or gastric cancer receive primary palliative treatment.[1] For patients receiving palliative treatment for oesophageal cancer the overall survival is less than 12 months, although for patients with advanced gastric cancer this may be up to 24 months.[2,3] This chapter describes the symptoms and signs of advanced oesophagogastric cancer, selection of patients for palliative treatment, clinical decision-making, and information provision, as well as surgical and endoscopic treatment modalities for symptom control. Chapter 8 focuses on palliative chemotherapy and radiotherapy, which has an increasing role to play in advanced oesophageal and gastric cancer.

SYMPTOMS AND SIGNS OF ADVANCED OESOPHAGEAL AND GASTRIC CANCER

TUMOURS OF THE OESOPHAGUS AND GASTRIC CARDIA

Dysphagia is the predominant symptom for most patients with tumours of the oesophagus, oesophagogastric junction, or gastric cardia. The progressive nature of malignant dysphagia is usually apparent. Initial difficulties in swallowing solid food may cause bolus obstruction and odynophagia. Solid food intake gradually reduces and, without treatment, patients may finally be unable to swallow saliva. Severe obstruction of the oesophagus may lead to aspiration pneumonia. Less than 5% of patients with oesophageal cancer develop an aero-digestive fistula, but this is generally associated with locally advanced disease and a very poor prognosis. Oesophageal tumours may also present with vomiting, haematemesis, or gastro-oesophageal reflux. Many patients present with other symptoms of advanced disease including fatigue, anorexia, abdominal pain (caused by ascites or liver metastases), or constipation. Rapid weight loss frequently occurs because of cancer cachexia exacerbated by poor oral intake. Hoarseness caused by tumour infiltration of the recurrent laryngeal nerves may result from advanced local disease or mediastinal recurrence after oesophagectomy.

TUMOURS OF THE GASTRIC BODY AND ANTRUM

Gastric cancer commonly has an insidious presentation, and some patients have few symptoms. Slow blood loss may result in symptoms of anaemia. Haematemesis may be the first symptom. Vague upper gastrointestinal problems, such as epigastric discomfort, early satiety, and gastro-oesophageal reflux, are common. Tumours of the distal stomach may cause outlet obstruction and patients describe epigastric fullness, reflux, and nausea, finally leading to effortless and copious vomiting. The presence of an epigastric mass, supraclavicular lymphadenopathy, jaundice, ascites, or pleural effusions all reflect advanced disease. Less commonly, bony pain and symptoms of increased intracranial pressure are seen related to metastatic spread. Symptoms of oesophageal and gastric cancer are listed in Box 9.1.

PATIENT SELECTION AND MULTIDISCIPLINARY TEAMS

In the UK it is mandated that treatment decisions for patients with cancer are made within the context of an upper gastrointestinal multidisciplinary team meeting. Guidelines for the constitution and processes for upper gastrointestinal multidisciplinary teams are used by national health services and the process is peer reviewed to maintain standards. Teams consist of specialist nurses, gastroenterologists, oncologists, pathologists, radiologists, administrators, palliative medicine experts, and surgeons. Additional members may include cytologists, dieticians, endoscopists, and researchers from clinical trials units. The aim of the team meeting is to comprehensively review available information for each new patient and make optimal treatment recommendations. Information about the cell type, disease stage, comorbidity, and patient choice is considered. Although team working has been widely implemented across the UK and is mandatory, it may not be routine in other international centres. In the United States, a 'multidisciplinary cancer case conference' is required for American College of Surgeons Commission on Cancer accreditation.[4] **Expert opinion: Evidence from several studies has been combined in a systematic review showing that multidisciplinary meetings frequently make changes to diagnostic and treatment decisions.[5] There is some evidence suggesting improved outcomes associated with discussion at a multidisciplinary meeting.[6]**

At first diagnosis, it is recommended that all patients are discussed at the multidisciplinary meeting, regardless of

Box 9.1 Symptoms of oesophageal and gastric cancer

Oesophageal cancer

Dysphagia
Odynophagia
Reflux
Chest pain
Haematemesis
Cough
Dyspnoea
Hoarseness
Weight loss
Fatigue

Gastric cancer

Dysphagia
Epigastric fullness/discomfort
Effortless vomiting
Haematemesis
Nausea
Reflux
Symptoms of anaemia
Weight loss
Fatigue

Metastatic disease

Upper abdominal pain
Epigastric fullness/discomfort
Anorexia
Bone pain
Constipation
Dyspnoea
Cough

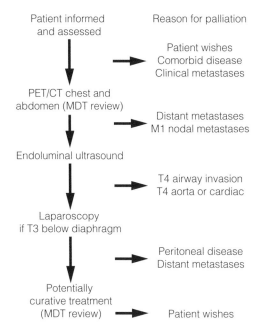

Figure 9.1 Algorithm for selection of palliative or curative treatment of oesophageal and junctional tumours. *CT*, Computed tomography; *MDT*, multidisciplinary team; *PET*, positron emission tomography.

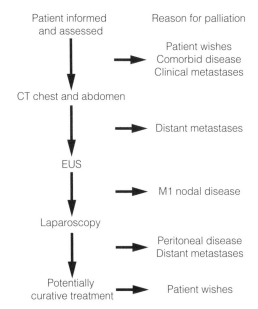

Figure 9.2 Algorithm for selection of palliative or curative treatment for cancers of the gastric body or antrum. *CT*, Computed tomography; *EUS*, endoscopic ultrasound.

initial treatment intent. However, there is uncertainty whether upper gastrointestinal multidisciplinary teams should routinely discuss patients who develop disease recurrence following radical treatment.[7] If this becomes mandatory in the UK the workload of teams could increase. Although optimising outcomes for patients with recurrence (especially after surgical resection) is very important, how they are best managed requires further consideration. Team working and teamwork training will continue to develop over the next decade; professionals may require specific skills and infrastructure to support these processes because high-quality information to inform clinical decisions is paramount to the process.

After establishing a diagnosis (see Chapter 3), new patients require careful assessment to decide whether treatment should be directed towards attempting a cure, or if palliation of symptoms is more appropriate. Careful patient selection has been shown to significantly influence results. Principal factors to consider are the type and stage of the tumour, physical and psychological well-being of the patient, and knowledge of patient preferences. Decisions should be considered in the knowledge of treatment outcomes, including impact on patients' health-related quality of life and expected functional recovery. Disease stage, age, and performance status influence outcomes and survival, although the effect of age may be largely due to increased comorbidity in older patients. Another recognised predictor of mortality is the length of the oesophageal tumour, mainly because this increases the likelihood of nodal involvement. All these factors need to be taken into consideration when planning treatment. Figs. 9.1 and 9.2 illustrate pathways that can be used to select patients for palliative treatment.

FITNESS FOR TREATMENT

The role of major oesophageal or gastric resection in many patients is often easily settled because of general debilitation or multiple coexistent medical problems. Age itself does not preclude octogenarians from surgery, but most older patients are carefully selected. In general, patients who are not fit enough for major surgery are also unable to tolerate a radical course of radiotherapy or definitive chemoradiation. On the whole, surgery for distal gastric tumours is better tolerated than oesophageal surgery by the elderly population, but patients still require careful preoperative assessment before undergoing major resection. Anaesthetic assessment for surgery is considered in more detail in Chapter 5.

STAGING INVESTIGATIONS

Accurate tumour staging plays a crucial part in any therapeutic protocol, enabling patients to be assigned appropriately to treatments with either curative or palliative intent. Clear evidence of haematogenous tumour spread or irresectability directs patients to palliative treatment. Palliative resection or bypass surgery to ameliorate bleeding or obstruction may be indicated for some patients with gastric cancer, even in the presence of haematogenous tumour spread. The decision to proceed with palliative surgery requires careful consideration as patients may rapidly deteriorate in the postoperative period. Chapter 3 describes details of staging protocols for patients with oesophageal and gastric cancer.

PATIENT PREFERENCES AND INFORMATION PROVISION

Information about the diagnosis and prognosis of oesophageal and gastric cancer should be offered to all patients and it is essential that a clinical nurse specialist is involved in this process whenever possible. The volume and type of information required will vary between individuals, although evidence from studies of patients' information needs performed in other disease sites generally show that patients wish to have as much information as possible and prefer the information to be provided by a health professional, as well as in other forms such as a booklet or video.[8] To gain informed consent for treatment (or best supportive care), it is important to provide sufficient information to allow patients to be able to understand the benefits and risks of each treatment option, including no treatment, and to inform them of the likely short- and long-term outcomes. In the UK, this requires discussion of risk that is specific to the individual patient's circumstances, such as their comorbidity or staging results, and exploration of the individual's own information needs.[9] Surveys of patients' information needs show that information about impact of treatments on health-related quality of life is considered important to many patients during treatment decision-making. Many oesophagogastric centres supplement information given by clinicians and nurse specialists with written information sheets. While these are helpful, systematic analysis of information sheets provided for oesophageal cancer shows that they are often inconsistent and incomplete.[10] Ensuring that consultations provide high-quality information in a way that is understood is important and in the UK it is recommended that all specialist cancer teams undergo training in advanced communication skills. There are also methods emerging to develop 'core information sets', which are the minimal baseline pieces of information that should be provided for patients in a particular clinical situation. Items within these 'information sets' may be selected through a rigorous method, incorporating views of patients and clinicians. Such information

sets will be effectively patient centred. One has been developed for oesophageal cancer surgery.[11] All clinicians will be faced with patients who demand every small chance of cure, despite its risks, and others who wish to receive minimal, dignified intervention. Communicating outcomes, providing adequate information, and listening to patients' views is necessary so that patients and their family have access to as much information and support as required.

PALLIATIVE TREATMENTS FOR CANCER OF THE OESOPHAGUS AND GASTRIC CARDIA

The provision of rapid relief of dysphagia for patients with advanced oesophageal and proximal gastric malignancies is the initial priority of palliative treatment for patients who are symptomatic, preferably with minimal intervention. A variety of approaches are available. These include insertion of self-expanding metal stents (SEMSs), endoscopic treatment with brachytherapy, chemical and thermal ablation, external beam radiotherapy (EBRT), and palliative chemotherapy. Treatments may be used individually or in combination. Palliative surgery is not indicated for oesophageal cancer due to the associated major complications and detrimental impact on patients' quality of life.[12] Patients do not have sufficient time to recover from the operation before they experience symptoms of metastatic disease. Non-surgical endoscopic interventions have the biggest role to play in palliation of malignant dysphagia and these are summarised in a recent Cochrane review which includes 51 trials.[13]

The Cochrane review did not find overall superiority of any one treatment over another and noted that only half of the included studies were of high quality. Key results were that SEMS insertion was associated with safer and quicker relief of dysphagia compared to rigid plastic stents. Radiotherapy or brachytherapy may be suitable alternatives and might provide additional survival benefit and improved quality of life.

The individual studies examining endoscopic methods of relieving luminal obstruction are considered in section 1, 'Endoscopic methods for relieving luminal obstruction', next and the other sections concentrate on treatments for palliation of other common problems in oesophageal or oesophagogastric junctional cancer. Medical oncological and radiation treatments are detailed in Chapter 8.

1. MANAGEMENT OF LUMINAL OBSTRUCTION

ENDOSCOPIC TREATMENTS

A tissue diagnosis is desirable prior to treatment of a malignant stricture and wherever possible should be undertaken as a planned procedure with informed consent. Endoscopic methods for relieving luminal obstruction include placement of stents, ablative techniques, and brachytherapy. Many modalities are complementary and no one method or combination is greatly superior to the rest in terms of relief of dysphagia.

Brachytherapy is a good alternative to stenting and may provide better long-term relief of dysphagia and improved quality of life compared to metal stent placement.[14,15]

Historically, dilatation and rigid plastic tubes were advocated for the palliation of malignant dysphagia. Because of the short-lived benefits of dilatation alone and the associated risks of perforation, its use nowadays is reduced to that of a preliminary measure before definitive management of dysphagia. Plastic tubes are also no longer used due to the risks of perforation and need for re-intervention. Minimal gentle oesophageal dilatation may be performed to allow insertion of a SEMS or to place a brachytherapy bougie. Guidelines on the use of dilatation in clinical practice recommend careful preparation, polyvinyl wire-guided bougies, or hydrostatic balloons.[16] Strictures with severe narrowing and angulation are best negotiated under X-ray screening.

ENDOSCOPIC STENTING

PLACEMENT OF OESOPHAGEAL STENTS

Intubation is probably the most widely used form of treatment for the palliation of malignant dysphagia. It allows rapid relief of dysphagia and is generally well tolerated. Prostheses may be placed endoscopically or radiologically and SEMSs are now routinely employed. Several trials have compared plastic stents with SEMS.

✓✓ Metal stents provided greater dysphagia improvement, reduced rates of recurrent dysphagia, fewer adverse events, and less procedure-related mortality compared to plastic tube insertion.[13]

Therefore, SEMSs have replaced rigid plastic tubes for the palliation of malignant dysphagia.

SELF-EXPANDING METAL STENTS

The design of SEMS has evolved since they were first introduced for the palliation of malignant dysphagia in the early 1990s. Modern stents have sutures or tags to allow removal or adjustment. SEMS are made from a flexible alloy mesh that expands for up to 48 hours after deployment. After expansion, an internal luminal diameter of 16 to 25 mm can be achieved. Problems with tumour ingrowth and stent migration have been reduced with newer materials and designs, although these may still occur. Stents may be fully or partially covered. There is no robust evidence of benefit of one stent type over another. Several randomised controlled trials (RCTs) have investigated the addition of a valve in the distal part of the stent to reduce acid reflux. However, because of differences in the reporting of primary and secondary outcomes, it has not been possible to synthesize the evidence.[13] A variety of antireflux stents are now available, and while some data suggest reduced symptoms of reflux (with comparable adverse event rates and effects on dysphagia), further research is required to confirm their effectiveness. Table 9.1 summarises trials of different types of SEMSs that randomised more than 50 patients. Smaller studies were excluded because they are less likely to influence practice. Even within the included studies, several may be at risk of selection bias because methods used to conceal the allocation sequence were unclear (i.e. intervention allocations could have been foreseen before or during enrolment).

METHOD OF INSERTION

SEMSs may be inserted endoscopically or radiologically, or by using a combination of the two. There are several designs with very similar delivery devices. Many companies employ an alloy of titanium and nickel, manufactured into a stent that has a shape 'memory' as well as superelastic behaviour. The stent is loaded in a small-diameter delivery catheter, constrained in a compressed form by a plastic membrane. Most stents incorporate flared ends for secure placement and to reduce the possibility of food entrapment. Comparative studies show that re-intervention rates for tumour ingrowth are higher with uncovered than covered stents. Other studies comparing SEMS with partial or full coverings show conflicting results, and although these trials may have design weaknesses, there is currently no good evidence that one design is superior to another in terms of morbidity or relief of dysphagia.

Contraindications to metal stent placement are tumours within 2 cm of the upper oesophageal sphincter. Placement of stents this high in the oesophagus risks proximal migration, laryngeal compression, intractable pain, and a globus sensation. Other contraindications to stent placement are more relative and dependent on operator expertise, but these include: total luminal obstruction; non-circumferential tumour growth prohibiting proper anchoring of the prosthesis; almost horizontal orientation of the malignant lumen; prior chemoradiation; and multiangulated lesions, particularly with tumours at the gastro-oesophageal junction. All of these situations render endoscopic intubation hazardous.

PREPARATION

Endoscopic prosthesis insertion is usually possible under intravenous sedation, although some endoscopists use general anaesthesia to completely protect the airway and prevent aspiration. Routine monitoring is required with intravenous sedation, as is continual attention to the airway. Saliva and regurgitated fluids should be constantly removed to prevent aspiration during the procedure.

ENDOSCOPIC INSERTION WITH FLUOROSCOPY

After endoscopic assessment and measurement of the tumour, a guidewire is passed into the stomach (after successful negotiation of the tumour with the endoscope or under fluoroscopic control). Occasionally dilatation may be required before passage of the delivery system over the guidewire. The proximal and distal extents of the tumour may be marked with radio-opaque skin markers or the tumour limitations injected with contrast. The slim delivery device is advanced over the guidewire until the radio-opaque markers of the compressed stent are correctly aligned with the tumour. Once in position the stent is deployed by retracting the covering sheath while maintaining stent position. It is possible to reposition some stents after partial deployment. The guidewire and delivery device are then carefully removed under fluoroscopic guidance. After release of the stent, the endoscope may be reinserted to check the final position. Balloon dilatation may be performed to improve expansion and prevent early migration, and this can also be performed up to several days after stent insertion.

RADIOLOGICAL INSERTION

Morphological imaging of the malignant stricture with oral contrast may be performed prior to stent insertion to assesses length and position of the tumour. A fine steerable

Table 9.1   Randomised controlled trials of self-expanding metal stents for the endoscopic palliation of malignant dysphagia (n > 50)

Author	n	Group 1	Group 2	Dysphagia	Clinical Outcomes	Health-Related Quality of Life*	Allocation Concealment†
Dua, 2019[23]	60	SEMS	SEMS with antireflux valve	No difference	No difference	No difference	B
Didden, 2018[24]	98	SEMS: fully covered Wallflex	SEMS: partially covered Wallflex	No difference	No difference	No difference	B
Persson, 2017[25]	95	SEMS: semi-covered Ultraflex	SEMS: fully covered Wallflex	No difference	No difference	No difference	A
White, 2015[26]	100	SEMS: semi-covered Ultraflex, 18/23mm diameter	SEMS: semi-covered Ultraflex, 23/28mm diameter	No difference	No difference	Not assessed	A
Zhu, 2014[27]	160	SEMS: covered	SEMS: covered with radio-iodine sheath	Favours group 2	Longer survival in group 2	Not assessed	A
Dai, 2013[28]	67	SEMS	SEMS: covered with radio-iodine sheath	Favours group 2	No difference	Not assessed	A
Javed, 2012[29]	84	SEMS: covered Ultraflex	External beam radiotherapy and SEMS: covered Ultraflex	Favours group 2 until 3 months, then no difference	Better survival in group 2	Favours group 1	A
Blomberg, 2010[30]	65	SEMS: Z-stent, Ultraflex or Wallstent	SEMS: Z-stent with Dua antireflux valve	Favours group 2	Favours group 2 (except for reflux)	No difference	A
Verschuur[±], 2008[31]	83	SEMS: Ultraflex	SEMS: Polyflex	Favours group 2	More stent migrations in group 2	Not assessed	B
Verschuur[±], 2008[31]	84	SEMS: Ultraflex	SEMS: Niti-S	Favours group 2	No difference	Not assessed	B
Fu, 2004[32]	53	SEMS	SEMS and chemotherapy or chemoradiotherapy	No difference	No difference	Not assessed	B
Sabharwal, 2003[33]	53	SEMS: Flamingo covered Wallstent	SEMS: covered Ultraflex	No difference	No difference	Not assessed	A
Siersema, 2001[34]	100	SEMS: Flamingo covered Wallstent	SEMS: covered Ultraflex or Gianturco Z-stent	No difference	No difference	Not assessed	B
Vakil, 2001[35]	62	SEMS: covered	SEMS: uncovered	No difference	Fewer re-interventions in group 1	Not assessed	A

±This RCT had three treatment arms and subsequently two comparisons.

†The risk of bias in the trial was judged as A=low, B=unclear, or C=high, using the Cochrane risk of bias tool assessing allocation concealment.[28] The tool allows an author to judge whether the randomisation process described in the study has clear evidence that the treatment allocation was concealed to the person randomising the patient before the patient is entered into the study.

*Health-related quality-of-life results reported from a valid multidimensional questionnaire.

Note: 30-day mortality rates were similar in all of the above trials.

SEMS, Self-expanding metal stent.

catheter is then negotiated over a guidewire through the stricture to the stomach and skin markers aligned. The proximal and distal ends of the tumour are marked (similar to endoscopic positioning). Cautious balloon dilatation may be performed if the stricture is very narrow. The stent insertion device is then passed safely and positioned radiographically over the guidewire and released according to the type of stent.

MANAGEMENT AFTER STENT PLACEMENT

After stent insertion the patient is instructed to sit upright. Oral fluids are usually allowed on the same day unless there is concern about complications such as perforation. Clinical and radiological examination may be performed to exclude perforation before oral fluids are commenced. Patients should receive written dietary information with advice to chew food carefully and drink regularly during and after meals. A daily intake of 10 mL hydrogen peroxide (20 vol.) or fizzy drinks is sometimes recommended to maintain stent patency.

COMPLICATIONS

Even in experienced hands, intubation with SEMSs has a procedure-related mortality of about 1–2% and early complication rates of between 0% and 30%. Complications are listed in Box 9.2.

1. Malposition of the stent may require insertion of a second or even third stent (if the tumour is long). This may overlap the malpositioned stent to adequately cover the tumour.
2. Incomplete stent expansion and early dysphagia may require balloon dilatation if no improvement is seen within 48 hours.
3. Early stent migration occurs in about 1% of patients and is more prone in stents placed at the oesophagogastric junction than in stents with both ends anchored within the oesophagus. Endoscopic retrieval may be performed safely, especially with the newer devices. Stents that have migrated into the stomach may also be safely left as they

rarely obstruct the pyloric channel or cause intestinal perforation.
4. Oesophageal perforation is the most serious complication and is more likely if the stricture has been dilatated before stent insertion, there has been prior use of radiotherapy and/or chemotherapy, if the tumour is sharply angulated, or if it extensively encases the oesophagus. Rapid development of subcutaneous emphysema, severe pain, radiological evidence of pneumomediastinum, air under the diaphragm or a pleural effusion should all raise suspicion. The extent of the leak is confirmed by contrast radiography. The most appropriate form of therapy depends on the time of detection and the extent of the leak. If recognised at endoscopy, the insertion of the prosthesis itself may seal off the perforation and prevent mediastinitis. Alternatively, the procedure may be abandoned and conservative treatment undertaken. This involves administration of broad-spectrum antibiotics, cessation of oral intake, acid suppression, and feeding either parenterally or by jejunostomy. An intercostal drain may need to be inserted if there is evidence of pleural contamination.
5. Severe upper gastrointestinal haemorrhage occasionally occurs. This is difficult to treat and only supportive measures may be possible.

LATE COMPLICATIONS

Long-term problems occur in at least 20% of patients and are most frequently related to eating. Problems often require hospital admission, further endoscopic manoeuvres, and occasionally replacement of the prosthesis.

1. Prostheses may block because of tumour overgrowth at either end of the stent or tumour ingrowth through the metallic stent latticework if an uncovered design is used. This leads to recurrent dysphagia and occurs in 5–30% of patients. Tumour ingrowth or overgrowth at either end may be successfully treated with placement of a further stent.
2. Food bolus obstruction occurs in metallic stents despite their wide diameter. Spontaneous resolution can occur or endoscopy may be required to retrieve or displace the impacted food bolus into the stomach.
3. Reflux of gastric acid occurs in all patients whenever the tube crosses the gastro-oesophageal junction. It may lead to oesophagitis and occasionally benign stricture formation above the device. This can be controlled by conservative measures, dilatation, and acid suppression therapy. The use of a stent with an antireflux valve may reduce reflux symptoms.
4. Pressure necrosis and late oesophageal perforation leading to mediastinal fistulation has been reported.
5. Stents can fracture or twist, leading to serious morbidity. These are rare problems as most patients do not live long enough. Operative removal of these tubes is only very occasionally required.
6. Eating difficulties may persist due to incomplete relief of dysphagia. Once a prosthesis is in place all food must pass through a tube with a fixed diameter. Patients therefore need appropriate nutritional support and advice.

Box 9.2 Complications of stent insertion

Early complications

Malposition/migration
Incomplete expansion
Oesophageal perforation
Upper gastrointestinal bleeding
Aspiration pneumonia
Pain

Late complications

Migration
Tumour ingrowth or overgrowth
Aspiration pneumonia
Pain
Reflux
Late perforation and fistulation
Disintegration of prosthesis
Stent torsion
Bleeding

Manufacturers continue to develop new designs to decrease the risk of migration, increase the ease of insertion, and enable stents to be repositioned or extracted. Despite the associated morbidity with stent insertion, the immediate relief of dysphagia in one endoscopy session has made intubation an attractively simple palliative treatment, particularly for patients with poor performance status whose life expectancy is short.

ENDOSCOPIC ABLATIVE TECHNIQUES

Several endoscopic ablative techniques (e.g. laser, argon beam, photodynamic therapy) have been attempted over the past four decades and these may be used alone or in combination. The principles of tumour ablation are successful recanalisation and relief of dysphagia, which may be achieved over several sessions. However, most patients will continue to manage only semisolid or liquid foods and the mean dysphagia-free interval is approximately 4–16 weeks. Repeated recanalisations can be performed as many times as necessary.

Although ablative techniques may be useful for non-circumferential, polypoid, or exophytic tumours, their use is generally diminishing because of wide access to SEMS and the ability of SEMSs to provide relief of dysphagia in a single treatment episode. There are some occasions where ablative and thermal interventions may be used in combination with a stent; for example, tumour overgrowth or ingrowth in patients with oesophageal stents. In tumours of the cervical oesophagus (where stents are difficult to place), ablative therapies may be the treatment of choice.

ENDOSCOPIC TECHNIQUE

Ablative treatments are usually carried out with intravenous sedation. If a malignant stricture is negotiable, the treatment is first applied to the distal end of the tumour. The scope is then withdrawn in a circular fashion into the more proximal tumour. If complete obstruction is encountered, tumours can either be treated in the antegrade direction or first dilated to allow passage of the endoscope. Antegrade therapy may be more dangerous because information about the luminal axis is lacking, and the area first treated rapidly becomes oedematous, impairing visualisation and access more distally.

EARLY COMPLICATIONS

1. Chest pain may result from extensive mucosal burning.
2. Oesophageal perforation. The risk is less than 5% and is said to be related to pre-dilatation rather than a direct complication of the ablative treatment.
3. A benign pneumoperitoneum or pneumomediastinum is sometimes detected. Contrast studies do not show a leak and patients usually make an uneventful recovery.
4. Gastric distension can be quite uncomfortable despite adequate decompression.
5. Haemorrhage is rare, occurring in about 1%.

LATE COMPLICATIONS

1. The main problem is tumour recurrence.
2. Delayed strictures can occur. They require dilatation and occasionally stent insertion.

3. Persistent dysphagia for solids despite recanalisation. This may be related to 'pseudoachalasia' that impairs swallowing. Residual intramural tumour may cause impaired oesophageal body motility and, together with progressive cachexia, this may make it impossible for some patients to take solid foods.

CHEMICALLY INDUCED TUMOUR NECROSIS

The use of intralesional injection of alcohol (usually ethanol) to induce tumour necrosis is a simple, cheap, and readily available palliative treatment, suitable for exophytic tumours and tumours in the proximal oesophagus. It is, however, rare to use this as a primary treatment for the palliation of malignant dysphagia.

ENDOSCOPIC TECHNIQUE

The alcohol injection is administered with intravenous sedation and flexible endoscopy. A sclerotherapy needle is used to inject 0.5- to 1-mL aliquots of alcohol into the protuberant part of the tumour. Endoscopic observation of the tumour blanching and swelling confirms needle position. It is best to start injections distally so that induced oedema does not impede the passage of the endoscope. There is no limit to the total volume injected in one session (1–36 mL has been reported).

OUTCOME

An improvement in dysphagia score is reported in most patients after treatment with absolute alcohol, although it may be made temporarily worse because of tumour oedema and swelling. Retrosternal chest pain and a low-grade pyrexia may occur. Perforation and fistula formation have been reported. The pattern of necrosis may be unpredictable and the main disadvantage is the need for repetitive treatments.

✓✓ Alcohol injection may provide similar relief of dysphagia to laser ablation, but is associated with increased pain post procedure, which may limit its widespread use.[13]

RADIOTHERAPY TREATMENTS

The usual aim of palliative radiotherapy is to inhibit local tumour progression, thereby delaying symptoms such as dysphagia. Radiotherapy may also be given to reduce tumour-related bleeding. Palliative radiotherapy may be delivered by external beam or an intraluminal source (brachytherapy).

EXTERNAL BEAM RADIOTHERAPY

EBRT is widely used because it is straightforward to plan and does not require admission to hospital. Initially, swallowing may deteriorate because of radiation-induced oedema and swelling of the tumour. For patients whose nutrition is at risk prior to treatment, a form of nutritional support may first be required (e.g. SEMS or enteral feeding). This is described in more detail in Chapter 8.

A recent well-designed multicentre RCT (Radiotherapy after Oesophageal Cancer Stenting, or ROCS) has challenged the utility of EBRT in this setting. After undergoing SEMS, a total of 220 patients were randomly assigned to receive usual care alone or EBRT (20 Gy in five fractions or 30 Gy in ten fractions) plus usual care.

Radiotherapy did not reduce dysphagia deterioration and there was no difference in median or overall survival between groups. However, the median time to first bleeding event or hospital admission for a bleeding event was reduced with EBRT.

✓✓ The authors therefore concluded that patients with advanced oesophageal cancer having SEMS insertion for management of dysphagia did not gain additional benefit from concurrent palliative radiotherapy and it should not be routinely offered. For a minority of patients clinically considered to be at high risk of tumour bleeding, concurrent palliative radiotherapy might reduce bleeding risk and the need for associated interventions.[17]

BRACHYTHERAPY (INTRACAVITARY IRRADIATION)

Over the past two decades the use of intracavitary radiation treatment for the palliative treatment of oesophageal cancer has increased. Placement of the radiotherapy source close to the tumour maximises the tumour radiation dose. The brachytherapy applicator can be placed endoscopically or under fluoroscopy. Precise measurements of the tumour are made and planning aims to incorporate a few centimetres of normal oesophagus at either end. The applicator is immobilised at the mouth or nose. The patient is then transferred to a protected treatment room and connected to the Selectron machine. Treatment may be repeated if required. The great merit of brachytherapy is that the radiation dose is highest to the tumour while adjacent normal tissues are relatively spared. It can be used in combination with other treatments. Complications associated with brachytherapy are similar to those of any endoscopic procedure (although uncommon if the tumour is not dilated). Other complications include the development of post-irradiation strictures or tracheo-oesophageal fistula.

Two well-designed multicentre randomised trials have compared single-dose brachytherapy (12 Gy) with SEMSs in patients unsuitable for curative treatment.[14,15] The main endpoint of both trials, which included a total of 274 patients, was dysphagia. Although SEMSs provided better short-term relief of dysphagia, this difference gradually diminished over time and there was a lower incidence of morbidity in the brachytherapy group. Survival was similar in both groups. Both trials also included a robust assessment of health-related quality of life and costs. In one trial, general health-related quality of life showed an overall significant difference favouring brachytherapy on four of five scales including emotional, cognitive, role, and social functioning.[14] In the other, differences were not significant.[14] There were only minor differences in costs between the two treatments.

✓✓ The synthesized results from these two trials conclude that brachytherapy provides good palliation of malignant dysphagia and may be associated with improved quality of life compared to SEMS.

PALLIATIVE CHEMOTHERAPY, RADIOTHERAPY, OR COMBINATION CHEMORADIOTHERAPY FOR OESOPHAGEAL CANCER

There is an increasing role of palliative medical, oncological, and radiation-based treatments for oesophageal and gastric tumours. Full consideration of these treatments is required for all patients presenting with locally advanced or metastatic disease and for patients with localised disease who are unable to receive radical treatments due to comorbidity. Discussions with appropriate specialists within the context of an upper gastrointestinal multidisciplinary team meeting are recommended and these are considered in detail in Chapter 8.

2. MANAGEMENT OF AERO-DIGESTIVE FISTULAS

Malignant fistulation between the gastrointestinal tract and airway is very serious. It leads to paroxysmal coughing fits associated with drinking and eating, and aspiration pneumonia. Untreated, death due to respiratory failure will occur usually within a few weeks. Fistulae occur in about 5% of patients with oesophageal cancer, either because of spontaneous necrosis of the tumour and/or local nodes through the oesophageal wall into the bronchial tree, or as a result of treatment. They can be diagnosed with endoscopy or imaging with oral contrast. These fistulas are difficult to treat, particularly those close to cricopharyngeus because of the risk of significant airway compromise. Endoscopic insertion of a SEMS prosthesis both within the airway and oesophagus is the treatment of choice. There are no clear benefits to chemotherapy in this context. The endoscopic placement of fibrin tissue glue has been tried, although results are poor. It is essential that patients with malignant aero-digestive fistulae receive full support from clinical nurse specialists and the palliative care team as appropriate.

3. MANAGEMENT OF RECURRENT LARYNGEAL NERVE PALSY

Recurrent laryngeal nerve palsy caused by tumour infiltration often results in eating difficulties, a weak voice, poor cough, and repeated chest infections because of aspiration pneumonia. Patients are usually hoarse and complain of swallowing difficulties in the oropharyngeal phase. Coughing and a sensation of choking are typical on consuming solids and liquids. The diagnosis is confirmed by laryngoscopy, and aspiration can be seen during the pharyngeal phase of swallowing on barium studies. Endoscopy may be required to exclude other problems contributing to dysphagia. The left nerve is more commonly involved because of its intrathoracic course.

4. MANAGEMENT OF BLEEDING

Bleeding from inoperable oesophageal and cardia tumours causes problems with refractory anaemia and occasionally acute upper gastrointestinal haemorrhage. It is often difficult to deal with because of the advanced nature of the tumour and it may be a terminal event. Symptoms may be controlled endoscopically using laser energy, adrenaline injection, or electrocoagulation. There is some evidence that external beam radiotherapy reduces bleeding in this setting.

PALLIATIVE TREATMENTS FOR GASTRIC CANCER

The role of palliative surgery for gastric cancer varies according to the location of the tumour. For tumours of the proximal stomach, body, and linitis plastica, palliative surgery is more controversial than for antral tumours. It probably has little to offer for those patients with peritoneal or liver metastasis or contiguous organ involvement, where life expectancy is very poor at around only 4 months. Even when disease is limited to the stomach or regional lymph nodes, patients with linitis plastica rarely survive beyond 12 months after total gastrectomy (performed with curative intent). Therefore, in the authors' unit palliative total gastrectomy is very rarely performed for linitis plastica. The role of distal gastrectomy for antral tumours is decreasing as endoscopic stent placement is becoming more common. Surgery may be considered to palliate the problems of chronic blood loss from gastric tumours that cannot be dealt with endoscopically, although this is rare. Radiotherapy may also be used to control chronic bleeding from gastric tumours, although there are no published data to support this practice. These treatments require very careful discussion with patients in the context of multidisciplinary teams because of the associated morbidity.

GASTRIC OUTLET OBSTRUCTION

Obstruction associated with distal gastric cancer presents with vomiting, reflux, and the symptoms of widespread disease, and can be difficult to manage. Many of the tumours extend proximally to involve extensive segments of the stomach, resulting in interference with both reservoir function and emptying, and influencing function even after the mechanical obstruction has been palliated.

Resection of the primary tumour may provide better symptomatic relief than bypass surgery, although there is a lack of well-designed and conducted trials comparing these two treatment options. The problem with palliative gastrectomy is that many patients are nutritionally depleted and frail. Surgical resection may therefore be best avoided, as patients never sufficiently recover from surgery to benefit from it during their remaining time alive (median survival < 12 months). There are also differing opinions about the type of palliative gastrectomy that should be performed in this situation (subtotal or total). In the Western world, where morbidity associated with total gastrectomy is high, gastric resections are not generally recommended for palliative purposes.

Gastrojejunostomy (laparoscopic or open) can be performed if distal gastric tumours are very advanced and symptomatic. A loop of jejunum is anastomosed close to the greater curve of the stomach. There is some evidence that laparoscopic gastrojejunostomy for palliation of incurable gastric outlet obstruction causes less morbidity than standard open surgery (Table 9.2).

Systematic reviews comparing gastrojejunostomy with endoscopic stenting suggest that stent placement may improve symptoms more quickly and reduce hospital stay, although there may be more re-interventions due to recurrence of symptoms secondary to stent blockage or migration. Stents may therefore be more favourable in patients with a very short life expectancy, whereas bypass may be preferable in patients with a prolonged prognosis.[18] The randomised trials examining these issues are small, however, and well-designed studies are still needed.[19–22] Generally, it is recommended to avoid surgery in the advanced setting and to focus treatment on reducing symptoms with minimal risks and side-effects. Wherever possible, endoscopic palliative treatment of obstructive symptoms and/or palliative chemotherapy are offered to these patients in combination with support from palliative care services.[3]

Table 9.2   Randomised controlled trials of the palliation of gastric outlet obstruction (gastrojejunostomy vs endoscopic duodenal stent insertion)

Author	n	Adverse Events	Time to Oral Intake	Hospital Stay	Health-Related Quality of Life	Survival	Allocation Concealment†
Jeurnink, 2010[19]	37	Favours surgery (mainly stent obstruction and dislodgement)	Favours stenting (5 vs 8 days)	Favours stenting (7 vs 15 days)	No difference	No difference	A
Mehta, 2006[20]	27	Favours stenting (surgery = 8, stent = 0)	Not assessed	Favours stenting (11.4 vs 5.2 days)	Favours stenting (physical health measured using SF-36)	No difference	A
Fiori, 2004[21,22] and 2013	18	Favours stenting (surgery = 2, stent = 1 dislodgement)	Favours stenting (most resumed liquid diet on day 1 vs day 5 in surgical group)	Favours stenting (3.1 vs 10 days)	No difference (patient satisfaction)	No difference	A

†The risk of bias in the trial was judged as A=low, B=unclear, or C=high, using the Cochrane risk of bias tool assessing allocation concealment.[28] The tool allows an author to judge whether the randomisation process described in the study has clear evidence that the treatment allocation was concealed to the person randomising the patient before the patient is entered into the study.

The insertion of nasogastric tubes, percutaneous endoscopically placed feeding tubes, and jejunostomies enables nutrition to be delivered to patients with inoperable tumours. However, these manoeuvres alone fail to palliate most of the patient's symptoms. Many believe that such palliation merely perpetuates suffering except in situations where they are used as an adjunct to recanalisation. They may be indicated to provide preliminary nutritional support in patients selected for palliative chemotherapy.

The role of palliative chemotherapy or radiotherapy in gastric cancer is very important and is described in detail in Chapter 8.

SUMMARY

The number of therapeutic options available for the palliation of patients with oesophageal and gastric cancer has increased over the past decade. No single treatment completely relieves all symptoms without side-effects and the median life expectancy for patients with either tumour type is between 6 and 12 months. Common clinical situations such as the management of fistulas, high oesophageal tumours, and bleeding inoperable gastric lesions continue to present formidable management problems. The introduction of SEMS, argon beam coagulation, brachytherapy, chemotherapy, and combination treatments offers new hope, although evidence of significant survival benefits or improvements in quality of life with new treatments have yet to be realised. The increasing centralisation of cancer services in order to provide high-technology specialised care may improve outcomes and increase recruitment into national randomised trials that focus on palliative treatments. There are still many patients who present with advanced disease who are severely debilitated and have a limited life expectancy. Such patients need to be identified early to prevent travelling long distances to a centre with specialised endoscopic facilities only to find that treatment has to be performed more than once. Genuine efforts should be made to see if patients with very short survival times (less than 4 weeks) can be identified and perhaps spared unnecessarily aggressive attempts at palliation.

There remains a need to define outcomes for patients with inoperable malignancies of the upper gastrointestinal tract. Although it would be useful to standardise dysphagia scores and improve audit, in the palliative setting the most important outcome should be patients' assessment of the benefits of treatment. The role of the specialist upper gastrointestinal nurse to support patients undergoing palliative treatment and to provide nutritional support is increasing, and links between palliative care and upper gastrointesinal cancer teams are very important.

The selection of palliation for patients with advanced disease is difficult. Every patient is unique with regard to tumour histology, stricture location, clinical stage, premorbid state, and emotional requirements. Choosing one technique over another must be justifiable on the grounds of treatment efficacy, ease of application, overall adaptability to other therapeutic areas, and patient acceptance, while minimising both complications and cost. Skilled multidisciplinary teams with a thorough understanding of all the available palliative treatments are needed and close liaison with palliative care services is essential to minimise suffering.

Key points

- Palliative treatment decisions should be taken in the context of a multidisciplinary team meeting and recommendations subsequently be shared with the patient. Patients require information that is imparted kindly but truthfully and it should include data about likely survival benefits and the impact of treatment on symptom relief and quality of life.
- Accurate tumour staging and assessment of patient comorbidity and choice play a critical part in any therapeutic protocol, enabling patients to be assigned appropriately to treatments with either curative or palliative intent.
- Surgery has a limited role to play in palliative treatments of cancer of the oesophagus and stomach. Subtotal gastrectomy may be useful to palliate outlet obstruction in patients with a reasonable prognosis. The role of palliative total gastrectomy is very limited.
- SEMS insertion provides quick, effective relief of malignant dysphagia. Single high-dose brachytherapy provides better long-term relief of dysphagia than SEMSs and survival benefit.
- Laser treatment or argon beam coagulation may be useful for non-circumferential, polypoid, or exophytic tumours, or for tumour overgrowth around a stent. Intubation is preferable in sclerotic stenosing tumours.
- Palliative chemotherapy has an increasingly important role to play in advanced oesophageal cancer and tumours of the oesophagogastric junction, although there is little evidence to show that this substantially influences survival (see Chapter 8).
- The median survival for patients with gastric cancer undergoing palliative treatment is poor; 50% of patients die within 8 months of diagnosis and the remainder within 2 years. Combination chemotherapy increases survival compared with best supportive care. This is described in Chapter 9.
- The selection of palliation for patients with advanced disease is difficult and requires skilled motivated input from multidisciplinary teams with a thorough understanding of all the available palliative treatments and awareness of the patient's individual needs.

 References available at http://ebooks.health.elsevier.com/

KEY REFERENCES

[1] National Oesophago-Gastric Cancer Audit 2019. London: The NHS Information Centre. Available at: https://www.nogca.org.uk/content/uploads/2019/12/REF150_NOGCA_2019-Annual-Report-FINAL_19Dec.pdf.
[13] Dai Y, Li C, Xie Y, et al. Interventions for dysphagia in oesophageal cancer. Cochrane Database Syst Rev 2014;10:CD005048.
    This systematic review did not find overall superiority of any one treatment for palliation of malignant dysphagia. Self expanding metal stents were associated with quicker and safer relief of dysphagia than plastic stents. Radiotherapy or brachytherapy were suitable alternatives that may have quality of life or potential survival benefits..
[18] Upchurch E, Ragusa M, Cirocchi R. Stent placement versus surgical palliation for adults with malignant gastric outlet obstruction. Cochrane Database Syst Rev 2018;(5):CD012506.
    Stent placement for palliation of malignant gastric outlet obstruction may improve symptoms more quickly and shorten hospital stay compared to surgical gastrojejunostomy bypass. However, stents were associated with more re-interventions.

Other oesophageal and gastric neoplasms

Matthew Forshaw | Andrew Macdonald

INTRODUCTION

Oesophageal adenocarcinoma, squamous cell carcinoma, and gastric adenocarcinoma are the commonest neoplasms affecting the oesophagus and stomach. This chapter deals with other less common tumours encountered in both the oesophagus and stomach (Tables 10.1 and 10.2). These can be classified as benign, malignant, or of uncertain malignant potential and can arise from epithelial or mesenchymal cells. The main neoplasms to be considered are gastrointestinal stromal tumours (GISTs), primary gastric lymphoma (PGL) and neuroendocrine neoplasms of the stomach. Over the last two decades, the terminology and management of these three conditions have evolved; new developments include the use of endoscopic ultrasound (EUS) in diagnosis, endoscopic surveillance, novel directed treatments, and changing indications for surgery. All other tumours in both the oesophagus and stomach are exceedingly rare, with information derived from either case reports or small case series in the surgical literature. Metastases to the oesophagus and stomach, principally from the lung, breast, and melanoma, have also been reported. Two other conditions (leiomyoma and leiomyosarcoma, both affecting the oesophagus) will be briefly discussed at the end of the chapter.

GASTROINTESTINAL STROMAL TUMOURS (GISTS)

PATHOPHYSIOLOGY

GISTs are soft-tissue sarcomas of mesenchymal origin that arise in the gastrointestinal (GI) tract; they are rare, representing 0.1–3% of all gut tumours and 5% of all soft-tissue sarcomas.[1] Historically, these tumours were considered to be of smooth muscle origin and were generally regarded as leiomyomas (benign) or leiomyosarcomas (malignant). Electron microscopy and immunohistochemical studies indicated, however, that only a minority of stromal tumours have the typical features of smooth muscle, with some having a more neural appearance and others appearing undifferentiated.[2] 'Gastrointestinal stromal tumour' was subsequently introduced as being a more appropriate term for these neoplasms, with the variable histological features (smooth muscle, neural, or undifferentiated) considered to be of little clinical relevance. GI autonomic nerve tumour (GANT) was also introduced to describe sarcomas with ultrastructural evidence of autonomic nervous system

differentiation[3]; these tumours are now recognised as a variant of GIST.[4] The discovery of CD34 expression in many GISTs suggested that they were a specific entity,[5] distinct from smooth muscle tumours. It was also observed that GISTs and the interstitial cells of Cajal (ICCs) express the receptor tyrosine kinase KIT (CD117).[6] This has led to the now widely accepted classification of mesenchymal tumours of the GI tract into GISTs, true smooth muscle tumours, and, far less frequently, true Schwann cell tumours.[7] A pathologist experienced in GI mesenchymal cancers should make the histopathological diagnosis of GISTs. Tumours may have a spindle cell, epithelioid, or mixed histological appearance. An immunohistochemical panel should include CD117, DOG-1, desmin, CD34, and smooth muscle antigen (SMA). Typically GISTs are positive for CD117 and DOG-1 and negative for desmin.[8] Around 85% of GISTs have activating mutations in either the KIT or PDGFRA genes, which are situated on the same chromosome. The most common KIT mutations are found in exons 11 and 9. GISTs with PDGFRA exon 18 D842V mutations are exclusively gastric in location and are resistant to the currently used tyrosine kinase inhibitors. About 15% of the GISTs are designated as 'wild type' with no mutations in KIT or PDGFRA genes and have distinctive clinical, biological, and molecular phenotypes. succinate dehydrogenase-deficient GISTs occur in young women and are almost exclusively gastric in their location.[9]

INCIDENCE AND MALIGNANT POTENTIAL

The estimated annual incidence of GISTs is around 15 per million,[10] which equates to approximately 900 new cases per year in the UK. Incidental microscopic gastric GISTs are commonly found in gastrectomy specimens[11] but not in other intestinal resections.[12] The size of the tumour, the symptoms at diagnosis, the organ of origin (small bowel GISTs have the worst prognosis), and mitotic count seem to be the most important factors when assessing prognosis.[13] An analysis of 1765 gastric GISTs showed that tumours <10 cm diameter or with a mitotic count <5/50 high-power fields (HPFs) had a 2–3% risk of having metastasised, whereas those >10 cm diameter or mitotic count >5/50 HPFs had an 86% risk of metastatic spread.[14] For non-gastric intestinal GISTs the risk of aggressive behaviour is highest for tumours >5 cm diameter and mitotic count >5/50 HPFs.[15]

✔ The size, mitotic count, and location are the most important prognostic factors for predicting GIST behaviour.[14,15]

Table 10.1   Epithelial tumours and cancer precursors of the oesophagus and stomach

	Oesophagus	Stomach
Benign epithelial tumours and cancer precursors	Barrett's dysplasia Squamous dysplasia	Polyps, e.g. hyperplastic, fundic gland Adenomas Epithelial (glandular) dysplasia
Malignant epithelial tumours	Adenocarcinoma of the oesophagus and OG junction Adenosquamous and mucoepidermoid carcinoma Adenoid cystic carcinoma Squamous carcinoma Undifferentiated carcinoma Neuroendocrine neoplasms	Adenocarcinoma Adenosquamous carcinoma Squamous carcinoma Undifferentiated carcinoma Neuroendocrine neoplasms Gastroblastoma

OG, Oesophagogastric.
Adapted from WHO Classification of Tumours. 5th ed. 2019.

Table 10.2   Non-epithelial tumours of the oesophagus and stomach

	Examples
Haematolymphoid tumours	Extranodal marginal zone lymphoma of mucosa-associated lymphoid tissue (MALT lymphoma) Diffuse large B-cell lymphoma (DLBCL) Other types of lymphoma are rare
Mesenchymal tumours	Gastrointestinal stromal tumours (GISTs) Adipose tissue and myofibroblastic tumours, e.g. lipoma Inflammatory myofibroblastic tumour, liposarcoma Smooth muscle tumours, e.g. leiomyoma, leiomyosarcoma Vascular and perivascular tumours, e.g. haemangioma, Kaposi's sarcoma, angiosarcoma Neural tumours, e.g. Schwannoma
Others	Melanoma Germ cell tumours

Reprinted from WHO Classification of Tumours, 5th Edition, 2019.

Table 10.3   Anatomical site of gastrointestinal stromal tumours

Site	Percentage
Stomach	60–70%
Small intestine	20–30%
Oesophagus, mesentery, omentum, colon or rectum	10%

PATIENT DEMOGRAPHICS AND ANATOMICAL DISTRIBUTION

No marked sex difference is apparent for GISTs. Two larger series of malignant GI sarcomas did, however, demonstrate a slight male predominance.[16,17] The age distribution appears to be unimodal with a median age at presentation of 58 years (range 16–94). The peak incidence in men occurs in the fifth decade, slightly before that in women, where it peaks in the sixth decade. Only 1–2% of GISTs present in patients before 30 years of age.[16]

Most GISTs arise in the stomach or small intestine, and infrequently in the oesophagus, mesentery, omentum, colon, or rectum[17,18] (Table 10.3). Approximately 10–30% of GISTs are overtly malignant at presentation[19]; the principal sites of metastasis are the liver and the peritoneal cavity, and spread to lymph nodes is very rare.[16]

PRESENTATION

The symptoms of GISTs are non-specific and depend on the size and location of the lesion. Small GISTs (2 cm or less) are usually asymptomatic and are detected during investigations or surgical procedures for unrelated disease. The vast majority of these are of low risk for malignancy.[20] In many cases the mucosa is normal so that endoscopic biopsies are unremarkable. Incidental discovery accounts for approximately one-third of cases.[21]

The most common symptom is GI bleeding which is present in approximately 50% of patients[22] (Table 10.4). Patients with larger tumours may experience abdominal discomfort or develop a palpable mass.[23] GISTs are often clinically silent until they reach a large size, bleed, or rupture. Most duodenal GISTs occur in the second part of the duodenum where they can cause obstructive symptoms or infiltrate into the pancreas.[24]

INVESTIGATION

Approximately 60% of GISTs are submucosal and grow towards the lumen where, if in the proximal GI tract, they may be visualised endoscopically as smooth submucosal projections. If a small submucosal mass is seen as an incidental finding at the time of endoscopy, EUS should be the first investigation as a proportion will be due to extrinsic impression from normal adjacent structures, e.g. gallbladder, spleen, or loaded colon. If this is the case, no further investigation is required. Other differentials to consider for submucosal lesions other than GISTs are gastric cancer, leiomyoma, soft tissue sarcoma, inflammatory fibrous polyps, pancreatic rest, and schwannoma. For larger palpable masses, or where the patients present with haemorrhage, abdominal pain, or obstruction, computed tomography (CT) is usually the first investigation after endoscopy both to assess the primary and to look for metastases.[25]

ENDOSCOPIC ULTRASOUND

The classical features are of a hypoechoic mass contiguous with the fourth (muscularis propria) or second (muscularis mucosae) layers of the normal gut wall, both of which are hypoechoic (Fig. 10.1).

✔ The accuracy of EUS in predicting GIST behaviour is controversial. EUS features most predictive of 'benign' tumours are regular margins, tumour size ≤30 mm, and a homogeneous echo pattern. Larger tumours with irregular extraluminal margins and cystic spaces may behave more aggressively.[26–28]

To further aid diagnostic accuracy it is possible to use a linear EUS scope through which needle aspirates and core biopsies can be taken without breaching surgical resection planes. EUS–fine-needle aspiration (FNA) in experienced hands has a diagnostic accuracy of up to 97% for GIST lesions,[29] is becoming more widely available, and should be considered in the diagnostic work-up of a possible GIST lesion if the result could change clinical management.

COMPUTED TOMOGRAPHY

GIST imaging by CT scanning typically shows an extraluminal mass, often with central necrosis, arising from the digestive tract wall.[21] Small tumours typically appear as sharply margined, smooth-walled, homogeneous, soft-tissue masses with moderate contrast enhancement.[30] Large tumours tend to have mucosal ulceration, central necrosis and cavitation, and heterogeneous enhancement following intravenous (IV) contrast.[30] As well as defining the presence and nature of a mass, if possible, the likely organ of origin should be defined.

Table 10.4   Symptoms of gastrointestinal stromal tumour at diagnosis[22]

Symptoms	Incidence
Abdominal pain	20–50%
Gastrointestinal bleeding	50%
Gastrointestinal obstruction	10–30%
Asymptomatic	20%

Multiplanar reconstruction can assist this, particularly with large masses. Negative oral contrast (e.g. tap water) and IV contrast for the assessment of gastric GISTs are recommended (Fig. 10.2). CT of the chest, abdomen and pelvis is recommended for staging of GIST, with the exception of small incidental tumours or when a patient presents as an emergency requiring urgent surgery. With regards to assessing treatment response, traditional CT criteria (Response Evaluation Criteria in Solid Tumours [RECIST] criteria) have been shown to be inaccurate for measuring GIST response to imatinib and the Choi criteria are recommended (10% reduction in size and 15% reduction in density).[31]

MAGNETIC RESONANCE IMAGING

In general, magnetic resonance imaging (MRI) offers no additional information regarding the intralesional tissue characterisation of primary GISTs. However, MRI provides excellent soft-tissue contrast resolution and direct multiplanar imaging, which can help delineate the relationships of the tumour and adjacent organs and is useful in anorectal disease.[30]

POSITRON EMISSION TOMOGRAPHY

Positron emission tomography (PET) scanning using a standard fluorodeoxyglucose (FDG)-PET technique has proven extremely useful in the prediction of tumour response to the tyrosine kinase inhibitor imatinib (Glivec®, Norvartis Pharma AG) now used in the treatment of unresectable and metastatic malignant GISTs.[32] Glucose uptake of the tumours decreases within a few hours to days of the start of treatment, which can be verified with FDG-PET.[20] The PET scan can be utilised to distinguish between tumour progression and increase in volume due to intratumoural bleeding. PET scan responses have also been demonstrated to predict subsequent tumour volume reductions found on CT or MRI.[33] However, PET-CT is not routinely used in staging of GISTs and is not recommended in any current guidelines for staging GISTs or assessing response to downstaging.

GIST SYNDROMES

Families have been reported with single-base 'gain of function' mutation in the kinase domain of KIT. The resultant effect is the development of multiple GISTs in the small bowel. Diffuse hyperplasia of spindle-shaped cells within the myenteric plexus at sites unaffected by GIST formation was also noted.[34,35] The association of three uncommon neoplasms – gastric GIST, functioning extra-adrenal paraganglionoma

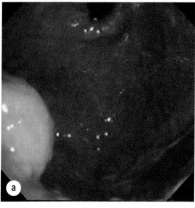
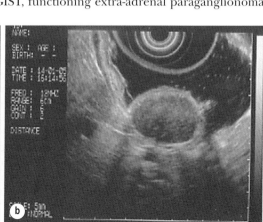

Figure 10.1 (a) Endoscopic view of a small incidental gastric gastrointestinal stromal tumour (GIST). (b) A 12-MHz EUS image of the incidental gastric GIST seen in (a), showing the lesion arising from the muscularis propria. (Courtesy of Richard Hardwick, Addenbrookes Hospital, Cambridge.)

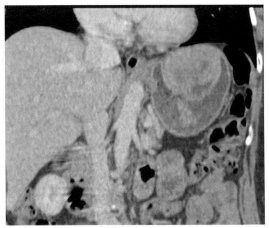

Figure 10.2 Coronal computed tomography scan of large gastric gastrointestinal stromal tumour arising from the fundus. (Courtesy of Richard Hardwick, Addenbrookes Hospital, Cambridge.)

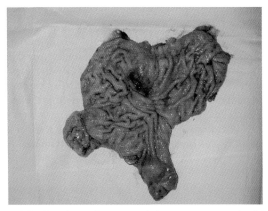

Figure 10.3 Specimen from completion gastrectomy for bleeding gastrointestinal stromal tumour (ulcer clearly visible) in a 34-year-old woman with Carney's triad. (Courtesy of Richard Hardwick, Addenbrookes Hospital, Cambridge.)

and pulmonary chondroma – was first reported in 1977 and has been recognised as 'Carney's triad' since (Fig. 10.3).[36] A subsequent review of 79 cases demonstrated that unlike isolated sporadic GIST, where no significant sex difference was noted, 85% were female.[37] Twenty-two per cent of the patients had all three tumours; the remainder had two of the three, usually the gastric and pulmonary lesions. Adrenocortical adenoma has since been identified as a new constituent of the disorder. The presence of two of the three main tumours is considered sufficient for the syndrome. GISTs may also occur in neurofibromatosis-1 patients, when they are often multicentric and found in the small intestine.[9]

TREATMENT AND PROGNOSIS (BOX 10.1)

A multidisciplinary specialist team is the optimal setting for the management of GISTs. A chest, abdominal and pelvic CT should be included in the preoperative assessment for all patients. If the tumour is located in the right or left upper quadrant then the patient should have an endocrine assessment to exclude a large functioning adrenal tumour. Male patients (under the age of 40 years) presenting with large centrally placed retroperitoneal tumours should have α-fetoprotein and β-HCG levels measured to exclude non-seminomatous germ cell tumour.

Percutaneous (ultrasound (US) or CT) or laparoscopically guided biopsies should not be used in resectable disease due to the risk of tumour rupture or seeding, unless it may result in a change of treatment.[20] Laparoscopy may be considered in the staging of large lesions to exclude peritoneal metastases but an exploratory laparotomy is usually required to decide whether a large primary tumour is technically resectable or not. In reality, if a gastric lesion looks readily resectable by a limited resection, it is not necessary to obtain histological diagnosis prior to surgery. However, if the lesion is close to the pylorus or gastroesophageal junction and a more major resection is required, histological confirmation is clearly advisable.

✔ The main goal of GIST management is complete macroscopic and microscopic removal of the tumour, that is, R0 resection. Complete excision offers a good chance of cure and must be attempted whenever possible.[38]

Box 10.1 Principles of GIST treatment

Locoregional disease

Principles of surgery

- A wide local resection with macroscopic and microscopic removal of the entire tumour is recommended (R0).
- The surgeon should aim to preserve function, but not at the expense of an R0 resection.
- Extended lymphadenectomy is normally not required.
- Some small tumours may be resected laparoscopically.
- Where adjacent organs are involved, en bloc resection is recommended whenever possible – input from other specialist surgeons should be considered prior to embarking on a resection.
- Endoscopic resection is not recommended.

Unresectable and/or metastatic disease

- Mutational analysis to assess sensitivity to imatinib is mandatory prior to starting treatment.
- Imatinib should be used as treatment for unresectable and/or metastatic GISTs.
- Unresectable GISTs may be rendered resectable after 6–12 months of imatinib.
- The recommended starting dose of imatinib is 400 mg/day.

The presence of a positive resection margin or tumour rupture leads to a significant reduction in survival.[39] In one study, only 11% of patients died of recurrent disease after R0 resection compared with 75% of those in whom the resection was R1 or R2, with a median follow-up of 2.2 years.[40]

At all sites the extent of resection is, therefore, dictated by the size of the tumour and its location in relation to, or invasion of, adjacent structures (Fig. 10.4). Oesophagectomy is the standard procedure for oesophageal GISTs but these are very rare and submucosal lesions in the oesophagus are much more likely to be leiomyomas. EUS-FNA core biopsy from these lesions is recommended to make a preoperative diagnosis so that surgical planning is appropriate.[29] Oesophageal GISTs and leiomyosarcomas require an oesophagectomy whereas leiomyomas can often be enucleated without removing the oesophagus.

In the stomach, R0 resection may involve a partial, subtotal or total gastrectomy, although 'wedge' excision and 'sleeve' resections are also frequently performed to preserve as much stomach as possible. Small gastric lesions lend themselves well to laparoscopic resection (Fig. 10.5). Resection of GISTs at the oesophagogastric junction creates particular problems as a poor quality of life may result from simple excision with anastomosis of stomach to oesophagus. Alternatively, reconstruction using a short jejunal interposition can be considered for these patients, i.e. the

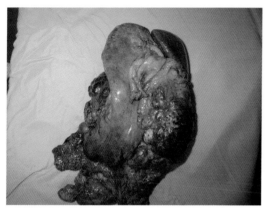

Figure 10.4   Operative specimen following en bloc total gastrectomy, splenectomy, and distal pancreatectomy for locally advanced gastrointestinal stromal tumour. (Courtesy of Richard Hardwick, Addenbrookes Hospital, Cambridge.)

'Merendino procedure' (Fig. 10.6)[41] as it results in a better quality of life compared to an oesophagogastric anastomosis.[42] An alternative to the Merendino procedure which is gaining favour is a proximal gastrectomy with double-tract reconstruction.[43]

The most important factors, as stated, are that the tumour is not ruptured and that negative resection margins are obtained. Simple enucleation of the tumour is inadequate as these lesions do not possess a true capsule. Direct invasion of adjacent structures occurs in 10–15% of GISTs, and surgery in such cases should include en bloc resection of involved adjacent organs.[16,40] Nodal metastases are extremely rare and routine extended lymph node dissection is therefore unjustified.[23]

Endoscopic therapy for GISTs has gained favour in some centres using endoscopic mucosal resection (EMR) and endoscopic submucosal dissection (ESD) but this is not widespread and surgical resection remains the mainstay of treatment.

Small asymptomatic GISTs <2 cm diameter with no concerning EUS features can safely be monitored with 6–12 monthly imaging.[44] In patients of borderline fitness for resection, or those who decline surgery at initial presentation, monitoring the lesion with EUS and/or CT for evidence of enlargement is acceptable so long as the results of surveillance influence the final management.

Endoscopic resections of GISTs has gained favour in some centres using endoscopic band ligation (EBL), ESD, endoscopic submucosal excavation (ESE), endoscopic full-thickness resection (EFTR), and submucosal tunnelling

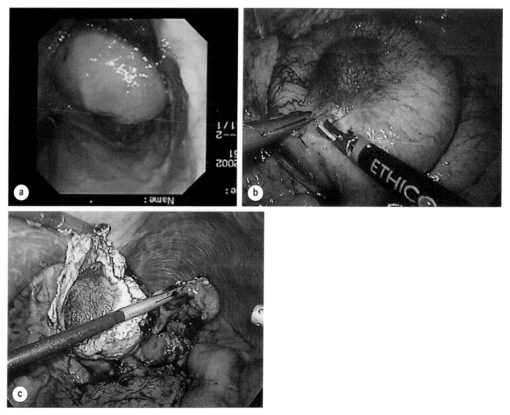

Figure 10.5   (a) Endoscopic view of a moderate-sized gastric fundal gastrointestinal stromal tumour (GIST). (b) Laparoscopic image of the lesion seen in (a). (c) Completed harmonic scalpel dissection of the gastric GIST in (a) prior to removal of specimen in a retrieval bag and closure of the resulting gastric defect with a linear EndoGIA stapler. (Courtesy of Richard Hardwick, Addenbrookes Hospital, Cambridge.)

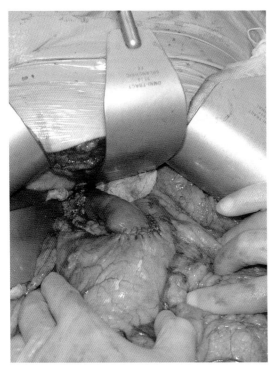

Figure 10.6 Completed Merendino procedure showing distal anastomosis between the jejunal interposition and the stomach. (Courtesy of Richard Hardwick, Addenbrookes Hospital, Cambridge.)

endoscopic resection (STER). This tends to be for small lesions less than 2 cm where resection is arguably not required.[45]

Surgical resection remains the mainstay of treatment for lesions over 2 cm. There may be a role for combined endoscopic and laparoscopic techniques in the future for 2–5-cm lesions but currently this practice is limited to enthusiasts and not widely adopted.

RISK STRATIFICATION OF RESECTED GISTS

The TNM classification is now not used for resected GISTs. Rather, risk stratification is calculated using a combination of tumour size, mitotic index, primary tumour site and the presence of rupture. This identifies patients using prognostic contour maps that are likely to be cured by surgery alone and identifies high-risk groups who may benefit from adjuvant therapy. Furthermore, molecular profiling, whilst not currently recommended in treatment guidelines, is likely to be included in the near future, particularly in tumours that contain deletions in the KIT exon codons that have a worse prognosis than point mutations or substitutions and may benefit from adjuvant chemotherapy.[46] Following neoadjuvant treatment with imatinib, it is difficult to assess the mitotic count post resection and this may affect use of risk stratification models.

IMATINIB

Imatinib mesylate is a receptor tyrosine kinase inhibitor that inhibits the constitutively activated tyrosine kinases of Abelson murine leukaemia viral oncogene homolog (including the stable transfection product fusion kinase breakpoint cluster region protein-Abelson murine leukaemia viral oncogene homolog [BCR-ABL] seen in chronic myeloid leukaemia), platelet-derived growth factor receptor (PDG-FR) and KIT. The drug is administered orally and its use, dosage, and side-effect profile are established following use in the treatment of chronic myeloid leukaemia. It has very little effect on normal cells, where the kinase is not constitutively active. Experiments on human tumour cell lines dependent upon the KIT pathway demonstrate that imatinib blocks the kinase activity of KIT, arrests proliferation, and causes apoptotic cell death.[44,47] Imatinib is generally well tolerated, although most patients experience some mild or moderate adverse events. Serious adverse events occur in around 20% of patients, the most serious of which is life-threatening tumour haemorrhage in approximately 5%.

UNRESECTABLE, METASTATIC OR RECURRENT DISEASE

Prior to the introduction of imatinib mesylate, patients with advanced GISTs faced severe morbidity and short life expectancy. Untreated, the median overall survival for unresectable or metastatic disease is around 12 months (ranging from 2 to 20 months).[48] Conventional chemotherapy and radiotherapy are ineffective in patients with metastatic GISTs.[49]

Early phase 1 studies of imatinib (then coded ST1571) took the oncology world by storm.[50] Never before had response rates of 80–90% been seen in metastatic sarcomas and a new era of 'smart' compounds was born. Over 50% of patients with metastatic or unresectable GISTs will survive more than 5 years if treated with imatinib.

In a randomised controlled trial of 147 patients with metastatic or unresectable GISTs the median survival was 54 months regardless of whether the 400-mg or 600-mg dose regimen of imatinib was used.[51]

A larger phase III trial recruited 746 patients and compared 400 mg with 800 mg imatinib and again found no difference in survival between the two doses but 33% of patients on the lower dose who progressed appeared to stabilise when transferred to the higher dose.[52] Similar results were obtained from an even larger randomised trial involving 946 patients although a longer progression-free survival was seen for patients on the higher dose of imatinib.[53]

Although 80% of GISTs respond to imatinib, 20% demonstrate initial resistance to the drug, and of those that respond initially, some will develop late resistance.[54] Neoadjuvant imatinib may be considered in patients with large GISTs to facilitate organ-conserving surgery or where the tumour lies close to the pylorus or gastroesophageal junction. The optimal duration of preoperative imatinib is between 6 and 12 months. Knowledge of mutational analysis results is mandatory before commencing neoadjuvant imatinib.

Ten per cent of all gastric GISTs contain a mutation in PDGFRA gene exon 18 codon 842, apartate substituted for a valane. These tumours can follow an aggressive clinical course but are resistant to imatinib even if the risk stratification is high. A new tyrosine kinase inhibitor avapritnib has demonstrated 90% durable response rates.[55]

For patients whose disease recurs or whose initial response to imatinib is not sustained, there is good evidence from randomised controlled trials for the use of sunitinib (second line)[56] and regorafenib (third line).[57]

ADJUVANT THERAPY POST RESECTION

✓✓ The role of imatinib in the adjuvant setting has now been investigated in randomised controlled trials in the USA, Europe, and Australasia. The ACOGSOG Z9001 study examined the role of adjuvant therapy for 12 months post curative resection for GISTs greater than 3 cm in diameter and found improvement in progression-free survival but not overall survival for those patients given imatinib versus placebo.[58] The SSG XVIII study randomised patients with high-risk resected GISTs to 12 months versus 36 months of adjuvant imatinib and found significant improvement in both progression-free and overall survival for the patients having the longer course of treatment.[59] Imatinib is now licensed in the USA and Europe for resected GIST patients deemed at high risk of recurrence and is standard treatment.

Surgery has a limited role in metastatic disease except when patients present with low-volume liver metastases; about a third of such patients may be cured by hepatic resection.[60] In selected patients with large incurable tumours, surgery may play an limited role in palliation of symptoms but whether to operate is best decided by a multidisciplinary team who have expertise in GIST management.[61] Downsizing of unresectable primary tumours and hepatic metastasis following treatment with imatinib can render lesions resectable, but long-term survival is uncommon, particularly if imatinib resistance has developed.[62] Randomised studies in the USA and Europe are ongoing to assess the value of neoadjuvant imatinib for unresectable GISTs which might be rendered resectable (and potentially curable).

PRIMARY GASTRIC LYMPHOMA (PGL)

INTRODUCTION

Gastric lymphoma accounts for approximately 5% of all primary gastric neoplasms.[63] The most common variant of lymphoma arising in lymphoid tissue outside the lymph nodes or spleen (i.e. extra-nodal sites) is represented by non-Hodgkin's lymphoma (NHL). The stomach is the most common extranodal site, representing between 30–40% of all extranodal lymphomas and 55–65% of all GI lymphomas.[64]

The incidence of PGL has been rising over the last few decades and it is most commonly seen in the 50–70-year-old age group; the incidence of developing PGL is two to three times higher in males than in females.[65,66] Potential risk factors identified in its pathogenesis include infection by *Helicobacter pylori*, HIV, Epstein-Barr virus, hepatitis B virus, and human T-cell lymphotropic virus 1. Other pathological conditions, such as coeliac disease and inflammatory bowel disease, including immunosuppressive drugs used in their treatment have also been associated with PGL.[67]

CLINICAL PRESENTATION

The initial symptoms of PGL are usually non-specific, mimicking gastritis, peptic ulcer disease, pancreatic disorders, or functional disorder of the stomach. The physical examination is unremarkable in 55–60% of cases, although epigastric tenderness, the presence of lymphadenopathy, and a palpable epigastric mass are occasionally found.[68] These non-specific findings can lead to a delay in diagnosis. The most common symptoms reported include dyspepsia, weight loss, nausea, vomiting, abdominal fullness, and indigestion.[69,70] Emergency presentations with upper GI bleeding, gastric outlet obstruction, and perforation are less common.

DIAGNOSIS

Diagnosis is by upper GI endoscopy and biopsy (Fig. 10.7). Endoscopic appearances are variable and range from minimal hyperaemic changes in gastric mucosa through diffuse or focal enlarged gastric folds to an exophytic ulcerated or polypoid mass.[71] For histological diagnosis, several biopsies must be obtained from the tumour area and additionally from the normal-looking antral mucosa so as to ascertain the presence of *H. pylori* and associated lesions such as atrophy and intestinal metaplasia.[72] The biopsies should be examined by a histopathologist with an interest in haemato-oncological malignancies and the biopsies should be repeated if the original biopsies are non-diagnostic.

✓✓ A systematic review of 2000 patients presenting with PGL showed a male preponderance, the absence of alarm symptoms in nearly 50% of patients, and the presence of *H. pylori* infection in nearly 90% of patients. PGL was diagnosed in a stage >I in one-third of the patients. At endoscopy, the ulcerative type was the most frequent presentation, although low-grade or mucosa-associated lymphoid tissue (MALT) lymphoma was diagnosed on normal/hyperaemic gastric mucosa in 9% of cases. Patients with high-grade or diffuse large B-cell lymphoma presented alarm symptoms, an exophytic or ulcerative lesion, a stage III–IV, and a *H. pylori* negative status more frequently than MALT lymphoma cases.[73]

HISTOPATHOLOGICAL CLASSIFICATION

The most common histological variants of NHL identified in the stomach are the marginal zone B-cell lymphoma of the mucosa-associated lymphoid tissue (MALT)–type lymphoma and the diffuse large B-cell lymphoma. Other histological

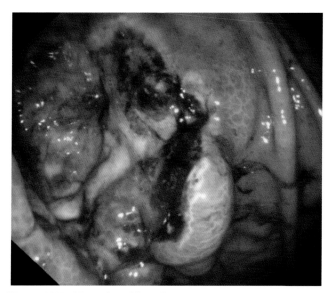

Figure 10.7 Ulcerating diffuse B-cell lymphoma arising on lesser curvature of stomach.

variants such as T-cell lymphoma, follicular lymphoma and Mantle lymphoma are all very rare.[74]

MALT lymphoma is usually a low grade lymphoma which arises from a proliferation of small B lymphocytes in marginal zone MALT in the gastric wall.[72] There is a strong relationship between chronic *H. pylori* infection and the development of MALT lymphoma.[75] The bacterial infection may trigger activation of CD4 T cells and indirectly stimulate B lymphocyte proliferation and subsequent malignant transformation.[76] However, not all cases of MALT lymphoma are associated with chronic *H. pylori* infection and in these cases, genetic and molecular alterations such as the chromosomal translocation t(11;18)(q21;q21) may be important.[77]

Conversely, diffuse large B-cell lymphoma is usually a high-grade lymphoma with a more aggressive course. The majority arise from a malignant proliferation of large B lymphocytes although some may evolve from transformed MALT lymphomas. Overexpression of the oncogene Bcl-6 (located on chromosome 3q27) is frequently identified.[67]

STAGING

Staging is essential for planning treatment and estimating prognosis. This should include a full physical examination and blood tests including lactate dehydrogenase (LDH) and *b*-2 microglobulin serum levels (high levels are related to a worse prognosis), as well as *H. pylori* serology. CT scanning of the chest, abdomen and pelvis permits assessment of any nodal involvement above and below the diaphragm and extension of the tumour outside the stomach. However, EUS has been established as more accurate than CT for assessing both the depth and invasion of the gastric wall and the involvement of regional lymph nodes.[78] This is of great importance since locoregional staging is one of the major factors that can predict the response to treatment thereby identifying patients whose disease is likely to be refractory to treatment or to recur. Additional staging investigations looking for distant spread may include bone marrow aspirate, ENT examination and lumbar puncture. The usefulness of a fusion PET/CT scan has been documented only for diffuse large B-cell lymphoma as MALT lymphomas are rarely PET avid (Fig. 10.8).

Clinical stage most commonly is expressed according to the Ann Arbor staging system modified by Musshoff (Table 10.5). Early-stage disease would be regarded as Stage IE–IIE1. The most important prognostic factor for PGL is the international prognosis index (IPI). This index includes age (> 60 years), poor performance status, elevated LDH and advanced stage.[67]

TREATMENT

The optimal frontline PGL treatment options depend upon the histological subtype and stage of the disease. MALT lymphomas have an 'indolent' clinical and biological behaviour pattern, with a tendency to stay localised at the onset site in 70% to 80% of cases. Regression of gastric MALT lymphoma can be achieved in the early stages of the disease by *H. pylori* eradication therapy and may be successful in over 70% of cases.[79] The choice of *H. pylori* eradication therapy should take account of local guidelines based upon *H. pylori* antibiotic resistance.[80] It is important to confirm *H. pylori* eradication and histological regression by means of repeat endoscopy and biopsy (culture and sensitivity may be required in resistant cases of *H. pylori* infection to guide second- and third-line therapies). Repeat endoscopy is advised at 6 monthly intervals to monitor response long-term. In cases of early-stage *H. pylori*–negative MALT lymphoma or persistent cases post *H. pylori* infection, moderate-dose radiotherapy (30 Gy) incorporating the stomach and surrounding lymph nodes offers good results, with a remission rate of over 90%.[81] Patients with either late-stage MALT lymphoma or those early-stage cases which did not respond to *H. pylori* eradication therapy or radiotherapy should be considered for immunotherapy with rituximab (an anti-CD20 monoclonal antibody) and chemotherapy (usually chlorambucil based).

The International Extranodal Lymphoma Study Group 19 (IELSG19) compared the outcomes from chlorambucil and rituximab alone and in combination in a three-arm randomised control trial. This showed the superior efficacy (improved progression-free survival with little added toxicity) of the combination therapy in the treatment of MALT lymphoma.[82]

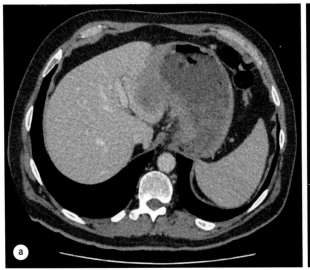
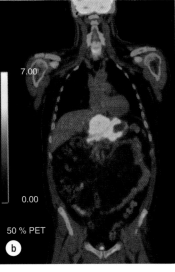

Figure 10.8 Diffuse B-cell lymphoma invading left lobe of liver (a) on computed tomography (CT) and (b) on positron emission tomography-CT.

The reference treatment for diffuse large B-cell lymphoma is an R-CHOP chemotherapy regimen combining rituximab with CHOP (doxorubicin, cyclophosphamide, vincristine, prednisone) for six or eight cycles every 3 weeks.[83] *H. pylori* eradication should be also be performed to treat those cases that may have evolved from *H. pylori*–positive MALT lymphomas.[72] In patients with early-stage disease or unfit for prolonged treatment, R-CHOP can be given for four cycles followed by involved field radiotherapy. PET-CT has a role at the end of treatment to look for residual or progressive disease to guide the use of second-line therapies including autologous stem cell transplantation.

✔✔ A randomised controlled trial of treatment with CHOP alone versus CHOP and rituximab in elderly patients with diffuse large B-cell lymphoma showed improved 5-year survival from 63% to 76%.[84] A large randomised controlled trial enrolled 589 patients with diffuse B-cell gastric lymphoma into four treatment arms: surgery alone, surgery with radiotherapy, surgery with CHOP, and CHOP alone. CHOP alone gave the best 10-year survival rates and had the lowest morbidity.[85]

The role of surgery in the management of PGL is now very limited and is usually restricted to the management of complications of treatment such as bleeding, obstruction, and perforation.

Table 10.5 Ann Arbor staging system for primary gastric lymphoma

Stage	Description
IE1	Confined to mucosa, submucosa
IE2	Confined to the stomach, invasion of the muscularis and/or serosa
IIE1	Involvement of the stomach and contiguous lymph nodes
IIE2	Involvement of the stomach and non-contiguous subdiaphragmatic lymph nodes
IIIE	Involvement of the stomach and lymph nodes on both sides of the diaphragm
IVE	Haematogenous spread

NEUROENDOCRINE NEOPLASMS OF THE STOMACH AND OESOPHAGUS

TERMINOLOGY

Neuroendocrine neoplasms can occur anywhere in the body but are most commonly found in the lungs and in the GI tract. These tumours arise from neuroendocrine cells such as the histamine producing enterochromaffin-like cells (ECL) in the gastric fundus and body and are defined by the expression of specific diagnostic biomarkers such as synaptophysin and chromogranin A (CgA).[86] The incidence of these neoplasms appears to be increasing and is most likely related to a greater access to endoscopy and imaging.[87]

Neuroendocrine neoplasms arising in the GI tract are referred to as gastroenteropancreatic (GEP) tumours and the World Health Organisation recently updated its classification of neuroendocrine neoplasms based upon histological grading, degree of differentiation, and proliferation rate (Table 10.6). The key point of difference is between the well-differentiated neuroendocrine tumours (NETs), which tend to be indolent in behaviour and of low metastatic potential, and the rarer poorly differentiated neuroendocrine carcinomas (NECs), which are aggressive in nature, often metastatic at presentation, and associated with a poor prognosis.[88]

GASTRIC NEUROENDOCRINE TUMOURS (G-NETS)

Gastric neuroendocrine neoplasms account for approximately 7% of all GI NETs and 3% of all gastric neoplasms.[89] The commonest form seen is the well-differentiated NETs (G-NETs), previously known as gastric carcinoids. The majority of G-NETs are non-functioning. Three types of G-NETs are recognised (Table 10.7 and Fig. 10.9).

TYPE 1

Type 1 G-NETs typically occur in the setting of pernicious anaemia-induced chronic atrophic gastritis (CAG). About 5% of autoimmune CAG patients will develop type I G-NETs; an association with chronic gastritis secondary to *H. pylori* infection has also been demonstrated.[87] In chronic gastritis, the destruction of parietal cells leads to achlorhydria. Gastric acid is normally produced by parietal cells when they are

Table 10.6 Classification and grading criteria for gastroenteropancreatic neuroendocrine neoplasms[88]

Terminology	Differentiation	Grade	Mitotic rate*	Ki67 index†
NET, G1	Well differentiated	Low	<2	<3%
NET, G2	Well differentiated	Intermediate	2–20	3–20%
NET, G3	Well differentiated	High	>20	>20%
NEC, small cell type	Poorly differentiated	High	>20	>20%
NEC, large cell type	Poorly differentiated	High	>20	>20%
MiNEN	Well or poorly differentiated	Variable	Variable	Variable

NEC, Neuroendocrine carcinoma; *NET,* neuroendocrine tumour; *MiNEN,* mixed neuroendocrine non-neuroendocrine neoplasm, i.e. a mixed tumour in which there are both neuroendocrine and non-neuroendocrine components.
*Mitotic rates are expressed as the number of mitoses/2 mm².
†The Ki-67 proliferation index value is determined by counting at least 500 cells in the regions of highest labelling (hot-spots), which are identified at scanning magnification.

Table 10.7 Classification of gastric neuroendocrine tumours according to type and general characteristics in endoscopic appearance, histology and prognostic indicators

	Type 1	Type 2	Type 3
Prevalence	70–80%	5–10%	10–20%
Background	Chronic atrophic gastritis and pernicious anaemia	Gastrinoma (Zollinger-Ellison syndrome); MEN1	Sporadic
Cell of origin	ECL	ECL	Endocrine
Stomach location	Fundus or body	Fundus or body	Anywhere in the stomach
Typical endoscopic and morphological characteristics	Often multiple (>60%), small (<1 cm); polypoid or submucosal	Often multiple, small (<1 to 2 cm); polypoid (sessile)	Single, large size (>2 cm); occasionally ulcerated
Surrounding gastric mucosa	Atrophic	Hypertrophic	Normal
Histology	Well differentiated (G1–2)	Well differentiated (G1–2)	Well differentiated, poorly differentiated or mixed tumours (G1, 2, 3 NET or NEC)
Fasting serum gastrin levels	Elevated	Elevated	Normal
Gastric pH	High	Low	Normal
Gastric wall invasion	Rare	More common	Common
Risk of metastases	2–5%	10–30%	50–100%
Prognosis	Excellent	Very good	Poor

Adapted from Ahmed,[87] Roberto et al.[90] and Exarchou et al.[91]

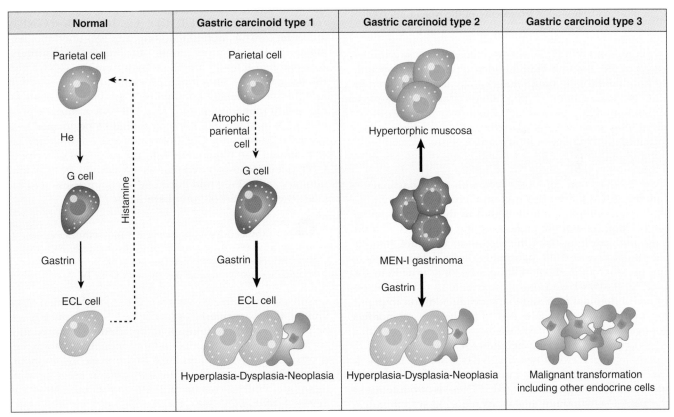

Figure 10.9 Pathogenesis of types 1–3 gastric neuroendocrine tumours.

stimulated by gastrin directly (secreted by the G cells in the gastric antrum) or by histamine released locally by ECL cells when these are stimulated by gastrin. Negative feedback is provided by D cells which release somatostatin when stimulated by rising intraluminal acid levels; somatostatin binds to G cells and ECL cells and inhibits the production of gastrin and histamine, respectively, hence reducing stimulation to parietal cells to produce acid. These feedback mechanisms are lost in chronic atrophic gastritis. The resulting hypergastrinaemia promotes hypertrophy and hyperplasia of the ECL cells, favouring the appearance of multiple small lesions.[90]

The vast majority of type 1 G-NETs are associated with an excellent prognosis. Annual endoscopic surveillance is recommended for small lesions <10 mm in diameter.[91] EUS is recommended for lesions >10 mm in diameter as this is associated with a greater risk of muscularis propria invasion and lymph node metastasis.[92] Endoscopic removal can be achieved by means of polypectomy, EMR or ESD for lesions >10 mm in diameter.

A meta-analysis of over 700 patients with type 1 G-NETs identified that size >10 mm and muscularis propria involvement were associated with a higher risk of lymph node metastasis. However, the overall rate of lymph node metastasis was low (3.3%) and the 5-year disease-specific survival for patients with and without lymph node metastases was 100% in most available studies irrespective of the type of intervention.[92]

Surgery in the form of wedge resection or gastrectomy is required for larger NETs with evidence of wall invasion and/or lymph node metastasis.[89] Surgery may also be required for multiple lesions or recurrence after endoscopic treatment. Antrectomy was previously advocated to reduce gastrin levels in these cases but a similar effect may be achieved using somatostatin analogues and so is no longer recommended.[93]

TYPE 2

Type 2 G-NETs are also associated with hypergastrinaemia but this is caused by the excessive production of gastrin from a gastrinoma (typically found in the 'gastrinoma triangle' composed of the junction of the cystic duct with the liver, the transition from the second to the third parts of the duodenum and the pancreatic neck).[94] This points to the presence of Zollinger-Ellison syndrome usually in the context of MEN-1 syndrome. These patients may also experience abdominal pain and diarrhoea in addition to peptic ulceration. Type 2 G-NETs tend to be slightly larger, affect younger patients, and have a slightly worse prognosis with a higher risk of lymph node metastases reaching up to 30%.[90]

The management of type 2 G-NETs is similar to type 1, except that the underlying gastrinoma will also need to be identified and surgically resected.[89] There is also interest in the use of somatostatin analogues reducing serum gastrin levels and regressing the type 2 G-NETs.[95]

TYPE 3

Type 3 G-NETs arise sporadically and are not associated with any underlying clinical condition. They occur most commonly in men over the age of 50 years in the presence of normogastrinaemia and a normal gastric mucosa. They develop from ECL cells in most cases in the absence of ECL hyperplasia and are not dependent on gastrin. Patients are often asymptomatic or may present with abdominal pain,

weight loss, and iron-deficiency anaemia.[87] Over 50% of patients present with metastases and the typical site is within the liver; rarely, this can lead to a carcinoid syndrome due to the systemic release of bioactive substances. Atypical carcinoid syndrome is due to histamine release and presents with a patchy cutaneous flush, oedema, watering eyes, bronchoconstriction, and headaches, whereas classical carcinoid syndrome presents with cutaneous flushing, bronchospasm, and diarrhoea and is probably due to circulating serotonin and tachykinins.[96] Pathologically, a mixture of well-differentiated NETs (Grades 1–3) and poorly differentiated NECs are seen.

The recommended treatment of non-metastatic type 3 G-NETs is surgical resection (subtotal or total gastrectomy) and regional lymphadenectomy.[97] This is usually accompanied by adjuvant chemotherapy, e.g. cisplatin/carboplatin and etoposide, although there is little evidence to support this approach. Recent studies have expanded the role of endoscopic resection in a selected group of type 3 G-NET patients: EMR or ESD can be used with curative intent in small (<20 mm), low-grade (G1/G2) lesions without evidence of local or distant metastases.[91]

PATIENT ASSESSMENT AND INVESTIGATION

All patients with a suspected G-NET should undergo a detailed assessment to ascertain the subtype of G-NET prior to referral to a dedicated NET MDT (Fig. 10.10). Most G-NETs are asymptomatic, non-functioning, and identified incidentally at endoscopy investigating other upper GI disorders. It is vital that biopsies are taken both from the G-NET and the background gastric mucosa looking for the presence of atrophic gastric mucosa. A full histological analysis incorporating differentiation, mitotic rate, Ki67 index, and the presence of lymphovascular invasion should be performed by a specialist pathologist. Gut hormones and a fasting gastrin level should also be measured. In the suspicion of a type 2 G-NET, it is recommended that serum calcium, gastrin, and pituitary and parathyroid hormone levels are assessed to exclude the possibility of MEN-1 syndrome.[90]

In a prospective study Gibril et al.[98] found the octreoscan to have a positive and negative predictive value of 63% and 97%, respectively, for the detection of G-NETs and so its use should be considered in all patients with G-NETs.

Conventional imaging such as CT scan and MRI may be of limited value particularly for small type 1 G-NETs but is more helpful for disease staging in more advanced neuroendocrine neoplasms. EUS is vital in locoregional evaluation, i.e. depth of wall invasion and local lymph node involvement. The current gold standard for somatostatin receptor scintigraphy is a nuclear medicine Tektroyd scan (also known as Tc99m HYNIC-TOC SPECT CT) which can be performed from a single attendance and fuses SPECT (single photon emission computed tomography) and CT data (Fig. 10.11); an alternative is a Gallium scan (also known as 68Ga-DOTA-NOC PET/CT). Both of these investigations can be useful in G-NETs as part of staging and perhaps also for directing therapy (99,100).[99,100]

TREATMENT OF METASTATIC DISEASE

The goal of metastatic G-NET therapy is to control symptoms by both reducing the level of circulating hormones

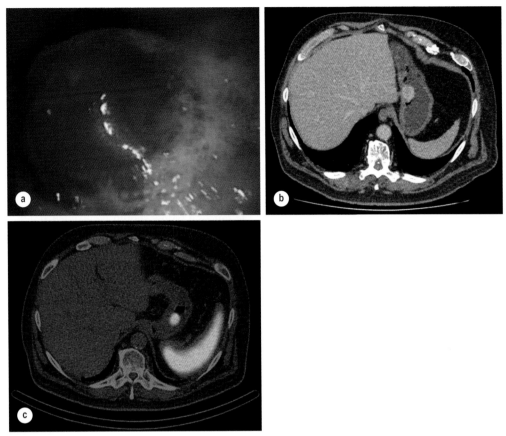

Figure 10.10   Type 1 grade 2 well-differentiated neuroendocrine tumour arising on the lesser curvature of the stomach on upper GI endoscopy (a), computed tomography (CT) (b), and nuclear medicine (NM) Tc99m HYNIC-TOC SPECT CT (c).

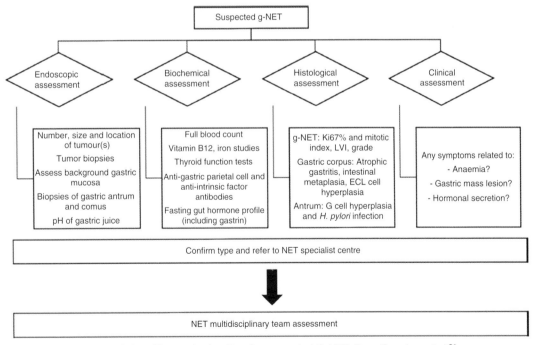

Figure 10.11   Diagnostic algorithm for suspected G-NET. From Exarchou et al.[91]

(when present) and tumour growth in order to improve quality of life and prolong survival. Important factors to be considered for the treatment of well-differentiated metastatic disease (Grades 1–3 NET) are the patient's performance status, the grade of tumour, the volume and extent of the metastatic disease, the expression of somatostatin receptors on functional imaging (octreoscan or ^{68}Ga-DOTATATE) and the presence or absence of a functioning syndrome.[90]

Options include somatostatin analogue therapy, molecular targeted agents (e.g. everolimus), targeted peptide receptor radionucleotide therapies (PRRTs) (e.g. ^{177}Lu-OctreoTate), transarterial chemoembolisation (TACE), or radiofrequency ablation (for symptomatic liver metastasis).[87]

✔✔ In patients with advanced GEP-NETs (predominantly from the pancreas, midgut or hindgut), the CLARINET study and its subsequent open label extension (OLE) study have demonstrated that lanreotide (a long-acting version of octreotide) is safe and well tolerated and extends progression-free survival.[101,102]

These results have been have extrapolated to G-NETs and so somatostatin analogues are usually the initial treatment of choice. In the presence of carcinoid syndrome (8% to 35% of G-NETs), the use of these drugs is mandatory to reduce symptoms and decrease the long-term risks of an uncontrolled carcinoid syndrome.

Systemic chemotherapy is usually reserved for metastatic Grade 3 NET or NECs for whom the prognosis is poor. For poorly differentiated tumours, first-line chemotherapy is based upon experience with small cell lung cancer and utilises a combination of cisplatin or carboplatin with etoposide. Second-line and experimental approaches include immunotherapy and PRRT.[103]

SMALL CELL CARCINOMA OF THE OESOPHAGUS

Neuroendocrine neoplasms affecting the oesophagus are extremely rare and are usually high-grade tumours. Neuroendocrine carcinoma of the oesophagus with a small cell type (previously referred to as just *small cell carcinoma*) is a rare, highly aggressive form of oesophageal malignancy accounting for less than 3% of all oesophageal malignancies.[104] Most patients present with lymph node and/or distant metastases and so median survival in most studies is less than 12 months.[105] The optimal treatment strategy for this rare cancer still needs to be defined as there are no randomised studies of treatment and so has been extrapolated from experience with small cell lung cancer. Patients with localised disease may benefit from oesophagectomy in combination with either chemotherapy (most regimens incorporate cisplatin/etoposide) or chemoradiotherapy. Patients with more advanced disease are treated with either chemotherapy or chemoradiotherapy.[105,106] There is interest in the use of immunotherapy for treating this disease but because of small patient numbers, clinical trial evidence is limited. However, immunotherapy has shown benefit in small cell lung cancer and has been approved for use in the first-line setting in this patient group.[107]

OTHER CLINICALLY RELEVANT RARE TUMOURS OF THE OESOPHAGUS

LEIOMYOMA

Oesophageal leiomyomas are the most common benign tumours of the oesophagus (70–80% of all benign tumours) and usually present in middle age.[108] They generally arise from the smooth muscle in the muscularis propria of the lower two-thirds of the oesophagus and present as an intramural or submucosal swelling in the oesophageal wall. Pathologically, they form bundles of well-differentiated spindle-shaped smooth muscle cells without clear demarcation or a well-formed capsule; immunocytochemistry is usually positive for desmin and SMA.[109] When small, they are usually asymptomatic and are found incidentally but when their diameter exceeds 5 cm, they become symptomatic with dysphagia, epigastric discomfort and indigestion, the commonest reported symptoms.[110] The key investigation is EUS which demonstrates characteristic features: the presence of a well-circumscribed, homogenous, hypoechoic mass with smooth borders, arising from the third submucosal layer without evidence of local lymphadenopathy. FNA via EUS imaging can be used to obtain cytology and immunohistochemical analysis and this can help to differentiate leiomyoma from GISTs and leiomyosarcoma.[111,112] Endoscopic mucosal biopsy should be avoided unless there is diagnostic doubt as this may compromise techniques for leiomyoma removal.[108] Treatment options depend upon size and symptoms. If the leiomyoma is small and asymptomatic, it may be followed with surveillance EUS imaging every 12 months as the risk of malignant transformation to leiomyosarcoma is very low. Whilst endoscopic techniques (EMR and ESD) have been described, surgical enucleation via a longitudinal myotomy currently remains the best option for symptomatic lesions with either thoracoscopic or laparoscopic approaches preferred over open surgery.[108,113] Oesophagectomy is still occasionally required for very large leiomyomas or where there is a suspicion of malignant transformation.

LEIOMYOSARCOMA

Oesophageal leiomyosarcoma is the most common sarcoma arising within the oesophagus albeit it accounts for less than 1% of all oesophageal malignancies.[114,115] Leiomyosarcoma arises from the muscular layer of the oesophageal wall and is characterised by spindle cell proliferation with associated cellular atypia, more than 10 mitoses per 10 HPFs or the presence of necrosis. On immunohistochemistry, leiomyosarcomas are positive for SMA (95%), muscle-specific actin (91%), calponin (88%), desmin (73%), caldesmon (66%), and myosin (64%) and negative for CD34, CD117, DOG1, and S100.[116] Leiomyosarcomas present in a similar fashion to leiomyomas but tend to be much larger at presentation and continue to enlarge at a much faster rate than leiomyomas. EUS-guided FNA or core biopsy of such a lesion should be attempted if leiomyosarcoma is suspected.[117] If confirmed or doubt continues after biopsy, oesophagectomy is recommended with good long-term survival results reported as metastasis tends to occur late.[115,118] Alternative treatment approaches include radiotherapy.[114]

ACKNOWLEDGEMENT

This chapter in the sixth edition was written by Mr Richard Hardwick and we are grateful to him for those parts of the chapter which we have kept in this edition. We would like to acknowledge the contribution of Dr David McIntosh, Consultant Oncologist at Beatson Oncology centre, Glasgow and Chair of West of Scotland NET MDT for his help with the section on neuroendocrine neoplasms of the oesophagus and stomach.

 References available at http://ebooks.health.elsevier.com/

Pathophysiology and investigation of gastro-oesophageal reflux disease

11

Anthony R. Hobson | Jordan J. Haworth

INTRODUCTION

Gastro-oesophageal reflux disease (GORD) is a common condition relating to the movement of stomach contents into the oesophagus, which can lead to unpleasant symptoms and a broad range of clinical complications. These associated symptoms and complications are highly eclectic and the pathophysiology of GORD is multifactorial, which can make an accurate diagnosis challenging. The current paradigm of GORD diagnosis is not based on specific pathophysiological mechanisms, but rather the severity of reflux seen on endoscopy and physiology testing.

Definition: GORD is defined by the World Gastroenterology Organization as 'troublesome symptoms sufficient to impair an individual's quality of life, or injury or complications that result from the retrograde flow of gastric contents into the oesophagus, oropharynx, and/or respiratory tract'.[1] It is the most common oesophageal disorder, yet disease manifestation may go beyond the oesophagus into the ear, nose, throat, mouth, and lungs.

ANATOMY AND PHYSIOLOGY OF REFLUX

There is a fine distinction between reflux and GORD. The former is a physiological phenomenon that occurs following meals and eructation, but the process whereby reflux results in troublesome symptoms or complications is a nuance of mechanisms relating to the oesophagogastric junction (OGJ), the oesophageal body, and the central nervous system.

THE OESOPHAGOGASTRIC JUNCTION

The OGJ is the principle antireflux barrier consisting of the lower oesophageal sphincter (LOS) and the crural diaphragm (CD), which are superimposed in health. The smooth muscles of the LOS are semi-circular fibres that form clasps around each other and bridge the gastric sling fibres, whereas the skeletal muscles of the CD form the external part of the antireflux barrier where the oesophagus passes through the right crus of the CD. Both the LOS and CD have an asymmetric pressure profile with inspiration producing a greater increase in OGJ pressure toward the greater curvature of the stomach, and the peak LOS pressure correlates with the maximum muscle thickness found on the greater curve where the gastric sling fibres are most dense.[2]

The CD produces a pinch-cock effect on the LOS, which results in an increase of 10 to 20 mmHg in OGJ pressure during inspiration. A type of biofeedback called diaphragmatic breathing has been shown in randomised controlled studies to augment LOS pressure, improve GORD-related quality-of-life scores, reduce the use of medications, and reduce physiological reflux.[3,4]

Reflux can occur when intragastric pressure exceeds the resting LOS pressure, forcing gastric contents up into the oesophagus. A hypotensive LOS is common in patients with GORD, but paradoxically, a hypertensive LOS in GORD is not uncommon.[5] Therefore, low LOS pressure cannot be the sole mechanism for reflux. When intragastric pressure increases, a 'yield' pressure is reached which triggers a transient lower oesophageal sphincter relaxation (TLOSR). This is a normal reflex mediated via vagal afferents, but if this reflex is hypersensitive, yield pressures are reduced and TLOSRs are triggered too frequently and are thought to have a stronger correlation with GORD than hypotensive LOS pressure.[2] Both LOS pressure and TLOSRs can be defined on high-resolution manometry (HRM) where the LOS pressure is < 10 mmHg (software dependant), and TLOSRs are LOS relaxations lasting greater than 10 seconds in the absence of swallowing and are associated with CD inhibition.[6]

TLOSRs are triggered by pharyngeal intubation, meal ingestion, upright posture, smoking, and hyperglycaemia,[2] although the primary trigger for TLOSRs is thought to be gastric distension following meals or aerophagia (excessive air swallowing). Gastric accommodation is the physiological response to gastric distension, which serves to offset a rise in intragastric pressure during meal intake. In patients with GORD and healthy controls, smaller changes in intragastric pressure (i.e. poor gastric accommodation) lead to an overall increased presence of TLSORs.[7] Hence, gastric accommodation likely plays a role in TLOSRs via mechanoreceptor signalling from the gastric wall. Moreover, this may explain why GORD frequently overlaps with conditions related to poor gastric accommodation, namely functional dyspepsia and gastroparesis.[8]

Delayed gastric emptying may contribute to increased TLOSRs since prolonged retention of contents leads to prolonged distension. Other gastric factors include cholecystokinin (CCK), which has been shown to induce a period of partial relaxation followed complete lower oesophageal sphincter (LOS) relaxation along with CD inhibition.[9] When nutrients enter the duodenum, CCK is released and prevents further emptying of the stomach. It should be noted that TLOSRs do have a physiological purpose, to allow gas venting from the stomach, whether that gas is ingested from air swallowing or carbonated drinks, or created by fermentation in the gut: excessive fermentation of poorly digested carbohydrates in the colon is associated with increased TLOSRs.[10]

HIATAL HERNIA

The OGJ antireflux barrier may become jeopardized following separation of the LOS and CD, resulting in a hiatal hernia (HH). This is a fundamental finding in GORD, and HH is associated with the presence and severity of oesophagitis, increased oesophageal acid exposure, and reflux episodes, but not increased TLSORs.[11] Instead, reflux episodes are increased during periods with low LOS pressure, straining, swallowing, and deep inspiration, which highlights the importance of the CD in protection against reflux. Impaired CD function can be assessed on HRM by inspiratory augmentation of OGJ pressure, and one study found that 37 out of 39 subjects with inspiratory augmentations of OGJ ≤ 0 mmHg had objectively pathological GORD.[12] This was the strongest predictor of GORD, even more so than LOS pressure and LOS-CD separation.

The prevalence of a HH is associated with increased age but the aetiology remains unclear. It is thought that repetitive elevation of intragastric pressure may force the hiatus upwards, or alternatively, age-associated myopathy may play a role. HHs are seen in up to 40% of obese individuals,[13] which supports the theory of increased gastric pressure. Furthermore, bariatric surgery can lead to increased intragastric pressure, namely sleeve gastrectomy and gastric band, for which worsening or new-onset GORD is more common compared to Roux-en-Y bypass.[14]

A HH can also promote reflux via an acid pocket where part of the stomach is positioned above the diaphragm. This stomach portion generates acid, particularly following meals, which can then pool and reflux more easily into the oesophagus. Healthy controls were shown to also have an unbuffered acidic segment in the proximal stomach; however, this is typically below the squamocolumnar junction (SCJ) whereas the acid pocket in patients with GORD and HH lies above the diaphragm.[15]

OESOPHAGEAL BODY

Defects in peristalsis may lead to impaired clearance of gastric refluxate and prolonged acid exposure. Indeed, hypomotility is common in GORD, but the cause and effect as to whether reflux causes hypomotility or vice versa is uncertain. Fundamentally, oesophageal peristalsis is required to counteract refluxate and this can be primary (swallow induced) or secondary (triggered by distension). Reflux elicits distension of the oesophageal lumen via activation of stretch receptors in the oesophageal wall, which triggers secondary peristalsis and volume clearance. However, this is not sufficient to neutralise acid. On the other hand, swallow-induced primary peristalsis contains bicarbonate saliva necessary to achieve chemical clearance and pH normalisation.

REFLUX OESOPHAGITIS

The traditional paradigm of GORD complications is that acid directly erodes the oesophageal mucosa leading to inflammation, oesophagitis, and more rarely, dysplasia. Noxious refluxate containing acid, pepsin, and bile salts is thought to damage the tight junction proteins between cells, such as claudins, occludins, and E-cadherin.[16] This leads to greater diametric separation between cells known as dilated intercellular spaces (DISs). DISs are seen in up to 100% of patients with erosive oesophagitis and up to 83% of patients with non-erosive reflux disease (NERD), and DISs reduce following proton pump inhibitor (PPI) therapy.[17] However, up to 30% of healthy controls have DISs as well as patients with NERD who are refractory to PPI.[17] Persistence of DISs may be consequent to bile acid or, indirectly, animal studies have shown that psychological stress induces DISs.[18]

Overall, DISs appear to reflect reflux burden, but immune response presents an alternative paradigm for complications of GORD. This was first proposed by Souza and colleagues, who demonstrated in an in vitro model that oesophagitis developed several days after acidified bile salt exposure.[19] Initial exposure triggered the increased presence of proinflammatory cytokines (interleukin-8 and interleukin-1β) that signal migration of T cells and neutrophils into the submucosa, which eventually progressed to the epithelial surface. More recently, biopsies from patients who discontinued PPIs 2 weeks before endoscopy showed T lymphocyte infiltration in areas without surface erosions.[20] Furthermore, in patients with reflux oesophagitis, biopsies showed increased hypoxia-inducible factor 2a, a proinflammatory cytokine that is induced by bile salts.[21]

Barrett's oesophagus (BO) relates to the histological change from normal stratified squamous epithelium lining the oesophagus to a metaplastic columnar epithelium with goblet cells, typically more reflective of the duodenum than the stomach.[22,23] BO is thought to be an intermediate step between oesophagitis and oesophageal adenocarcinoma (OAC), and is more common in GORD than the general population. The risk of BO progressing to OAC is significantly reduced with adequate PPI therapy, which demonstrates the pathophysiology of gastric acid in BO progression, but there are likely immunological mechanisms akin to reflux oesophagitis. While these mechanisms remain unclear, *FoxP3*, a gene associated with poor prognosis for oesophageal cancer, is greatly expressed in BO.[23,24]

SYMPTOM PERCEPTION

The means by which reflux triggers symptoms is still not well understood and highly paradoxical. First, patients with BO often report fewer symptoms compared to patients with no objective evidence of reflux. Second, symptoms respond variably to acid-suppression medications, which suggests other mechanisms than gastric acid alone. Indeed, pain receptors called transient receptor potential vanilloid-1 (TRPV1), present in oesophageal sensory afferents, are activated in response to several stimuli including heat, low pH, protons, lipid derivatives, and the principle compound in chilli peppers, capsaicin.[25] In one study, researchers injected the oesophageal submucosa of healthy volunteers with acid and capsaicin, which only capsaicin triggered severe sensations of heartburn and chest pain.[26] Patients will often report that spicy foods cause reflux, but capsaicin has not been shown to induce LOS dysfunction nor increase TLOSRs.[27] Rather, enhanced symptom perception is likely due to direct effects on oesophageal sensation. TRPV1 may be the primary afferent pathway for reflux symptoms since it is upregulated in patients with erosive oesophagitis and NERD.[28] Evidence to support this was objectively demonstrated in a study by Hobson et al. that showed that oesophageal afferent pathway sensitivity negatively correlated with acid exposure in NERD patients, meaning that equivalent symptoms could be generated by lower levels of acid exposure dependent on the sensitivity of oesophageal afferent nerves.[29]

The advent of pH-impedance monitoring has revealed that symptom perception is multifactorial owing to acidity, composition (liquid, gas, or mixed), impaired reflux bolus clearance, and the proximal extent or volume of reflux.[30] In NERD patients, spontaneous acid reflux enhances subsequent reflux perception regardless of activity or composition.[31] Clearly, sensitization of the oesophagus from acidic and weakly acidic events primes the oesophagus. Additionally, mental fatigue may play a fundamental role in perception. Schey and colleagues showed that sleep deprivation led to heightened sensitivity and a greater intensity response to oesophageal acid exposure.[32]

EPIDEMIOLOGY AND RISK FACTORS FOR GORD

Defining GORD epidemiology is not straightforward because symptoms are entirely subjective and objective evidence of GORD is seldom reported in epidemiological studies, which makes understanding the true impact of GORD challenging.

According to a systematic review published in 2020, the pooled prevalence of GORD in the UK was 14.53% and the economic cost is approximately £760 million/year, whereas the US was 21.04% and an estimated $24 billion/year.[33] GORD is a significant health and financial burden that will continue to escalate, since the all-age prevalence of GORD increased by 18.1% between 1990 and 2017, while in the same time frame, years lived with disability related to GORD increased by 67.1%, reflecting the increased prevalence in older age groups and a generally ageing population.[34] A systematic review from 2014 found that the adult incidence was approximately 5 per 1000 person-years in the UK and USA, but the overall incidence was 0.84 per 1000 person-years for paediatrics in the UK, which further reflects the adult-onset nature of GORD.[35] Indeed, age is one of the strongest predictors for GORD, with a lower prevalence in 18–34 years (8.70%) versus 35–59 years (14.53%; odds ratio [OR] 1.17 and relative risk [RR] 1.15) and ≥ 60 years (13.12%; OR 1.20 and RR 1.17).[33]

Obesity is another strong risk factor for GORD, with an OR around 1.7 for a body mass index (BMI) ≥ 30.[33,36] Increased abdominal pressure plays a significant role in the pathophysiology of GORD in obese patients.[37] Other risk factors for GORD include low education level, urban habitation, and nonsteroidal anti-inflammatory drug (NSAID) use, but not alcohol intake or smoking.[33] A review from 2018 confirmed that GORD prevalence is not significantly different between alcohol and non-alcohol users.[36] However, in this study, smoking had an OR of 1.26 compared to non-smokers. Typically, smokers will make poorer lifestyle

choices, but it is thought that reflux is induced by deep inspiration and coughing.[38] In any case, patients who report smoking should be encouraged to quit since it is strongly associated with OAC independent of GORD.[39]

Interestingly, according to marital status, the prevalence of GORD in divorced/separated/widowed individuals was significantly greater than single individuals (22.95% vs 12.85%, respectively), which suggests a contributory role for emotional stress in GORD. Data on the effect of diet, food, and drink are somewhat limited, but those with moderate/high intake of carbonated drinks had greater risk (OR 1.29 and RR 1.24), which may be attributed to the gas-provoked mechanism of refluxate. Also, moderate/high intake of coffee/tea was associated with greater risk (OR 1.47 and RR 1.38), which may be consequent to caffeine-induced oesophageal dysfunction, resulting in a decrease in basal LOS pressure and distal oesophageal contraction.[40]

The GBD 2017 Gastro-oesophageal Reflux Disease Collaborators used data from the Global Burden of Diseases, Injuries, and Risk Factors Study (GBD) 2017 to assess the global burden of GORD.[34] The age-standardised prevalence was highest (> 11,000 cases per 100,000 population) in the USA, Middle East, North Africa, Eastern Europe, and several Latin America countries, while it was lowest (< 7000 cases per 100,000 population) in East Asia and several European countries. Overall, the global age-standardised prevalence of GORD was relatively stable between 1990 and 2017. However, the all-age prevalence of GORD increased by 18.1% and years lived with disabilities related to GORD increased by 67.1%, which suggests that the global burden of GORD will continue to escalate along with an ageing and expanding population.

INVESTIGATION AND DIAGNOSIS

HISTORY, QUESTIONNAIRES, AND AN EMPIRIC PROTON PUMP INHIBITOR TRIAL

Typical GORD symptoms (i.e. heartburn and regurgitation) respond better to medical and surgical treatment than atypical symptoms, which emphasises the value of a good clinical history.[41] According to the Montreal Consensus, atypical symptoms include non-cardiac chest pain and extraoesophageal symptoms; i.e. laryngeal or pulmonary complaints,[42] although chest pain, discomfort, and burning may be indistinguishable to some patients. In any case, an empiric trial of PPI therapy is often the first step, but up to 40% of patients will experience persistent symptoms despite PPI use.[43] In addition, a large proportion of these patients do not demonstrate conclusive evidence of GORD on endoscopy or pH monitoring.[44,45]

When compared to endoscopy and pH monitoring, expert history by a gastroenterologist has only a sensitivity and specificity of 70% and 67%, respectively. Questionnaires share similarly limited sensitivity and specificity of 62% and 67% for the Reflux Disease Questionnaire (RDQ),[46] and 65% and 71% for the GerdQ, respectively.[47] Trial with PPIs is even more limited with a sensitivity of 71% and specificity of 44%,[46,48] yet PPI trials are cheap, pragmatic, and recommended by societal guidelines.[49] This has undoubtedly led to the overuse of PPIs, which although they appear to be safe,[50] may have detrimental consequences to the gut microbiome.[51,52] Ultimately, history, questionnaires, and PPI trials are of limited value in the diagnosis of GORD, highlighting the need for further investigation in most cases.

✓ There is a contretemps over PPI use based on several large observational studies that showed an association between PPIs and medical complications – including death. However, a large observational study in 1.9 million US seniors found that PPI use is not associated with increased risk after accounting for comorbidities and protopathic bias; for example, a patient starts PPI for cough but dies from pneumonia.[50] The only clear complication from PPI use is changes to the gut microbiota to one that is predisposed to enteric infections and populated with oropharyngeal flora.[51,52] The effects of PPI on the microbiome are more prominent than the effects of antibiotics or other commonly used drugs.[51]

ENDOSCOPY AND BIOPSY

Upper endoscopy (OGD) is advised when symptoms of GORD do not respond to empiric PPI therapy, or if there are concomitant alarm symptoms including dysphagia, unexplained weight loss, and persistent vomiting.

✓✓ The Lyon Consensus was published in 2018 to standardise the objective diagnosis of GORD.[53] Conclusive evidence for GORD requires high-grade erosive oesophagitis (LA grades C and D), long-segment Barrett's mucosa, or peptic strictures on endoscopy or distal oesophageal acid exposure time (AET) > 6% on ambulatory pH monitoring. Alternatively, GORD can be excluded if endoscopy is normal, distal AET is < 4% and < 40 reflux episodes on pH-impedance monitoring off PPI therapy. Of note, there is no recommendation for the use of DeMeester score in the diagnosis of GORD.

However, erosive oesophagitis is found in fewer than 10% of patients already taking PPIs.[54] In addition, oesophagitis is typically low grade, and with significant interobserver variability, pH-metry evidence of GORD is most often required prior to antireflux surgery.[55] Overall, endoscopy has a low sensitivity in GORD diagnosis.

OGD should also exclude eosinophilic oesophagitis (EoE), as well as heterotopic gastric mucosa within the cervical oesophagus, also known as an inlet patch. The prevalence of an inlet patch is approximately 3% in those undergoing OGD.[56] While the clinical significance remains unclear, studies have shown that ablation therapy may result in improvement of laryngopharyngeal reflux (LPR) symptoms.[57,58]

AMBULATORY REFLUX MONITORING

Ambulatory reflux monitoring is the most reliable means of identifying GORD in patients with a normal or inconclusive endoscopy and is a prerequisite for antireflux surgery to quantify GORD if endoscopic reflux oesophagitis is unequivocal; i.e. LA grade A or B.[53] Hence, reflux monitoring demonstrates the true ramification of GORD pathophysiology, evident by an excessive distal oesophageal AET and/or excessive number of reflux episodes. In addition, the relationship between reflux episodes and symptoms can be assessed, which is especially valuable in patients with atypical symptoms.

There are three well-established techniques for reflux monitoring: wireless pH, transnasal pH, and transnasal pH-impedance monitoring. The primary outcome for 24-hour pH monitoring is the AET and extending to 48 hours or more increases diagnostic yield.[59] Wireless pH monitoring is useful for those who cannot tolerate the transnasal catheter. However, wireless pH monitoring is expensive, requires endoscopy for placement, and lacks impedance measurements. In addition, detachment of the wireless pH capsule occurs in 10% of cases, requiring the test to be repeated.[60] Ideally, pH-impedance monitoring is preferred since it detects all reflux (liquid, gas, or mixed) and can determine if refluxate is acidic (pH < 4), weakly acidic (pH 4–7), or alkaline (pH > 7). The addition of impedance sensors defines the direction of flow and assists diagnosis of rumination and belching disorders, which can mimic GORD. Moreover, impedance testing improves the sensitivity and the false-negative rate from pH monitoring alone, which is unable to detect non-acid or gaseous events. Thus, pH-impedance monitoring is considered the gold standard.

Reflux monitoring can be performed 'on' or 'off' PPI therapy. However, the Lyon Consensus proposes that testing should always be performed off therapy to demonstrate baseline AET in 'unproven GORD'; i.e. no (or low-grade) oesophagitis and no recently positive pH study.[53] Conversely, patients with 'proven GORD' (prior LA grade C or D oesophagitis, long-segment BO, or abnormal pH testing) should be evaluated on therapy, ergo they should remain on optimised-dose PPI therapy to establish the association between refractory symptoms and reflux episodes. The patient should also record the time of taking PPIs to exclude poor compliance as a cause of persistent symptoms. This must be performed with pH impedance, since most reflux episodes on PPI therapy are weakly acidic. In addition, pH impedance should use multichannel pH sensors, with one located in the gastric lumen to exclude inadequate acid suppression.

✓✓ Ambulatory pH or pH-impedance monitoring should be performed off PPI therapy to demonstrate a baseline acid exposure.[53] Only patients with proven GORD should be tested on PPI (i.e. high-grade oesophagitis, long-segment BO, or a previously abnormal pH study). When testing on PPI, pH impedance is mandatory to determine non-acidic reflux events. Also, patients should report when PPIs were taken to assess for compliance and optimisation.

ACID EXPOSURE TIME

Oesophageal AET is the most salient metric on pH monitoring and most predictive of a positive response to medical and surgical therapy.[61] The Lyon Consensus proposes that AET < 4% be considered definitively normal (physiological) and > 6% be considered definitively abnormal.[53] Intermediate values should be considered inconclusive and therefore adjunctive measures are necessary to support a diagnosis of GORD. While the decision for antireflux surgery is typically bolstered by an abnormal AET, physicians should carefully consider the caveat of an unusually high AET on pH monitoring in the event of artefact, such as slipping of the transnasal pH catheter or dislodgement of the wireless pH capsule into the stomach (Fig. 11.1).

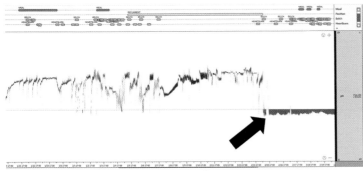

Upright AET 42.5% | Supine AET 0.3% | Total AET 21.2%
Reflux episodes 38 | Longest episode 93.1 min | DeMeester 54.3

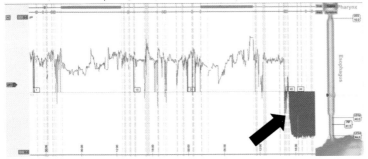

Upright AET 18.0% | Supine AET 0.0% | Total AET 10.3%
Reflux episodes 27 | Longest episode 93.1 min | DeMeester 54.3

Figure 11.1 Don't be fooled... 24-hour pH monitoring (top) and wireless 48-hour pH monitoring (bottom) demonstrating pathological gastro-oesophageal reflux disease with an excessive acid exposure time. However, the transnasal catheter and wireless capsule appear to have slipped into the stomach *(black arrow)* towards the last period of the tests. Otherwise, the rest of the studies appeared normal and these periods should be excluded from analysis or studies repeated. Always scrutinise the longest episode if there is no image of the trace.

REFLUX EPISODES

The total number of reflux episodes can quantify excessive reflux where pH impedance is required for the detection of acidic, weakly acidic, and weakly alkaline events. Reviewers should consider the caveat of impedance reflux episodes being overestimated by the automated analysis software[62] or exasperated by behavioural disorders, such as rumination or supragastric belching (Fig. 11.2). The Lyon Consensus proposes that < 40 reflux episodes per 24 hours is physiological while > 80 is definitively abnormal.[53] Intermediate values should be considered inconclusive. The clinical value of an abnormal number of reflux episodes is not clear-cut, although improvement in regurgitation severity was consistent with a reduction in reflux episodes following magnetic sphincter augmentation.[63] Therefore, this should be considered an adjunctive measure secondary to AET, and it is not unlikely that patients will have both an inconclusive AET (4–6%) and number of reflux episodes (n = 40–80). Ultimately, there is no justification for such stringent cut-off values, nor have they been validated. Moreover, elevated AET or reflux episodes does not necessarily prove that a patient's symptoms are consequent to reflux.

REFLUX-SYMPTOM ASSOCIATION

The reflux-symptom association is paramount to determine if symptoms are indeed related to reflux episodes, especially for patients with a physiological or inconclusive AET to distinguish reflux hypersensitivity. Reflux-symptom association describes the temporal relationship between reflux episodes and symptoms with acute onset (e.g. heartburn, chest pain, regurgitation, cough, or belching). Every logged symptom event on reflux monitoring is preceded by a time window, optimally set at 2 minutes.[64] The Symptom Index (SI) is the percentage of symptom events preceded by reflux episodes, with the optimal SI threshold of ≥ 50% for heartburn.[65]

SI = (Number of reflux-related symptom episodes) / Total number of symptom episodes) × 100%.

A major limitation of the SI is that the total number of reflux episodes is not accounted for, leading to the possibility of a chance association; for example, a patient has frequent reflux, but only reports one symptom so may get a 100% SI if that symptom is related. Therefore, a minimum of three symptoms is required to avoid chance association. The Symptom Association Probability (SAP) expresses the relationship between symptoms and reflux episodes, using a more complex probability approach to determine that the observed association is not due to chance. The 24-hour data is divided into consecutive 2-minute segments, and a 2 × 2 contingency table is calculated for each segment comprised with and without symptoms and with and without reflux. A P value of < 0.05 in considered positive, or an SAP of > 95%.[66]

Interpretation of SI and SAP are complementary; the SI is a measure of effect size and the SAP is a measure of probability; i.e. the SAP tells you if reflux affects the patient while the SI tells you how much it affects them. A combination of a positive SI and SAP provides the best evidence of a clinically relevant association between reflux episodes and symptoms.[53] Both the SI and SAP are predictive of a symptomatic response to antireflux surgery independent of AET.[67,68]

The Ghillebert Probability Estimate (GPE) is an additional post hoc method that considers the total pH-impedance study duration and total AET. Similar to SAP, the GPE determines if the temporal relationship between reflux episodes

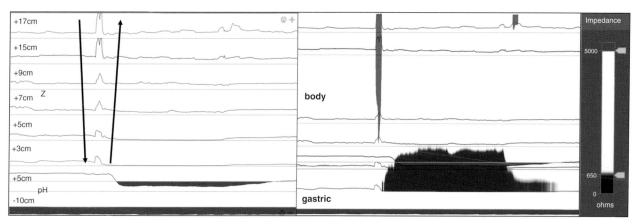

Figure 11.2 Supragastric belch followed by an acid reflux episode on pH-impedance monitoring. Air is sucked into the oesophagus and then rapidly expelled, seen as a rapid antegrade rise in impedance (Z) followed by a retrograde rise in impedance (black arrows). The right image shows the same event on impedance contour with > 5000 Ω (i.e. air) in blue and < 650 Ω in (i.e. reflux) in purple. Supragastric belching can precipitate reflux episodes and result in overestimation of gastro-oesophageal reflux disease.

and symptom events occurring by chance is less than 5%.[69] SI and SAP remain the most widely used indices, but all have the caveat that patients may not report symptoms appropriately. Extending the study to 48 or 96 hours was shown to increase the reported symptoms by 5.2%, but the SAP is also affected as the study duration increases.[59]

GASTRO-OESOPHAGEAL REFLUX DISEASE PHENOTYPES

Phenotyping of GORD can be determined by pH-impedance monitoring. When patients demonstrate a positive reflux-symptom association in the presence of physiological AET and no evidence of endoscopic mucosal disease, then a diagnosis of reflux hypersensitivity may be considered according to Rome IV criteria.[70] Reflux hypersensitivity describes a disease of heightened visceral sensitivity in the oesophagus and therapy includes a trial of neuromodulation. Reflux hypersensitivity accounts for a large proportion of patients presenting with typical GORD symptoms refractory to high-dose PPI therapy.[66] Interestingly, a positive reflux-symptom association for regurgitation was independently associated with small intestinal bacterial overgrowth (SIBO) in patients under consideration for antireflux surgery.[71] Thus, SIBO may play a role in the development and/or perception of reflux.

✅✅ The SI and SAP are complementary and should both be positive to outline a strong correlation between symptoms and reflux.[53] A positive reflux-symptom association provides supplementary evidence for GORD when AET is inconclusive (4–6%), but additionally determines if and which symptoms are indeed caused by acid reflux.[66] Ideally, pH impedance should be used because weakly acidic refluxes have a major role in the pathogenesis of PPI-refractory GORD.

Another phenotype, although not considered to be GORD, is functional heartburn, which relies on a negative reflux-symptom association in the presence of a physiological AET and normal endoscopy. In addition, the Rome IV diagnostic criteria for functional heartburn requires 1)

retrosternal burning, discomfort, or pain; 2) inadequate symptom relief despite optimal antisecretory therapy; 3) absence of GORD or EoE; and 4) absence of major oesophageal motor disorders.[70] The pathophysiology of functional heartburn is puzzling, as some studies suggest lower perception thresholds for pain while others show delayed or no hypersensitivity to chemical or mechanical stimuli.[72] Currently, treatment focuses on neuromodulation and psychological intervention, but further investigations are warranted before functional heartburn should be diagnosed, especially in the presence of concomitant dyspeptic symptoms.

✅ GORD can be phenotyped into three distinct groups: erosive reflux disease when patients have reflux oesophagitis or BO; NERD when patients have pathological acid exposure without mucosal disease, and reflux hypersensitivity when symptoms are related to reflux but acid exposure is normal.[53] Functional heartburn describes no pathological reflux and no association of reflux with symptoms, and is not considered an entity of GORD despite similar symptomatic presentation.

NOVEL METRICS FOR GASTRO-OESOPHAGEAL REFLUX DISEASE

There are two novel impedance metrics that have been investigated within GORD phenotypes that may help to discriminate GORD from functional heartburn.[53] These are the postreflux swallow peristatic wave (PSPW) index and baseline impedance.

POSTREFLUX SWALLOW PERISTATIC WAVE

The PSPW index represents chemical clearance of the oesophagus whereby reflux episodes trigger primary peristalsis to neutralise acid refluxate via salivary bicarbonate. This is evident as an antegrade drop in impedance of 50% occurring within 30 seconds of a reflux episode (Fig. 11.3). The PSPW index is determined by the proportion of reflux

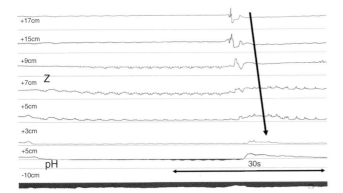

Figure 11.3 Postreflux swallow peristatic wave (PSPW) demonstrated on pH-impedance tracing as an antegrade drop in impedance ≥50% starting in the proximal most impedance (Z) channel and occurring within 30 seconds of a reflux episode. PSPW reflects primary peristalsis containing salivary bicarbonate to neutralise acid refluxate.

episodes followed by a PSPW on pH-impedance monitoring. Studies have shown that the PSPW index is significantly lower in patients with reflux oesophagitis and NERD compared to functional heartburn and controls.[73,74] However, calculation of the PSPW index is laborious as it is not integrated into the analysis software.

BASELINE IMPEDANCE

The baseline impedance reflects the permeability of the oesophageal mucosa and is related to acid exposure.[75] Acid degrades tight junction proteins between oesophageal epithelial cells resulting in DISs (termed spongiosis), which make the epithelium more permeable and baseline impedance decreases.[16] Therefore, baseline impedance is a marker of mucosal integrity and suggestive of long-term reflux burden. The mean nocturnal baseline impedance (MNBI) is measured during sleep on pH-impedance monitoring because there are fewer swallows and reflux events. Progressively lower MNBI values are seen in GORD phenotypes of erosive oesophagitis, NERD, and reflux hypersensitivity compared to healthy controls.[73,76] Low MNBI (< 2292 Ω) can predict symptomatic response to antireflux therapy in patients with an inconclusive (4–6%) AET.[77] The MNBI can also provide complimentary evidence to AET, as normal AET values have been detected in up to 30% of patients with erosive oesophagitis.[78] The baseline impedance can also be measured on HRM with impedance (HRIM).[79]

Direct measurement of mucosal integrity during endoscopy can distinguish EoE from GORD as there is a significant overlap between these two oesophageal syndromes with heartburn reported in up to 63% of patients with EoE.[80] This novel technique for the assessment of oesophageal epithelial integrity is employed by mucosal impedance (MI). Patients with GORD or EoE have DIS between oesophageal epithelial cells related to spongiosis and/or eosinophilia. MI measurements have been shown to correlate with histopathology, i.e. the degree of spongiosis and eosinophilia,[81] and normalise following treatment.[82] The MI pattern along the oesophageal axis differs significantly in patients with GORD (erosive or non-erosive reflux disease) or EoE compared to

patients without GORD or patients with achalasia.[82] In addition, the MI pattern had high positive-predictive values for EoE during endoscopy without the need for histology, with a sensitivity and specificity of 100% and 96%, respectively.[83]

☑☑ Baseline impedance is a highly advantageous metric for the diagnosis of GORD, especially when no mucosal disease is obvious on endoscopy. Baseline impedance highlights the long-term burden of reflux because acid leads to DIS in the oesophageal epithelium, which in turn lowers impedance. Baseline impedance can be assessed by HRM in conjunction with impedance or pH-impedance monitoring via MNBI. The MNBI is especially helpful when acid exposure is equivocal (4–6%) to provide supportive evidence for GORD and predict successful symptom outcomes.[77] Alternatively, MI can be directly measured on endoscopy with specialised impedance probes, which can differentiate EoE from GORD with high a diagnostic accuracy of 100% sensitivity and 96% specificity.[83]

An innovative balloon MI measurement device, as shown in Fig. 11.4, can accurately discriminate patients with GORD, EoE, or non-GORD during endoscopy, and only adds around 2 minutes to the procedure time.[84] The use of 180° impedance sensors mounted on an inflated balloon allows precise opposition of the sensor to the mucosal lining, which reduces the interobserver variability due to 360° design of single channel MI catheters.[85] Long-term outcome studies are needed to see if changes in mucosal integrity detected by balloon MI better predict response to medical or surgical therapy in patients with GORD compared to ambulatory pH testing. However, MI can be a surrogate marker of histology and intuitive MI topography patterns can reliably diagnose EoE, which can often overlap with GORD (see Fig. 11.4).

HIGH-RESOLUTION MANOMETRY

Oesophageal manometry assesses oesophageal motility by measuring the amplitude of contractility in the oesophagus and its sphincters over time. HRM catheters typically have five to six times more pressure sensors than conventional manometry catheters. Moreover, HRM data are recorded and displayed seamlessly on oesophageal pressure topography plots. The value of HRM in oesophageal motility disorders has been defined by the Chicago working group classification.[86] However, HRM is also valuable in the work-up of GORD.

There are three primary reasons for HRM in the setting of GORD: first, to measure the distance from the nares to the proximal LOS in order to accurately place pH catheters; second, to exclude any major motility disorders, or with the addition of impedance, rumination syndrome; third, to assess the current state of peristaltic function prior to antireflux surgery.

OESOPHAGOGASTRIC JUNCTION MORPHOLOGY

The most ubiquitous abnormality in GORD is an incompetence of the OGJ barrier both physiologically and structurally with the presence of TLOSRs and hiatal defects,

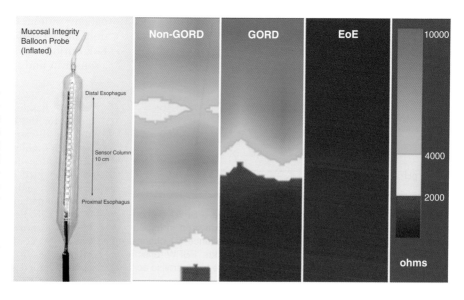

Figure 11.4 A balloon catheter can be introduced into the oesophagus during endoscopy to assess mucosal integrity via impedance values on a topography plot. Low impedance *(red)* reflects loss of mucosal integrity and is seen distally in both gastro-oesophageal reflux disease (GORD) and eosinophilic oesophagitis (EoE), but the mucosal impedance (MI) values remain low in EoE proximally (due to panoesophageal involvement) compared to GORD. Non-GORD patients have minimal loss in mucosal integrity, resulting in normal MI values *(green and blue)*. (Courtesy of MiVu™, Diversatek Healthcare, Milwaukee, WI, USA.)

respectively. A comparative study against open surgery found that HRM is superior to endoscopy and radiology for the detection and classification of HHs.[87] There are three subtypes of OGJ morphology on HRM, as demonstrated in Fig. 11.5.[53]

✓✓ The size of a HH is associated with reflux severity. HHs can be diagnosed by endoscopy or barium oesophagogram, but these are subjective and indirect evaluations of OGJ components. HRM can better define axial dislocation and was shown to have superior diagnostic sensitivity and specificity to OGD and barium oesophagogram when compared to open surgery.[87] HH can be categorised into three subtypes on HRM: type 1 where the LOS and CD are superimposed (no HH); type 2 with partial separation of the LOS and CD < 3 cm (small HH); and type 3, complete separation of the LOS and CD ≥ 3 cm (moderate-large HH), but the respiratory inversion point (RIP) remains at the level of the CD in Type 3a or elevated to the level of the LOS pressure band in Type 3b.

On HRM, OGJ barrier function may be further assessed at rest via the LOS pressure and oesophagogastric junction contractile integral (OGJ-CI), as shown in Fig. 11.6. The OGJ-CI is a quantification of OGJ contractility using the distal contractile integral (DCI) box to encompass the LOS and CD over a period of three respiratory cycles. However, the total OGJ-CI, measured over 10 swallows, can predict reflux better than the resting LOS pressure and OGJ-CI.[88] However, assessment of total OGJ-CI is often difficult due to frequent swallows and may be overestimated by increased pressure from coughing or vascular artefact. The Lyon Consensus concludes that OGJ-CI is a promising metric, but the data for normal values varies considerably based on software and methodology. It requires further standardisation, although it has been outlined in the Chicago Classification v4.0 for motility disorders.[86]

MOTILITY

Assessment of oesophageal motility is mandatory before antireflux surgery.[55] Typically, oesophageal peristalsis is weak in GORD and categorised as ineffective oesophageal motility.[89] However, the most recent iteration of the Chicago

Classification (v4.0) recommends stricter criteria for ineffective motility, with > 70% of 5-mL test swallows being weak or fragmented, or > 50% failed contractions.[86] Failed contractions are more predictive of an abnormal AET compared to weak swallows,[90] and reflux burden is greatest in absent oesophageal motility.[91] However, a diagnosis of ineffective or absent motility is not always a contraindication for antireflux surgery. Provocative tests on HRM, such as solid swallows or multiple rapid swallows (MRS), can demonstrate improved peristalsis that responds to challenge. Post-MRS contractions are indicative of peristaltic reserve function, whereas the post-MRS contraction is greater than that during 5-mL test swallows (Fig. 11.7). The absence of peristaltic reserve is predictive of dysphagia and subsequent benefit from dilation following antireflux surgery.[92,93]

✓✓ The Chicago Classification v4.0 is the latest working group classification for oesophageal motility disorders using HRM.[86] Provocative testing, specifically 5 × 2-mL MRS, can identify peristaltic reserve in patients with absent or ineffective motility. The lack of contraction reserve following MRS is associated with an increased likelihood of postoperative dysphagia in patients following antireflux surgery. The working group recommends at least three attempts of the MRS if no augmented contraction is observed.[86]

POSTPRANDIAL HIGH-RESOLUTION MANOMETRY

HRM with impedance assessment can include a test meal for postprandial identification of pathophysiological mechanisms in GORD: TLOSR-related reflux episodes were significantly increased in patients with NERD compared to controls.[94] Postprandial HRIM can also detect reflux episodes consequent to rumination syndrome or supragastric belching.[95] Since HRIM is not widely available, any suspicion of rumination or supragastric belching disorders can also be determined by pH-impedance monitoring.

FUNCTIONAL LUMEN IMAGING PROBE

The functional lumen imaging probe (FLIP) is a novel, catheter-based device that uses impedance planimetry to

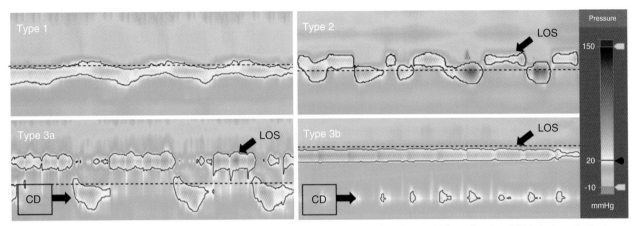

Figure 11.5 High-resolution manometry characterisation of the oesophagogastric junction and hiatus hernias (HHs). In type 1, the lower oesophageal sphincter (LOS) and the crural diaphragm (CD) are superimposed (no HH); in type 2, partial separation of the LOS and CD < 3 cm (small HH); in type 3, complete separation of the LOS and CD ≥ 3 cm (moderate-large HH), but the respiratory inversion point (RIP) remains at the level of the CD in type 3a and the RIP is elevated to the level of the LOS pressure band in type 3b.

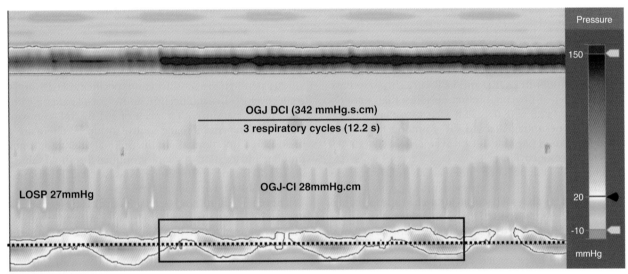

Figure 11.6 High-resolution manometry assessment of oesophagogastric junction (OGJ) contractility at rest. Basal lower oesophageal sphincter (LOS) pressure *(dashed line)* and oesophagogastric junction contractile integral (OGJ-CI) *(black box)*. OGJ-CI is measured above the gastric baseline using the distal contractile integral (DCI) box over to cover the proximal and distal OGJ margin over three respiratory cycles. The DCI is then divided by the duration of three respiratory cycles.

assess the distensibility of hollow organs. Specifically, FLIP allows for easier measurement of OGJ distensibility and cross-sectional area. OGJ distensibility was shown to be two to three times greater in patients with GORD compared to controls.[96] Smeets and colleagues showed that preoperative OGJ distensibility was predictive of objective treatment outcome (i.e. reduced acid exposure), but not for clinical outcome (i.e. symptom improvement), after transoral incisionless fundoplication.[97] However, more data are needed to understand if FLIP can assist in GORD diagnosis and tailoring of surgical techniques.

LARYNGOPHARYNGEAL REFLUX

LPR describes extraoesophageal symptoms associated with retrograde bolus transit into the proximal oesophagus and pharynx. The diagnosis of LPR is less straightforward, since

the pathogenesis of extraoesophageal symptoms can be multifactorial and affect the entire upper aerodigestive mucosa, which is sensitive to pepsin, bile salts, and other gastroduodenal proteins. Hence, LPR was recently defined as an inflammatory condition of the upper aerodigestive tract tissues related to the direct (i.e. refluxate composition) and indirect (i.e. neuroreflexive signalling and compensatory vagal responses) effects of gastroduodenal content reflux, which may induce morphologic changes.[98]

Akin to GORD, questionnaires such as the Reflux Symptom Index (RSI) and empiric PPI trials are extremely limited for the diagnosis of LPR. In fact, a multicentre, double-blind, randomised, placebo-controlled trial showed no evidence of benefit with twice-daily PPI for 4 months in patients with troublesome throat symptoms.[99] This calls into question the use of empiric PPI treatment for throat symptoms, especially in those presenting without heartburn or regurgitation. Nonetheless, GORD and LPR may be dichotomous and

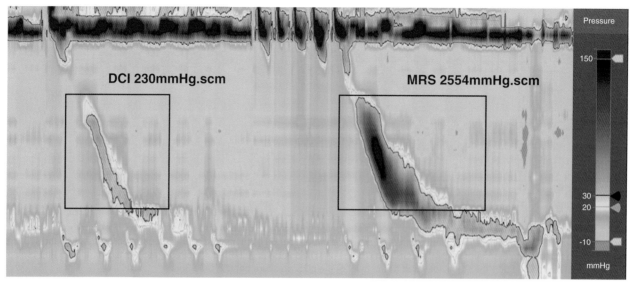

Figure 11.7 The distal contractile integral (DCI) measures the vigour of smooth muscle contraction according to length, duration, and amplitude of contraction. Following multiple rapid swallows (MRS), an augmented DCI higher than the mean DCI from single swallows is evidence of contraction reserve.

investigation with multichannel pH-impedance monitoring is warranted to objectively measure reflux with proximal extent. Patients with both GORD and LPR were shown to have a higher number of proximal reflux episodes than patients with LPR alone (42.3 ± 48.0 vs 24.8 ± 25.4, respectively),[100] and those with oesophageal and LPR symptoms have lower proximal MNBI compared with LPR symptoms only (2500.0 Ω vs 3689.7 Ω, respectively).[101]

Multichannel pH-impedance catheters can indirectly assess LPR via the number of reflux episodes with proximal extent or, more directly, with a pH sensor located in the proximal oesophagus 1–2 cm above the Upper oesophageal sphincter (UOS) (Fig. 11.8). Given that pharyngeal events are almost obsolete in asymptomatic controls, only one proximal reflux episode is thought to be required for a diagnosis of LPR regardless of AET time and DeMeester score,[102] although there is no consensus on these data. Other novel techniques for the diagnosis of LPR include oropharyngeal pH monitoring, which consists of a single Dx-pH sensor in the hypopharynx designed to measure the pH of aerosolized droplets. In addition, the Dx-pH sensor is not prone to drying artefact, unlike traditional catheters with a pH sensor above the UES. When compared to simultaneous multichannel pH-impedance monitoring, oropharyngeal pH monitoring has been shown to reliably capture reflux episodes and have a greater positive-predictive capability of response to PPI therapy.[98] However, LPR and GORD may be separate entities based on synchronous oesophageal and oropharyngeal pH monitoring.[103,104] A Ryan score greater than 9.4 upright and/or 6.8 supine is considered abnormal on oropharyngeal pH testing.[105] In patients with an inconclusive or borderline oesophageal pH-metry, oropharyngeal pH monitoring may add value in the prediction of outcome for patients with atypical symptoms following antireflux surgery,[106,107] but these studies are limited based on small sample sizes.

The contents of gastroduodenal refluxate including pepsin, bile salts, and trypsin make for intriguing diagnostic biomarkers in the diagnosis of LPR. Pepsin is most active at pH 2 and becomes enzymatically inactive at pH 6.5. However, pepsin remains stable until pH 8 and for at least 24 hours in the laryngeal epithelia after a reflux event.[108] A meta-analysis found that salivary pepsin had a sensitivity and specificity of 64% and 68%, respectively.[109] In a multicentre study, 75% of patients with LPR had salivary pepsin, with a mean of 131 ng/mL compared to 0 g/mL in an asymptomatic control group.[110] There are many unanswered questions about the optimal timing for sampling, number and location of samples, optimal threshold values, and impact of diet for pepsin testing. However, if all other tests have been exhausted then salivary pepsin may be useful.

Ultimately, there is no gold standard diagnosis or consensus for LPR, but the use of pH impedance in combination with oropharyngeal pH monitoring may be useful to detect whether LPR and GORD coexist. More outcome data are needed to outline the clinical relevance of oropharyngeal pH testing and salivary pepsin levels, but these can be considered complementary tests in the work-up of GORD and LPR.

✔✔ PPI use was not shown to be effective for persistent throat symptoms in a multicentre, double-blind, randomised, placebo-controlled trial.[99] Clearly, acid is not the primary cause of throat symptoms, but the throat is sensitive to other noxious refluxate such as bile salts and pepsin. A comprehensive review defined LPR as an inflammatory condition of the upper aerodigestive tract tissues related to the direct and indirect effects of gastroduodenal content reflux.[98] Standardisation of LPR testing and diagnosis needs to be ascertained.

OVERLAP BETWEEN GASTRO-OESOPHAGEAL REFLUX DISEASE, GASTROPARESIS, AND FUNCTIONAL GASTROINTESTINAL DISORDERS

In the work-up of GORD, other contributing pathophysiology of the foregut should be considered. The relationship between gastroparesis and GORD is multifactorial but centred around delayed gastric emptying: prolonged retention

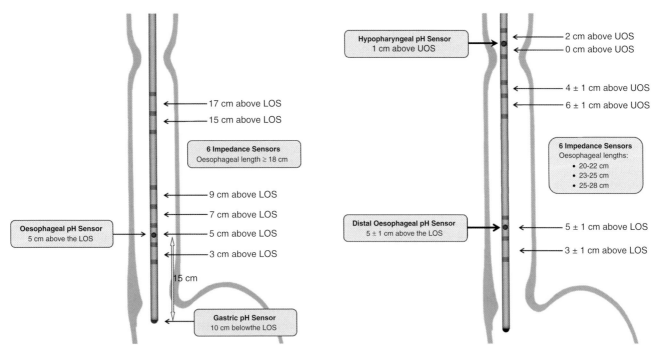

Figure 11.8 Multichannel intraluminal pH-impedance catheter schematics. The left probe has one pH sensor 10 cm below the lower oesophageal sphincter (LOS) (gastric) and one 5 cm above the LOS. While there is no pH sensor in the pharynx, the proximal extent of reflux episodes can be assessed on impedance as an indirect measurement of the LPR. The right probe has one pH sensor 1 cm above the upper oesophageal sphincter (UOS) (hypopharyngeal) and one 5 ± 1 cm above the LOS (dependant on oesophageal length). This a more direct method of assessing laryngopharyngeal reflux to detect pH events in the hypopharynx.

of material in the stomach can precipitate reflux via an increase in gastric pressure, gastric volume, and gastric acid secretion. Indeed, delayed gastric emptying is seen in around 50% of patients with GORD, especially proximal retention, while patients with functional dyspepsia and GORD have greater distal retention.[111] Additionally, up to 20% of patients with gastroparesis have pathological reflux.[8]

Gastroparesis is a disorder of gastrointestinal motility and requires objective evidence of delayed gastric emptying in the absence of mechanical obstruction.[8] Gastroparesis can be interchangeable with functional dyspepsia since they are both manifested by symptoms of nausea, vomiting, early satiety, postprandial bloating, and epigastric discomfort. The only distinction between these two disorders is an abnormal gastric emptying study in patients with gastroparesis.[70] There are several investigations for gastric emptying including scintigraphy, C^{13} breath testing, and wireless motility capsule (WMC). Each have their own pros and cons: scintigraphy is considered the gold standard but exposes the subject to radiation; C^{13} breath testing is inert and cheap but less sensitive than scintigraphy, and WMC provides additional information on whole gut transit but is expensive and not widely available. Delayed gastric emptying prior to antireflux surgery is not a contraindication, but patients are more likely to report gas-bloat symptoms postoperatively.[55] Recent introduction of electrogastography (EGG) could provide useful information on the aetiology of idiopathic gastroparesis, which accounts for 39.4% of cases in the UK.[112]

EGG indirectly assesses antro-pyloric-duodenal motility via extrapolation of patterns of gastric myoelectrical activity (GMA). Cutaneous electrodes are placed on the abdominal skin to measure GMA before and after a water load satiety test. GMA is approximately three cycles per minute (cpm): Koch and colleagues used EGG to evaluate pyloric dysfunction and found that of 33 patients with normal 3-cpm GMA, 78% had a symptomatic response to pyloric therapy (Botox injection or pyloric balloon dilation) for gastroparesis symptoms.[113] A more recent study by Koch and colleagues showed that the increased GMA in the normal 3-cpm range was decreased significantly following pyloroplasty in line with a reduction in gastric emptying time.[114] These symptomatic and physiological responses to pyloric therapy suggest that normal or hypernormal 3-cpm GMA is characteristic of intact gastric pacemaker activity and that gastroparesis is likely due to mechanical or functional outlet obstruction at the pylorus. EGG may be a valuable tool in selecting patients for pyloric intervention and future studies should determine if symptoms of GORD improve following pyloric therapy.

GORD can overlap functional gastrointestinal disorders (FGIDs), namely functional dyspepsia and irritable bowel syndrome (IBS). Around one in four patients with functional dyspepsia have an abnormal AET on pH monitoring,[115,116] while a meta-analysis found that the prevalence of GORD symptoms in patients with IBS was 42%.[117] GORD, functional dyspepsia, and IBS are separate entities, yet FGIDs should be considered in the diagnostic work-up of GORD, especially in the presence of gas-related symptoms such as belching and bloating. More than half of the patients referred for antireflux surgery present with gas-related symptoms, and these patients are more likely to have intestinal dysbiosis, i.e. SIBO.[71] The gut microbiome may play a confounding role in FGIDs.[118] Since PPIs are shown to cause changes to the intestinal microbiome,[51,52] this should be considered in all patients presenting for antireflux surgery, who have likely been taking PPIs for many years. There is also a post-infectious paradigm of FGIDs relating to previous or ongoing bacterial, protozoal, and viral infection. Thus, an inevitable surge in FGIDs should be expected following the COVID-19 pandemic.[119]

✓✓ The most common FGID is IBS and a meta-analysis published in 2012 found the prevalence of GORD symptoms in patients with IBS was 42% and the pooled OR for symptoms of GORD in those with IBS was 4.17 compared to those without, which suggests that patients with IBS are four times more likely to report reflux symptoms. FGIDs should be considered in the work-up of GORD.

DIAGNOSTIC PATHWAY FOR GASTRO-OESOPHAGEAL REFLUX DISEASE (FIG. 11.9)

INVESTIGATION OF SYMPTOMS FOLLOWING ANTIREFLUX SURGERY

Antireflux surgery is generally more effective than medical management, at least in the short-to-medium term, with greater patient satisfaction and GORD-related quality of life following laparoscopic antireflux surgery.[120] Nevertheless, antireflux surgery is not without risks or complications, but a thorough diagnostic work-up can help to minimise these. Indeed, this includes emotional assessment given that patients with concomitant psychological disorders report much lower satisfaction rates postoperatively.[121]

The most common complaints following antireflux surgery are dysphagia, recurrence of GORD, and gas-bloat syndrome. In some cases this can lead to redo-surgery, albeit repeat surgery is associated with increased complications and reduced satisfaction.[122] Recurrent reflux and dysphagia are the most frequent indications for repeat surgery (45.7% and 20.6%, respectively), followed to a much lesser extent by anatomical abnormalities and gas-bloat syndrome (2.5% and 0.7%, respectively).[122] There is no consensus on how to select patients for reoperation, but reinvestigation is warranted. Evidence for further investigation could be based on postoperative PPI dependency or unsatisfactory quality-of-life scores.

DYSPHAGIA

Dysphagia is an early yet expected manifestation of antireflux surgery reported in around half of patients postoperatively. It is likely consequent to oedema and inflammation of the tissue, but generally mild and resolves within 3 months. Preoperative dysphagia and a lack of peristaltic reserve on HRM are predictors of late postoperative dysphagia.[123] Remember, in patients with hypomotility, MRS provocation can clarify intact peristaltic reserve, which is required to overcome the surgically competent OGJ.

For those with persistent dysphagia, OGD and contrast radiology are the first steps to exclude structural complications. During endoscopy, retention of bolus in the oesophagus and difficulty passing the endoscope may indicate disruption of the fundoplication or stenosis at the wrap. The addition of novel FLIP during endoscopy may be useful to document abnormal distensibility of the OGJ, but it is

not widely available. A barium oesophagogram can better identify anatomy, such as a paraesophageal or HH, which suggests migration of the wrap. In addition, a barium oesophagogram can provide information on oesophageal emptying and clarify distal obstruction. Indeed, distal obstruction created by the surgery can increase the contraction amplitude of the oesophageal body on HRM, which can differentiate mechanical from functional obstruction based on the second or third segment, respectively.[124] Furthermore, intrabolus pressurisation and OGJ basal pressures on HRM can identify functional outlet obstruction secondary to hiatal stenosis or a wrap that is too tight or too long, and the addition of impedance allows for assessment of oesophageal clearance. In all patients with persistent or progressive postoperative dysphagia, HRM should be considered to exclude undiagnosed oesophageal motility disorders such as achalasia, distal oesophageal spasm, or hypercontractile oesophagus. Ayazi et al. found a stepwise increase in the rate of persistent dysphagia following magnetic sphincter augmentation that was correspondent to an increase in preoperative DCI from > 4000 mmHg.s.cm.[125] A DCI at the upper end of normal pre-operatively may be suggestive of outflow obstruction and challenge swallows with increased liquid volumes and solids should be carried out to elucidate this.[86]

RECURRENCE OF REFLUX

Recurrence of reflux symptoms accounts for up to 26.8% of primary postoperative complaints.[126] Recurrent GORD is the primary indication for reintervention and is more common among females, older patients, and patients with comorbidities. Antireflux surgery is highly effective for regurgitation, and moderate-severe regurgitation should raise suspicion of wrap failure and be investigated with radiology and pH monitoring to determine acid exposure. Additionally, failure may be inclined from postoperative heartburn and/or chest pain, especially if the patient is dependent on PPIs. Repeating HRM and pH-impedance monitoring could be useful for indistinguishable heartburn or chest pain to exclude newly acquired oesophageal dysmotility and non-acidic or gaseous reflux, respectively.

GAS-BLOAT SYNDROME

Gas-bloat syndrome is characterised by symptoms of bloating, flatulence, and the inability to belch. Interestingly, these symptoms are more commonly reported at 5 years postoperatively than heartburn, chest pain, and dysphagia.[126] In addition, outcomes of bloating and the inability to belch are regarded as less acceptable than dysphagia by patients considering antireflux surgery.[127] It is thought that gas-bloat syndrome is related to an inability of the OGJ to relax in relation to distension and consequent to a super-competent fundoplication. This may explain why gas-bloat symptoms are less frequent following magnetic sphincter augmentation compared to fundoplication.[128] However, this does not explain the cause for excessive gas production in the first place.

Aerophagia describes the excessive swallowing of air and is a behavioural habit often acquired in patients with GORD as a coping mechanism for severe reflux, but it is also associated with increased anxiety. Outlining aerophagia prior to antireflux surgery is important because while surgical intervention

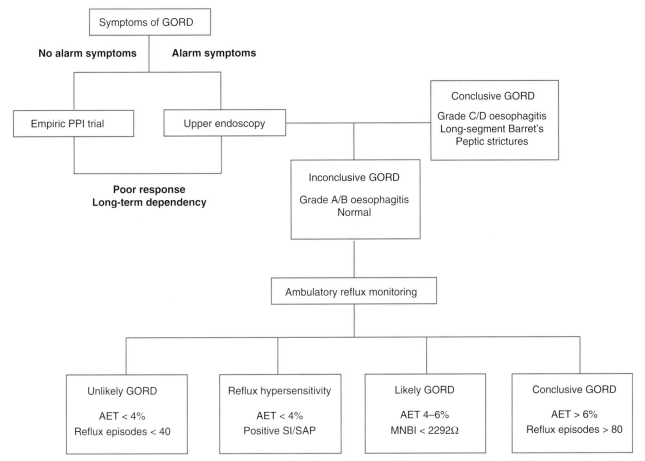

Figure 11.9 The diagnostic pathway for gastro-oesophageal reflux disease (GORD). *AET*, Acid exposure time; *MNBI*, mean nocturnal baseline impedance; *PPI*, proton pump inhibitor; *SI*, symptom index; *SAP*, symptom association probability.

will likely remove the underlying physiological problem, it does not address the hardwired behavioural problem. Epigastric discomfort from surgical intervention may also lead to the development of aerophagia. HRIM or pH-impedance monitoring can detect aerophagia, which can easily be resolved with biofeedback therapy, namely diaphragmatic breathing.

Around 60% of patients referred for antireflux surgery were shown to have intestinal dysbiosis (SIBO and/or intestinal methanogen overgrowth) according to hydrogen and methane breath testing.[71] These patients were more likely to report gas-related symptoms prior to antireflux surgery. In a separate study, patients with Nissen's fundoplication who also tested positive for SIBO had inferior quality-of-life scores, namely gas-bloat symptoms.[129] Therefore, hydrogen and methane breath testing could be a useful investigation of gas-bloat syndrome following antireflux surgery and should be part of the preoperative work-up for patients under consideration for antireflux surgery with gas-related symptoms.[71]

DYSPEPSIA AND GASTROPARESIS

Symptoms of dyspepsia and gastroparesis are the most prevalent early manifestations following antireflux surgery, with up to 88% of patients reporting early satiety.[130] Antireflux surgery may resolve or induce delayed gastric emptying in 18% and 12% of patients, respectively.[131] Post-surgical

gastroparesis is often due to sensory and motor changes in the proximal stomach or vagus nerve injury during fundoplication. However, assessment of vagal function is limited. EGG can be of value for two reasons: firstly, the water load satiety test prior to electrical measurement can determine poor gastric accommodation, and secondly, hyponormal GMA may be suggestive of vagal injury whereas hypernormal GMA may identify pyloric outlet dysfunction. FLIP is also useful for assessing pyloric sphincter distensibility.[132] Khajanchee and colleagues found that patients with delayed gastric emptying who underwent concomitant Nissen fundoplication and pyloroplasty had fewer symptoms of dyspepsia postoperatively compared to those who had fundoplication alone.[133] Drug-induced gastroparesis should also be excluded, such as anticholinergics or more commonly opioid narcotics, especially given their use for pain relief following surgery and high addiction risk.

SUMMARY

GORD is a complex condition that can have significant health and quality-of-life effects. Treatment of GORD beyond lifestyle changes and empirical medication requires careful history taking and clinical investigation. In recent years, advances in technology, publication of internationally accepted guidelines and standards, and the advent of novel treatments have moved the field on considerably. Regardless of these advances, GORD is still underserved generally, and the establishment of reflux-focussed multidisciplinary teams to aid decision-making can be essential in ensuring that the correct decisions are made for the long-term management of these challenging patients.

Key points

- The primary mechanism of gastroesophageal reflux is TLOSRs, which may be precipitated by hiatal defects, impaired gastric function, or excessive fermentation in the proximal colon. These can be investigated by complementary tests including high resolution manometry, gastric emptying studies, electrogastrography, and hydrogen-methane breath testing.
- According to the Lyon Consensus, conclusive evidence of GORD on endoscopy includes long-segment Barret's oesophagus, severe (grade C/D) oesophagitis, and peptic strictures.
- Multichannel-impedance pH monitoring is the gold standard investigation to identify GORD and its subtypes due to the availability of adjunctive measures, including baseline impedance, postreflux swallow peristaltic wave, and proximal extent of reflux.
- High resolution manometry is more than a tool to assess oesophageal motility prior to antireflux surgery: it can distinguish GORD mimicking disorders, such as rumination and achalasia, as well as define a hiatus hernia better than endoscopy or barium oesophagogram.
- Laryngopharyngeal reflux does not respond well to PPIs and is likely related to other gastroduodenal content, such as pepsin and other proteases. Hypopharyngeal pH-impedance monitoring may be useful to detect LPR, but most LPR events are belch related, which can lead to prolonged bolus exposure, especially at night time when swallowing is reduced.

 References available at http://ebooks.health.elsevier.com/

KEY REFERENCES

[1] Hunt R, Armstrong D, Katelaris P, Afihene M, Bane A, Bhatia S, et al. World gastroenterology organisation global guidelines: GERD global perspective on gastroesophageal reflux disease. J Clin Gastroenterol 2017;51(6):467–78

This is the second World Gastroenterology Guideline (WGO) published on GORD. It is intended to highlight appropriate, context-sensitive, and resource-sensitive management options for GORD in all geographical regions, regardless of whether they are considered to be 'developing,' 'semi-developed,' or 'developed.'

[3] Eherer AJ, Netolitzky F, Högenauer C, Puschnig G, Hinterleitner TA, Scheidl S, et al. Positive effect of abdominal breathing exercise on gastroesophageal reflux disease: a randomized, controlled study. Am J Gastroenterol 2012;107(3):372–8

This study randomised 19 patients with NERD or healed oesophagitis to receive diaphragmatic breathing training or control. The 10 in-training group (limited small sample size) demonstrated a significant reduction in AET (9.1% ± 1.3 vs 4.7% ± 0.9; P < 0.05) but there was no change in the control group. In addition, quality-of-life scores and PPI use were significantly decreased at 9-months' follow-up in the training group.

[4] Halland M, Bharucha AE, Crowell MD, Ravi K, Katzka DA. Effects of diaphragmatic breathing on the pathophysiology and treatment of upright gastroesophageal reflux: a randomized controlled trial. Am J Gastroenterol 2021;116(1):86–94

This study examined diaphragmatic breathing in 23 patients with proven GORD on pH-metry and 10 healthy controls. Postprandial diaphragmatic breathing reduced the number of postprandial reflux events in patients and healthy controls compared to observation. During 48-hour ambulatory reflux monitoring, diaphragmatic breathing reduced reflux episodes on day 2 compared to observation on day 1, but not total acid exposure (10.2% ± 7.9 vs 9.4% ± 6.2; P = 0.804). However, in patients randomised to diaphragmatic breathing or sham, postprandial acid exposure was significantly reduced in the 2-hour period following standardised meal (11.8% ± 6.4 vs 5.2% ± 5.1; P = 0.015) This study also looked at the potential mechanism, showing an increase in the difference between LES and gastric pressure on HRM during diaphragmatic breathing.

[34] Dirac MA, Safiri S, Tsoi D, Adedoyin RA, Afshin A, Akhlaghi N, et al. The global, regional, and national burden of gastro-oesophageal reflux disease in 195 countries and territories, 1990–2017: a systematic analysis for the global burden of disease study 2017. Lancet Gastroenterol Hepatol 2020;5(6):561–81

A comprehensive systematic review looking at the global burden of GORD over 27 years across 195 countries and territories by using data from the GBD 2017 Data Resources website and 112 studies. Methods used a novel, complex Bayesian mixed-effects meta-regression tool that incorporates predictive covariates and adjustments for differences in study design in a geographical cascade of models. The review primarily looked at the age-standardised prevalence of GORD, all-age prevalence of GORD, and years lived with disabilities (YLDs). YLDs estimation is the prevalence (specific to year, age, sex, and location) of specific health states that can result from the disease, generally at different levels of severity. YLDs increased by 67·1% (95% CI 63.5–70.3) between 1990 and 2017, from 3.60 million (1.93–6.12) in 1990 to 6.01 million (3.22–10.19).

[50] Baik SH, Fung K-W, McDonald CJ. The mortality risk of proton pump inhibitors in 1.9 million U.S. seniors: an extended cox survival analysis. Clin Gastroenterol Hepatol 2021;20:E671–81

A retrospective cohort study used data from 1 930 728 Medicare fee-for-service beneficiaries aged 65 years or over to assess whether protopathic bias could explain the association between PPI use and death that has been reported in prior observational studies. Overall, without accounting for protopathic bias, PPIs were weakly associated with mortality (adjusted hazard ratio [HR] 1.10; 95% CI 1.08–1.12), but, when including the lag time of 90 days and look-back windows to reduce protopathic bias, PPIs were not associated with mortality (adjusted HR 1.01; 95% CI 0.99–1.02).

[51] Imhann F, Bonder MJ, Vich Vila A, Fu J, Mujagic Z, Vork L, et al. Proton pump inhibitors affect the gut microbiome. Gut 2016;65(5):740–8

The gut microbiome of 1815 individuals in The Netherlands was sequenced with 211 of these identified PPI users. Oral bacteria and potential pathogenic bacteria including Enterococcus, Streptococcus, Staphylococcus, and Escherichia coli were increased in the gut microbiota of PPI users. On the population level, microbial alterations in the gut associated with PPI use was more profound than with antibiotics, especially in relation to increased risk of Clostridium difficile infection.

[52] Jackson MA, Goodrich JK, Maxan ME, Freedberg DE, Abrams JA, Poole AC, et al. Proton pump inhibitors alter the composition of the gut microbiota. Gut 2016;65(5):749–56

The gut microbiome of 1827 healthy twins was sequenced with 229 of those prescribed PPIs, although the actual number of current PPI users at time of testing was not clear. The microbial diversity was lower in PPI users with significant increase in oral commensals, particularly Streptococcaceae as similarly shown by Ihmann et al.[51]

[53] Gyawali CP, Kahrilas PJ, Savarino E, Zerbib F, Mion F, Smout AJPM, et al. Modern diagnosis of GERD: the Lyon consensus. Gut 2018;67(7):1351

These consensus guidelines from an international working group went beyond the previous classifications to define GORD. The Lyon Consensus outlines when testing should be performed 'on' or 'off' PPI and conclusive evidence for GORD on endoscopy (grade C and D oesophagitis, long-segment Barrett's mucosa, or peptic strictures) or ambulatory pH or pH-impedance monitoring (distal AET > 6%). Adjunctive measures are recommended for the diagnosis of GORD when AET is inconclusive including novel impedance metrics such as MNBI and the value HRM for hypomotility and OGJ barrier function.

[66] Kamal AN, Clarke JO, Oors JM, Smout AJ, Bredenoord AJ. The role of symptom association analysis in gastroesophageal reflux testing. Am J Gastroenterol 2020;115(12)

An up-to-date review on the relationship between symptoms and acid reflux events including statistical analysis, interpretation of symptom association, and practical issues that can arise during symptom analysis.

[77] Rengarajan A, Savarino E, Della Coletta M, Ghisa M, Patel A, Gyawali CP. Mean nocturnal baseline impedance correlates with symptom outcome when acid exposure time is inconclusive on esophageal reflux monitoring. Clin Gastroenterol Hepatol 2020;18(3):589–95

This retrospective study from a European and US cohort of 371 patients with treatment-refractory symptoms of GORD looked at the relationship between MNBI and AET, and found that when AET is inconclusive, or 4–6% according to the Lyon Consensus,[53] a low MNBI (< 2292 ohms) identifies patients who respond better to antireflux therapy.

[83] Choksi Y, Lal P, Slaughter JC, Sharda R, Parnell J, Higginbotham T, et al. Esophageal mucosal impedance patterns discriminate patients with eosinophilic esophagitis from patients with GERD. Clin Gastroenterol Hepatol 2018;16(5):664–71.e1

A retrospective analysis of 91 patients with upper GI symptoms who underwent endoscopy with biopsies and MI measurements at 2, 5, and 10 cm from the SCJ, and ambulatory pH monitoring. MI measurements at 5 cm could discern patients with normal versus abnormal mucosa with 83% sensitivity and 79% specificity, and patients with EoE versus GORD with 84% sensitivity and 70% specificity; these measurements differentiated the patient populations with the highest level of accuracy of any of the six measurements tested. When validated against a series of 49 patients undergoing upper endoscopy for dysphagia, the MI patterns were able to identify EoE with 100% sensitivity and 96% specificity.

[86] Yadlapati R, Kahrilas PJ, Fox MR, Bredenoord AJ, Prakash Gyawali C, Roman S, et al. Esophageal motility disorders on high-resolution manometry: Chicago classification version 4.0. Neuro Gastroenterol Motil 2021;33(1):e14058

The latest iteration of the Chicago Classification for the utility of HRM in oesophageal motility disorders, which included standardisation of the manometric protocol to include provocative tests, specifically the 5 × 2-mL MRS for the assessment of peristaltic reserve in patients with GORD.

[87] Tolone S, Savarino E, Zaninotto G, Gyawali CP, Frazzoni M, de Bortoli N, et al. High-resolution manometry is superior to endoscopy and radiology in assessing and grading sliding hiatal hernia: a comparison with surgical in vivo evaluation. United European Gastroenterol J 2018;6(7):981–9.

A comparative study to assess the diagnostic accuracy of HRM in detecting HH compared to barium oesophagogram and upper endoscopy against in vivo measurement: distance between the OGJ and crural diaphragm proximal border. 53 of 100 patients had a HH, and HRM performed with superior sensitivity and specificity (94.3% and 91.5%, respectively). 92.6% had a predictive value of a positive test and 93.5% a predictive value of a negative test. The kappa value for HRM and in vivo evaluation was 0.85 compared to 0.72 for endoscopy and 0.66 for barium oesophagogram.

[98] Lechien JR, Akst LM, Hamdan AL, Schindler A, Karkos PD, Barillari MR, et al. Evaluation and management of laryngopharyngeal reflux disease: state of the art review. Otolaryngol Head Neck Surg 2019;160(5):762–82

There is currently no consensus for the diagnosis and management of laryngopharyngeal reflux (LPR). This comprehensive review aimed to provide a clear definition of LPR and outline the most appropriate diagnostic tests available, specifically multichannel intraluminal pH-impedance monitoring in addition to pepsin and bile salt detection.

[99] O'Hara J, Stocken DD, Watson GC, Fouweather T, McGlashan J, MacKenzie K, et al. Use of proton pump inhibitors to treat persistent throat symptoms: multicentre, double blind, randomised, placebo controlled trial. BMJ 2021;372:m4903

This double-blind, placebo-controlled, randomised trial included 346 patients from ear, nose, and throat clinics in the UK with persistent throat symptoms. After 16 weeks, the mean RSI score was similar between lansoperazole 22.0 (95% CI 20.4–23.6) and placebo 21.7 (95% CI 20.5–23.0). Lansoprazole showed no benefits over placebo for any secondary outcome measure, including quality of life and RSI scores at 12 months.

[117] Lovell RM, Ford AC. Prevalence of gastro-esophageal reflux-type symptoms in individuals with irritable bowel syndrome in the community: a meta-analysis. Am J Gastroenterol 2012;107(12)

This meta-analysis of 49 939 participants found the prevalence of GORD symptoms in those with IBS to be 42.0%. The pooled OR for GORD symptoms in individuals with IBS was 4.17 (95% CI 2.85–6.09), meaning patients with IBS are four times more likely to report concomitant reflux symptoms. The degree of overlap between GORD and IBS varied from 14.2% to 26.7% using the Rome II and Manning criteria, respectively, although the prevalence of IBS would likely be lower using more recent and stringent Rome IV criteria.

12 Treatment of gastro-oesophageal reflux disease

David I. Watson | Sarah K. Thompson

INTRODUCTION

Gastro-oesophageal reflux is common, affecting between 10% and 40% of the population of most Western countries.[1] It is caused by excessive reflux of gastric contents, which contain acid and sometimes bile and pancreatic secretions, into the oesophageal lumen. Pathological reflux leads to symptoms such as heartburn, upper abdominal pain, and the regurgitation of gastric contents into the oropharynx. Gastro-oesophageal reflux is associated with a range of contributing factors, and a multifactorial aetiology is likely. First is hiatus herniation, which is found in approximately half of patients who undergo surgical treatment.[2,3] This results in widening of the angle of His, effacement of the lower oesophageal sphincter, and loss of the assistance of positive intra-abdominal pressure acting on the lower oesophagus. Second is the reduced lower oesophageal sphincter pressure which is often found, although in many patients with reflux the resting lower oesophageal sphincter pressure is normal. Reflux in these patients results from an excessive number of transient lower oesophageal sphincter relaxation events. Other factors that might contribute to the genesis of reflux include abnormal oesophageal peristalsis (which causes poor clearance of refluxed fluid) and delayed gastric emptying.

The treatment of reflux is usually incremental, commencing with various levels of medical measures, surgery being reserved for patients with more severe disease who either fail to respond adequately to medical treatment, those who are intolerant of medical therapy, or those who do not wish to take lifelong medication. Non-operative therapy treats the effects of reflux, as the underlying reflux problem is not corrected, and therapy for most patients must be continued indefinitely. Surgical procedures, however, aim to be curative, preventing reflux by reconstructing an antireflux valve at the gastro-oesophageal junction. In the past, surgery has tended to be reserved for patients with complicated reflux disease or those with very severe symptoms. However, since the introduction of laparoscopic surgical approaches, some surgeons advocate utilising surgery at earlier stages in the course of reflux disease. Endoscopic (transoral) antireflux procedures have also been developed, although the outcomes following these treatments have generally been disappointing.

MEDICAL TREATMENT

SIMPLE MEASURES

A variety of simple measures can be helpful for the management of patients who experience mild symptoms. These include simple antacids, the avoidance of precipitating factors such as spicy foods, and the avoidance of alcohol. Additional measures include weight loss (when appropriate), avoiding cigarette smoking, modification of the timing and quantity of meals (e.g. avoiding going to bed with a full stomach), and raising the bed head. Unfortunately, these measures are rarely effective for patients with moderate-to-severe disease, and most patients who present for surgery cannot be adequately treated with these measures.

HISTAMINE TYPE 2-RECEPTOR ANTAGONISTS

The first effective non-operative treatment for reflux was the development of medications that reduced the production of acid by the stomach. The histamine type 2 (H_2)-receptor antagonists sometimes relieve mild-to-moderate reflux symptoms. When first used in the 1970s they revolutionised the medical approach to duodenal ulcer disease. However, they were less effective for reflux disease and few patients achieve complete relief of reflux symptoms with these medications. Even so, in milder forms of the disease they can reduce symptoms. When medications are ceased, however, symptoms usually return and treatment has to be recommenced. With the current widespread availability of proton pump inhibitors (PPIs), H_2-receptor antagonists are now rarely used as first-line medical therapy.

PROTON PUMP INHIBITORS

PPIs (omeprazole, lansoprazole, pantoprazole, rabeprazole, and esomeprazole) were introduced into clinical practice in the late 1980s. These agents are much more effective for the relief of symptoms and achieve better healing of the oesophagitis than H_2-receptor antagonists. However, patients with higher grades of oesophagitis (e.g. Los Angeles grade C or D) have a higher failure rate with these medications,[4] and in addition many patients who initially achieve good symptom control go on to develop 'breakthrough' symptoms at a later date, usually requiring an increased dose of medication to maintain symptom control.

It is presumed that failure is due to inadequate acid suppression, although in some cases the presence of bile or duodenal fluid in the refluxate may play a role. In patients who respond well to PPIs, symptoms usually recur rapidly (sometimes in less than 24 hours) following cessation of medication, and for this reason lifelong medical treatment is likely to be required, unless surgery is performed. The long-term use of PPIs is generally considered to be safe, although associations have been shown between PPI consumption and small increases in the rates of community-acquired pneumonia and hip fractures.[5,6] Other studies have shown associations between long-term use and the development of atrophic gastritis with intestinal metaplasia in patients with concurrent *Helicobacter pylori* infection, as well as parietal cell hyperplasia.[5] The latter phenomenon may be the reason why symptoms recur rapidly in some patients on cessation of therapy, and may be another reason why some patients require escalating dosages of PPIs to control their symptoms.

SURGICAL TREATMENT

The principle underlying the surgical management of gastro-oesophageal reflux disease is the creation of a mechanical antireflux barrier between the oesophagus and stomach. This works independently of the composition of the refluxate. While medical therapy is effective in relieving symptoms for many patients with acid reflux, only surgery achieves effective control of duodeno-gastro-oesophageal reflux.

SELECTION CRITERIA FOR SURGERY

As a general rule, all patients who undergo antireflux surgery should have objective evidence of reflux. This may be the demonstration of erosive oesophagitis on endoscopy or an abnormal amount of acid reflux demonstrated by 24-hour pH monitoring. Neither of these tests is sufficiently reliable to base all preoperative decisions on their outcome,[7] as a number of patients with troublesome reflux will have either a normal 24-hour pH study or no evidence of oesophagitis at endoscopy (and, very occasionally, both). For this reason, the tests have to be interpreted in light of the patient's clinical presentation, and a final recommendation for surgery should be based on all available clinical and objective information.[7] More recently, impedance monitoring (in combination with pH monitoring) has been used to measure 'volume' reflux, although the additional information obtained from this investigation probably only influences surgical decision-making in a small cohort of patients.[8]

Patients selected for surgery fall into two general groups: 1) patients who have failed to respond (or have responded only partially) to medical therapy; and 2) patients whose symptoms are fully controlled by medications, but who have developed side-effects or do not wish to continue medications throughout their lives. The first group represents the large majority of patients presenting for surgery, whereas the latter group are less common and more likely to be younger patients who face decades of acid suppression to alleviate their symptoms. In the first group, the response

to surgery is usually more certain if the patient has had a good response to acid suppression in the past, or at least has had some symptom relief from medication. In patients who have had no response to PPIs, particularly those presenting with atypical symptoms, their symptoms are often due to something other than reflux, despite concurrent objective evidence of reflux (which can be asymptomatic). Such patients will usually not benefit from antireflux surgery.

Failure of medical treatment can be defined as: 1) continuing symptoms of reflux while on an adequate dose of acid suppression; or 2) ongoing erosive oesophagitis on maximal medical therapy (regardless if asymptomatic). This usually means at least a standard dose of a PPI for a minimum period of 3 months, although in some individuals escalation to a higher dose of a PPI can achieve symptom control and can be considered before progressing to surgery. PPIs are generally more effective for the control of the symptom of heartburn than volume regurgitation, and it is the latter symptom that is often the dominant problem in patients who have failed on medical therapy.

A further classification of patients who undergo surgery for gastro-oesophageal reflux disease can be made into two groups: 1) patients who have complicated reflux disease; and 2) patients who have straightforward disease without complications.

PATIENTS WITH COMPLICATED REFLUX DISEASE

Reflux with stricture formation

The treatment of peptic oesophageal strictures has been greatly altered since PPIs became available, and this is one area where the role of surgery has declined. In the past, surgery was the only effective treatment for strictures, and when the stricture was densely fibrotic this even meant resection of the oesophagus. Fortunately, patients with refractory strictures are now rare. Most patients who develop strictures can be successfully managed by PPIs and endoscopic dilatation. Rarely, strictures in young and fit patients might be best treated by antireflux surgery and dilatation.

Reflux with respiratory complications

When gastro-oesophageal regurgitation spills over into the respiratory tree, this can cause chronic respiratory illness such as recurrent pneumonia, asthma, or bronchiectasis. This is an indication for antireflux surgery, as the predominant action of PPIs is to block acid secretion and the volume of reflux is not greatly reduced.

Reflux with throat symptoms

Such problems as halitosis, chronic cough, chronic laryngitis, chronic pharyngitis, chronic sinusitis, and loss of enamel on the teeth are sometimes attributed to gastro-oesophageal reflux. While there is little doubt that on occasions such problems do arise in refluxing patients, these problems in isolation are not reliable indications for surgery. Whether or not these symptoms will be relieved following surgery is often unpredictable. If symptoms are associated with typical reflux symptoms such as heartburn and/or regurgitation, then response rates of approximately 80% are reported, whereas throat symptoms in the absence of typical reflux symptoms respond poorly to surgery, with success rates of less than 50% reported.[9]

Columnar-lined (Barrett's) oesophagus

Barrett's oesophagus in itself is probably not an indication for antireflux surgery, but it is evidence that the patient has gastro-oesophageal reflux disease. Patients with Barrett's oesophagus who have reflux symptoms should be selected for surgery on the basis of their symptoms and their response to medications, not simply because they have a columnar-lined oesophagus.[10] There is some experimental evidence to suggest that continuing reflux may be deleterious in regard to malignant change in oesophageal mucosa, and one prospective randomised trial has suggested that antireflux surgery gives superior results to drug therapy in this patient group.[11] However, PPIs were introduced into the medical arm of that trial only in its later years.

There is also evidence that abolition of symptoms with proton pump inhibition does not equate to 'normalising' the pH profile in a patient's oesophagus.[12] Since antireflux surgery does usually abolish acid reflux, this may become a further reason to recommend surgery in patients with Barrett's oesophagus. However, there is limited evidence to support the contention that either surgical or medical treatment of reflux in patients with Barrett's oesophagus consistently leads to regression of the columnar lining. A report from Gurski et al.[13] suggests that although fundoplication is not followed by a reduction in the length of Barrett's oesophagus, it can be followed by 'histological' regression. In 68% of patients in this study with low-grade dysplasia there was regression to non-dysplastic Barrett's mucosa. A more recent study by the author's group evaluated 50 patients with Barrett's oesophagus using Bravo pH monitoring and endoscopy. Histological regression of Barrett's oesophagus was seen in 40% of patients, and a significant association was found between regression and an intact fundoplication (assessed using Bravo pH monitoring).[14] Other studies have also shown that a combination of medical or surgical therapy with argon-beam plasma coagulation, photodynamic therapy, or radiofrequency ablation of the columnar lining achieves complete or near complete reversion to squamous mucosa.[15–17] Longer term follow-up from a randomised trial of ablation versus surveillance in patients with Barrett's oesophagus who had undergone a fundoplication showed a reduction in the length of Barrett's oesophagus in both study groups, although to a greater extent following ablative therapy.[16] There is currently insufficient evidence to support the contention that antireflux surgery reduces the risk of Barrett's oesophagus progressing to cancer.

PATIENTS WITH UNCOMPLICATED REFLUX DISEASE

Medical therapy, in the form of PPIs, is very effective and the majority of patients get substantial or complete relief of their symptoms using these agents. Despite this, patients continue to present for antireflux surgery for reasons already discussed. An additional proposed indication for antireflux surgery is the rising incidence of adenocarcinoma of the oesophagus associated with gastro-oesophageal reflux disease. Whether antireflux surgery is more effective than long-term proton pump inhibition at preventing the development of columnar-lined oesophagus and subsequently carcinoma of the lower oesophagus is controversial. If duodenal fluid has

a role in the pathogenesis of adenocarcinoma of the oesophagus, then antireflux surgery would be preferable to acid suppression alone in patients with Barrett's oesophagus, and of course it may also prevent the development of Barrett's oesophagus in the first place. However, this hypothesis has not been adequately tested, and evidence to support a position that antireflux surgery should be performed to prevent subsequent malignant transformation is lacking.

MEDICAL VERSUS SURGICAL THERAPY

The issue of the most appropriate treatment for gastro-oesophageal reflux disease has been the subject of disagreement between surgeons and gastroenterologists. While most would agree that a single management strategy is unlikely to be appropriate for all patients, disagreements arise when interpreting comparative data for medical versus surgical therapy. Ten randomised trials have investigated this issue, although five of these commenced before the availability of both laparoscopic antireflux surgery or PPI medication.[11,18–26] In general, the protocol for these trials entailed recruiting patients who had reflux symptoms that were well controlled by medical therapy. For the latter trials this entailed complete symptom control with a PPI at trial commencement, and patients with uncontrolled symptoms were excluded. Hence, the surgical groups in these trials excluded the patients who represent the majority of those currently selected for surgery, i.e. patients with a poor response to a PPI.

Spechler et al.[19] reported the first large trial in 1992. A total of 247 patients (predominantly men) were randomised to either continuous medical therapy with an H_2-blocker, medical therapy for symptoms only, or an open Nissen fundoplication. Overall patient satisfaction was highest following surgery at 1 and 2 years follow-up. However, neither the surgical approach nor the medical treatment investigated would now be considered to be optimal. The longer term outcomes from this study were published in 2001, with a median follow-up of approximately 7 years, and PPIs now used for the medically treated patients.[27] Follow-up was not complete and only 37 (45%) surgical patients were available for late follow-up, with 23% of the original surgical group lost to follow-up, and 32% died during follow-up. The late results did, however, show reasonable outcomes in both the medically and surgically treated groups. However, 62% of the surgical patients consumed antireflux medications at late follow-up, although when these medications were ceased in both the study groups the surgical group had significantly fewer reflux symptoms than the medical group, suggesting that most of the surgical patients did not actually need the medications!

In 2003 Parrilla et al.[20] reported a trial that randomised 101 patients with Barrett's oesophagus. Medical therapy was initially an H_2-blocker and later a PPI. A satisfactory clinical outcome was achieved at 5 years follow-up in 91% of each group, although medical treatment was associated with a poorer endoscopic outcome. Progression to dysplasia was similar in both groups.

In 2000 Lundell et al. reported a trial of PPI medication versus open antireflux surgery.[28] A total of 310 patients were randomised, and antireflux surgery achieved a better outcome at up to 3 years follow-up. Later reports of

7 years follow-up in 228 patients, and 12 years follow-up in 124 patients, confirmed that surgery still achieved better reflux control than medication, although dysphagia and various wind-related side-effects were more common after fundoplication.[28]

Rhodes et al. reported the first randomised trial to compare PPI medication with laparoscopic Nissen fundoplication; 217 patients were enrolled. Surgery was followed by less oesophageal acid exposure 3 months after treatment, and better symptom control at 12 months.[21] A similar study from Anvari et al. enrolled 104 patients into a trial of PPI therapy versus laparoscopic Nissen fundoplication.[22] Follow-up at 12 months and 3 years demonstrated better control of reflux and better quality of life in the patients who underwent surgery.

Two large, randomised trials were reported in 2009. Lundell et al.[23] reported the outcomes on a multicentre study of laparoscopic Nissen fundoplication versus esomeprazole PPI (20–40 mg per day) which enrolled 554 patients. Similar success rates of approximately 90% were reported for each treatment at up to 3 years follow-up. A subsequent report of objective follow-up at 5 years demonstrated greater reductions in oesophageal pH following surgery.[28] The other trial, reported by Grant et al., utilised a pragmatic design, randomising 357 participants to a PPI versus fundoplication (Nissen or partial).[25] At 5 years follow-up fundoplication achieved better reflux symptom control and appeared to yield a better overall outcome.

A more recent trial reported by Spechler et al. randomised 78 patients with PPI refractory reflux symptoms to fundoplication versus ongoing PPI use versus a strategy of escalating PPI dosing. Predictably, this study showed that fundoplication provided significantly better symptom control than the two PPI strategies.[26]

✓✓ It can be contended from the results of randomised trials that surgery achieves better control of reflux than medical therapy in some patients. When medical therapy fails to control symptoms, fundoplication should be offered. Further, the majority of patients who have gastro-oesophageal reflux sufficient to require a PPI should also be offered the opportunity to consider surgical correction of their reflux irrespective of whether symptoms are well controlled by medication or not. The clinical trials all support an ongoing and important role for surgery in the treatment of reflux, and potentially a wider role in the management of reflux if offered to PPI-dependent patients with symptoms that are well controlled by medication.

PROS AND CONS OF ANTIREFLUX SURGERY

ADVANTAGES

The advantages of surgery are clear. The operation is the only treatment that actually cures the problem, i.e. stops gastric contents from refluxing into the oesophagus. Hence, patients treated by surgery can usually eat whatever foods they choose, can lie flat and bend over without reflux occurring, and importantly they do not need to take any tablets.

DISADVANTAGES

The first disadvantage is the morbidity associated with the operation (see discussion of complications later). While laparoscopic surgery has meant that the pain of the open operation has been greatly reduced, most patients have some difficulty in swallowing in the early postoperative period, although in the great majority this is only temporary. The time taken to for this to resolve is variable, although for most individuals no more than 3–6 months are required.[3] Furthermore, the great majority of patients feel full quickly after eating even small meals, and this often leads to some postoperative weight loss.[3] In patients who are overweight at the time of surgery, this might be seen as an advantage. This restriction on meal size also usually disappears after 3–6 months.

Because fundoplication produces a one-way valve, swallowed air that has passed into the stomach usually cannot pass back through the valve. Thus, patients have to be forewarned that they may not be able to belch effectively after the operation, especially in the first 6–12 months after surgery, and hence they should be cautious about drinking gassy drinks. This applies particularly to patients who undergo a Nissen (total) fundoplication. For similar reasons, patients will be unable to vomit after an effective procedure, and should be informed of this. As swallowed gas is often not belched effectively, the majority of patients are aware of increased bloating and passage of wind after the procedure. Although patients who undergo a partial fundoplication (particularly anterior) have a lower incidence of these problems,[2] difficulties can still occur. Despite these possible disadvantages, the overwhelming majority of patients claim that the disadvantages are far outweighed by the advantages of the operation. To date it has not been possible to predict preoperatively those patients who will develop problems following surgery.

OPERATIONS AVAILABLE

To the non-surgeon, it might seem that there is a bewildering array of operations available for the treatment of reflux. The fundoplication introduced by Rudolf Nissen in 1956, or some variant of it, remains the most popular antireflux operation in the world today. Total fundoplications, such as the Nissen, or partial fundoplications, whether anterior or posterior, probably all work in a similar fashion,[29] and that is largely mechanical, as it has been demonstrated that these procedures are effective even when placed in the chest in vivo,[30] and also on the benchtop, i.e. ex vivo.[29] The principles of fundoplication are to mobilise the lower oesophagus, wrap the fundus of the stomach, either partially or totally, around the oesophagus, and then stabilise this new anatomy long term. When the oesophageal hiatus is enlarged, it is narrowed with sutures to prevent paraoesophageal herniation postoperatively and to prevent the wrap migrating into the chest (Fig. 12.1). Complications of reflux such as fibrotic stricturing with shortened oesophagus are now seen rarely compared to the past. In the circumstance of true oesophageal shortening, an oesophageal lengthening (Collis) procedure can be undertaken to provide a long enough oesophagus to reach the abdomen. The upper lesser curvature of the stomach is used to produce the new oesophagus and the gastric fundus is then wrapped around this. In the authors' experience the Collis procedure is rarely indicated or required during a primary antireflux procedure, although some other surgeons hold a different view and apply the Collis procedure more liberally.

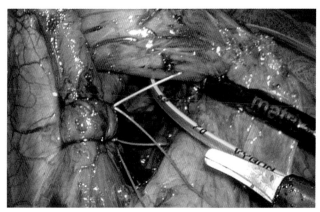

Figure 12.1 Dissected oesophagus with the hiatus repaired with posteriorly placed sutures, and the posterior vagus nerve separated from the oesophagus.

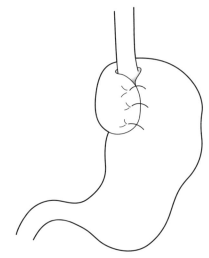

Figure 12.2 Nissen fundoplication.

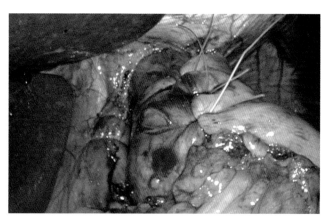

Figure 12.3 Laparoscopic view of a completed Nissen fundoplication.

MECHANISMS OF ACTION OF ANTIREFLUX OPERATIONS

The mechanisms of action of an antireflux operation integrate several principles. Proposed mechanisms include:

1. The creation of a floppy valve by maintaining close apposition between the abdominal oesophagus and the gastric fundus. As intragastric pressure rises, the intra-abdominal oesophagus is compressed by the adjacent fundus.
2. Exaggeration of the flap valve at the angle of His.
3. Increase in the basal pressure generated by the lower oesophageal sphincter.
4. Reduction in the triggering of transient lower oesophageal sphincter relaxations.
5. Reduction in the capacity of the gastric fundus, thereby speeding proximal and total gastric emptying.
6. Prevention of effacement of the lower oesophagus (which effectively weakens the lower sphincter).

Since the procedures seem to work, even ex vivo, it seems likely that the first two mechanisms account for the efficacy of the majority of antireflux procedures. The increase in lower oesophageal sphincter pressure following surgery is not important, and in some partial fundoplication procedures there is very little increase in pressure yet reflux is well controlled.[2,31] The trend towards increasingly looser and shorter total fundoplications or greater use of partial fundoplication procedures suggests that there is no such thing as a fundoplication that is 'too loose'.

TECHNIQUES OF ANTIREFLUX SURGERY

A range of antireflux operations are currently performed and all have their advocates. No one procedure currently yields perfect results, i.e. 100% cure of reflux and zero side-effects. Despite this, published reports can be found that support every known procedure, and it is probably better to consider results from randomised trials when assessing the merits of these procedural variants (see later) rather than relying on uncontrolled outcomes reported by advocates of a single procedure. It should also be recognised that the experience of the operating surgeon is of great importance for achieving a good postoperative outcome.[32] Variability can be reduced, but not eliminated, by detailed technical descriptions and effective surgical training. Laparoscopic approaches are the standard for primary antireflux surgery.

NISSEN FUNDOPLICATION (FIGS. 12.2 AND 12.3)

This is probably the most commonly performed antireflux operation worldwide. Nissen originally described a procedure that entailed mobilisation of the oesophagus from the diaphragmatic hiatus, reduction of any hiatus hernia into the abdominal cavity, preservation of the vagus nerves and mobilisation of the posterior gastric fundus behind the oesophagus, without dividing the short gastric vessels, and suturing of the posterior fundus to the anterior wall of the fundus using non-absorbable sutures, thereby achieving a complete wrap of stomach around the intra-abdominal oesophagus.[33] The original fundoplication was 5 cm in length and an oesophageal bougie was not used to calibrate the wrap.

✔ Because the original Nissen fundoplication was associated with an incidence of persistent postoperative dysphagia, gas bloat syndrome, and an inability to belch, the procedure has been progressively modified in an attempt to improve the long-term outcome. Most surgeons agree that calibration of the wrap with a large (e.g. 52–60 Fr) intraoesophageal bougie, and shortening the fundoplication to 1–2 cm in length, achieves a better outcome.[34] Furthermore, while the need for routine hiatal repair was uncertain in the era of open surgery, most surgeons routinely include this step during laparoscopic antireflux surgery. Omission of this step is associated with a higher incidence of postoperative hiatal herniation.[35] The hepatic branch of the vagus nerve is usually preserved during this procedure.

Controversy remains about the need to divide the short gastric vessels to achieve full fundal mobilisation. The so-called floppy Nissen procedure originally described by Donahue and Bombeck[36] relies on extensive fundal mobilisation. On the other hand, the modification of the Nissen fundoplication using the anterior fundal wall alone, also first described by Nissen and Rossetti,[33,37] does not require short gastric vessel division to construct the fundoplication. This simplifies the dissection, although more judgement and experience may be required to select the correct piece of stomach to use for the construction of a sufficiently loose fundoplication. Both procedures have their advocates, and good results (90% good or excellent long-term outcome) have been reported for both variants.[34,37] Nevertheless, strong opinions are held about whether the short gastric vessels should be divided or not, and this controversy was heightened by the introduction of laparoscopic fundoplication.

POSTERIOR PARTIAL FUNDOPLICATION (FIG. 12.4)

A variety of fundoplication operations have been described in which the fundus is wrapped partially round the back of the oesophagus, with the aim of reduction of the possible side-effects of total fundoplication due to overcompetence of the cardia, i.e. dysphagia and gas-related problems. Toupet described a posterior partial fundoplication in which the fundus is passed behind the oesophagus and sutured to the left lateral and right lateral walls of the oesophagus, as well as to the right diaphragmatic pillar, creating a 270° posterior fundoplication.[38] A very similar procedure was described by Lind et al.[39] This entails a 300° posterior fundoplication, which is constructed by suturing the fundus to the oesophagus at the left and right lateral positions, and additionally anteriorly on the left, leaving a 60° arc of oesophageal wall uncovered. The hiatus is repaired if necessary.

ANTERIOR PARTIAL FUNDOPLICATION

Several anterior partial fundoplication procedures have been described, and all purport to reduce the incidence of dysphagia and other side-effects. The Belsey Mark IV procedure, popular in thoracic practice up to the early 1990s, entailed a 240° anterior partial fundoplication that was usually performed through a left thoracotomy approach.[40] This procedure is no longer used and is largely of historical interest.

The Dor procedure is an anterior hemifundoplication that involves suturing of the fundus to the left and right sides of the oesophagus, as well as the right hiatal pillar.[41] The Dor procedure is commonly used in combination with an abdominal cardiomyotomy for achalasia as it is unlikely to cause dysphagia, and it may reduce the risk of gastro-oesophageal reflux following cardiomyotomy.[42]

A 120° anterior fundoplication has also been described.[31] This entails reduction of any hiatus hernia, posterior hiatal repair, suture of the posterior oesophagus to the hiatal pillars posteriorly, suture of the fundus to the diaphragm to accentuate the angle of His, and creation of an anterior partial fundoplication by suturing the fundus to the oesophagus on the right anterolateral aspect. Satisfactory medium-term reflux control following open surgery was reported for this procedure, with a low incidence of gas-related problems.

The authors have reported the results from prospective randomised trials of laparoscopic anterior 180° partial fundoplication and laparoscopic anterior 90° partial fundoplication versus a Nissen procedure[2,43–48] (see later). The anterior 180° fundoplication procedure entails hiatal repair, suture of the distal oesophagus to the hiatus posteriorly, and construction of an anterior fundoplication that is sutured to the oesophagus and the hiatal rim on the right and anteriorly (Figs. 12.5 and 12.6). The anterior 90° partial fundoplication procedure entails hiatal repair, posterior oesophagopexy, narrowing of the angle of His, and construction of a limited anterior fundoplication that covers the left anterolateral aspect of the oesophagus (Fig. 12.7). These variants of anterior fundoplication control reflux in most patients and compare favourably with Nissen fundoplication in randomised trials.

OTHER ANTIREFLUX PROCEDURES

Hill procedure

Hill described a procedure that is often regarded as a gastropexy rather than a fundoplication.[49] However, it also plicates the cardia and when examined endoscopically the

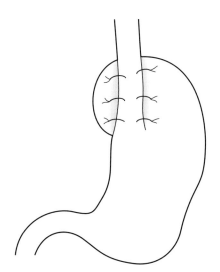

Figure 12.4 Posterior partial fundoplication.

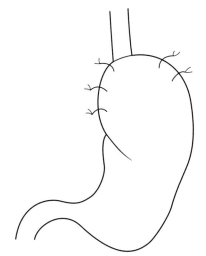

Figure 12.5 A 180° anterior partial fundoplication.

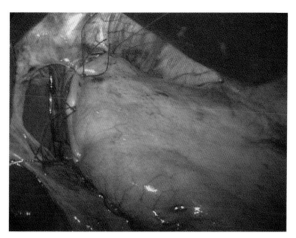

Figure 12.6 Laparoscopic view of a completed 180° anterior partial fundoplication.

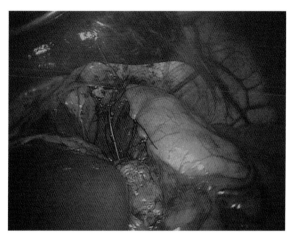

Figure 12.7 Laparoscopic view of a completed anterior partial fundoplication. This particular fundoplication was fashioned as a 90° wrap, leaving an area of exposed oesophagus on the right side.

intragastric appearances are similar to a fundoplication. The procedure entails suturing the anterior and posterior phreno-oesophageal bundles to the pre-aortic fascia and the median arcuate ligament. While excellent results have been reported by Park et al.,[50] it has not been applied widely because most surgeons have difficulty understanding the anatomical principles and, in particular, the so-called phreno-oesophageal bundles are not clear structures. Hill also emphasises the need for intraoperative manometry. This is not widely available, limiting the dissemination of his technique.

Collis procedure (Fig. 12.8)

The Collis procedure is useful for patients whose oesophagogastric junction cannot be reduced below the diaphragm.[51] However, this situation is very uncommon in current practice with sufficient mediastinal dissection. The Collis procedure entails the construction of a tube of gastric lesser curve to recreate an abdominal length of oesophagus, around which a fundoplication can then be constructed to help with oesophageal shortening. Laparoscopic and thoracoscopic techniques for this procedure have been described.[52] A disadvantage is that the gastric tube does not have peristaltic

activity and furthermore it can secrete acid. This leads to a poorer overall success rate for this procedure, although some of this could be due to the end-stage nature of the reflux disease that led to the choice of this procedure in the first place.

Magnetic lower oesophageal sphincter augmentation (Linx)

In 2010 Bonavina et al.[53] described a novel approach to surgery for gastro-oesophageal reflux which entailed augmentation of the lower oesophageal sphincter with an implantable string of interlinked titanium beads with magnetic cores. This device (Linx Reflux Management System; Torax Medical, Shoreview, MN) is placed laparoscopically around the oesophagogastric junction and aims to control reflux but still allow normal swallowing and belching. Success rates of approximately 90%, as measured by both clinical scores and pH monitoring, have been reported at short-term follow-up, and this appears similar to the success rate following fundoplication. However, experience remains limited to a small number of predominantly North American centres, and cases are often selected to avoid patients with large hiatus hernias or more severe reflux disease. This procedure is yet to enter wide clinical practice across the world. Asti et al. reported outcomes from a study comparing 135 patients who underwent magnetic sphincter augmentation versus 103 who underwent a Toupet fundoplication.[54] Quality-of-life and symptom outcomes were similar at follow-up, ranging from 1 to 7 years. Reynolds et al. compared 62 patients undergoing sphincter augmentation versus a matched group undergoing Nissen fundoplication and reported comparable outcomes at 12 months, with better preservation of belching after the sphincter augmentation procedure.[55] As the magnetic sphincter augmentation approach entails placing a foreign body around the distal oesophagus, it is perhaps not surprising that erosion of the device into the oesophageal lumen has been reported,[56] with rates of up to 2.4% at 3 years follow-up described.

Electrical stimulation of the lower oesophageal sphincter

In 2013 Rodríguez described laparoscopic implantation of electrodes to stimulate the lower oesophageal sphincter (EndoStim LES Stimulation System; EndoStim BV, The Hague, The Netherlands).[57] Early data demonstrated improvement in reflux symptoms, a reduction in oesophageal acid exposure, and reduced use of PPI medication. Two-year follow-up data in 21 of 23 patients confirmed similar results; oesophageal pH data were normalised in 71%, and 76% stopped PPIs.[57] This procedure has not reached the mainstream, and longer term data in larger patient cohorts will be needed to support its wider use.

COMPLETE OR PARTIAL FUNDOPLICATION?

Because fundoplication is associated with an incidence of postoperative dysphagia, gas bloat and other gas-related symptoms such as increased flatulence, the relative merits of the Nissen fundoplication procedure have been debated for many decades. The introduction of laparoscopic approaches only served to heighten this controversy. It is generally accepted that the Nissen procedure produces an

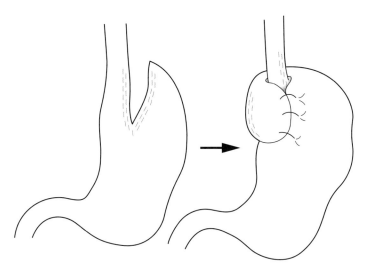

Figure 12.8 Collis gastroplasty, with subsequent Nissen fundoplication.

overcompetent oesophagogastric junction, which contributes to the problems of dysphagia and gas bloat following surgery. Partial fundoplication variants reduce the risk of overcompetence and have been proposed as strategies to reduce side-effects, and improve overall outcomes, but this might be at the expense of a less durable antireflux repair.

The rationale behind the newer procedures described earlier (Linx and EndoStim) is similar to the rationale for partial fundoplication. These procedures also aim to reduce side-effects while maintaining good reflux control. Partial fundoplications can be constructed using operating equipment that is available in most modern operating theatres, thereby offering a solution that can be applied by any surgeon undertaking surgery for reflux, whereas newer procedures that involve implanting devices require expensive implants and equipment that is not readily available for the majority of surgeons. Furthermore, the novel devices are yet to be tested in well-designed randomised trials, whereas data are available from many prospective randomised trials of Nissen versus partial fundoplication.

NISSEN VERSUS POSTERIOR FUNDOPLICATION

A total of 14 randomised trials have compared a Nissen with a posterior partial fundoplication. Some of the trials contribute little to the pool of evidence as they are small and underpowered, or only reported very short-term outcomes.[58–62]

Lundell et al. reported the outcomes of the first large trial of Nissen versus a posterior (Toupet) partial fundoplication; 137 patients were enrolled.[61,62] The early outcomes at 6 months follow-up were similar. At 5 years follow-up[63] reflux control and dysphagia rates were also similar, although flatulence was more common after Nissen fundoplication at 2 and 3 years but not at 4 or 5 years follow-up. Re-operation was more common following Nissen fundoplication, with one patient in the posterior fundoplication group undergoing further surgery for severe gas bloat symptoms and five of the Nissen group undergoing re-operation for postoperative paraoesophageal herniation. A reanalysis of the data from this trial sought to answer the question of whether a tailored approach to antireflux surgery should be applied. There were no demonstrable disadvantages for the Nissen procedure in

those patients who had manometrically abnormal peristalsis before surgery. In 2011, a minimum follow-up of 18 years was reported.[63] The outcomes at this very late follow-up were equivalent, with success rates of more than 80% reported for both procedures and no significant differences in the incidence of side-effects at late follow-up, suggesting that the mechanical side-effects following Nissen fundoplication progressively improve with very long-term follow-up.

Zornig et al.[64] reported a trial that enrolled 200 patients to either total fundoplication with division of the short gastric vessels or posterior fundoplication. In total, 100 patients had normal preoperative oesophageal motility and 100 had 'abnormal' motility. At 4 months follow-up an overall good outcome was obtained in about 90% of patients in each group and reflux control was equivalent. Short-term dysphagia was less common following posterior partial fundoplication and no correlation was seen between preoperative oesophageal motility and outcome, providing no support for the selective application of a partial fundoplication in patients with abnormal preoperative motility. The 2-year follow-up outcomes were similar.[65] In each group, 85% was satisfied with their clinical outcome, and dysphagia remained significantly more common after Nissen fundoplication (19 vs 8 patients).

A study by Guérin et al.[66] enrolled 140 patients. At 3 years follow-up 118 patients were evaluated and no outcome differences could be identified. Similarly, Booth et al.[67] enrolled 127 patients in a trial of Nissen versus Toupet fundoplication, Khan et al.[68] enrolled 121 patients in another trial, and Shaw et al.[69] enrolled 100 patients. Each of these trials showed no differences in reflux control 1 year after surgery. Although dysphagia was more common following Nissen fundoplication in Booth et al.'s trial, there were no differences in the prevalence of side-effects in the other trials. Subgroup analysis in the Booth et al. and Shaw et al. trials did not reveal any differences between patients with or without poor preoperative oesophageal motility.

A much larger trial of laparoscopic Nissen versus posterior partial fundoplication that enrolled 456 patients was recently reported Håkanson et al.[70] Less dysphagia was seen following the partial fundoplication at earlier follow-up to 12 months, but not beyond.

- If one combines all the data of the Nissen versus posterior fundoplication trials together, the available evidence supports the view that side-effects are less common following a posterior partial fundoplication, particularly for wind-related problems. The hypothesis that dysphagia is less of a problem following a posterior partial fundoplication has been substantiated by only three of the 14 trials.

NISSEN VERSUS ANTERIOR FUNDOPLICATION

Eleven trials have evaluated anterior partial fundoplication variants. In 1999 the author's group reported the first prospective randomised trial to compare a Nissen fundoplication with an anterior partial fundoplication technique.[2] Both procedures were performed laparoscopically. This study enrolled 107 patients to undergo either a Nissen or anterior partial fundoplication. The partial fundoplication variant entailed a 180° fundoplication that was anchored to the right hiatal pillar and the oesophageal wall (Figs. 12.5 and 12.6). While no overall outcome differences between the two procedures were demonstrated at 1 and 3 months follow-up, at 6 months patients who underwent an anterior fundoplication were less likely to experience dysphagia for solid food, were less likely to be troubled by excessive passage of flatus, were more likely to be able to belch normally, and the overall outcome was better. The outcomes at 5 years confirmed the results of the initial report.[43] Reflux control was slightly better after total fundoplication, but this was offset by significantly less dysphagia, less abdominal bloating, and better preservation of belching, resulting in a greater proportion of patients reporting a good or excellent overall outcome 5 years after anterior fundoplication (94% vs 86%). At 10 years follow-up, however, there were no significant outcome differences for the two procedures, with equivalent control of reflux, and no differences for side-effects,[46] a similar outcome to the very late follow-up for Lundell and colleagues' trial of Nissen versus posterior partial fundoplication.[63] Recently, good outcomes at 20 years were reported from this trial, with a good overall outcome achieved in approximately 90% of patients after each procedure, but with a trade-off between better reflux control after Nissen fundoplication versus fewer side-effects after anterior 180° partial fundoplication.[71]

Baigrie et al. reported a 2-year follow-up from a similar study in which 161 patients underwent either a Nissen or anterior 180° partial fundoplication.[72] This trial demonstrated equivalent control of reflux symptoms and less dysphagia following anterior 180° partial fundoplication, although the incidence of re-operation for recurrent reflux was higher after anterior fundoplication. Long-term results also confirm the early report.[73] Cao et al. reported 5-year outcomes for a similar trial that enrolled 100 patients.[74] Reflux control was similar for the two procedures and flatulence was less common after anterior 180° partial fundoplication. Raue et al. reported equivalent outcomes at 18 months' mean follow-up in a smaller trial that enrolled 64 patients.[75]

Djerf et al. reported 1- and 10-year outcomes from a trial that randomised 72 patients to undergo an anterior 120° partial or Nissen fundoplication.[76] Both procedures achieve effective reflux control, but with less dysphagia and better preservation of belching at 10 years after the anterior partial fundoplication.

Two further trials have compared a laparoscopic anterior 90° partial fundoplication with a Nissen fundoplication. In the first of these, 112 patients were enrolled in a multicentre randomised trial conducted in six cities in Australia and New Zealand.[44,47] Side-effects were significantly less common following anterior 90° fundoplication, although this was offset by a slightly higher incidence of recurrent reflux at 6 months follow-up.[44] At 5 years the outcomes were similar for side-effects, although reflux was worse after the partial fundoplication.[47] Satisfaction with the overall outcome was similar for both fundoplication types. Similar outcomes were reported from a parallel single-centre randomised trial that enrolled 79 patients – fewer side-effects offset by more reflux.[45] A recent meta-analysis of these two trials provided a 10-year follow-up for 191 patients, demonstrating comparable overall success rates but a similar trade-off between reflux control versus fewer side-effects to that seen in the late outcomes following anterior 180° versus Nissen fundoplication.[48]

ANTERIOR VERSUS POSTERIOR PARTIAL FUNDOPLICATION

Four randomised trials have directly compared anterior versus posterior partial fundoplication. Hagedorn et al.[77,78] randomised 95 patients to undergo either a laparoscopic posterior (Toupet) or anterior 120° partial fundoplication. Their results showed better reflux control but more side-effects following posterior partial fundoplication. Unfortunately the clinical and objective outcomes following anterior 120° fundoplication in this trial were much worse than the outcomes from other randomised and non-randomised studies. The average exposure time to acid (pH <4) was 5.6% following anterior fundoplication in their study, whereas in other studies this figure is reported to be around 2.5%,[2,44] suggesting that the procedure performed in the study by Hagedorn et al. was less effective and therefore different to that performed in other studies. Later clinical follow-up at 5 years confirmed similar outcomes, with poorer control of reflux after the anterior partial fundoplication.[78]

Khan et al.[79] reported 6 months' follow-up from a trial that enrolled 103 patients to undergo anterior 180° versus posterior partial fundoplication. Reflux control was also better after posterior partial fundoplication but offset by more side-effects. Similar outcomes were reported at 12 months follow-up by Daud et al. in a trial enrolling 47 patients,[80] whereas Roks et al. recently reported equivalent reflux control but fewer side-effects after anterior 180° partial fundoplication in a trial enrolling 94 patients.[81]

✓✓ Currently, the overall results from the 11 trials that included an anterior fundoplication suggest that anterior fundoplication variants achieve satisfactory control of reflux, a reduced incidence of post-fundoplication dysphagia and other side-effects, and a good overall clinical outcome. However, the reduced incidence of troublesome side-effects is, to some extent, offset by a higher risk of recurrent reflux (Fig. 12.9). Nevertheless, excellent long-term outcomes and good reflux control have been reported in a series of 548 patients who underwent anterior 180° partial fundoplication, with approximately 90% of patients highly satisfied with the clinical outcome at up to 10 years follow-up.[82]

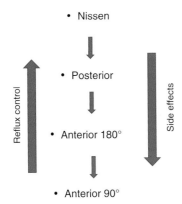

Figure 12.9 Outcomes from randomised trials suggest a balance of reflux control versus side-effects varying across a spectrum of fundoplication types.

THE CONTROVERSY OF DIVISION/NO DIVISION OF SHORT GASTRIC VESSELS

Routine division of the short gastric vessels during fundoplication, to achieve full fundal mobilisation and thereby ensure a loose fundoplication, is thought by some to be an essential step during laparoscopic (and open) Nissen fundoplication.[32] This opinion was popularised by the publication of studies that compared experience with division of the short gastric vessels with historical experience with a Nissen fundoplication performed without dividing these vessels.[34,36,83] Other uncontrolled studies confuse the issue further, as good results have been reported whether these vessels were divided or not.[34,37]

Six randomised trials have been reported that investigate this aspect of technique, Luostarinen et al.[84] reported the outcome of a small trial of division versus no division of the short gastric vessels during open total fundoplication. Fifty patients were entered into this trial and outcomes following median 3-year follow-up have been reported. Both procedures effectively corrected endoscopic oesophagitis. However, there was a trend towards a higher incidence of disruption of the fundoplication (5 vs 2) and reflux symptoms (6 vs 1) in patients whose short gastric vessels were divided, and 9 out of 26 patients who underwent vessel division developed a postoperative sliding hiatus hernia compared to only 1 out of 24 patients whose vessels were kept intact. The likelihood of long-term dysphagia or gas-related symptoms was not influenced by mobilising the gastric fundus.

In 1997 the author's group reported a randomised trial that enrolled 102 patients undergoing a laparoscopic Nissen fundoplication to have a procedure either with or without division of the short gastric blood vessels.[3] No difference in overall outcome was demonstrated at initial follow-up of 6 months and the trial failed to show that dividing the short gastric vessels during laparoscopic Nissen fundoplication reduced the incidence or severity of early postoperative dysphagia, or the outcome of any objective investigations. At 5, 10, and 20 years follow-up[85,86] both procedures were equally durable in terms of reflux control and the incidence of postoperative dysphagia. At 5 and 20 years follow-up, division of the short gastric vessels was associated with more flatulence and bloating, and greater difficulties with belching.

Mardani et al.[87] reported the outcome of a similar trial that enrolled 99 patients. At 12 months and 10 years follow-up,

this study also showed that dividing the short gastric vessels did not improve the outcome. A recent meta-analysis of a larger data set with 12 years follow-up, generated by combining the raw Adelaide and Swedish data, confirmed equivalent reflux control, but more bloating after division of the short gastric vessels.[88]

Farah et al.,[89] Kösek et al.,[90] and Chrysos et al.[91] all reported trials that showed equivalent reflux control of postoperative dysphagia irrespective of whether the short gastric vessels were divided or not. However, as with the Adelaide and Swedish data, they also demonstrated an increased incidence of bloating symptoms after division of the short gastric vessels.

✓✓ The belief that dividing the short gastric vessels will improve the outcome following laparoscopic total fundoplication is not supported by the results of any published trials. Furthermore, dividing the vessels increases the complexity of the procedure and actually produced a poorer outcome in three of the six trials due to an increase in the incidence of bloating symptoms, and this persists with follow-up now to 20 years.

LAPAROSCOPIC ANTIREFLUX SURGERY

RESULTS AND COMPLICATIONS FOLLOWING LAPAROSCOPIC FUNDOPLICATION

Laparoscopic Nissen fundoplication was first reported in 1991 and rapidly established itself as the procedure of choice for reflux disease. The results of large series with long-term clinical follow-up have confirmed that laparoscopic Nissen fundoplication is effective, and that 10 years or longer after surgery it achieves an excellent clinical outcome in more than 85–90% of patients.[92]

However, several complications unique to the laparoscopic approach have been described (see later). In the 1990s it was suggested that dysphagia might be more common following laparoscopic fundoplication, although this probably reflected the more intense nature of the prospective follow-up applied in many centres. Furthermore, in the author's experience dysphagia has been less of a problem after fundoplication than it was before surgery, with a reduction in the incidence from approximately 30% before surgery to less than 10% at 12 months following surgery,[2,3] and for the majority of these patients dysphagia has not been troublesome in the long term.

Up to 10% of patients are dissatisfied and a proportion of the dissatisfaction encountered is due to poor case selection. In others, dissatisfaction follows a complication of the original surgery. This has usually followed the development of recurrent reflux or a paraoesophageal hernia, or because of continuing troublesome dysphagia (with either the wrap or the hiatus being too tight). Some patients are dissatisfied, however, even though their reflux has been cured and they have not had any complications. This is usually because they do not like the flatulence that can follow the procedure. It is also important to recognise that there is a learning curve associated with this form of surgery, and it has been demonstrated that the first 20 patients in an individual surgeon's experience are associated with a higher complication rate, and as experience increases the re-operation rates fall to below 5%.[32] There are no specific contraindications to the laparoscopic approach, and the repair of giant hiatal hernias and re-operative antireflux surgery are both feasible (although technically more demanding). Differences in management after laparoscopic and open fundoplication procedures are primarily due to the accelerated recovery following laparoscopic surgery allowing early mobilisation, reintroduction of oral intake, and discharge.

LAPAROSCOPIC VERSUS OPEN ANTIREFLUX SURGERY

Ten randomised controlled trials have been reported that compare a laparoscopic fundoplication with its open surgical equivalent.[93–98] Nine of these investigated a Nissen fundoplication and one study compared laparoscopic versus open posterior partial fundoplication.[98] The early reports that described follow-up extending up to 12 months confirmed advantages for the laparoscopic approach, albeit less dramatic than the advantages expected from the results of non-randomised studies. Longer term outcomes from some studies have been reported.[99–102]

Early reports from smaller trials[93,94] that each enrolled 20–42 patients demonstrated equivalent short-term clinical outcomes, shortening of the postoperative stay by about 1 day (3 vs 4 median), longer operating times (extended by approximately 30 minutes), and an overall reduction in the incidence of postoperative complications following laparoscopic Nissen fundoplication. The reduction in the length of the postoperative hospital stay by only 1 day was unexpected. This was achieved entirely by a shorter hospital stay following open fundoplication, suggesting that at least some of the apparent benefits of the laparoscopic approach followed a general change in management policy to encourage earlier oral intake, avoid nasogastric tubes, and encourage earlier discharge from hospital.

Chrysos et al.[95] reported 12 months' follow-up for a trial that enrolled 106 patients. There was effective reflux control in both groups, post-fundoplication dysphagia was similar, and the laparoscopic approach had fewer complications, a quicker recovery, and fewer symptoms of epigastric bloating and distension. Similar 12-month outcomes were demonstrated by Ackroyd et al.[99] in a trial that enrolled 99 patients.

Håkanson et al.[98] enrolled 192 patients in a trial of laparoscopic versus open posterior partial fundoplication. Their results were similar to the trials of laparoscopic versus open Nissen fundoplication. Early complications were more common after open surgery, the length of the hospital stay was longer (5 vs 3 days) and return to work was slower (42 vs 28 days). However, this was offset by a higher incidence of early side-effects and recurrent reflux in the laparoscopic group. At 3 year-follow-up, there were no outcome differences, satisfaction with surgery was similar for the two groups, and the need for re-operative surgery of any sort was not influenced by the choice of technique.

Laine et al.[93] reported 110 patients randomised to undergo laparoscopic or open Nissen fundoplication. As with the other trials, hospital stay was halved from 6.4 to 3.2 days and patients returned to work quicker (37 vs 15 days), but the operating time was prolonged by 31 minutes. Subsequent reports from this group[100] described up to 15 years follow-up in 86 patients. While symptom control and side-effects were similar at late follow-up and 82% of the laparoscopic surgery group were satisfied with the late outcome, the incidence of wrap disruption at endoscopic assessment was significantly higher following open surgery (40% vs 13%) and there were 10 incisional hernias, all following the open technique. Nilsson et al. reported similar outcomes in a smaller trial that followed patients for 5 years.[101]

A study that created significant controversy was a multicentre study of 103 patients published by Bais et al. in 2000.[96] The early (3 months) results of this trial showed a disadvantage for the laparoscopic approach and the trial was stopped early because of an excess of adverse endpoints. The investigators were criticised for terminating the trial prematurely, as the decision to stop the trial was based primarily on postoperative dysphagia within the first 3 months. Other studies reported that most patients who undergo a Nissen fundoplication still have some dysphagia 3 months after surgery,[3,97] but that this usually subsides with time. Hence, a follow-up period of 3 months was too short for the endpoint of dysphagia to be adequately assessed. Subsequent reports of 5- and 10-year follow-ups from this trial[102] confirmed the validity of this critique. With further enrolment boosting the number of patients to 177, no differences in symptoms or subjective outcome could be demonstrated at late follow-up. In addition, 24-hour pH monitoring confirmed equivalent reflux control. At 10 years follow-up, there was a higher rate of surgical reintervention following open surgery, mainly due to an excess of incisional hernias. Ultimately, the late results of this trial actually supported the application of laparoscopic antireflux surgery!

✓✓ If the overall results of trials are synthesised, it is clear that laparoscopic antireflux surgery has short- and long-term advantages over the open approach in terms of reduced overall morbidity, quicker recovery, and fewer incisional hernias. In addition, control of reflux and risk of side-effects at late follow-up (up to 15 years) is not influenced by the choice of a laparoscopic approach. For these reasons, the laparoscopic approach has superseded the open approach for all patients undergoing primary antireflux surgery.

SYNTHESIS OF THE RESULTS FROM PROSPECTIVE RANDOMISED TRIALS

The results of randomised trials can be assessed together to facilitate the development of guidelines for antireflux surgery (Box 12.1). Some of these will meet with wide acceptance as they support the current body of thought of the international surgical community. However, others are controversial, as they do not support the opinions of the majority of experts in the field.

Most surgeons performing surgery for reflux agree that the laparoscopic approach has been a major advance in surgical technique for antireflux surgery and that this has led to surgery becoming a more attractive management option. Controversy, however, will be raised by conclusions drawn about division of the short gastric blood vessels, and the place of partial fundoplications in the surgeon's armamentarium.

Box 12.1   Evidence from prospective randomised trials for antireflux surgery

- Laparoscopic Nissen fundoplication is associated with fewer complications overall and a shorter recovery than open Nissen fundoplication
- The longer term outcome following laparoscopic Nissen fundoplication is at least as good as the equivalent open surgical procedure
- Division of the short gastric blood vessels does not improve the outcome following Nissen fundoplication
- The incidence of recurrent reflux is similar following posterior partial fundoplication and Nissen fundoplication
- The incidence of dysphagia is probably less following posterior partial fundoplication compared to Nissen fundoplication
- The incidence of dysphagia and 'gas-related' complications is reduced following anterior partial fundoplication
- Partial fundoplications are associated with fewer wind-related problems than total fundoplication
- Anterior partial fundoplications are associated with fewer side-effects but more reflux than posterior partial fundoplication

Box 12.2   Unique or common complications following laparoscopic antireflux surgery[102]

- Pneumothorax
- Pneumomediastinum
- Pulmonary embolism
- Injury to major vessels
- Paraoesophageal hiatus hernia
- Hiatal stenosis
- Bilobed stomach
- Oesophageal perforation
- Gastric perforation
- Cardiac laceration and tamponade

The longer term outcomes from published trials that have investigated division of the short gastric vessels clearly support the position that this manoeuvre is not necessary for the creation of a satisfactory Nissen fundoplication and that it actually increases the likelihood of bloating side-effects.

Evidence from the larger trials of posterior versus Nissen fundoplication demonstrates advantages for the posterior partial fundoplication technique. While the combined data from the reported trials can be confusing, with most of the smaller trials showing no advantages for posterior partial fundoplication, the larger trials do support the proposition that this technique reduces the risk of gas-related side-effects and might reduce the risk of post-fundoplication dysphagia. However, the magnitude of these differences is probably less than for anterior partial versus Nissen fundoplication. Eight of 11 randomised trials support the anterior partial fundoplication approach, although poor results were reported in one study.[77] Longer term results for anterior partial fundoplication techniques confirm their efficacy as antireflux procedures.[43,82]

COMPLICATIONS OF LAPAROSCOPIC ANTIREFLUX SURGERY

As laparoscopic approaches for antireflux surgery became standard practice with experience, complications unique to the laparoscopic approach emerged (Box 12.2). These include postoperative paraoesophageal hiatus hernia, reoperation for dysphagia, and gastrointestinal perforation. Nevertheless, the risk of complications should be balanced against the advantages of the laparoscopic approach as the overall complication rate is reduced following laparoscopic surgery.[102] The likelihood of complications can be influenced by a number of factors, including surgeon experience and expertise, operative technique, and perioperative care. Furthermore, the final outcome of some complications can be moderated by applying appropriate early management strategies.

COMPLICATIONS THAT ARE MORE COMMON FOLLOWING LAPAROSCOPIC ANTIREFLUX SURGERY[103]

Paraoesophageal hiatus hernia

Paraoesophageal hiatus herniation was thought to be an uncommon finding following open fundoplication, usually presenting in the late follow-up period, although its frequency was probably underestimated in the past. Most large series of laparoscopic procedures report the occurrence of paraoesophageal herniation following surgery (Fig. 12.10), particularly in the immediate postoperative period. The incidence of this complication ranged up to 7% in older published reports, and it seems that this was exacerbated by some factors inherent in the laparoscopic approach. These include a tendency to extend laparoscopic oesophageal dissection further into the thorax than during open surgery, an increased risk of breaching the left pleural membrane, and the effect of reduced postoperative pain. Loss of the left pleural barrier can allow the stomach to slide more easily into the left hemithorax, and less pain permits more abdominal force to be transmitted to the hiatal area during coughing, vomiting, or other forms of exertion in the initial postoperative period, pushing the stomach into the thorax, as the normal anatomical barriers have been disrupted by surgical dissection. Early resumption of heavy physical work has also been associated with acute herniation. Strategies are available that can reduce the likelihood of herniation. Routine hiatal repair has been shown to reduce the incidence by approximately 80%. Sutures placed to close the space between the anterior oesophagus and the hiatal rim might also reduce this risk. In addition, excessive strain on the hiatal repair during the early postoperative period should be avoided by the routine use of antiemetics, as well as advising patients to avoid excessive lifting or straining for about 4–8 weeks following surgery.

Dysphagia

Nearly all patients, including those who undergo a partial fundoplication, experience dysphagia requiring dietary modification in the first weeks to months following laparoscopic surgery. However, it is dysphagia that is severe enough to need further surgery that is of most concern. Early severe dysphagia requiring surgical revision has been reported in many series. Conversion of a Nissen fundoplication to a partial fundoplication has been performed for troublesome dysphagia following both open and laparoscopic techniques, usually with success.

Perhaps more common with the laparoscopic approach, however, has been the problem of a tight oesophageal diaphragmatic hiatus causing dysphagia (Figs. 12.11, 12.12, and 12.13). Several factors may cause this problem: over-tightening of the hiatus during hiatal repair, excessive perihiatal scar tissue formation, and construction of a fundoplication that results in excessive angulation of the oesophagus and gastro-oesophageal junction. Many surgeons use an intraoesophageal bougie to distend the oesophagus, to assist with calibration of the hiatal closure. However, this will not always prevent over-tightening from occurring. In addition, we prefer to use a permanent, monofilament suture for the hiatal closure rather than a braided suture and/or mesh, which can cause increased perihiatal scar formation. If a problem does arise in the immediate postoperative period, it can usually be corrected by early laparoscopic reintervention with release of one or more hiatal sutures. Later narrowing of the oesophageal hiatus due to postoperative scar tissue formation in the second and third postoperative weeks, even in patients not undergoing initial hiatal repair, has also been described. In the authors' experience, endoscopic dilatation with standard bougies usually provides only temporary relief of symptoms rather than a long-term solution for this problem. Correction often requires surgical widening of the diaphragmatic hiatus. This can be achieved by a laparoscopic approach, with anterolateral division of the hiatal ring and adjacent diaphragm until the hiatus is sufficiently loose. An alternative strategy, which is sometimes successful, is pneumatic balloon dilatation (using a 30-mm diameter balloon).

Pulmonary embolism

Pulmonary embolism was more common in some of the early reports of laparoscopic Nissen fundoplication and in particular following conversion of cases to open surgery, suggesting that prolonged operating times might be an important aetiological factor. In addition, several mechanical factors inherent in the laparoscopic antireflux surgery environment create a scenario in which venous thrombosis is more likely. The combination of head-up tilt of the operating table, intra-abdominal insufflation of gas under pressure, and elevation of the legs in stirrups greatly reduces venous flow in the leg veins, potentially predisposing to deep venous thrombosis. This problem is now rare and is minimised by the routine use of anti-thromboembolism prophylaxis.

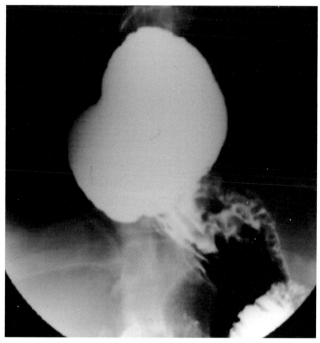

Figure 12.10 Barium meal X-ray demonstrating a large paraoesophageal hiatus hernia 3 months after laparoscopic fundoplication.

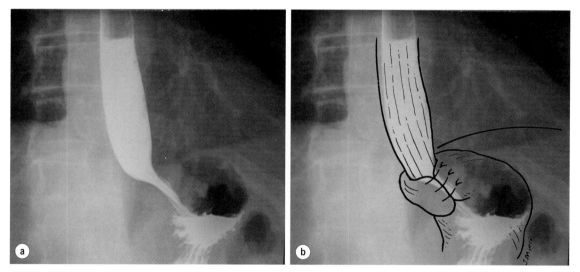

Figure 12.11 Contrast swallow X-ray demonstrating the usual appearance following laparoscopic Nissen fundoplication. The gastro-oesophageal junction is lifted anteriorly by the stomach placed behind the distal oesophagus. (a) Contrast swallow. (b) Contrast swallow with overlay of configuration of Nissen fundoplication. (Republished with permission of the British Institute of Radiology, © 2012 from; Raeside MC, Madigan D, Myers JC, et al. Post-fundoplication contrast studies: Is there room for improvement? Br J Radiol 2012;85:792-9.)

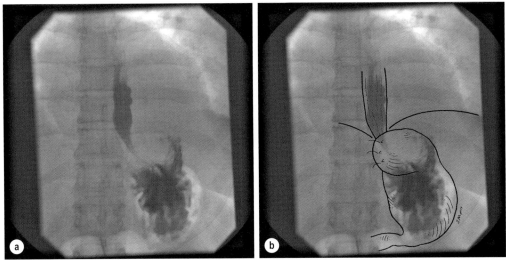

Figure 12.12   Contrast swallow X-ray demonstrating the usual appearance following laparoscopic anterior partial fundoplication. The gastro-oesophageal junction remains in an anatomical position. (a) Contrast swallow. (b) Contrast swallow with overlay of configuration of anterior partial fundoplication. (Republished with permission of the British Institute of Radiology, © 2012 from; Raeside MC, Madigan D, Myers JC, et al. Post-fundoplication contrast studies: Is there room for improvement? Br J Radiol 2012;85:792-9.)

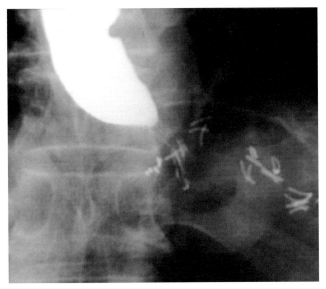

Figure 12.13   Day 2 postoperative barium meal in a patient with total dysphagia following Nissen fundoplication due to a tight oesophageal hiatus. This was corrected by widening the hiatus by removing the hiatal repair sutures.

COMPLICATIONS UNIQUE TO LAPAROSCOPIC ANTIREFLUX SURGERY

Bilobed stomach

A technical error that was described during early experiences with laparoscopic Nissen fundoplication is the 'bilobed stomach'. This problem occurs when too distal a piece of stomach is used to form a fundoplication, usually the gastric body rather than the fundus, resulting in a bilobular-shaped stomach (Fig. 12.14). While this error is most likely to be made when constructing a Nissen fundoplication, it is possible when constructing other fundoplication types. While most patients are asymptomatic, in extreme cases it is possible for the upper part of the stomach to become obstructed at the point of constriction in the gastric body resulting in

postprandial abdominal pain, which requires surgical revision (Fig. 12.15). Checking carefully to ensure that the correct piece of stomach (the fundus) is used for construction of the fundoplication prevents this problem from arising.

Pneumothorax

Intraoperative pneumothorax occurs in up to 2% of patients due to injury to the left pleural membrane during retro-oesophageal dissection, particularly if dissection is directed too high within the mediastinum. This is more likely to occur during dissection of a large hiatus hernia. Careful dissection behind the oesophagus, ensuring that the tips of instruments passed from right to left behind the oesophagus do not pass above the level of the diaphragm, and experience with laparoscopic dissection at the hiatus reduces its likelihood. The occurrence of a pneumothorax does not usually require the placement of a chest drain, as CO_2 gas in the pleural cavity is rapidly reabsorbed at the completion of the procedure, allowing the lung to re-expand rapidly.

Vascular injury

Vascular injury to the inferior vena cava, left hepatic vein, and the abdominal aorta have all been reported. These problems may be associated with aberrant anatomy, inexperience, the excessive use of monopolar diathermy cautery dissection, the incorrect application of ultrasonic shears, or a combination of several of these. Intraoperative bleeding more commonly follows inadvertent laceration of the left lobe of the liver by a laparoscopic liver retractor or other instrument, and haemorrhage from poorly secured short gastric vessels during fundal mobilisation. A rare complication is cardiac tamponade. This has been reported twice due to laceration of the right ventricle by a liver retractor and/or injury of the cardiac wall from a suture needle. Certainly the proximity of the heart, inferior vena cava, and aorta to the distal oesophagus make potentially life-threatening injuries a possibility if surgeons are unfamiliar with the hiatal anatomy as seen via the

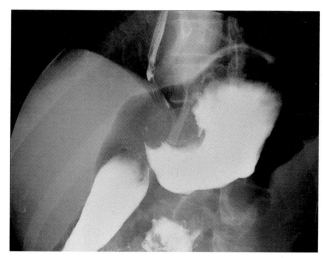

Figure 12.14   Barium meal image of a 'bilobed' stomach. This patient continues to have an excellent clinical result at 7 years follow-up.

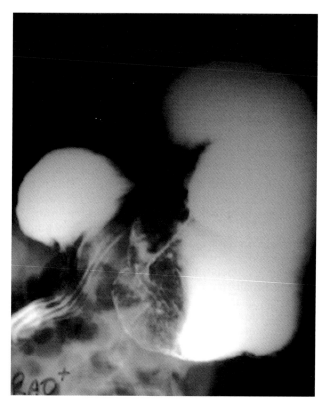

Figure 12.15   Barium meal image of a more severe 'bilobed' stomach. This patient developed gastric obstruction and required surgical revision.

laparoscope. Nevertheless, the overall risk of perioperative haemorrhage during and after antireflux surgery and the likelihood of splenectomy is reduced by the laparoscopic approach.

Perforation of the upper gastrointestinal tract

Oesophageal and gastric perforation are specific risks, with an incidence of approximately 1% reported in some larger series. Gastric perforation is usually an avulsion injury of the gastric cardia due to excessive traction by the surgical

assistant. Perforation of the back wall of the oesophagus usually occurs during dissection of the posterior oesophagus. The anterior oesophageal wall is probably at greatest risk when a bougie is passed to calibrate the tightness of a Nissen fundoplication or the oesophageal hiatus. These injuries can all be repaired with sutures provided they are identified intraoperatively. Awareness that injury can occur enables surgeons to institute strategies that reduce the likelihood of damage. Furthermore, injury is less likely with greater experience.

Mortality

Deaths have been reported following laparoscopic antireflux procedures. Causes include peritonitis secondary to duodenal perforation, thrombosis of the superior mesenteric artery and the coeliac axis,[104] and infarction of the liver. However, death is rare, and the overall mortality of elective laparoscopic surgery for reflux is certainly less than 0.1%.

AVOIDING COMPLICATIONS FOLLOWING LAPAROSCOPIC ANTIREFLUX SURGERY AND MINIMISING THEIR IMPACT

To avoid or minimise complications following a laparoscopic antireflux procedure, a range of strategies should be considered and applied whenever possible. In individuals likely to have an enlarged fatty liver, a very low-calorie diet for 2 weeks before surgery can reduce liver bulk and subjectively improve visualisation of the hiatus, a manoeuvre that some surgeons find helpful in selected patients. In addition, surgeons should use a surgical technique that will reduce the likelihood of an adverse outcome arising. Most agree that the oesophageal hiatus should be narrowed or reinforced with sutures irrespective of whether a hiatus hernia is present or not.[35] However, as complications will occur in a small number of patients, one strategy is to perform a contrast swallow X-ray examination on the first postoperative day to confirm that the fundoplication is in the correct position and that the stomach is entirely intra-abdominal. If there is any uncertainty, endoscopic examination may clarify the situation. If the appearances are not acceptable, or if other problems such as severe dysphagia or excessive pain occur, then early laparoscopic re-exploration should be performed. Early laparoscopic reintervention is associated with minimal morbidity and usually delays recovery by only a few days.[105] Most complications requiring reintervention can be readily dealt with laparoscopically within a week of the original procedure. Beyond this time, however, laparoscopic re-operation becomes difficult, and for this reason a relatively low threshold for laparoscopic re-exploration in the first postoperative week is advised if problems arise.

If complications become apparent at a later stage, laparoscopic re-operation is often still feasible if the surgeon is experienced. However, the likelihood of success is reduced in the intermediate period following the original procedure. Waiting, if possible, until scar tissue has matured (i.e. at least 3–6 months) simplifies subsequent laparoscopic dissection and increases the likelihood of completing the procedure laparoscopically.

Box 12.3   Endoscopic antireflux procedures

Procedures that narrow the oesophagogastric junction

Radiofrequency
- Stretta procedure

Polymer injection
- Enteryx
- Gatekeeper
- PMMA (Plexiglas microspheres)

'Suturing'
- EndoCinch
- NDO Plicator

Procedures that aim to create a partial fundoplication
- EsophyX endoluminal fundoplication procedure
- MUSE endoluminal fundoplication procedure

ENDOSCOPIC THERAPIES FOR REFLUX

Over the past two decades, various endoscopic procedures for the treatment of reflux have emerged. These procedures highlight the possibility of curative procedures for reflux without the need for abdominal wall incisions, and such approaches have been appealing to both patients and physicians, although outcomes have been generally disappointing. These approaches can be broadly categorised into four types (Box 12.3). Three types of procedures aim to narrow the oesophagogastric junction. This has been done by using either radiofrequency energy,[106] injection of an inert substance,[107] or endoscopic suturing.[108] In the early 2000s these procedures were applied with enthusiasm in some centres, particularly in the USA. However, none of these treatments applied the established principles that underpin the efficacy of antireflux surgery (see 'Mechanism of action of antireflux operations' section earlier) and the clinical outcomes were predictably disappointing. More recently, however, techniques have been described that use a totally endoscopic (transoral) technique to construct a partial fundoplication.[109] Because the latter approaches aim to fix the fundus of the stomach to a length of intra-abdominal oesophagus, first principles suggest that these approaches should be more successful, although the clinical reality has again been disappointing.

RADIOFREQUENCY

The Stretta procedure[106] uses a purpose-built device to apply radiofrequency energy to the muscular layer of the oesophageal wall at the oesophagogastric junction. The device comprises a 30-mm diameter balloon, four 5.5-mm long retractable stylet electrodes, and a mucosal irrigation system. It is passed over an endoscopically placed guidewire and positioned at the oesophagogastric junction. The electrodes are deployed to puncture the oesophageal wall, and radiofrequency energy is applied to cauterise the oesophageal muscle. The Stretta procedure probably generates

fibrosis in the muscle layer and this aims to tighten the oesophagogastric junction. In general, patients are only selected for this treatment if they have mild grades of reflux. While short-term follow-up of case series suggests reduced reflux symptoms and reduced oesophageal acid exposure, the magnitude of the reduction in acid exposure has been disappointing, and most patients continue to have abnormal reflux after treatment.[110] A randomised trial that compared the Stretta procedure with a sham endoscopy showed no differences at 6 months follow-up.[111] This trial demonstrated a large placebo effect in the sham controls, and this should be remembered when considering the outcomes of any antireflux therapy! The company that originally made the device closed in 2006. However, the technology has been acquired by another company, and this procedure is now available again, albeit with limited efficacy compared to antireflux surgery.

POLYMER INJECTION

Polymer injection (and similar procedures) aimed to add bulk to the oesophagogastric junction, thereby narrowing it, to reduce reflux. The most popular of these procedures was Enteryx.[107] The procedure entailed endoscopic injection of 5–8 mL of a bioinert polymer into the plane between the circular and longitudinal muscle of the distal oesophagus, to create a ring of polymer just above the oesophagogastric junction. Initial reports suggested success rates of 70–80% at 12 months follow-up.[107] However, the results from a randomised sham-controlled trial were also unimpressive, with no difference in acid exposure (11.2% vs 12.7%) at 3 months follow-up, with this trial also demonstrating a significant placebo effect. A total of 41% of the sham-treated patients were able to cease PPI medication compared to 68% of the treated group.[112] Unfortunately, there were also some catastrophic complications, including deaths,[113] and the manufacturer withdrew the procedure. A similar product, the Gatekeeper reflux repair system, was also withdrawn from clinical use.

ENDOSCOPIC SUTURING

ENDOCINCH

The EndoCinch (Bard Endoscopic Technologies, Murray Hill, NJ) procedure entailed the endoscopic placement of two 3 mm-deep sutures into adjoining gastric mucosal folds immediately below the oesophagogastric junction, to create pleats to narrow this region. The sutures were not deep enough to include the underlying muscle. Case series demonstrated improvements in symptoms and distal oesophageal acid exposure (15.4–8.7%).[114] However, as with the other endoscopic procedures, reflux was cured in only a minority and 90% of sutures disappeared within 12 months.[115] In a randomised sham-controlled trial, oesophageal acid exposure was similar in the treated and sham groups and the results of this trial also failed to compare well with the outcomes for laparoscopic antireflux surgery.[115]

NDO PLICATOR

The NDO Plicator (NDO Surgical, Mansfield, MA) represented the first attempt to perform a more 'surgical' procedure via a transoral approach. A screw device penetrated and retracted the oesophagogastric junction, and a full-thickness plication of the cardia was fashioned to narrow the oesophagogastric junction. This was secured with a pre-tied pledgeted suture. For the first time, a sham-controlled trial[116] actually showed a significant reduction in oesophageal acid exposure (measured by ambulatory pH monitoring) from 10% to 7% at 3 months following treatment. However, acid exposure was not restored to normal in most patients, and the degree of improvement was inferior to the 0–2.5% expected following laparoscopic fundoplication.[2] At 3 months follow-up, 50% of patients were able to cease PPI medication compared to 25% of the sham-treated patients. Again, these results were inferior to those of laparoscopic antireflux surgery and the company making this device closed in 2008.

ENDOSCOPIC FUNDOPLICATION

Unlike the previous procedures, the EsophyX (Endogastric Solutions, Redmond, WA) procedure, or transoral incisionless fundoplication (TIF) aims to construct an actual fundoplication.[117] The procedure requires general anaesthesia and two operators. A standard endoscope is passed through the device (Figs. 12.16 and 12.17) and both are passed transorally into the stomach. The endoscope is retroflexed for vision and a screw device anchors tissue at the oesophagogastric junction to retract it caudally. A plastic arm (tissue mould) then compresses the fundus against the side of the oesophagus, and polypropylene fasteners are passed between the oesophagus and the gastric fundus to anchor these structures. Multiple fasteners are applied to fashion a 200–300° anterior partial fundoplication.

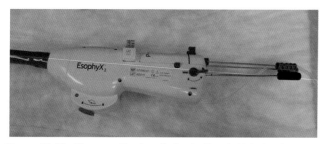

Figure 12.16 The operating handle for the EsophyX device for endoluminal anterior partial fundoplication.

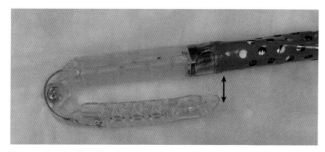

Figure 12.17 The distal end of EsophyX device. The tip is sited within the stomach and the shaft in the distal oesophagus. The two components close together as indicated (arrow) to allow the fasteners to be deployed.

Some cases series have reported promising short-term outcomes, with claimed success rates of 55–80% at up to 2 years follow-up, but lower success rates for normalisation of oesophageal acid exposure.[116] In general, however, this procedure has been restricted to patients with milder degrees of reflux, i.e. no circumferential ulcerative oesophagitis, Barrett's oesophagus, hiatus hernia ≥ 3 cm or a body mass index > 30. While most patients recover uneventfully, significant complications have also been reported, including bleeding, pneumoperitoneum, and oesophageal perforation. Cadière et al. reported a series of 86 patients, followed for 12 months.[117] A total of 81% of patients were not using PPI medication and 56% claimed cure of their reflux. Postoperative pH monitoring, however, revealed that only 37% of patients had a normal pH study following the EsophyX procedure. The results from this experience suggest that in some patients a fundoplication can be constructed, but perhaps not as reliably as with a laparoscopic approach. Other experience is also less than satisfactory. In a three-centre experience of 19 EsophyX procedures, only five patients were able to stop antireflux medication, whereas 10 underwent laparoscopic fundoplication within 12 months for a failed EsophyX procedure.[118] A sham-controlled trial reported outcomes at 6 months follow-up.[119] pH outcomes were improved but not normalised (mean 9.3% before vs 6.3% after), and regurgitation was eliminated in 67% of treated patients versus 45% of controls. Overall, the published literature suggests EsophyX is less effective than any type of partial fundoplication,[4] with less than half of patients treated showing objective evidence that reflux has been cured.

A similar approach has also been pursued by Medigus (Omer, Israel), who developed a stapling endoscope for the construction of an anterior partial fundoplication (MUSE procedure). In a series of 37 patients followed for 4 years, reflux symptoms were improved at up to 4 years follow-up, and 84% were off PPI medication at 6 months and 69% at 4 years. However, normalisation of acid exposure was only achieved in 37% of patients.[120]

Unfortunately, reflux control following both EsophyX and MUSE procedures appears to be inferior to that achieved by laparoscopic fundoplication approaches, and for now it seems that a durable partial fundoplication is not reliably fashioned using an endoscopic approach. This might be because the endoscopic approaches fail to repair a hiatus hernia and also fail to anchor the fundus to the diaphragm, both important steps for constructing a stable partial fundoplication.

OVERVIEW OF ENDOSCOPIC ANTIREFLUX SURGERY

✓✓ None of the endoscopic approaches to the treatment of gastro-oesophageal reflux have achieved outcomes that are comparable to those of a surgical fundoplication, and some of the earlier procedures that were initially applied enthusiastically have been withdrawn from clinical use, either because of safety concerns, lack of efficacy, or both. For many of these procedures, this is not surprising, as the initial endoscopic procedures ignored the principles that underpin antireflux surgery, i.e. accentuation of the angle of His, and maintaining a close anatomical relationship between the fundus of the stomach and the intra-abdominal oesophagus.

The newer procedures that aim to perform an anterior partial fundoplication appear to be based on more sound principles. However, the results remain disappointing, and this might be because some key steps used routinely during antireflux surgery cannot be replicated when undertaking this approach. It is hard to see how an endoscopic approach can be modified to include repair of a hiatus hernia, or accurate anchorage of the fundoplication to the hiatal rim, and for these reasons endoscopic treatments are unlikely to offer a viable alternative to laparoscopic antireflux surgery for the majority of patients considering surgery for gastro-oesophageal reflux and hiatus hernia.

Lessons can be learnt from the experience with failed endoscopic antireflux treatments. Before any new endoscopic or surgical treatment for reflux is made widely available, it should first be evaluated in well-designed clinical trials. An appropriate endoscopic procedure must be as effective as a conventional fundoplication, it should apply the same principles that underpin an effective antireflux operation, and it should be equally safe or safer. Surgeons will also need to have an appropriate strategy to deal with patients who develop recurrent reflux after these procedures, and any procedure that makes a subsequent laparoscopic fundoplication procedure more difficult or more dangerous will be a problem, particularly if there is a substantial risk of the primary endoscopic procedure failing.

CONCLUSION

For patients with moderate-to-severe symptoms of gastro-oesophageal reflux disease which are poorly controlled by PPI medication, a laparoscopic fundoplication, either Nissen or partial, offers effective treatment, and will achieve a good outcome for approximately 85–90% of patients at long-term follow-up. The Nissen procedure continues to offer the most effective reflux control, but this is offset by a significant risk of side-effects. Partial fundoplications also offer good reflux control, but with fewer side-effects, although the evidence from randomised trials supports a trade-off between the risk of recurrent reflux versus side-effects across a spectrum of fundoplications types, from Nissen to posterior to anterior partial fundoplication variants. In an effort to reduce the risk of side-effects novel devices have been developed, including implantable devices and endoscopic approaches. As these new procedures all require a patented device, they are generally more expensive than a conventional laparoscopic fundoplication, and arguably a more practical and cost-effective approach to reducing side-effects, applying readily available technology found in most operating theatres, is a partial fundoplication.

Key points

- The treatment of reflux is usually incremental, commencing with various levels of medical measures. Surgery is reserved for patients with more severe disease who either fail to respond adequately to medical treatment or who do not wish to take lifelong medication.
- A single management strategy is unlikely to be appropriate for all patients. Surgical therapy achieves better control of reflux in patients with moderate-to-severe reflux.
- A recommendation for antireflux surgery must be based on all available clinical and objective information.
- Barrett's oesophagus alone is not an indication for antireflux surgery. Patients with Barrett's oesophagus should be selected for surgery on the basis of their reflux symptoms and their response to medications, not because a columnar-lined oesophagus is associated with an increased risk of cancer.
- The overwhelming majority of patients with moderate-to-severe gastro-oesophageal reflux who are selected for surgery claim that the disadvantages of an antireflux operation (temporary dysphagia, early fullness, increased flatulence, and inability to belch and vomit) are significantly outweighed by the advantages of the operation.
- Total fundoplications and partial fundoplications (whether anterior or posterior) probably all work in a similar fashion. No one procedure currently yields perfect results, i.e. 100% cure of reflux and no side-effects.
- The available evidence appears to support the view that the main difference in outcome between total and posterior fundoplication is in wind-related problems.
- Long-term reflux control is better after total compared with anterior fundoplication, but this is offset by significantly less dysphagia, less epigastric bloating, and better preservation of belching.
- The results of randomised trials of open versus laparoscopic surgery confirm advantages for the laparoscopic approach.
- Most large series of laparoscopic procedures report the occurrence of paraoesophageal herniation following surgery, particularly in the immediate postoperative period. Routine hiatal repair has been shown to reduce the incidence by approximately 80%.
- None of the currently reported endoscopic procedures achieve the level of reflux control associated with fundoplication.

 References available at http://ebooks.health.elsevier.com/

RECOMMENDED VIDEOS

- Nissen fundoplication with short gastric vessel division – https://tinyurl.com/y9mvw7rv
- Posterior partial (Toupet) fundoplication – https://tinyurl.com/yaoc9xcs
- Anterior 180° partial fundoplication and repair of hiatus hernia – https://youtu.be/KqliPobUKgc
- Anterior 180° fundoplication without hiatus hernia – https://youtu.be/4OBHAN76nMM
- EsophyX endoscopic fundoplication procedure – https://youtu.be/P_j5FaDBZYI
- MUSE procedure – https://tinyurl.com/y9fqtlvs
- Linx procedure – https://tinyurl.com/y7yc46lc
- Endostim procedure – https://tinyurl.com/ybh72bsj

KEY REFERENCES

[2] Watson DI, Jamieson GG, Pike GK, et al. A prospective randomised double blind trial between laparoscopic Nissen fundoplication and anterior partial fundoplication. Br J Surg 1999;86:123–30. PMID: 10027375
  The first published randomised trial to compare an anterior partial fundoplication with the Nissen procedure.

[3] Watson DI, Pike GK, Baigrie RJ, et al. Prospective double blind randomised trial of laparoscopic Nissen fundoplication with division and without division of short gastric vessels. Ann Surg 1997;226:642–52. PMID: 9389398
  A randomised trial of 102 patients who underwent a total fundoplication with versus without division of the short gastric vessels.

[23] Lundell L, Attwood S, Ell C, et al. Comparing laparoscopic antireflux surgery with esomeprazole in the management of patients with chronic gastro-oesophageal reflux disease: a 3-year interim analysis of the LOTUS trial. Gut 2008;57:1207–13. PMID: 18469091
  The largest randomised trial of medical versus surgical therapy for gastro-oesophageal reflux.

[24] Lundell L, Miettinen P, Myrvold HE, et al. Comparison of outcomes twelve years after anti-reflux surgery or omeprazole maintenance therapy for reflux esophagitis. Clin Gastroenterol Hepatol 2009;7:1292. 8. PMID: 19490952
  Long-term results of a randomised trial of PPIs versus open antireflux surgery.

[26] Spechler SJ, Hunter JG, Jones KM, et al. Randomized trial of medical versus surgical treatment for refractory heartburn. N Engl J Med 2019;381:1513–23. PMID: 31618539
  Randomised trial of medical versus surgical therapy demonstrating better outcomes following surgery for patients with refractory gastro-oesophageal reflux.

[46] Cai W, Watson DI, Lally CJ, et al. Ten-year clinical outcome of a prospective randomized clinical trial of laparoscopic Nissen versus anterior 180° partial fundoplication. Br J Surg 2008;95:1501–5. PMID: 18942055
  Longer term follow-up from a randomised trial of anterior versus Nissen fundoplication.

[48] Hopkins RJ, Irvine T, Jamieson GG, et al. 10 year follow-up of laparoscopic Nissen vs anterior 90 degree partial fundoplication –two double-blind randomised controlled trials. Br J Surg 2020;107:56–63. PMID: 31502659
  Long-term outcomes from randomised trials of anterior 90° versus Nissen fundoplication.

[63] Mardani J, Lundell L, Engström C. Total or posterior partial fundoplication in the treatment of GERD: results of a randomized trial after 2 decades of follow-up. Ann Surg 2011;253:875–8. PMID: 21451393
  Longer term follow-up from a randomised trial of Nissen versus posterior partial fundoplication.

[72] Baigrie RJ, Cullis SN, Ndhluni AJ, et al. Randomized double-blind trial of laparoscopic Nissen fundoplication versus anterior partial fundoplication. Br J Surg 2005;92:819–23. PMID: 15898129
  Largest randomised trial of anterior versus Nissen fundoplication.

[86] Kinsey-Trotman SP, Devitt PG, Bright T, et al. Randomized trial of division vs non-division of short gastric vessels during Nissen fundoplication - 20 yr outcomes. Ann Surg 2018;268:228–32. PMID: 29303805
  A 20-year follow-up from a randomised trial of Nissen fundoplication with versus without division of the short gastric blood vessels.

[88] Engström C, Jamieson GG, Devitt PG, et al. Meta-analysis of two randomized controlled trials to identify long-term symptoms after division of short gastric vessels during Nissen fundoplication. Br J Surg 2011;98:1063–7. PMID: 21618497
  Meta-analysis of original data from two randomised trials of division versus no division of the short gastric vessels during Nissen fundoplication. Vessel division associated with significantly more abdominal bloating symptoms.

[100] Salminen PT, Hiekkanen HI, Rantala AP, et al. Fundoplication: a prospective randomized study with an 11-year follow-up. Ann Surg 2007;246:201–6. PMID: 17667497
  Long-term follow-up from a randomised trial of laparoscopic versus open Nissen fundoplication.

[102] Broeders JA, Rijnhart-de Jong HG, Draaisma WA, et al. Ten-year outcome of laparoscopic and conventional Nissen fundoplication: randomized clinical trial. Ann Surg 2009;250:698–706. PMID: 19801931
  Long-term follow-up from a randomised trial of laparoscopic versus open Nissen fundoplication demonstrating less surgical reintervention following laparoscopic surgery.

[111] Corley DA, Katz P, Wo JM, et al. Improvement of gastroesophageal reflux symptoms after radiofrequency energy: a randomized, sham-controlled trial. Gastroentrol 2003;125:668–76. PMID: 12949712
  A randomised trial of sham endoscopy versus endoscopic application of radiofrequency energy to the gastro-oesophageal junction.

[115] Schwartz MP, Wellink H, Gooszen HG, et al. Endoscopic gastroplication for the treatment of gastro-oesophageal reflux disease: a randomised, sham-controlled trial. Gut 2007;56:20–8. PMID: 16763053
  A randomised trial of sham endoscopy versus endoscopic mucosal suturing at the gastro-oesophageal junction.

[116] Rothstein R, Filipi C, Caca K, et al. Endoscopic full-thickness plication for the treatment of gastroesophageal reflux disease: a randomized, sham-controlled trial. Gastroenterology 2006;131:704–12. PMID: 16952539
  A randomised trial of sham endoscopy versus endoscopic full-thickness plication of the gastro-oesophageal junction.

[119] Hunter JG, Kahrilas PJ, Bell RC, et al. Efficacy of transoral fundoplication vs omeprazole for treatment of regurgitation in a randomized controlled trial. Gastroenterology 2015;148:324–33. PMID: 25448925
  A randomised trial of sham endoscopy versus endoscopic transoral partial fundoplication.

Revisional oesophagogastric surgery

13

Mark Smithers | Iain Thomson

INTRODUCTION

Following the assessment of a patient with a primary functional upper gastrointestinal (GI) problem or malignancy, it is likely there will be high-level evidence for the appropriate intervention, guiding the clinician and the patient. This is not the case when assessing patients with functional problems after upper GI surgery, whether the initial operation be for benign or malignant disease. This chapter will deal with the role of surgery for this group of patients, specifically for the more chronic problems, and not acute issues such as bleeding, anastomotic leakage, or acute conduit complications. Nearly all the information and data come from observational studies, reviews, and some meta-analyses, with the level of evidence for most statements and recommendations being level III and IV.

Typically the role of surgery is being explored because of the impact of the symptoms on the patient's quality of life, when there has been a failure of medical management. Revisional oesophagogastric surgery can be very complex, being more complex than the primary procedure and more complex than major resectional oesophagogastric surgery. There is often higher morbidity than the first operation, as well as a reduced potential for optimal outcomes compared with the primary surgery. Thus, in making the decision to consider surgery, the surgeon and the patient need to weigh up the risks of the surgery, as well as the potential for the operation to affect the symptoms. Surgeons should consider their personal and institutional experience with both the primary surgery and the specific types of revision. It seems reasonable to consider that, for revisional surgery, those managing a high volume of the primary surgery are more likely get better outcomes with lower morbidity, although there is a lack of evidence to support this.

REVISIONAL HIATAL SURGERY

Following straightforward antireflux surgery, the rate of recurrence will increase with time, with the likelihood of further surgery occurring in fewer than 10% of these patients. Table 13.1 outlines the most common symptoms, reported in two large reviews, of revisional surgery.[1,2] Dysphagia is the most common reason for revision in the early postoperative phases,[3,4] but overall the recurrence of reflux symptoms will lead to a consideration of further surgery, with many patients having a combination of symptoms. There are patients that develop unusual symptoms that are attributed to

the previous antireflux surgery, such as nausea, pain after eating, and vomiting. It is important to assess the temporal development of these symptoms as a component to the investigation, aiming to assess whether the problem is related to the previous surgery or not. Recurrent symptoms are more likely to occur after more complex hiatal surgery, such as para-oesophageal hernia repair, or previous hiatal operations for recurrence. Patients who have undergone surgery for a para-oesophageal hernia are more likely to develop a recurrent hiatus hernia (HH) and, because of the extent of the previous dissection around the hiatus and into the mediastinum, will often have more complex pathology around the hiatus. In addition, patients who have had more than one redo hiatal procedure have a reduced potential to achieve satisfactory results and have a higher rate of intraoperative complications.[5]

The more complex hiatal surgery recipients, including those who have had multiple operations, have a higher risk of vagal injury and gastroparesis. In New York State, a study of 5 656 patients who had hiatal surgery from 2005 to 2010 reported the incidence of gastroparesis requiring treatment to be 3.8% after a primary fundoplication and 4.4% after a para-oesophageal hernia repair.[5] The risk was higher in diabetic patients, especially if they had diabetic complications, and the more times there has been surgery at the hiatus.[6] In a randomised trial comparing patients who had had direct hiatal repair or a repair with mesh support, 19% had food in the stomach after a 6-hour fast at a routine gastroscopy performed as part of the follow-up. The incidence reduced with time.[7]

INVESTIGATIONS

Where there are recurrent upper GI symptoms or unusual symptoms following hiatal surgery, the following investigations should be considered:

- Obtain the previous operative notes – assess the extent of oesophageal mobilisation; were the vagus nerves identified; were the short gastric vessels divided; was the hiatus closed and, if so, how; was mesh used; type of fundoplication.
- Oesophagogastroscopy – assess for oesophagitis; the position of the oesophagogastric junction (OGJ); on retroflexion the appearance of an intact fundoplication; the site of the hiatus; evidence of HH, which may be obvious or a subtle slip of fundus into the hiatus (Fig. 13.1).
- Contrast swallow – assess the anatomy of the lower oesophagus and OGJ; site of the OGJ; flow of contrast; the

Table 13.1 Reviews of revisional hiatal surgery: indications for surgery; cause of the recurrent symptoms; outcomes

		Furnee et al., 2009[1]	Van Beek et al., 2011[2]
Number of patients		4 509	1 167
Number of studies		81	17
Indications for surgery			
	Recurrent reflux	42%	59%
	Dysphagia	17%	30%
	Both dysphagia and reflux	4%	
	Gas bloat	0.7%	4.6%
	HH		2.2%
	Miscellaneous	3.2%	3.2%
Cause for symptoms			
	Intrathoracic wrap migration	28%	44%
	Para-oesophageal HH	6%	
	Wrap disruption	23%	16%
	Telescoping	14%	
	Slipped wrap		12%
	Hiatus disruption		5%
	Improper wrap position		4%
	Tight wrap	5%	
	Wrong diagnosis	1.5%	
Conversion[a]		8.7%	7.4%
– laparoscopic to open			
Intraoperative complications		15.6%[b]	18.6%
Mortality		0.9%	
Success – patient		81%	81%
– Objective		78%	

HH, Hiatus hernia.
[a]Operations commenced laparoscopically.
[b]Perforation of the oesophagus or stomach, 76% of this group.

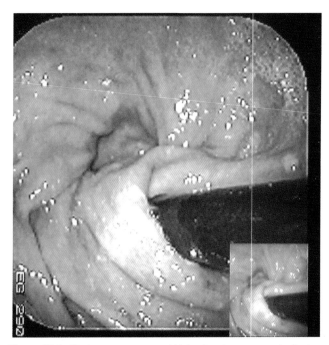

Figure 13.1 Endoscopy – recurrent hiatus hernia seen on retroflexion.

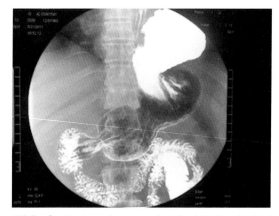

Figure 13.2 Contrast meal – wrap migration into the chest.

- Selective manometry – patients with new-onset dysphagia with no cause found or patients with worsening dysphagia, present preoperatively, and who did not have manometry.
- Selective 24-hour pH monitoring – unusual symptoms with normal anatomy and no objective signs of reflux on investigations.
- Radionucleotide gastric emptying studies with solid phase – suspicion of gastroparesis.

From the investigations there should be some clarity with respect to the anatomy of the problem and the ability to

presence of HH or not; the presence of reflux; delayed gastric emptying (Fig. 13.2).
- Computed tomography (CT) scan of the chest and upper abdomen – if a significant recurrent HH is suspected, to define anatomy and exclude other causes.

match the clinical picture with the investigations. The presence of an anatomical change does not demand surgery. The patient symptoms and the impact on quality of life should be the major consideration when discussing the role of surgery. Having some idea of the pathology offers insights into the potential difficulties, and outcomes, for the patient, which can be discussed prior to considering surgery.

A good classification of the pathophysiology of abnormal hiatal anatomy in patients with recurrent symptoms has been offered by Suppiah et al. and shown in Fig. 13.3.[6] In that report the reasons for redo surgery were:

i) Wrap intact/hiatus intact – typically dysphagia with fibrosis ± tight hiatus
ii) Wrap disruption only – intact hiatus and intra-abdominal position
iii) 'Telescope' or 'slipped' fundoplication – the fundoplication has 'slipped' onto the cardia such that there is stomach above the wrap (Fig. 13.3a).

iv) Para-oesophageal HH – typically lateral (left) to posterior defect with migration of a portion of the fundus into the lower mediastinum. The crura are intact (including the previous posterior suture) but there is a defect. The slip may be small or large (Fig. 13.3b).
v) Crural failure with intact wrap – herniation into the lower mediastinum (Fig. 13.3c).
vi) Crural failure with wrap disrupted – herniation into the lower mediastinum.

Assessing the pathology with time, the authors found that 'telescoping' was the most common problem in the first year. Over subsequent years crural failure with degrees of fundal herniation were more common, likely reflecting the temporal sequence of events that leads to a recurrent hernia.

Hiatal recurrence after repair of a giant HH is common,[6–8] with one randomised controlled trial reporting a 5-year recurrence, of any size, to be more than 40%. Although the recurrent hernia may increase the risk of symptoms[9] many

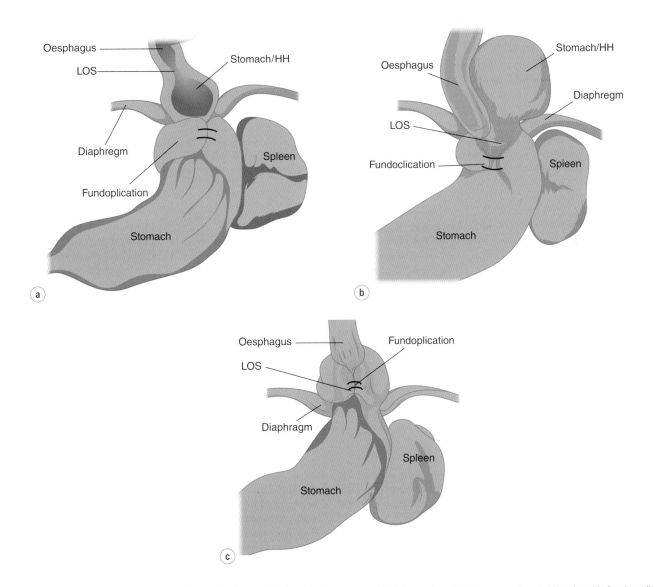

Figure 13.3 Anatomy of a recurrence after antireflux and hiatus hernia surgery. (a) Telescoping. (b) Para-oesophageal hernia with fundus slip into lower mediastinum. (c) Crural failure with fundoplication migration into the lower mediastinum.

patients will have no symptoms and those with symptoms are often controlled medically. One study assessed 115 patients without symptoms 6 months and 5 years after a giant HH repair and reported 41 patients to have a hernia, with only two proceeding to revisional surgery.[9] The low rate of revisional surgery for recurrent hernia after giant hiatus hernia repair has been confirmed in a number of studies.[8,10,11]

✓✓ In spite of the higher rate of recurrent HH after para-oesophageal hernia repair, very few patients require revisional surgery.[8–11]

REVISIONAL SURGERY POST HIATAL SURGERY FOR HERNIA OR REFLUX

Indications for an operation include: upper GI symptoms considered relevant to the previous operation; a correctable disorder defined in the investigations and symptoms affecting quality of life, for which medical therapy does not work or cannot be tolerated. Where the previous surgery was performed through an open approach, the potential for a successful laparoscopic approach is reduced. In spite of this, it is reasonable to approach the first revisional operation laparoscopically, in experienced hands, accepting and counselling the patient that there is a high potential to convert to an open approach. In patients who had a primary laparoscopic approach, the conversion risk is 7–9% (Table 13.1).

The principles are to take the previous operation down, define the pathology, close the hiatus around the oesophagus, and redo a fundoplication. This will entail clearing the adhesions around the cardia, liver, and diaphragm, with definition of both crura of the diaphragm, and then the lower oesophagus, looking for the vagus nerves, with the aim of preservation. Where there was a recurrent HH there is often elongation of the left crus and attenuation of the central tendon anteriorly.[6] This will need repair, typically including an anterior suture. The fundoplication is then performed and fixed to the crura, aiming to reduce migration. There is a school of thought that this group should have mesh supplementation of the hiatal repair. The evidence is mixed, both with respect to the use of mesh, what type of mesh, and where it should be placed and, thus, its use will relate to local preferences and experience.

SPECIFIC ISSUES

Dysphagia – if present in the first few weeks consider reoperation. If tight at hiatus, an anterior slit may be required. If no cause is found change to a lesser fundoplication.[12] The use of dilatation has been reported to be successful in selected patients where there is no anatomical defect or mechanical obstruction on investigations.[13] Revision would be reasonable if little or no response to dilatation.

Bloat – Where intractable, and surgery considered reasonable, aim to convert to a lesser fundoplication. The rate of functional symptoms has been shown to be reduced with fundoplications such as anterior 90 degree and 180 degree [14] and in analyses that have compared 270 degree with a 360-degree fundoplication.[15]

Delayed gastric emptying/gastroparesis – symptoms such as anorexia, nausea, dry retching, post-prandial bloat, and colic may indicate this diagnosis, although vomiting may not be a major issue due to the action of the fundoplication. Food present in the stomach after a 6-hour fast suggests a diagnosis of delayed gastric emptying. If early, after the operation, there is the potential for improvement with time. In the longer term, with persistent symptoms the surgical procedures performed to address this diagnosis include pyloroplasty, pyloromyotomy, gastroenterostomy, or distal gastrectomy with either a Billroth II or Roux-en-Y reconstruction. Pyloroplasty/myotomy are the least invasive. Bile reflux gastritis may occur, but is more prevalent following a gastro-enterostomy or Billroth II operations. More recently, there has been the introduction of per-oral endoscopic myotomy of the pylorus – GPOEM. A meta-analysis and systematic review reported equivalent efficacy for this procedure compared with pyloroplasty, with 85% and 84% improvement, respectively, on gastric emptying studies and similar outcomes when the gastroparesis cardinal symptom index score was assessed.[16] GPOEM is not widely performed at this time and requires special expertise.

MORE THAN ONE HIATAL OPERATION

There will be a need to consider alternative approaches other than a further revisional fundoplication. The same operation repeated is likely to lead to the same outcome, i.e. a poor functional outcome.[17] The options include: a Collis gastroplasty, a Roux-en-Y bypass, or an oesophagogastrectomy.

Collis gastroplasty – For recurrent 'telescoping', one should consider that there may be shortening of the oesophagus. If likely, it is reasonable to consider a Collis fundoplication with creation of a neo-oesophagus using the gastric cardia. This segment sits below the hiatus with a partial fundoplication placed around it.[18]

Roux-en-Y bypass with or without gastric resection – Following multiple hiatal procedures, there is a role for a gastric bypass with Roux-en-Y anastomosis for a patient without dysphagia but with recurrent reflux, where the potential to create a fundoplication is reduced or impossible. This procedure is especially relevant if there is also associated gastroparesis.[19] In the past this operation typically included a distal gastric resection; however, using the bariatric principles for the creation of the bypass, the excluded stomach may be left in place. In a study in an experienced centre, 87 patients had a Roux-en-Y bypass performed after reducing the fundal hernia and repairing the crura using a 50-cc pouch, reporting a 12.6% recurrence rate at a median of 3 years follow-up.[20]

Oesophagogastric resection – Where the proximal stomach cannot be used or retained, consideration for an oesophagogastrectomy may be necessary.[21] Typically, this is the secondary plan when operating, aiming for a lesser procedure, but it becomes apparent that resection is the safest and most definitive procedure. Whether the approach is via an abdominal approach or a thoracic approach will be dependent upon the previous surgery, the defined pathology, but most probably, on the expertise of the treating surgeon. The abdominal approach allows assessment generally around the hiatus and the supracolic regions, aiming for non-resectional treatments, and is preferred by non-thoracic surgeons. With a left thoracic approach, dissection around the hiatus will still be required, reducing any HH. The incision may need to be extended into the abdomen, across the diaphragm, to gain adequate intra-abdominal access.

ROLE OF MESH AT THE HIATUS

The use of mesh to reinforce the hiatus after HH repair has become common practice. A survey of European surgeons in 2015 reported that 67% use mesh in all or selected cases.[22] The reported indications included large defect, tension in hiatal sutures, and weak muscle.[22] These factors may be more prevalent at the time of revisional hiatal surgery. However, the risk of recurrence must be weighed up against the risk of mesh complications, which have been reported to occur more frequently following revisional hiatal surgery.[23] Which mesh to use and the optimal placement position at the hiatus are also not clear, so the choice to use mesh and decide which mesh will be surgeon related and focused on the individual case.[22,23]

Complications from mesh at the hiatus – Potential complications from mesh at the hiatus include erosion and oesophageal stenosis. One series reported the mesh erosion rate to be 5% in a series of 122 patients where the mesh encircled the hiatus.[23] The rate was higher in patients who had revisional surgery. Management will be individualised and may include observation, endoscopic removal of the mesh, and surgical removal of the mesh, which, in severe cases, may include resection of the OGJ. Patients requiring surgery for mesh complications need to be aware of the potential for a major resection, with one series reporting a 6.8-times risk following revisional surgery compared to patients who did not have a mesh present.[24]

INTRAOPERATIVE COMPLICATIONS FOLLOWING REVISIONAL HIATAL SURGERY

Conversion from a laparoscopic approach will typically be required due to dense adhesions, mesh adhesions, bleeding, and visceral injury. The rate of complications has been reported to be 16–19%, with the most common being injury to the oesophagus or the stomach (Table 13.1). One large study[6] reported a 19.7% rate with the stomach requiring repair, or a wedge resection of the tip in 9.5%, oesophageal perforation in 2%, and bleeding in 3%

POST-PAEDIATRIC OESOPHAGEAL ATRESIA SURGERY

The survival rate of children with oesophageal atresia exceeds 90%. There are limited long-term data relating to functional outcomes in this group of patients who have required surgery, with or without reconstruction. Dysphagia is common and associated with oesophageal dysmotility, with reported rates of 18–65%. Manometric studies demonstrate uncoordinated peristalsis with low amplitudes above a normally relaxing lower oesophageal sphincter. Reflux and regurgitation symptoms are reported in 18–63% (mean 40%), with the incidence of Barrett's metaplasia ranging from 1 to 11% (mean 6%). New or progressive symptoms of dysphagia in adulthood will require exclusion of a stricture secondary to reflux. The rate of oesophageal cancer in this group is low, with two studies reporting a range of 0.8–2.6%.[25,26]

When reconstruction was required, the conduit will have been either a gastric tube or the colon. Patients with a gastric tube in adulthood may suffer from reflux, with a risk of stricture formation requiring intervention such as dilatation. In addition, aspiration may occur in these patients due to oesophageal dysmotility, a stricture, or both. Children who have had a colon pull-up may develop redundancy of the colon, causing problems with reflux, regurgitation, aspiration, or obstruction. The incidence has been reported to be around 20% in a group of patients with a mean follow-up of 10 years. It is less frequent if the colon was placed retrosternally.[27] Options for treatment will be discussed further in this chapter.

OESOPHAGEAL REPLACEMENT AND CONDUIT DYSFUNCTION

A gastric pull-up is the most common conduit after oesophageal resection. There are occasions when an alternative is required such as gastric conduit necrosis, previous gastrectomy, and caustic damage to the stomach making it unsuitable. The alternative options include the colon or jejunum. In a small group of patients with benign disease, for example, end-stage achalasia, an argument can be made to leave the stomach in place and use an alternative conduit, such as the colon, to replace the oesophagus. When the posterior mediastinum is unavailable due to previous surgery, the conduits can be passed proximally, retrosternally, or subcutaneously to reach the neck for anastomosis to the remnant oesophagus or pharynx.

Severe dysfunction of an oesophageal replacement conduit, requiring intervention, is rare but does occur. If there is a decision to reoperate on these patients, this should be undertaken in high-volume centres with expertise in upper GI, thoracic, and microvascular surgery. Being mindful that most interventions are not for life-threatening issues and more related to improvement of quality of life, patients require in-depth counselling. Also, there needs to be consideration of the options for reconstruction that would be available if there was a vascular injury causing necrosis of a segment or all of the conduit.

GASTRIC CONDUIT

Severe gastric conduit dysfunction, requiring intervention, is uncommon. The incidence in two studies with large numbers of patients was 2%.[28] The most common causes were: excess conduit above the diaphragm, with the stomach in a horizontal position above the right diaphragm causing delayed emptying; mechanical obstruction due to pyloric dysfunction or at the hiatal aperture (half the patients); a twisted conduit; and the development of a 'sigmoid-shaped' conduit without outflow obstruction.[29] Another potential cause for obstruction at the hiatus is the presence of a HH beside the conduit.

Symptoms of a dysfunctional conduit may include dysphagia, severe postprandial fullness, nausea, regurgitation, and vomiting. In extreme cases, patients may suffer from aspiration pneumonia and/or significant weight loss. Investigations should include upper GI endoscopy; a contrast study to assess the site of the pylorus as well as the gastric conduit emptying into the duodenum; and a CT scan to assess the anatomy and exclude a para-conduit HH. Abnormal radiology includes distended conduit, poor emptying, air-fluid levels, and a horizontal course through the chest leading to angulation at the diaphragm.[28]

When conservative measures have failed, revision will be considered where patients are aspirating or have intractable regurgitation and/or vomiting that is having a major impact on their quality of life. If delayed gastric emptying appears to be a significant issue, balloon dilatation of the pylorus should be considered.[30] For persistent dysfunction in patients who have not had a pyloromyotomy or pyloroplasty, Botox injection should be considered to assess its impact. If there is evidence of improvement, then a formal pyloroplasty is an option.

Conduit revision may be considered if it is dilated and redundant, and there are severe symptoms. The aim is to have a vertical conduit without redundancy. If there is redundancy above the right diaphragm the conduit should be mobilised with refashioning of the anastomosis, if a low anastomosis was the problem. If the site of the anastomosis is appropriate, mobilisation of the conduit should be performed, aiming to reduce some of the conduit into the abdomen.[29] For a dilated, redundant conduit that is not horizontal, the options include plication or longitudinal resection along the lesser curve, aiming for a 5 cm-wide conduit. On-table endoscopic assessment should be performed.[28]

COLON CONDUIT

The colon conduit may be the left colon based on the ascending branch of the left colic artery or the right colon based on the middle colic artery. Both conduits require an intact marginal artery. A recent systematic review of 1 849 patients reported the left colon placed in the retrosternal position to be the safest option, with lower mortality and morbidity compared with the use of the right colon.[31] In patients with benign disease such as achalasia, a vagus-sparing oesophagectomy has been described, with the colon anastomosed to the stomach in the abdomen.[32]

There is a paucity of quality data on the surgical management of dysfunctional colon conduits. One large series reported the need for intervention to be 8%.[33] Redundancy of the colon with a sump effect or kinking with partial obstruction were the most common problems, leading to consideration for intervention. Distal obstruction at the hiatus or at the site of the anastomosis of the colon to the GI tract should be excluded. Redundancy was seen more commonly in long-segment colon interpositions. Patients may present with regurgitation, dysphagia, aspiration pneumonia, or postprandial pain or discomfort. Investigations should be focused to assess the anatomy and the functional status of the conduit, and should include upper GI endoscopy, a contrast swallow, and CT scanning of the chest and upper abdomen. Surgery is considered when the symptoms are severe and the patient's quality of life is significantly compromised.

The surgery should be tailored to the identified cause of the problem. Surgical options include resection of a redundant segment or longitudinal 'sleeve' resection along the anti-mesenteric border where there is generalised dilatation and redundancy or a combination of both. Access to the dilated conduit may require redo thoracotomy for intrathoracic conduits, a careful sternotomy for retrosternal conduits, or a laparotomy if the dysfunctional segment is in the abdomen. The conduit must be approached carefully, ensuring the vascular pedicle is not damaged and where resection is performed the vessels are divided staying close to, or on, the colon wall.[34,35] The aim is to have a conduit that is narrower and passes more directly to the hiatus and to the distal bowel anastomosis. Gastrocolonic reflux may be another indication for late revision and can be managed with conversion to a Roux-en-Y colojejunostomy.

✓✓ The need for revision of gastric or colonic conduits for functional symptoms is rare.[28,33] The surgery is complex with the potential for loss of the conduit and should be performed in specialist centres by experienced surgeons.

JEJUNAL CONDUIT

Short segments of the lower oesophagus and OGJ can be bridged by jejunal interposition. Originally the technique was described for complex strictures requiring resection, and more recently used in the context of localised oesophagogastric resection for cancer at this site.[36] This operation can be considered for a severe benign stricture or if a local OGJ resection was required in conjunction with hiatal mesh removal. The original technique used a pedicled segment of jejunum. A recent report described a Roux-en-Y reconstruction with the formation of an oesophagojejunostomy and subsequent end-to-side anastomosis of the gastric remnant to the efferent limb 10–15 cm below the oesophageal anastomosis. This so-called 'double tract' operation has nutritional and functional advantages over a total gastric resection with Roux-en-Y reconstruction.[37]

Jejunal conduits may be the only option in patients where the stomach or colon is not available. The length of the mesentery determines the effective length of the conduit. A length up to 30cm can be derived from a single jejunal branch pedicle. 'Supercharging' the proximal segment using microvascular anastomosis to the jejunal artery and vein, at the proximal cut edge, has been described to allow the jejunum to reach the neck for a proximal anastomosis.[38]

For both colon pull-up and jejunal pull-up to the neck, it is recommended that the thoracic inlet be expanded by resection of the left hemi-manubrium, clavicular head, and medial first rib, being careful not to damage the deep anterior mediastinal vessels. This procedure also provides access to the internal mammary vessels as well as the cervical vasculature for microvascular supercharging of the colon or jejunal pull-up, if considered necessary.

HIATUS HERNIA POST-OESOPHAGECTOMY

A large European survey assessing the outcome on 6 608 patients reported the rate for hiatal herniation to be 1.2%. One in five will be diagnosed in the first 90 days and 68% of this group will present as an emergency. The rate was twice as high after laparoscopic gastric mobilisation.[39] The approach to these hernias will depend on the presentation and the context, that is, a life-threatening problem, symptomatic hernia, or a hernia found incidentally on follow-up imaging. In this series laparoscopy or laparotomy was used to reduce and seal the hiatus in 79% of patients, with 31% requiring a thoracotomy.

REVISIONAL SURGERY FOLLOWING BENIGN OR MALIGNANT GASTRIC SURGERY

With the reduction in peptic ulcer surgery, there has been a reduction in the incidence of the functional problems that occurred in this patient cohort. More recently, with gastric resectional procedures becoming more prevalent for bariatric surgery, there may be an increase in some of these problems. Thus for this group, and for patients requiring major gastric resections for malignant disease, where medical management has failed we are somewhat reliant on the information from historic observational surgical series regarding the potential outcomes from surgical approaches. The surgical options used in these patients were commonly reported without long-term follow-up, and as such many patients exchanged one set of symptoms for another or increased their functional problems. Thus, in this group of patients, if surgery is ever considered one should look at a simple approach that makes anatomical sense.

The functional problems occur as a result of division of the vagus nerve and/or the destruction or removal of the gastric pyloric mechanism, as well as issues surrounding reconstruction after gastric resection. Patients will have rapid or slow transit syndromes.

RAPID TRANSIT SYNDROMES

Post vagotomy diarrhoea – The rate of diarrhoea after a truncal vagotomy has been reported to be as high as 25%.[40] However most times this will be self-limiting, with improvement over time. A few patients will require regular antidiarrhoeal medication. In modern times there would be very few, if any, patients where surgery would be considered. The historic approach was to use a 10-cm reversed segment of jejunum inserted 100 cm from the ligament of Treitz.[41]

Dumping syndrome – This consists of vasomotor and GI symptoms that have the potential to have a major impact on a patient's quality of life. These symptoms tend to improve with time. When a patient's quality of life is significantly affected and the symptoms are resistant to medical management, patients and their doctors become desperate and may seek a surgical solution. The most common operation in the past was a pyloric reconstruction with reversal of whatever pyloroplasty had been used. This was followed by reversed segments of jejunum inserted to reduce the intestinal transit times.[42] The outcomes from these procedures were variable but there were some patients who benefited; however, the literature does not guide selection.

SLOW TRANSIT SYNDROMES

Following a gastric resection, there will be an afferent or bilio-pancreatic limb and an efferent or alimentary limb.

Alkaline reflux gastritis – This occurs when bile and pancreatic enzymes pool in the stomach to cause pain, often constant, which may be associated with nausea and intermittent vomiting. The diagnosis is considered following an endoscopy, which includes findings such as severe gastric mucosa inflammation, usually with thickened folds, and typically with bile seen washing over the mucosa or refluxing into the stomach. Most commonly, this occurs following a gastric resection with reconstruction to the duodenum (Billroth 1, BI) or a gastro-enterotomy (Billroth II, BII). Delayed gastric emptying or gastroparesis needs to be considered as a differential diagnosis or as a component of the syndrome. A hepatobiliary iminodiacetic acid (HIDA) scan may assist by showing pooling of the tracer in bile in the stomach. If delayed gastric emptying is considered, a formal radionucleotide gastric emptying should be performed. Conversion of a BI or BII reconstruction to a Roux-en-Y reconstruction with a 60-cm efferent jejunal loop has been shown to be beneficial.[42] If gastroparesis is present, with a large gastric remnant revision to a smaller pouch should be performed.

Afferent loop syndrome – This is a manifestation of an obstruction in this limb, occurring with an incidence between 0.2% and 1%, with a lower incidence when a Roux-en-Y anastomosis has been performed.[43] When acute it is due to obstruction at the anastomosis, kinking, or internal herniation. There is the risk of duodenal 'blow out' following a gastric resection. The definitive treatment is laparotomy and, if relevant, revision of the anastomosis if Billroth II or conversion to a Roux-en-Y reconstruction. Where the problem is chronic, there is typically a partial obstruction. The presentation may be insidious, ranging from bacterial overgrowth syndrome to pain, nausea, and vomiting, which is typically voluminous due to a sudden release of accumulated biliary and pancreatic fluid into the stomach, giving complete relief of the pain and nausea. The diagnosis is made from a CT scan, and when considered appropriate, a magnetic resonance cholangiopancreatography (MRCP) will help define the biliary and pancreatic anatomy. The definitive treatment is to revise the anastomosis or to anastomose the proximal limb to the efferent limb, usually as a Roux-en-Y conversion. Endoscopic treatment with dilatation of the anastomosis, pigtail catheters, or metallic stents have been described, but are more relevant to a patient not fit for surgery or in the presence of malignant obstruction.[43]

Efferent loop syndrome (Roux stasis syndrome) – With this condition, patients will not tolerate oral intake and in particular solid food. This may be associated with pain, usually colic, epigastric fullness, regurgitation, vomiting, and,

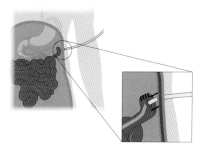

Figure 13.4 Rouy-en-Y feeding jejunostomy.

when severe, weight loss and malnutrition. In a study performed at the Mayo clinic it was felt to be present in 30% of 202 patients after a gastrojejunostomy and 2 (6%) of 32 patients after an oesophagojejunostomy.[44] It was felt to be more prevalent after a partial gastrectomy because of the involvement of the gastric pouch with delayed emptying. A study using manometry after a total gastrectomy in asymptomatic patients, at a median time of 74 months postoperatively, reported normal oesophageal peristalsis but abnormal jejunal peristalsis in most patients.[45] The severe form is very rare but when treatment with prokinetics has failed resection of the gastric remnant has been recommended. If there is no gastric remnant, to maintain nutrition, a nasogastric feeding jejunostomy tube may be required.[42] If a long-term solution is required a procedure used in children who require long-term feeding can be considered. This is a surgical jejunostomy with the tube placed into a modified Roux-en-Y jejunojejunostomy to keep the cutaneous connection out of the enteric stream. (Fig. 13.4).[46] Following a total gastrectomy the use of a jejunal pouch has been advocated by some; however, the evidence for benefit is conflicting[47] and there is no evidence for its use for efferent loop syndrome.

CONCLUSION

The vast majority of the literature published on revisional surgery comes from observational studies from large tertiary specialist centres. There will be publication bias favouring studies with positive outcomes where complex surgery has been applied. For many revisional operations there is a 'law of diminishing returns'. Second revisions have the added complexity of pathology put there by the previous surgery and, in general, even the good results of specialist centres are never quite up to their outcomes for primary surgery. The problems tend to be functional and the issue is the impact on a patient's quality of life, with a few rare instances of surgery required for life-threatening problems. Thus, with the focus on quality of life, one has to undertake an assessment of the risk balance aiming to achieve this goal. In considering further revision, it is often worth asking if the patient is failing nutritionally, with inexorable weight loss, and whether there is a correctable problem that is likely to continue to deteriorate if a procedure is not undertaken. For instance, is there a risk that an overflowing dilated oesophagus causing aspiration pneumonitis likely to lead to respiratory failure? If the answer to these questions is 'no', the surgeon should exercise considerable caution before advising further surgery.

Key points

- Revisional oesophageal and gastric surgery is often complex and high risk, and is not warranted in patients with mild symptoms and in those whose quality of life is not significantly affected.
- Ensure correlation between symptoms and the objective findings and that the identified abnormalities are amenable to a surgical solution.
- Surgery for recurrent reflux and dysphagia will usually result in satisfactory outcomes.
- Second and later revisions are always complex operations and should only be undertaken when symptoms are severe, the patient cannot maintain adequate nutrition, or when there are perceived risks that might pose a threat to life.
- Replacement of the oesophagus with colon may be appropriate in benign disease or when the stomach is unavailable. The constructed graft based on the left colic artery is reliable in a variety of lengths.
- Jejunal grafts are suitable as short oesophageal replacements. Long jejunal grafts can be performed but will likely need additional microvascular reconstruction.
- Severe conduit dysfunction in a gastric or colon pull-up is uncommon, with surgery reserved for those with severe disability, accepting the significant risks including loss of the conduit and operative mortality.
- The need for revisional surgery for functional problems postgastrectomy is uncommon.
- Despite a lack of evidence, most revisional surgery should be confined to specialist centres.

References available at http://ebooks.health.elsevier.com/

KEY REFERENCES

[1] Furnee EJ, Draaisma WA, Broeders IA, Gooszen HG. Surgical re-intervention after failed antireflux surgery: a systematic review of the literature. J Gastrointest Surg 2009;13(8):1539–49.

[2] van Beek DB, Auyang ED, Soper NJ. A comprehensive review of laparoscopic redo fundoplication. Surg Endosc 2011;25(3):706–12.
Comprehensive reviews of indications for revisional hiatal surgery, including outcomes.

[6] Suppiah A, Sirimanna P, Vivian SJ, O'Donnell H, Lee G, Falk GL. Temporal patterns of hiatus hernia recurrence and hiatal failure: quality of life and recurrence after revision surgery. Dis Esophagus 2017;30(4):1–8.
Good classification of the anatomical features of recurrent HH pathology, with information on the outcomes for each pattern.

[22] Huddy JR, Markar SR, Ni MZ, Morino M, Targarona EM, Zaninotto G, et al. Laparoscopic repair of hiatus hernia: does mesh type influence outcome? A meta-analysis and European survey study. Surg Endosc 2016;30(12):5209–21.
Large European study reporting the use of mesh for hiatal repair.

[25] Connor MJ, Springford LR, Kapetanakis VV, Giuliani S. Esophageal atresia and transitional care—step 1: a systematic review and meta-analysis of the literature to define the prevalence of chronic long-term problems. Am J Surg 2015;209(4):747–59.
Assessment of the long-term outcomes following treatment for children with oesophageal atresia.

[31] Brown J, Lewis WG, Foliaki A, Clark GWB, Blackshaw G, Chan DSY. Colonic interposition after adult oesophagectomy: systematic review and meta-analysis of conduit choice and outcome. J Gastrointest Surg 2018;22(6):1104–11.
Large review of the outcomes from colonic conduits using either the right or left colon.

[38] Marks JL, Hofstetter WL. Esophageal reconstruction with alternative conduits. Surg Clin North Am. 2012;92(5):1287–97.
Outline of possible options when a gastric conduit is not available after oesophagectomy.

[41] Sawyers JL. Management of postgastrectomy syndromes. Am J Surg 1990;159(1):8–14.
A review of postgastrectomy disorders and the role of revisional surgery. Mainly historic relevance.

The management of achalasia and other motility disorders of the oesophagus

14

Jimmy Bok-yan So

INTRODUCTION

With the development of high-resolution manometry (HRM) and new treatment paradigms such as peroral endoscopic myotomy (POEM), patients with achalasia and other oesophageal motility disorders are increasingly being diagnosed and treated. Our understanding of motility disorders and their treatment has also increased rapidly in the last decade. In this chapter, we will consider the management of these disorders and highlight recent studies pertaining to the treatment of achalasia and related diseases.

ACHALASIA

Achalasia is derived from the Greek word '*khalasis*', which means 'unable to relax'. It is the most common primary motility disorder of the oesophagus, with an incidence of about 1 in 100,000 people per year. It affects both males and females equally. The mean age of diagnosis is over 50 years old, but it can present in children or the elderly. Although it is a benign disease, it can cause debilitating symptoms that adversely affect patients' quality of life. Achalasia is also a risk factor for oesophageal malignancy.

PATHOPHYSIOLOGY

Achalasia results from the loss of myenteric neurons at the lower oesophageal sphincter (LOS) and distal oesophagus that leads to failure of relaxation of the LOS and ineffective oesophageal peristalsis. The exact aetiology of the loss of myenteric plexus is unknown, but autoimmune dysfunction after exposure to viral infections such as herpes simplex, human papillomavirus, and measles are postulated.[1] In Chicago type 1 or 2 achalasia the mesenteric ganglia are replaced with fibrosis, but in type 3 achalasia the mesenteric ganglia are infiltrated with chronic inflammatory cells such as lymphocytes. This may account for the spastic contraction and chest pain that patients experience in type 3 achalasia. A large-scale genetic association study revealed significant abnormality at the major histocompatibility (MHC) region on chromosome 6; its protein products form the receptors of antigen-presenting cells. The findings imply that immune-mediated processes are involved in the pathophysiology of achalasia.[2]

While most cases of achalasia are idiopathic, the disappearance of the myenteric plexus can occasionally be due to malignant infiltration, which is called pseudoachalasia, or due to *Trypanosoma* infection in Chagas disease. Pseudoachalasia is an important cause of secondary achalasia, especially in the elderly. It accounts for 2–4% of patients with suspected achalasia. It behaves like achalasia, with dilation of the proximal oesophagus and narrowing at the LOS. It is caused by submucosal infiltration of neoplastic cells or autoimmune damage from a reaction to tumour cells at the LOS, and the findings on barium oesophagogram and manometry might be similar to true achalasia. In a recent systemic review, the mean age of patients with pseudoachalasia was 60 years and the most common cause was gastric cancer, followed by oesophageal cancer and small-cell lung cancer.[3] Many of the patients were mistakenly treated as having achalasia. Repeat endoscopy, computed tomography (CT) scan, and endoscopic ultrasound were found to be useful in the diagnosis of pseudoachalasia. A high index of clinical suspicion and correct interpretation of investigations is important to exclude this serious condition.

CLINICAL FEATURES

Dysphagia and regurgitation are the cardinal symptoms of achalasia, and these symptoms tend to be chronic. Many patients could be misdiagnosed as having gastro-oesophageal reflux disease (GORD) due to the presenting symptoms. Other symptoms include weight loss and chest pain. For patients with type 3 (or spastic) achalasia, chest pain is the predominant symptom. The Eckardt score is a composite symptom score that includes dysphagia, regurgitation, chest pain, and weight loss. This is commonly used for achalasia to grade the severity of disease and quantify treatment outcomes.[4] As highlighted earlier, it is important to exclude pseudoachalasia before embarking on treatment.

INVESTIGATIONS

Upper endoscopy is usually the first diagnostic test for achalasia, given the presenting symptoms. It is used to exclude oesophageal or gastric neoplasm. In achalasia, the proximal oesophagus may appear dilated with food or saliva retention and occasionally, candidiasis is identified. Abnormal oesophageal body contractions can be seen, especially for type 3 achalasia. The LOS will be tight and there is often difficulty passing the standard endoscope through. However, if a patient has been previously treated, there might be minimal resistance encountered.

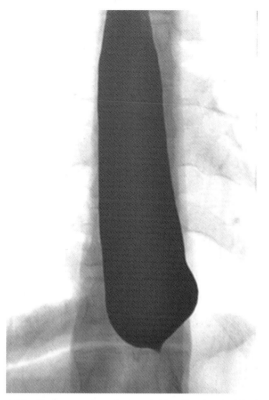

Figure 14.1 Barium swallow demonstrating the classical features of achalasia with 'bird's beak' and dilatation of the oesophagus.

A barium swallow study may show hold-up of the contrast, with a tapering stricture in the distal oesophagus often described as a 'bird's beak' (Fig. 14.1). The oesophagus is dilated proximally. However, the findings of a barium study are non-specific and additional tests are required to confirm the diagnosis. Recently, a timed barium swallow (or timed oesophagogram) was described in which the height of barium was measured 5 minutes after the ingestion of barium. It is used to assess the emptying of the oesophagus and can also be adopted as a simple objective method to monitor treatment response.[5]

MANOMETRY AND HIGH-RESOLUTION MANOMETRY (HRM)

Manometry is recommended to confirm the diagnosis of achalasia (Fig. 14.2). In conventional manometry, the cardinal features are a hypertensive non-relaxing LOS and the absence of oesophageal peristalsis. More recently, HRM is increasingly being used for diagnosis. In HRM, catheters with 36 or more sensors are placed 1 cm apart along the oesophagus, which allow a much more detailed pressure recording from the pharynx to the stomach.

✔✔ HRM is more sensitive than conventional manometry to diagnose motility disorders and is regarded as the gold standard for the diagnosis of achalasia.[6] The use of HRM has also led to the subclassification of achalasia based on the pattern of contractility in the oesophageal body, which forms the basis for the Chicago classification[7] (Fig. 14.3).

Integrated relaxation pressure (IRP) is the mean post-swallow LOS pressure of a 4-second period. Achalasia is typically diagnosed when IRP is higher than the upper limit of

normal. It is subclassified as type 1 when there is complete loss of contractility of the oesophageal body with no evidence of pressurisation, type 2 when there is pressurisation or compression in the distal oesophagus over 30 mmHg, and type 3 when there are two or more premature spastic contractions in the oesophageal body.

✔✔ Type 1 and 2 achalasia responds well to all forms of treatment. Type 2 has the best prognosis as it may represent the early stages of achalasia with the presence of residual body contractions. Type 3 or spastic achalasia classically responds less favourably after Heller myotomy or pneumatic dilation. Peroral endoscopic myotomy or POEM is currently the recommended treatment for Type 3 achalasia, as this technique allows for more proximal division of the affected muscle fibres.[8]

TREATMENT MODALITIES

There are many treatment options available for achalasia. However, these options are non-curative in nature as they are unable to restore neuromuscular function, including normal peristalsis. Most treatments target the LOS by lowering its resting pressure, and the goal of treatment is symptom control and quality of life improvement. The management of patients' expectations is an important aspect of counselling for treatment.

MEDICAL TREATMENT

The two most commonly used medications for achalasia are nitrates and calcium channel blockers. However, their use is limited by adverse drug events such as headache and postural hypotension. A Cochrane review identified only two randomised studies on nitrates in achalasia but no recommendations were given.[9] Another pharmacological agent used is botulinum toxin A, which is a neurotoxin that blocks the release of acetylcholine from nerve endings. It is injected via a sclerotherapy needle into the LOS in four or eight quadrants. Unfortunately, its effects are temporary and repeated treatment is often necessary; however, repeated injections have been shown to make subsequent myotomy more difficult due to fibrosis. At least five randomised studies comparing botulinum injections with pneumatic dilation and one study comparing botulinum with surgical myotomy have been published.[10] All showed comparable results in symptom relief initially but rapid recurrence of dysphagia with botulinum toxin subsequently. Hence, pharmacological treatment is only reserved as a bridge before definitive treatment or in high-risk patients who are not suitable for definitive treatment.[11]

PNEUMATIC DILATATION

Pneumatic dilatation (PD) is usually performed with an air-filled balloon (30–40 mm in diameter) under endoscopic and fluoroscopic guidance. An upper endoscopy is performed and a guidewire is inserted into the stomach. Under fluoroscopy, the balloon mounted on a flexible catheter is placed over the guidewire across the LOS and the balloon is gradually inflated until the waist is flattened. PD is effective for achalasia, with symptom relief observed in 74–90%

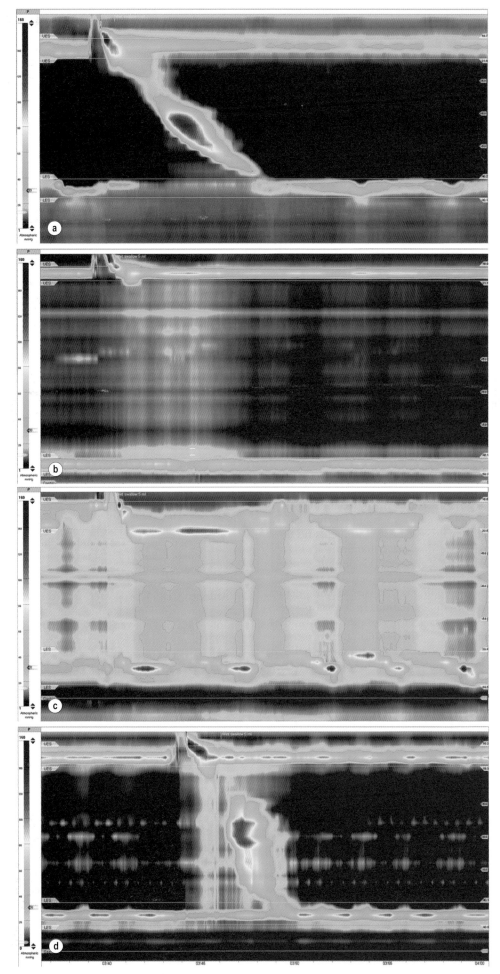

Figure 14.2 High-resolution manometry.

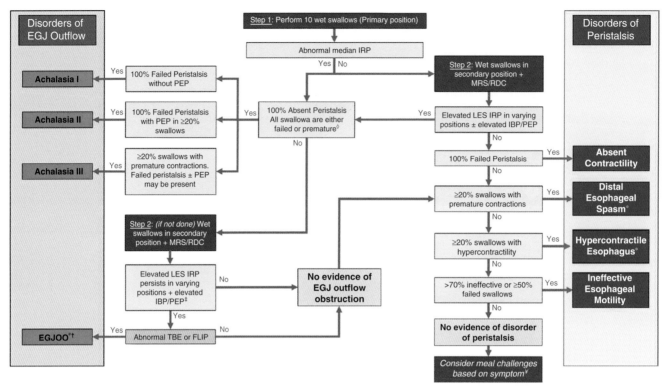

Figure 14.3   The Chicago classification.

of patients.[12] In the long term, one-third of patients will require repeated treatment due to symptom recurrence.[13] Patients who are older than 40 years of age, women, and those with type 2 achalasia have the best outcomes with PD.[13,14] The most serious adverse event after PD is oesophageal perforation, which occurs in 0–16% of patients.[15] About 50% will require surgery depending on the size of the perforation and the degree of contamination. In a recent systemic review, the risk of oesophageal perforation with modern techniques was less than 1%.[16] Perforation occurs more often during initial dilatation, especially with larger balloons (35 mm), older patients, and when there is difficulty keeping the balloon in position.[14] GORD is another potential complication of PD, but these episodes tend to be mild and usually improve with proton pump inhibitors. The addition of botulinum toxin A injection does not appear to improve outcomes.[17]

HELLER MYOTOMY

Heller myotomy, first described by German surgeon Ernest Heller in 1913, has been a standard treatment for achalasia for more than a century. The original method involved the division of muscle fibres of the distal oesophagus and LOS on both the anterior and posterior sides. Nowadays, it has been modified to include an anterior myotomy only. Laparoscopy is the preferred surgical approach compared to thoracoscopic, with better efficacy and a reduced incidence of postoperative gastroesophageal reflux.[18]

✔✔ The addition of a fundoplication is recommended at the time of laparoscopic Heller myotomy (LHM) to reduce the risk of reflux. A partial fundoplication is preferred to Nissen fundoplication as the latter is associated with a higher risk of postoperative dysphagia.[19,20]

Anterior (Dor) or posterior (Toupet) partial fundoplication have similar outcomes after LHM, but the former is simpler because it avoids dissection behind the oesophagus and division of short gastric vessels.[21]

✔✔ LHM with partial fundoplication is the current standard surgical treatment for achalasia. A myotomy with a length of 6 cm on the lower oesophagus and 2–3 cm on the gastric cardia is usually performed.[22]

LHM is safe, with a reported mortality risk of 0.1%.[18] Intraoperative endoscopy is useful to assess the adequacy of myotomy and the most important surgical complication is perforation. Hence, a leak test is usually performed after myotomy with air insufflation through endoscopy (Fig. 14.4). If a leak is detected, the perforation can be repaired with sutures without any consequence. The mean success rate of LHM was about 90% but it reduces to 65–85% after 5 years.[11,18,23] Favourable predictive factors for LHM include young age, type 2 achalasia, and a LOS resting pressure > 30 mmHg.[19,24] Patients with type 3 achalasia or sigmoid oesophagus have poorer functional outcomes after LHM.[8]

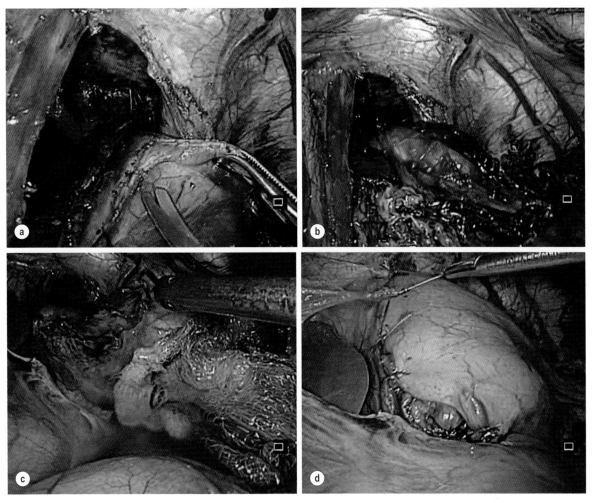

Figure 14.4   Leak test performed after myotomy with air insufflation through endoscopy.

PERORAL ENDOSCOPIC MYOTOMY (POEM)

POEM is the latest treatment for achalasia that was first performed by Professor Haruhiro Inoue in 2010.[25] It is a so-called natural orifice surgery. The procedure is performed under general anaesthesia using CO_2 insufflation during endoscopy. It involves a mucostomy and the creation of a submucosal tunnel from the oesophageal body to the gastric cardia. A myotomy is then performed, followed by the closure of the mucostomy (Fig. 14.5). This procedure has gained wide popularity as it is less invasive to patients.[26,27] It also allows a long myotomy and hence is recommended, especially for type 3 spastic achalasia and diffuse oesophageal spasm (DOS), when the proximal oesophageal muscle is affected.[8] Many studies have confirmed its efficacy in relieving the symptoms of achalasia.[27-32] Operative complications are uncommon. The most significant postoperative side-effect of POEM is gastroesophageal reflux, which happens in 10–50% of patients.[28-33] Unlike Heller myotomy, there is no anti-reflux procedure after POEM. Recently, Inoue et al. performed endoscopic partial fundoplication with clips and loops or sutures during POEM, but the long-term result of this procedure is unknown.[34]

COMPARATIVE TRIALS RESULTS

PNEUMATIC DILATATION VERSUS LAPAROSCOPIC HELLER MYOTOMY

There were at least three randomised studies comparing PD with LHM.[14,35,36]

The largest study is the European Achalasia Trial, in which patients were randomly assigned to Rigiflex dilatation ($n = 94$) or laparoscopic myotomy with Dor fundoplication ($n = 103$).[14] The results showed that their efficacy was similar: 90% for LHM and 86% for PD in 2 years. However, 4% of patients with PD developed oesophageal perforations. Among patients with LHM, 12% had mucosal tears, which were repaired during the procedure without complication. In the long term, although patients who were treated with PD were considered to have equivalent results to LHM patients, 25% required up to three series of repeat dilatations over the 5-year period to maintain their clinical response.

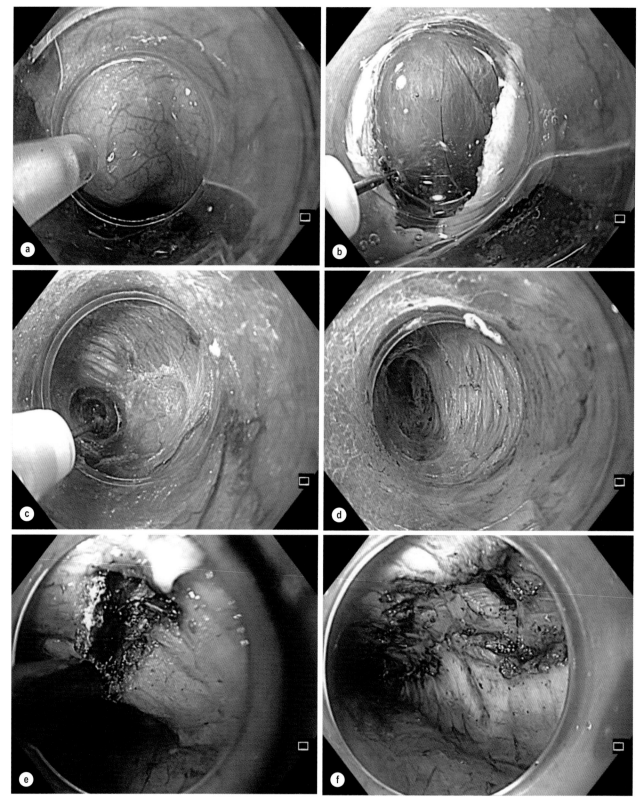

Figure 14.5   (a-g) Peroral endoscopic myotomy.

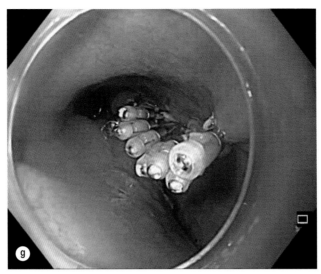

Figure 14.5, cont'd

PERORAL ENDOSCOPIC MYOTOMY VERSUS PNEUMATIC DILATATION

✅✅ In a recent multicentre randomised study comparing POEM ($n = 67$) with PD ($n = 66$), treatment success (defined as an Eckardt score ≤ 3 and the absence of severe complications or re-treatment) at 2 years was 92% in the POEM group compared with 54% in the PD group ($P < 0.001$).[30]

Two serious complications, including one perforation, occurred after PD, while no patients with POEM suffered any serious adverse events. Reflux esophagitis, however, was more common among patients with POEM compared with PD (41% vs 7%, $P = 0.002$). The study supported POEM as an initial treatment option for patients with achalasia.

PERORAL ENDOSCOPIC MYOTOMY VERSUS LAPAROSCOPIC HELLER MYOTOMY

In a recent large multicentre trial in Europe, 221 patients with achalasia were randomised into POEM or LHM with Dor fundoplication.[31] The primary endpoint was clinical success (defined as an Eckardt score ≤ 3) at 2 years. The results showed that the clinical success for POEM and LHM was similar (83% and 81.7%, respectively, $P < 0.007$ for noninferiority). In terms of secondary endpoints, severe adverse events occurred in 2.7% of patients in the POEM group and 7.3% in the LHM group. No patient in the POEM group required surgical repair, but two patients in the LHM group required re-surgery due to perforation. No significant difference was found between the two groups in terms of improvements in oesophageal function, as measured by integrated relaxation pressure of the LOS and the Gastrointestinal Quality of Life Index. On the other hand, reflux esophagitis, as assessed by endoscopy, was higher in the POEM group compared with the LHM group (57% and 20% at 3 months and 44% and 29% at 2 years, respectively).

✅✅ –The authors of a recent large, multicentre randomised trial concluded that the less invasive POEM is non-inferior to LHM in controlling symptoms of achalasia but may result in a higher incidence of gastroesophageal reflux.[31] These results are important for clinicians in decision-making and counselling for patients with achalasia.

SIGMOID OESOPHAGUS

Sigmoid oesophagus is characterised by a grossly dilated (> 6 cm) and tortuous oesophagus, which is considered to be an advanced stage of achalasia. Oesophagectomy is the treatment of choice as a last resort.[22] Laparoscopic Heller myotomy was found to have satisfactory results, even in sigmoid esophagus.[37] A 'pull-down' technique using sutures to straighten the lower oesophagus was described with good outcomes.[38] Recently, POEM has been applied on sigmoid oesophagus and the results have also been promising in selective patients.[39,40] Being a less invasive treatment, POEM can be offered as first-line treatment for sigmoid oesophagus. Surgery can be reserved as a salvage procedure for patients with intractable symptoms.

REVISION PROCEDURES AND THE ROLE OF OESOPHAGECTOMY

Achalasia is a chronic disease and treatment is usually not curative. Up to 20% of patients may require additional treatment regardless of the modality used to treat the disease. Repeat endoscopy and manometry with or without a 24-hour pH-impedance study is useful to identify the cause of recurrent symptoms. Conventionally, repeated pneumatic dilatation or re-do LHM has been used to treat the recurrence. Repeat LHM can be challenging due to previous adhesions, which results in a relatively high perforation rate of 1.5–20%.[41] Recently, POEM was described as an excellent rescue procedure, as the direction of myotomy could be tailored to avoid the scar tissue from the previous myotomy.

✓✓Although there is no head-to-head comparison, a recent meta-analysis showed that POEM was safe and effective for treating patients with achalasia with previous surgical myotomy, with a 90% clinical success rate.[42] Repeat POEM can also be performed in patients who have failed a prior POEM procedure with reasonable success.

Up to 6–20% of treated patients may have progressive dilation due to mega-oesophagus or end-stage achalasia. Oesophagectomy is reserved as a final option in patients with severe oesophageal dilatation and symptoms not responding to dilatation and myotomy. Miller et al. reported good or excellent results in 37 patients with achalasia who underwent oesophagectomy.[43] However, the operation can be technically challenging due to oesophageal dilatation, inflammation, and enlarged paraoesophageal vessels.[44]

OTHER OESOPHAGEAL MOTILITY DISORDERS

DIFFUSE OESOPHAGEAL SPASM

DOS is a rare oesophageal motility disorder characterised by dysphagia and/or chest pain. It is usually diagnosed by HRM, which demonstrates abnormal body contraction (similar to spastic or type 3 achalasia) but with a normal LOS (Fig. 14.6). Barium swallow may show a classical corkscrew appearance. The disease may be self-limiting and reassurance is important. Nitrates, calcium channel blockers, and botulinum toxin A injections have been used. A long myotomy by thoracoscopic technique or more recently by POEM may be required for severe cases.[45] In addition, it is logical that the myotomy can be tailored to the area of spasticity when there are more localised findings at HRM. A concern about long myotomy is that disrupting the oesophageal muscle layer may cause a severely dilated oesophagus in 15–20 years postoperatively. The clinical outcomes of treatment are variable, particularly the response to pain symptoms. It

seems prudent that long myotomy or POEM is considered for patients who have severe symptoms that are refractory to medical treatments. The counselling process should explain the paucity of evidence in the long-term results of these approaches.

NON-SPECIFIC OESOPHAGEAL MOTILITY DISORDERS

With the increasing use of HRM, many non-specific findings are identified such as isolated spasms, high amplitude contractions, or peristaltic waves that do not fulfil the criteria for a normal swallow. Most of these abnormalities are incidental and unlikely to be of clinical significance, and often related to physiological changes associated with ageing. HRM results need to be interpreted cautiously and in consultation with gastroenterologists who have a special interest in motility disorders.[46] Many rheumatological disorders can cause oesophageal dysmotility. The most significant is systemic sclerosis or scleroderma, where patients develop dysphagia with almost no peristaltic activity or LOS tone seen on manometry. These patients can develop reflux and are to be considered for partial fundoplication.

OESOPHAGEAL DIVERTICULAE

Oesophageal diverticula can occur anywhere in the oesophagus and most are acquired rather than congenital. 'False' diverticulae only include mucosa and submucosa herniates, and are most commonly caused by an underlying motility disorder. 'True' diverticulae (usually traction diverticulae) are uncommon and secondary to the oesophagus becoming tethered to an adjacent structure, such as a mediastinal lymph node infected by tuberculosis or histoplasmosis. The tethering leads to a *traction* effect, which causes the diverticulum. The most useful classification is by location, and this also gives a clue as to their aetiology. Upper oesophageal diverticulae or a 'Zenkers diverticulum', are secondary to a hypertensive cricopharyngeus muscle, which causes a pharyngeal pouch to form.

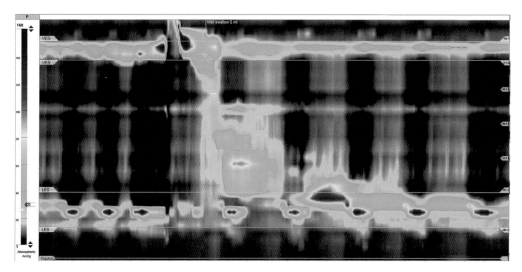

Figure 14.6   High-resolution manometry demonstrating abnormal body contraction with a normal lower oesophageal sphincter.

The diverticulum occurs through 'Killian's triangle' – the area between the thyropharyngeus and cricopharyngeus. The pharyngeal pouch usually forms on the left side of the oesophagus posteriorly. Treatment, if the diverticulum is large enough to be symptomatic (cervical dysphagia, aspiration, regurgitation of undigested food, voice changes, and halitosis), is directed at dividing the hypertensive cricopharyngeus.[47] An open approach is suited to any size diverticulum, the pouch is excised or plicated, and a myotomy is performed. An endoscopic approach can be taken for larger pouches (> 3 cm) where a surgical stapler is used to simultaneously divide the cricopharyngeus and lay the pouch open. Mid-oesophageal diverticulae are traditionally described as traction diverticulae, but with the decrease in tuberculosis most are now secondary to a motility disorder. Epiphrenic diverticulae tend to arise from the posterolateral wall of the oesophagus on the right. The most important part of managing these is identifying the underlying motility disorder – usually achalasia – as excising a diverticulum without addressing the underlying cause is usually futile. A laparoscopic approach can be used with stapled excision of the diverticulum, cardiomyotomy, and a partial fundoplication.

Key points

- With advances in diagnostic investigations, oesophageal motility disorders are increasingly being diagnosed.
- Achalasia is the most common primary oesophageal motility disorder.
- High-resolution manometry has become the gold standard for the diagnosis and classification of achalasia. However, pseudoachalasia needs to be excluded, especially in elderly patients.
- PD, LHM with partial fundoplication, and more recently POEM have evolved as the standard treatment options for achalasia.
- POEM is an effective and less invasive treatment for achalasia, especially in patients who are elderly, with Type III achalasia, or DOS.
- POEM is associated with an increased risk of gastroesophageal reflux compared with LHM or PD. Preoperative counseling and postoperative follow-up is essential.

 References available at http://ebooks.health.elsevier.com/

RECOMMENDED VIDEOS

- Video of Heller cardiomyotomy with a Dor patch for achalasia.

https://www.youtube.com/watch?v=JGzBTQgjNfs

- POEM

https://www.youtube.com/watch?v=dmxpFcAdBFE

- Laparoscopic diverticulectomy + Dor patch

https://www.youtube.com/watch?v=maqN9A7GMI4

ACKNOWLEDGEMENTS

This chapter in the sixth edition was written by Peter Hamer and Peter Lamb, and I am grateful to them for those parts of the chapter that have been retained for this edition. I would also like to thank Dr Jarrod Tan Kah Hwee and Dr Lim Tian Zhi for editing the operation videos.

KEY REFERENCES

[6] Roman S, Huot L, Zerbib F, et al. High-resolution manometry improves the diagnosis of esophageal motility disorders in patients with dysphagia: a randomized multicenter study. Am J Gastroenterol 2016;111(3):372–80. PMID: 26832656.

[7] Yadlapati R, Kahrilas PJ, Fox M, Bredenoord AJ, et al. Esophageal motility disorders on high-resolution manometry: the chicago classification of esophageal motility disorders, v4.0. Neuro Gastroenterol Motil 2021;33(1):e14058.

[8] Kahrilas PJ, Katzka D, Richter JE. Clinical practice update: the use of per-oral endoscopic myotomy in achalasia: expert review and best practice advice from the AGA institute. Gastroenterology 2017;153(5):1205–11.

[14] Boeckxstaens GE, Annese V, des Varannes SB, et al. Pneumatic dilation versus laparoscopic heller's myotomy for idiopathic achalasia. N Engl J Med 2011;364(19):1807–16.

[20] Rebecchi F, Giaccone C, Farinella E, et al. Randomized controlled trial of laparoscopic heller myotomy plus Dor fundoplication versus nissen fundoplication for achalasia: long-term results. Ann Surg 2008;248(6):1023–30.

[22] Zaninotto G, Bennett C, Boeckxstaens G, et al. The 2018 ISDE achalasia guidelines. Dis Esophagus 2018;31(9). https://doi.org/10.1093/dote/doy071.

[30] Ponds FA, Fockens P, Lei A, et al. Effect of peroral endoscopic myotomy vs pneumatic dilation on symptom severity and treatment outcomes among treatment-naive patients with achalasia: a randomized clinical trial. JAMA 2019;322(2):134–44.

[31] Werner YB, Hakanson B, Martinek J, et al. Endoscopic or surgical myotomy in patients with idiopathic achalasia. N Engl J Med 2019;381(23):2219–29.

[42] Huang Z, Cui Y, Li Y, et al. Peroral endoscopic myotomy for patients with achalasia with previous heller myotomy: a systematic review and meta-analysis. Gastrointest Endosc 2021;93(1):47–56. e5.

15 Diaphragmatic hernias and gastric volvulus

Graeme W. Couper

INTRODUCTION

The chapter for this edition has been extended to include three types of diaphragmatic hernias: congenital diaphragmatic hernias, hiatus hernias and the management of gastric volvulus, and traumatic diaphragmatic hernias. All conditions require an understanding of the anatomy and interpretation of appropriate investigations to allow timely and appropriate management.

EMBRYOLOGY AND ANATOMY

The earliest element of the embryological diaphragm, the septum transversum, forms in the cervical region and descends inferiorly. The pleuroperitoneal membranes are a pair of membranes which during week 6 grow medially and ventrally. Their free edges fuse with the dorsal mesentery of the oesophagus and with the septum transversum to separate the pleural and pericardial cavities. Closure of the openings is further enhanced by growth of the liver and muscle tissue extension into the membranes. The right-sided opening closes before that of the left. As a consequence of the origin of the septum transversum, the phrenic nerve supplying the diaphragm originates from the cervical spinal cord at the C3–C5 levels and descends either side of the pericardium. The peripheral portions of the diaphragm send sensory afferents via the intercostal (T5–T11) and subcostal nerves (T12).

The diaphragm is a C-shaped structure made up of peripheral muscle and a central fibrous tendon that separates the thoracic cavity from the abdomen (Fig. 15.1). Anteriorly its fibres insert into the xiphoid process and along the costal margin. Laterally, insertion is into the sixth to twelfth ribs and posteriorly into the twelfth thoracic vertebra. Two appendages, the right and left crus, descend and insert into the lumbar vertebrae, L1–L3 on the right and L1 and L2 on the left. There are two large openings in the diaphragm, as strictly speaking the aorta does not pierce the diaphragm but passes behind it between the left and right crus with the arcuate ligament situated anteriorly. The caval opening passes through the central tendon of the diaphragm. It contains the inferior vena cava and some branches of the right phrenic nerve. The oesophageal hiatus is situated in the posterior part of the diaphragm and is formed by elements of the right diaphragmatic crus.[1] The fibres of the left crus take no part in the boundaries of the oesophageal hiatus. The muscle fibres of the right crus form two bundles separated by connective tissue that diverge to form the right and left pillars of the oesophageal

hiatus. The lateral fibres of each pillar insert directly into the central tendon of the diaphragm while the medial fibres cross each other anterior to the oesophagus. The oesophageal hiatus contains the oesophagus and anterior and posterior vagal trunks.

The oesophagus is fixed to the diaphragm by the phreno-oesophageal ligament. This is formed from the fascia transversalis on the under surface of the diaphragm and fused elements of the endothoracic fascia, and inserts circumferentially into the oesophageal musculature close to the squamocolumnar junction. With increasing age the elasticity of the phrenoesophageal ligament declines, increasing the risk of developing a hiatal hernia.

CONGENITAL DIAPHRAGMATIC HERNIAS

BOCHDALEK HERNIAS

Bochdalek hernias, first described by Bochdalek in 1848, are characterised by a congenital defect on the posterolateral region of the diaphragm that does not contain a hernial sac. Closure of the pleuroperitoneal canal occurs around the eighth week of gestation.[2] Failure of closure results in a characteristic defect through the posterior lumbocostal triangle. Since the right canal closes before the left canal, most Bochdalek hernias (85%) are left sided. Although the majority of these will present in early childhood, congenital defects can present in adulthood.[3] The incidence of adults with asymptomatic Bochdalek hernias has been estimated to be between 0.17% and 6%, although some are suggested to have been acquired during adulthood.[4] The diagnosis of a Bochdalek hernia in adults is not easy and it is commonly misdiagnosed. Unlike infants, who present with respiratory distress in early life, the most frequent symptoms in adults are chest and/or abdominal pain (in 66%) or symptoms of ileus (in 38%).[5] 25% of adult patients are asymptomatic. A variety of abdominal organs may be present in the thorax, which may lead to hypoplasia of the left lung. Retroperitoneal structures including pancreas and kidney may also be present. On chest X-ray Bochdalek hernias may be diagnosed by the presence of gas-filled loops of bowel or a soft tissue mass above the level of the diaphragm (Fig. 15.2). Correct interpretation may however be difficult, as the appearance can be similar to other thoracic pathologies or the more common condition of a paraoesophageal hernia. Computed tomography (CT) of the chest and abdomen allows clear visualisation of the location of the diaphragmatic defect and the herniated abdominal organs (Fig. 15.3). In symptomatic patients surgical repair must be considered.[3] In patients with suspected obstruction or strangulation, an abdominal approach allows reduction and inspection of

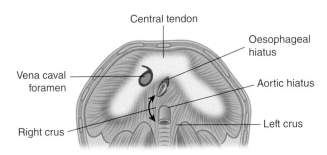

Figure 15.1   Anatomical features of the diaphragm.

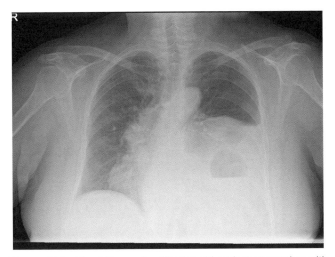

Figure 15.2   Chest X-ray of a 62-year-old patient presenting with worsening symptoms of breathlessness, chest pain, and vomiting. Appearances are of abdominal viscera within the left chest.

the abdominal viscera. It is the author's experience that the margins of the defect are usually of good quality and allow approximation with minimal tension using a non-absorbable suture. If mesh is felt to be necessary to reinforce the repair, a composite form should be considered. A transthoracic repair has been proposed if the bowel does not display signs of strangulation or necrosis due to its technical simplicity in comparison to a midline laparotomy.[3]

FORAMEN OF MORGAGNI HERNIA

In 1769 Morgagni described the herniation of abdominal contents through a triangular diaphragmatic defect between the muscle fibres of the diaphragm that originate from the xiphisternum and the costal margin and insert on the central tendon of the diaphragm.[6] A natural weakness in this retrosternal area arises due to the passage of the internal mammary artery as it becomes the superior epigastric artery with its associated vein and lymphatics. The majority of Morgagni hernias are right sided, with only rare left-sided occurrences because of the protection provided by the pericardial sac. Herniation of abdominal contents is typically caused by an increase in intra-abdominal pressure secondary to trauma, pregnancy, or obesity. Foramen of Morgagni hernias account for 3% of all surgically treated diaphragmatic hernias.[7] In a study of 50 cases, Comer reported that 70% of the patients were female, 90% of the hernias were right sided, and 92% of the hernias had hernia sacs.[8] The most common contents of the hernia were omentum, with 60% containing transverse colon and 12% containing stomach. Only 28% of patients were symptomatic, with symptoms including upper abdominal discomfort, fullness, bloating, vomiting, and bouts of large-bowel obstruction. Investigation is with CT, which may show contrast-filled bowel in the chest or a solid-appearing mass that can be confused with a lipoma. Fine curvilinear or linear densities within the mass

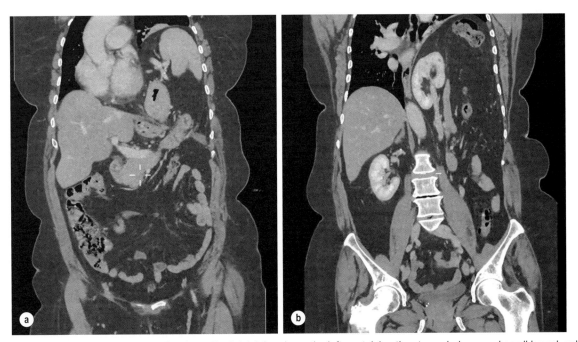

Figure 15.3   Computed tomography scan showing a Bochdalek hernia on the left containing the stomach, large and small bowel, spleen, and left kidney. The patient underwent uncomplicated repair through the abdominal approach. The diaphragm was repaired using Ethibond sutures (Ethicon, New Jersey, USA) without the need for mesh reinforcement.

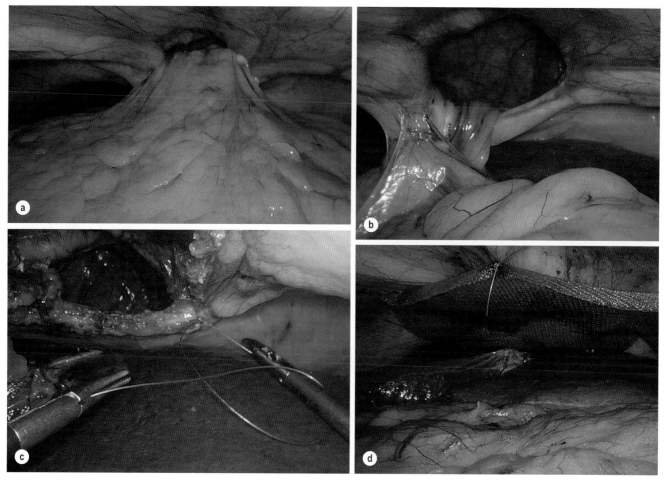

Figures 15.4 (a–d) Laparoscopic repair of a right-sided foramen of Morgagni hernia. The sac contained omentum. (c) The defect was closed with interrupted 2/0 Novafil sutures (Medtronic, Minneapolis, USA) and a (d) composite mesh used to reinforce the repair.

most likely represent vessels within the omentum and confirm the diagnosis.[9] Once confirmed, these hernias should be referred for surgical repair. A laparoscopic abdominal approach is recommended, allowing reduction of the hernia contents, assessment of the abdominal viscera, and repair of the defect (Fig. 15.4). This is achieved with the insertion of non-absorbable sutures and placement of mesh, if required. Resection of the hernia sac is not universally performed.

HIATUS HERNIA

Epidemiology

It is estimated that hiatal hernias occur in approximately 10% of the population, with approximately 15% of these being paraoesophageal hernias. Risk factors include age greater than 50 years, body mass index greater than 25 kg/m^2, and male sex.[10] There is also a familial occurrence that confers a 20-fold increased risk in the younger siblings of children with a hiatal hernia.[11]

Classification of hiatal hernias

Hiatal hernias are classified into four types (Fig. 15.5).

Type I (sliding hiatal hernia)
  Type I hiatus hernias are the most common type and are often diagnosed in patients undergoing investigation for reflux disease. An increase in the diameter of

the oesophageal hiatus and an associated laxity of the phreno-oesophageal membrane allows the upper portion of the gastric cardia to herniate upwards. Although thinned, the phreno-oesophageal membrane remains intact and the herniated gastric cardia is contained within the posterior mediastinum.

Type II, III, and IV (varieties of paraoesophageal hernias)
  These less common types are all varieties of paraoesophageal hernias and account for 5–15% of all hiatal hernias. In addition to reflux, patients often present with chest pain, dysphagia, intermittent vomiting, and worsening respiratory symptoms. True type II hernias are rare and result from a localised defect in the phreno-oesophageal membrane that allows the gastric fundus to herniate upwards. The oesophagogastric junction (OGJ) remains in its normal position fixed to the preaortic fascia and the median arcuate ligament. Type III hernias have elements of both types I and II hernias. With progressive enlargement of the hernia through the hiatus, the phreno-oesophageal membrane stretches, displacing the OGJ above the diaphragm and thereby adding a sliding element to the type II hernia. Type IV hiatus hernia is associated with a large defect in the phreno-oesophageal membrane, allowing other organs such as the colon, spleen, pancreas, and small intestine, to enter the hernia sac.

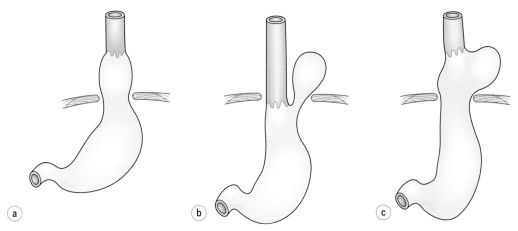

Figure 15.5 Classification of hiatal hernias.

The natural history of a type II hernia is progressive enlargement so that the entire stomach eventually herniates with the pylorus juxtaposed to the gastric cardia, forming an upside-down intrathoracic stomach. Paraesophageal hernias are associated with abnormal laxity of structures which act to prevent displacement of the stomach; the gastrosplenic and gastrocolic ligaments. As the hernia enlarges, the greater curvature of the stomach rolls up into the thorax. Because the stomach is fixed at the OGJ, the herniated stomach tends to rotate around its longitudinal axis, resulting in an organoaxial volvulus. Gastric volvulus may lead to acute gastric obstruction, strangulation, and perforation.

SYMPTOMS AND DIAGNOSIS

Approximately half of all paraoesophageal hernias are clinically silent and become apparent on imaging studies obtained for another indication. Symptomatic hernias may present with epigastric or chest pain, heartburn, postprandial fullness, regurgitation, or dysphagia. Many of the signs and symptoms are non-specific and may mimic those of acute myocardial infarction, gastric ulcer, or pneumonia. The condition may be identified in patients undergoing upper gastrointestinal (GI) endoscopy for investigation of iron-deficiency anaemia. This may be due to chronic blood loss from erosions of the gastric mucosa caused by repeated movement across the hiatus, a phenomenon originally described by Collis in 1961.[12] Cameron lesions/ulcers represent linear gastric erosions and ulcers on the crests of mucosal folds in the distal neck of the hiatus hernia.[13] A chest X-ray may be diagnostic, demonstrating a retrocardiac air-fluid level within a paraoesophageal hernia or intrathoracic stomach (Fig. 15.6). Barium contrast studies are almost always diagnostic and attention should focus on the position of the OGJ in order to differentiate type II and III hernias (Fig. 15.7). Upper GI endoscopy is required to inspect for gastric ischaemia, ulceration or erosion. If a gastric ulcer is present, elective surgery should be delayed until after the ulcer is healed, or after at least 6 weeks of proton pump inhibitor treatment. If manometry is considered, it may not be technically possible due to difficulties positioning the catheter beyond the lower oesophageal sphincter. The lack

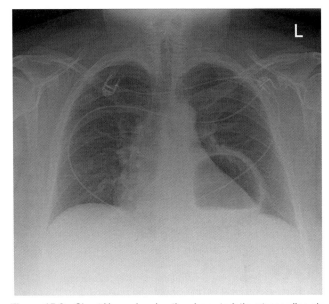

Figure 15.6 Chest X-ray showing the characteristic retrocardiac air-fluid level within a paraoesophageal hernia.

of evidence of the influence of manometry on postoperative outcomes means this is not an essential investigation in these patients.[14,15]

OPERATIVE INDICATIONS

Repair of all symptomatic paraoesophageal hernias is recommended in patients who are medically fit for surgery.[16] Symptoms include those of gastro-oesophageal reflux, vomiting suggestive of gastric outlet obstruction, anaemia, or concern for possible gastric strangulation with patients describing intermittent severe chest pain. The overall condition of the patient clearly influences the decision to operate. The decision on whether to operate on asymptomatic patients is more difficult. Stylopoulos et al. developed a decision analytic model to track a hypothetical cohort of patients with asymptomatic or minimally symptomatic paraesophageal hernias and reflect the possible clinical outcomes associated with two treatment strategies: elective laparoscopic paraesophageal hernia repair (ELHR) or

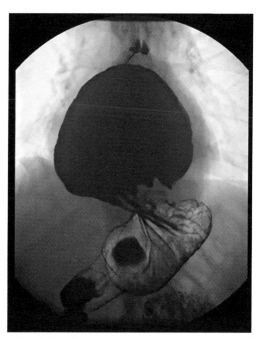

Figure 15.7   Barium swallow and meal showing a large sliding hiatus hernia, with the gastro-oesophageal junction, cardia, fundus, and proximal half of the gastric body lying in the thorax.

watchful waiting (WW).[17] The model predicted that WW was the optimal treatment strategy in 83% of patients, with ELHR in the remaining 17%. The annual probability of developing acute symptoms requiring emergency surgery with the WW strategy was 1.1%, with an associated mortality of 5.4% in comparison to a mortality rate of 1.4% in ELHR. Using similar modelling, Jung et al. reached a similar conclusion with almost identical results.[18]

✓✓ The current recommendation is that all symptomatic paraoesophageal hernias should be repaired.[16] In the case of an elderly, frail patient with significant comorbidities, it may be appropriate to decide on a course of watchful waiting due to the increased risks associated with surgical repair in these patients.[17]

SURGERY FOR PARAOESOPHAGEAL HERNIA

With the laparoscopic technique of paraoesophageal hernia repair now well established and excellent results reported, a transthoracic approach is now rarely advocated. The principles of surgery are: (1) to fully reduce the hernia contents; (2) to excise the hernia sac from the mediastinum; (3) to mobilise the oesophagus to obtain at least 2.5 cm of intra-abdominal oesophagus; (4) to approximate the oesophageal hiatus; and (5) to construct a fundoplication.

REDUCTION OF THE HERNIA CONTENTS

In the majority of patients the hernia contains the proximal stomach and this can be easily reduced at the start of the

procedure (Fig. 15.8a). In patients presenting acutely with distension of the intrathoracic component of the stomach, a period of decompression with an NG tube will reduce the existing oedema and increase the ease with which the stomach can be reduced. This should also increase the likelihood of the procedure being completed laparoscopically.[19,20] CT imaging can demonstrate the sac contents, but the indications to operate should be based on patient symptoms and risk rather than what has actually herniated through the diaphragm. If the contents of the sac cannot be easily reduced, then mobilising the sac at the neck and dissecting the sac free within the mediastinum will allow the sac and its contents to be reduced. Any adhesions between the sac and its contents can then be divided.

DISSECTION OF THE SAC

This should begin at the neck of the sac at the level of the diaphragm. An electrosurgical device such as a harmonic scalpel (Johnson & Johnson), Thunderbeat (Olympus), or other similar device can be useful. Entry into the correct dissection plane allows easy and bloodless dissection of the sac. This can be achieved by clear identification of the muscle fibres on the right or left pillar at the start of dissection. The sac is separated by sweeping the muscle fibres laterally (Fig. 15.8b). With division of the neck of the sac, the majority of the intrathoracic component can be easily mobilised using predominantly blunt dissection. Care must be taken when mobilising the sac from the front wall of the oesophagus, as a traction injury or ischaemia may result in perforation (Fig. 15.8c). Particularly in elderly patients with poor-quality tissues, the surgeon may choose to leave the sac attached to the oesophagus and divide it on either side. The posterior component of the sac must be dissected free to allow approximation of the pillars and achieve an adequate length of intra-abdominal oesophagus (Figs. 15.8d and e).

MOBILISATION OF THE OESOPHAGUS AND OESOPHAGEAL LENGTHENING

In most cases the oesophagus can be easily mobilised within the chest cavity without a significant risk of ischaemia or stricturing. A shortened oesophagus is defined as a OGJ that does not lie more than 2.5 cm below the diaphragmatic hiatus without undue tension, despite adequate surgical mobilisation. The pathophysiology underlying this finding is most probably multifactorial. The original description of a technique creating a functional 'lengthening of the oesophagus' by performing a vertical gastroplasty in order to create a tubular length of neo-oesophagus created from the gastric fundus was made by Collis in 1957.[21] The procedure gained further support following the exceptional results published by the Toronto group on the long-term follow-up outcomes in a group of 500 patients all treated with a cut gastroplasty tube and 360-degree fundoplication, referred to as a total fundoplication gastroplasty.[22] In a follow-up period ranging from 6 to 60 months, 2 patients had proven recurrence (0.4%) and none had reflux. Excellent results occurred in

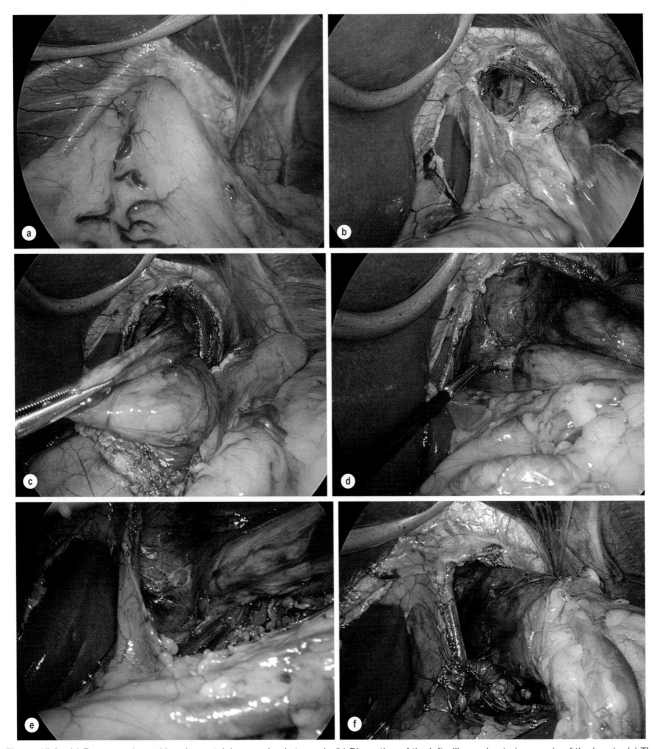

Figure 15.8   (a) Paraoesophageal hernia containing proximal stomach. (b) Dissection of the left pillar and anterior margin of the hernia. (c) The hernial sac is gently dissected from the anterior oesophageal wall. (d) Dissection of the posterior component of the hernia sac. (e) Completed dissection with an adequate length of intra-abdominal oesophagus. (f) Insertion of posterior non-absorbable sutures.

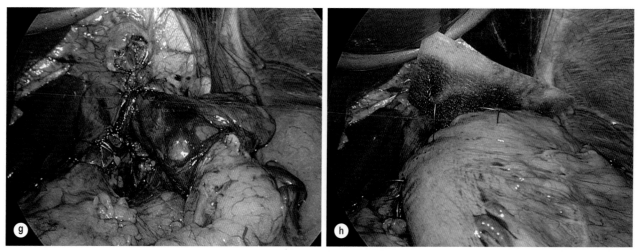

Figure 15.8 Cont'd   (g) Anterior sutures placed. (h) Insertion of an inverse-C biodegradable mesh. (BioA, Gore, Newark, Delaware, USA) and formation of anterior fundoplication.

93.4% (467 patients), improvement in 5% (25 patients), and poor results in 1.6% (8 patients). Repeat operation was necessary in 0.4% (2 patients) for recurrence and in 0.8% (4 patients) for severe dysphagia. In the laparoscopic era different techniques have been described to allow formation of a gastroplasty. An initial paper described a circular stapler technique.[23] This involved the firing of a 25-mm circular stapler 3 cm inferior to the angle of His, adjacent to a 48-Fr intraoesophageal bougie to create a sealed hole through both walls of the stomach. A linear stapler is then inserted through the hole and fired up to the angle of His to create a vertical staple line. Another lengthening technique is the wedge gastroplasty or wedge fundectomy.[24] A point 3 cm below the angle of His and adjacent to a 45–48-F intraoesophageal bougie is marked and an articulated stapler is fired one to three times, starting from the greater curve of the stomach, until the mark is reached. At this point the stapler is oriented upwards and parallel to the intragastric bougie and a final staple line is created. The resulting 'wedge' of gastric fundus is then removed. Oesophageal lengthening has been felt necessary to perform in up to 28% of patients in some series, with this figure increasing to 45% in patients with paraoesophageal hernias.[25]

CLOSURE OF THE OESOPHAGEAL HIATUS

Ideally the hiatus should be approximated without tension to reduce the risk of recurrence. Despite a plethora of techniques, the long-term recurrence rate in several studies is reported to be between 30% and 50%. Reduction in axial tension related to oesophageal shortening can be achieved with adequate mobilisation or a lengthening procedure. Radial tension, due to wide separation of the pillars, is more common and may be more difficult to assess using a laparoscopic approach as opposed to an open technique. Various techniques of closure have been used, and with the wealth of published literature on the subject support can be found for most techniques that are chosen. Simple closure with non-absorbable sutures has been used for both open and laparoscopic repairs (Fig. 15.8f and g). The addition of pledgets to reduce the risk of the sutures tearing out of the pillars has

been reported.[26,27] These can be of a non-absorbable material such as Teflon or a biodegradable material. While the use of pledgets to reinforce hiatal sutures has been reported to show a low early recurrence rate compared to other methods, there are reports of the development of oesophagogastric fistulas due to pledget erosion.[26,27]

The use of mesh around the hiatus remains controversial. The use of a permanent mesh around the hiatus is a concern for many surgeons, with several reports of patients experiencing significant dysphagia and oesophageal erosion following insertion.[28,29] The hiatal region is a dynamic area and movement of the bowel adjacent to a fixed mesh may result in migration of mesh through the bowel wall. As a consequence, the patients may require an oesophagectomy or gastrectomy for correction. Mesh should never be used to bridge a gap in the hiatus when closure of the pillars cannot be achieved as the resulting edge can produce a sawing motion, increasing the risk of erosion.

Several studies have reported initially good short-term results with the introduction of mesh reinforcement of the hiatal closure, but longer follow-up periods often demonstrate comparable results to simple suture closure.[30–34] Due to concerns regarding the use of permanent mesh, trials of alternatives have been reported.[35] Zehetner et al. reported on 35 patients who had reinforcement of crural repair using absorbable Vicryl mesh secured with BioGlue.[36] Follow-up assessment at 1 year or more after surgery was reported for 21 patients. This demonstrated two recurrences (9.5%), with only one of them symptomatic. A similar, larger study of 190 patients who underwent laparoscopic repair of large paraoesophageal hernias with insertion of an absorbable polyglactin mesh secured with BioGlue reported recurrences in 17 patients (15.3%), with a median time to recurrence of 23 months (8–67 months).[37] The estimated recurrence rate at 60 months was 29.5% ± 7.9%. It was noted that the rate of recurrence plateaus over time, with the majority of recurrences being small-to-moderate asymptomatic hernias. A recent review of the use of absorbable meshes in laparoscopic hernia repair concluded that despite high recurrence rates, their use is increasingly accepted due to the majority of recurrences remaining asymptomatic and patients reporting good quality-of-life scores[35] (Fig. 15.8h). A recent publication of a multicentre, prospective, double-blind, randomised controlled trial (RCT) of three methods of hiatus hernia repair – sutures versus absorbable mesh versus non-absorbable mesh – contradicts this conclusion.[31] Of the 126 patients enrolled, 41 had insertion of absorbable mesh, and while no benefit was achieved in terms of recurrence, the side effects of chest pain, diarrhoea, and bloat symptoms were more common after repair with absorbable mesh. Recurrence rates at 5 years follow-up remained high at 39.3% after suture repair, 56.7% in the absorbable mesh group, and 42.9% in the non-absorbable mesh group. A more recent meta-analysis of seven RCTs comparing mesh augmented (non-absorbable mesh: $n = 296$; absorbable mesh: $n = 92$) with sutured repair ($n = 347$) reported no significant differences for short-term hernia recurrence (defined as 6–12 months, 10.1% mesh versus 15.5% sutured, $P = 0.22$), long-term hernia recurrence (defined as 3–5 years, 30.7% mesh vs 31.3% sutured, $P = 0.69$), functional outcomes, and patient satisfaction.[38] The only statistically significant difference was that the mesh repair required a longer operation time ($P = 0.05$, odds ratio [OR] 2.33, 95% CI 0.03–24.69). The report concluded that mesh repair for hiatus hernia does not offer any advantage over sutured hiatal closure.

The long-term risk of recurrence does not appear to be improved with the insertion of mesh. Although recurrence rates remain high, the recurrences often do not cause the severe preoperative symptoms that these patients experience.[38]

RELAXING INCISIONS

Concern regarding the placement of mesh adjacent to the oesophagus has driven some surgical teams to develop alternative strategies to achieve hiatal closure when excessive tension is encountered.[25,39,40] Crespin et al. preferentially chose a right-sided diaphragmatic relaxing incision but performed a left-sided incision if the right pillar was of very poor quality.[39] An incision was made 2 cm lateral to the edge of the crus. After successful approximation, a biologic mesh was sutured in place in a C configuration prior to creation of a fundoplication. Although the rate of recurrence was similar between patients with diaphragmatic relaxing incisions and patients who underwent primary hiatal closure, those who had relaxing incisions were the group with excessive tension. An important point was highlighted in that biologic mesh should not be used to patch a left-sided relaxing incision due to the risk of developing a diaphragmatic hernia. A similar, selective approach to the use of relaxing incisions was reported 2 years previously by Alicuben et al.[25] A combination of techniques were used to try and minimise tension on the hiatal closure. Three patients (4%) had evidence of recurrence at a median follow-up of 5 months. Bradley et al. identified four different hiatal shapes (slit, teardrop, 'D', and oval) that appeared to influence tension and the need for a relaxing incision.[40] A tension gauge was used to measure the tension after hiatal dissection and after relaxing manoeuvres were performed. Tension was reduced by 35.8% after a left pleurotomy (12 patients), by 46.2% after a right crural relaxing incision (15 patients), and by 56.1% if both manoeuvres were performed (6 patients). Long-term

results were not reported. A recent study used a Digital Force Gauge for measuring the tension of crural closure during laparoscopic repair of hiatal hernia.[41] The results suggested that crural closure tension up to approximately 4 N could be the permissible tension threshold for suture cruroplasty, as higher tension often resulted in muscle splitting during cruroplasty.

If performing a relaxing incision on the left side, the defect should not be repaired with a biological mesh due to the risk of developing a diaphragmatic hernia at that site.[39]

CONSTRUCT A FUNDOPLICATION

There are now several studies comparing short- and long-term outcomes of the various fundoplications, and overall there is no agreement on which is superior.[42–44] There is a gathering body of evidence that 'tailoring the wrap' based on preoperative evidence of oesophageal dysmotility does not influence outcome and the author would recommend choosing and performing a single type of fundoplication and doing it well.[14,15] Whichever wrap is utilised, fixation to the diaphragm and oesophagus at various points is recommended with non-absorbable sutures.

RCTs and meta-analyses of RCTs would suggest that no one particular fundoplication is superior to another.[42–44]

POSTOPERATIVE COMPLICATIONS

EARLY RECURRENCE

While longer term recurrence rates remain high at around 40% in some studies and are possibly unavoidable in many cases, early or immediate recurrence represents a life-threatening situation, with patients at risk of aspiration, respiratory compromise, or gastric ischaemia. These recurrences are due to technical issues and may occur in patients where the hiatal defect has not been fully closed, the fundoplication has not been sutured adequately, or the sutures have pulled through poor-quality tissue. The diagnosis can be confirmed on contrast swallow (Fig. 15.9) and patients require an immediate return to theatre. The failure to achieve an adequate repair laparoscopically requires most of these patients to undergo laparotomy. The stomach should be examined for any evidence of ischaemia after reduction from the chest and an open hiatal repair and fundoplication performed. It is the authors' routine practice to pexy the stomach at several points to the anterior abdominal wall after hiatal repair and fundoplication. A previous study that reported on 89 patients undergoing laparoscopic repair without mesh for large hiatus hernias reported a recurrence rate of 15.7% overall.[45] Three factors were associated with hernia recurrence: the absence of an anterior gastropexy, younger patients, and history of abdominal surgery. The authors observed that 10.8% and 50% of recurrences occurred in patients with and without anterior gastropexy, respectively ($P = 0.0028$). In the knowledge that most recurrences are on

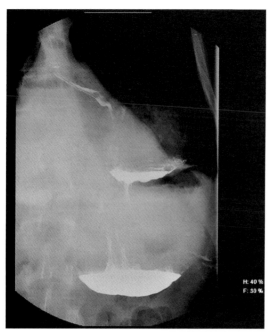

Figure 15.9 Contrast study first day post-laparoscopic repair of the intrathoracic stomach showing reherniation of the stomach into the chest cavity. The operating team returned the patient to theatre for open reduction and repair.

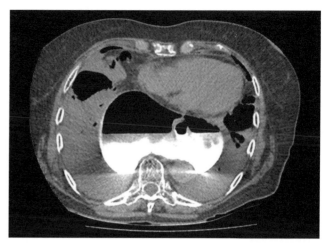

Figure 15.10 Contrast computed tomography scan 48 hours post-laparoscopic repair of an intrathoracic stomach demonstrating a defect in the oesophageal wall with leakage of contrast into the mediastinal cavity. This was felt to be ischaemic in origin. The patient underwent a left thoracotomy with closure of the defect over the t-tube and drainage.

the left side, closure of the phreno-oesophageal ligament as part of the operation has been shown to reduce recurrence rates in the paediatric population.[46] It is the author's routine practice to suture the left pillar to the oesophagus prior to formation of the fundoplication using a continuous non-absorbable suture.

✓✓ Closure of the phreno-oesophageal ligament in the paediatric population has been shown to reduce recurrence rates following fundoplication by over 50%.[46]

OESOPHAGEAL INJURY

As mentioned in the operative section, injury to the oesophageal wall can occur during repair. This may be due to a traction injury on the oesophagus, an effect from an electrosurgical device or diathermy, or ischaemia resulting from removal of the sac from the oesophageal wall (Figs. 15.10 and 15.11). In order to reduce the risks of this occurring, the author does not routinely sling the oesophagus to avoid a traction injury and does not remove the sac from the oesophageal wall if the quality of tissues is felt to be poor. This is most likely to occur in elderly patients.

POST-TRAUMATIC DIAPHRAGMATIC HERNIA

Post-traumatic diaphragmatic hernia (PTDH) can occur after blunt or penetrating trauma.[47] Road traffic accidents are responsible for up to 90% of cases in some series and occurs in 1–7% of patients after major blunt trauma.[48,49] The majority are left sided and are thought to be due to the protective effect of the liver on the right and the reduced strength of the diaphragmatic tissue on the left. The excessive forces

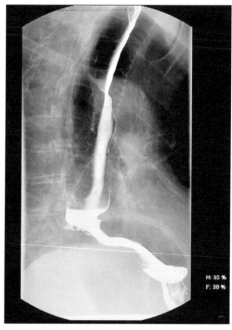

Figure 15.11 Predischarge contrast study showing a healed oesophagus. The patient remains well at 8 years.

required to rupture the diaphragm are associated with injuries to other organs in up to 100% of cases in some reported series.[50] Right-sided ruptures have associated liver injuries in 93% of cases. A significant diaphragmatic breach at the time of injury may result in respiratory distress or be evident on initial imaging. Bilateral and injuries extending into the central tendon of the diaphragm are rare, occurring in only 2–8% of patients.[51] An initial chest X-ray performed in the emergency department may not demonstrate any abnormality (Fig. 15.12). Imaging is with CT of the chest and abdomen with reported sensitivities of 78% for left-sided hernias and 50% for right-sided hernias.[52] Various studies

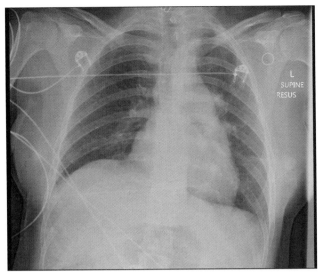

Figure 15.12 Trauma series chest X-ray (CXR) on a patient run over by a car. Computed tomography (CT) imaging demonstrated liver laceration, right kidney laceration, and complex pelvic fracture. No evidence of diaphragmatic injury is seen on CXR or CT.

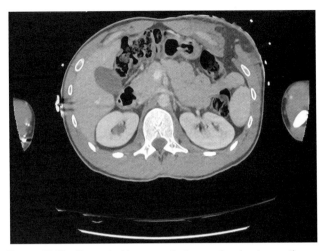

Figure 15.13 Computed tomography image showing traumatic rupture of the diaphragm and costal margin after a high-speed fall onto bike handlebars. Repair was achieved with a direct approach through the costal margin.

have revealed CT to have a variable sensitivity and specificity of 61–87% and 72–100%, respectively, for the diagnosis of diaphragmatic rupture.[53] There are three classical changes which may be evident on CT following blunt trauma: (1) The collar sign (hourglass sign) is a waist-like constriction of the herniated viscera at the margins of the defect (2) The dependant viscera sign. This is seen when the upper third of the liver abuts the posterior ribs on the right and on the left if the stomach or bowel abuts the posterior ribs. This does not normally occur as an intact diaphragm maintains a significant costophrenic angle posteriorly. (3) Discontinuity of the diaphragm sign. Present if there is visualisation of direct discontinuity of the diaphragm along with segmental non-visualisation of the diaphragm.

Penetrating traumatic diaphragmatic injuries can be diagnosed by following the trajectory of the weapon and looking for contiguous injuries to structures on both sides of the diaphragm, commonly a haemothorax or lung injury coupled with a liver injury on the right side or spleen or gastric injury on the left.[53,54] The characteristic CT changes evident following blunt trauma are often not present following penetrating injury. The dependent viscera sign is rarely seen in patients with penetrating injuries. This has been attributed to the small size of the defect and its variable location. For similar reasons the collar sign, which is dependent on the presence of intrathoracic herniation, is often absent in penetrating trauma. Thickening of the diaphragm is a non-specific sign but should suggest a possibility of diaphragmatic injury even if it is the only abnormality present.

Surgical repair is mandatory when a ruptured diaphragm is identified.[55,56] Repair in the acute setting is achieved through an abdominal approach in the majority of cases (Fig. 15.13). Injuries can be missed during exploratory surgery, with one series reporting 14% missed at initial laparotomy.[57] This may be in part due to the difficulty in visualising the hemidiaphragms and the smaller injuries seen in penetrating trauma. Small defects can be closed primarily

with non-absorbable sutures.[51] Larger defects may require a prosthetic mesh to achieve a tension-free closure. If the field is contaminated, alternative methods include the use of biologic mesh, vascularised tissue flaps, or a temporary absorbable mesh with plans for a delayed reconstruction. Insertion of an intercostal drain above the repair is recommended, as patients may develop a reactive pleural effusion. Patients with small tears may have a delayed presentation and present with delayed herniation of intra-abdominal contents (Fig. 15.14a-d). Such patients often present with GI complaints relating to volvulus or incarceration of the abdominal viscera.

✔✔ CT appearances differ between blunt and penetrating diaphragmatic injury.[53] Repair of a traumatic diaphragmatic rupture is mandatory. This should be through an abdominal approach.[51]

GASTRIC VOLVULUS

Gastric volvulus occurs when the stomach rotates > 180 degrees around either its longitudinal axis (organoaxial volvulus) or its horizontal axis (mesenteroaxial volvulus) (Fig. 15.15). Organoaxial volvulus is more common, occurring in two-thirds of cases. The underlying cause in both forms is the elongation of the attachments to the stomach (gastrosplenic, gastroduodenal, and gastrocolic ligaments) to its adjacent structures. While this may occur with the stomach positioned entirely within the abdominal cavity (primary gastric volvulus), it more commonly occurs in patients with a pre-existing paraoesophageal or diaphragmatic hernia (Fig. 15.16). In some patients the finding of a gastric volvulus will be incidental during radiological imaging for unconnected symptoms. The intermittent nature of the condition can make accurate diagnosis difficult, but patients may give a history of abdominal distention/bloating, epigastric or chest pain, heartburn, dysphagia, and early satiety. Patients presenting with acute gastric volvulus have sudden onset of severe epigastric or chest pain and retching but often without significant vomiting. In 1904 Borchardt described

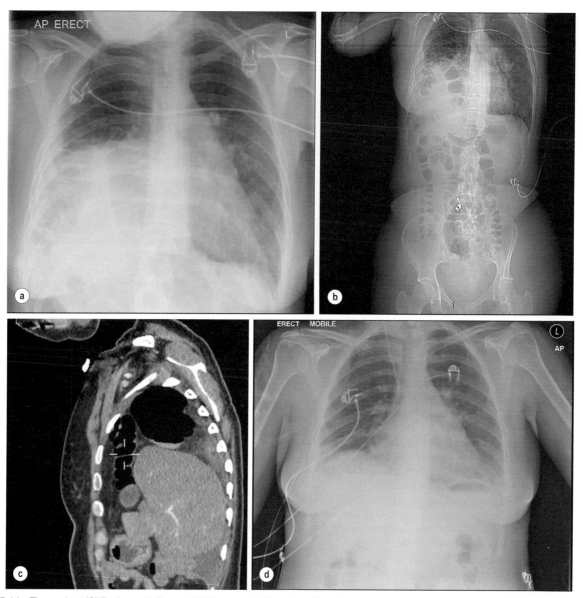

Figure 15.14 The patient (CXR shown in figure 15.12) presented 6 weeks after the accident with sudden onset of right-sided chest pain and breathlessness. Chest X-ray (CXR) on this occasion shows herniation of the intra-abdominal contents through the right side of the diaphragm (a). CT (b and c) shows herniation of the colon and liver with dependant viscera sign. The defect was closed using Ethibond sutures and a composite mesh (Ventralite) to reinforce. (d) Postoperative CXR shows satisfactory appearances.

the three main clinical signs of gastric volvulus, then named the 'Borchardt triad': unproductive retching, localised epigastric distension, and inability to pass a nasogastric tube.[58]

Management of the condition depends on the severity of the symptoms, urgency of presentation, and patient comorbidities. In elderly patients with long-standing mild symptoms, the condition may be managed conservatively. Those patients with severe, acute symptoms need urgent management. The major concern is the development of gastric ischaemia, which may be partly due to the physical twisting of the stomach but also caused by increased intragastric pressure caused by obstruction of the inlet and outlet of a portion or the whole of the stomach. For this reason urgent decompression of the stomach is essential to prevent further injury. The insertion of a nasogastric (NG) tube can prove

difficult due to the twist that has occurred within the stomach. If an NG tube cannot be correctly positioned urgent upper GI endoscopy,decompression and NG insertion must be arranged in the operating theatre. Patients commonly have a raised lactate on presentation and, if after successful NG decompression the patient is well and the lactate improves, endoscopy can be performed later to assess mucosal ischaemia. A period of 48 hours following successful decompression will help reduce the oedema in the stomach and surrounding tissues and increase the chances of performing the required surgery laparoscopically.[19,20]

All patients presenting with acute gastric volvulus should be offered surgery if medically fit. The aim of surgery is to prevent further volvulus and may require repair of the underlying condition in addition to fixation of the stomach.

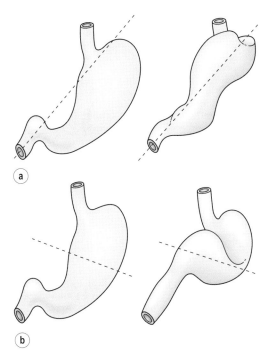

Figure 15.15   Mechanisms of gastric volvulus. (a) Organoaxial rotation. (b) Mesenteroaxial rotation.

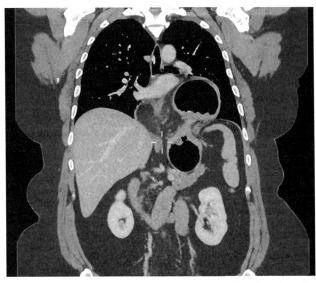

Figure 15.16 Computed tomography scan showing intrathoracic herniation of the stomach. The gastric antrum lies within the thorax, consistent for mesenteroaxial gastric volvulus. The gastrooesophageal junction is subdiaphragmatic.

In patients who are frail, fixation of the stomach to the anterior abdominal wall can be achieved using a double percutaneous endoscopic gastrostomy (PEG) technique.[59] Two PEG tubes are placed, one in the body and one in the antrum of the stomach. In order to achieve this the stomach must be within the abdominal cavity and the colon safely displaced. A combined laparoscopic/endoscopic technique can be utilised when the stomach cannot be endoscopically reduced safely.

Laparoscopic repair of existing paraoesophageal or diaphragmatic hernias should ideally be performed using techniques discussed earlier in the chapter. In addition to creating a fundoplication, the stomach can be sutured to the anterior abdominal wall at several points along the greater curvature and antrum using non-absorbable sutures.[60] Gastropexy alone can be considered in patients deemed unsuitable for a prolonged anaesthetic.[61]

Patients with full-thickness ischaemia need urgent surgery. In some cases the affected portion of the stomach is localised and can be excised with a wedge or sleeve excision. In the rare situation where the majority of the stomach is ischaemic, all non-viable tissue must be excised but any healthy portion of the stomach must be retained to improve the chances of successful future reconstruction. Immediate reconstruction is not always advised and in this situation the distal oesophagus should be taken back to healthy tissue and a Foley catheter placed distally within the oesophagus. This should be pursestringed and exteriorised through the left upper quadrant. To not achieve drainage distally confines the patient to a period of prolonged and uncomfortable NG drainage until reconstruction occurs. If the distal stomach remains viable this can be used as a route for enteral feeding by the insertion of a gastrostomy tube, or if no safe portion of the stomach is available a feeding jejunostomy should be inserted. Subsequent reconstruction should be with a Roux-en-Y reconstruction.

Key points

- Bochdalek hernias can present in adulthood, often with pain or symptoms of obstruction. If symptomatic they should be repaired.
- Foramen of Morgagni hernias should be surgically repaired and this can be achieved with a laparoscopic approach. They are predominantly right sided and most commonly contain omentum.
- Paraoesophageal hernias should be repaired in medically fit, symptomatic patients to prevent the development of potentially life-threatening complications.
- WW is an acceptable management strategy in most asymptomatic individuals, especially the elderly or those with significant comorbidities.
- A shortened oesophagus is defined as a OGJ that does not lie more than 2.5 cm below the diaphragmatic hiatus without undue tension, despite adequate surgical mobilisation. A gastroplasty can be performed if sufficient length cannot be produced by dissection alone.
- In patients with a hiatal defect that cannot be closed without excessive tension, a right-sided diaphragmatic relaxing incision can be performed with a left-sided incision if the right pillar is of very poor quality.
- Mesh reinforcement of the crural closure has not been shown to be of benefit over simple suture closure.
- The majority of PTDHs occur after blunt trauma. Most are left sided and due to the protective effect of the liver on the right and the reduced strength of the diaphragmatic tissue on the left. The excessive forces required to rupture the diaphragm are associated with injuries to other organs in up to 100% of cases in some reported series. Right-sided ruptures have associated liver injuries in 93% of cases.
- Acute gastric volvulus requires urgent decompression via NG tube insertion on presentation to avoid life-threatening complications of gastric strangulation, infarction, and perforation.
- When gastric decompression of acute gastric volvulus can be obtained preoperatively, delaying surgery to allow reduction of inflammation will increase the chances of performing the repair laparoscopically.

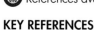 References available at http://ebooks.health.elsevier.com/

KEY REFERENCES

[16] Kohn GP, Price RR, DeMeester SR, et al. SAGES Guidelines Committee. Guidelines for the management of hiatal hernia. Surg Endosc 2013;27(12):4409–28.
A systematic review of published literature with recommendations for the management of hiatal hernias.
[17] Stylopoulos N, Gazelle GS, Rattner DW. Paraesophageal hernias: operation or observation? Ann Surg 2002;236(4):492–501.

A decision analytic model predicted that WW was the optimal treatment strategy in 83% of patients and ELHR in the remaining 17%. The annual probability of developing acute symptoms requiring emergency surgery with the WW strategy was 1.1% with an associated mortality of 5.4% in comparison to a mortality rate of 1.4% in ELHR.
[38] Petric J, Bright T, David S Liu DS, et al. Sutured versus mesh-augmented hiatus hernia repair: a systematic review and meta-analysis of randomized controlled trials. Ann Surg 2021. https://doi.org/10.1097/SLA.0000000000004902. Online ahead of print.
A meta-analysis of seven RCTs comparing mesh-augmented with sutured repair of hiatus hernias. No significant differences in short-term hernia recurrence (defined as 6–12 months, 10.1% mesh vs 15.5% sutured, P = 0.22), long-term hernia recurrence (defined as 3–5 years, 30.7% mesh vs 31.3% sutured, P = 0.69), functional outcomes, and patient satisfaction were reported.
[39] Crespin OM, Yates RB, Martin AV, et al. The use of crural relaxing incisions with biologic mesh reinforcement during laparoscopic repair of complex hiatal hernias. Surg Endosc 2016;30(6):2179–85.
Study comparing the outcomes of primary closure of the hiatus, primary closure with biologic mesh reinforcement, and relaxing incision with biologic mesh reinforcement.
[42] Broeders JA, Roks DJ, Jamieson GG, et al. Five-year outcome after laparoscopic anterior partial versus Nissen fundoplication. Four randomized trials. Ann Surg 2012;255(4):637–42.
[43] Broeders JA, Roks DJ, Ali UA, et al. Laparoscopic anterior versus posterior fundoplication for gastroesophageal reflux disease. Systematic Review and Meta-Analysis of Randomized Clinical Trials. Ann Surg 2011;254:39–47.
[44] Broeders JA, Mawitz FA, Ali UA, et al. Systematic review and meta-analysis of laparoscopic Nissen (posterior total) versus Toupet (posterior partial) fundoplication for gastro-oesophageal disease. BJS 2010;97:1318–30.
Three publications that lend support to the evidence that no single fundoplication has superiority over another.
[46] St Peter SD, Valusek PA, Calkins CM, et al. Use of esophagocrural sutures and minimal esophageal dissection reduces the incidence of postoperative transmigration of laparoscopic Nissen fundoplication wrap. J Pediatr Surg 2007;42(1):25–9.
A study of 249 children undergoing Nissen fundoplication, 130 patients without oesophagocrural sutures and 119 with repair of phreno-oesophageal ligament. The wrap migration rate reduced from 12% to 5% with closure.
[51] Ties JS, Peschman JR, Moreno A, et al. Evolution in the management of traumatic diaphragmatic injuries: a multicenter review. J Trauma Acute Care Surg 2014;76(4):1024–8.
A total of 454 patients were included, 87% were men. Minimally invasive repairs increased over the study time period. Complex repairs (mesh, transposition) were required in only three patients. In-hospital mortality was 15% and 4% for blunt and penetrating traumatic diaphragmatic injury, respectively (P < 0.001).
[53] Panda A, Kumar A, Gamanagatti S, et al. Traumatic diaphragmatic injury: a review of CT signs and the difference between blunt and penetrating injury. Diagn Interv Radiol 2014;20(2):121–8.
The discontinuous diaphragm sign was the most common sign. Organ herniation was observed more often in blunt trauma. Contiguous injury on either side of the diaphragm was observed more often in penetrating trauma.

Specialist oesophagogastric emergencies

16

Shajahan Wahed

INTRODUCTION

This chapter focuses on the diagnosis and management of injuries to the oesophagus and stomach from a variety of different insults, resulting in a spectrum of damage. It will deal with perforations of the oesophagus as a grouped entity, caustic injuries to the oesophagus and stomach, management of foreign body ingestion, and difficult gastroduodenal perforation. It will not deal with the management of routine gastroduodenal perforations or upper gastrointestinal bleeding. These topics will be covered in the companion series volume *Core Topics in General and Emergency Surgery*. Management of acute gastric volvulus and paraoesophageal hernia is covered in Chapter 15 in this volume.

PERFORATION OF THE OESOPHAGUS

Most clinicians gain limited exposure to patients with oesophageal injury due to its rarity. Misdiagnosis, incorrect investigations, and inappropriate and delayed management are common as a result. The difficulty in accessing the oesophagus, its unusual blood supply, the lack of a strong serosal layer, and the proximity of vital structures make clinicians wary. The clinical experience is compounded by a lack of evidence for management, with much of the published literature limited to observational studies. Diagnostic and treatment strategies vary widely.[1] Mortality rates with oesophageal injury have improved but remain high. Management in centres dealing with higher volumes of oesophageal-related problems can improve the chances of a successful outcome.[2]

The management of such injuries is actually straightforward to a clinician who regularly accesses the oesophagus and stomach, and is familiar with the basic principles to minimise morbidity and mortality. Hopefully the outcomes from these injuries will improve with the ongoing reconfiguration of services for patients with upper gastrointestinal disease and the provision of dedicated specialist units.

Partial- and full-thickness perforations of the oesophagus can result from a spectrum of conditions. The underlying aetiology influences the type of disruption and the degree of contamination. Mediastinal and pleural contamination can give rise to a massive systemic inflammatory response and sepsis.

Iatrogenic injuries continue to be the most common aetiology, particularly given the increase in therapeutic endoscopic interventions. The key to diagnosing an oesophageal injury is to have a high index of suspicion following any endoscopic oesophageal procedure and recognise the possibility at the time of the event. It is far better for the patient if the clinician errs on the side of caution and instigates appropriate management if a perforation is suspected. This can always be stepped down if subsequent investigations exclude a full-thickness perforation.

The rare, eponymous Boerhaave's syndrome of spontaneous perforation of the oesophagus occurs in the absence of pre-existing pathology. Minor differences in management can lead to major outcome improvements. Penetrating and blunt injuries to the oesophagus are similarly uncommon and misdiagnosis often compounds any injury.

AETIOLOGY AND PATHOPHYSIOLOGY

IATROGENIC PERFORATION OF THE OESOPHAGUS

Iatrogenic damage to the oesophagus leading to full-thickness disruption occurs from within in 60–70% of cases, such as during endoscopic instrumentation, or from without, such as during paraoesophageal or thoracic lung surgery. Diagnostic flexible endoscopy remains a safe procedure when performed by appropriately trained individuals. However, the sheer numbers of endoscopies performed have led to an overall increase in perforations. Flexible endoscopy (0.03% perforation risk) has almost totally replaced rigid oesophagoscopy (0.11% perforation risk).[3] There are very few indications to perform a rigid endoscopy and there is no longer a role for food bolus removal with rigid oesophagoscopy given the safer flexible endoscopic techniques.

Intubation of the oesophagus can cause proximal perforation, with the risk increased by hyperextension of the neck and the presence of arthritic cervical osteophytes or an oesophageal diverticulum. However, in 75–90% of diagnostic perforation cases trauma is sustained to the distal oesophagus, often in conjunction with an abnormality.

The majority of oesophageal full-thickness perforation occurs during endoscopic interventions (Table 16.1).[4] Balloon or Savary–Gilliard dilatation of strictures accounts for most perforations. This risk is increased in patients with a malignant stricture, previous radiotherapy, or chemotherapy. The risk from self-expanding metal stents for palliating malignant strictures is lower. Stents placed for other reasons such as attempted treatment of anastomotic disruption or benign strictures can erode through the oesophagus at other sites. Stents not placed for palliation of malignancy should therefore be removed in a timely manner to avoid such situations. Endoscopic mucosal and submucosal resection for

Table 16.1   Risk of iatrogenic oesophageal disruption through instrumentation

Medical Instrumentation	Percentage Risk of Iatrogenic Oesophageal Disruption
Dilatation	0.5
Dilatation for achalasia	2
Endoscopic mucosal resection	2
Stent placement	2
Endoscopic thermal therapy	1–2
Treatment of variceal bleeding	1–6
Endoscopic laser therapy	1–5
Photodynamic therapy	5
Stent placement	5-25

dysplastic or intramucosal adenocarcinoma also carries a perforation risk of up to 2%.

Treatment for achalasia with pneumatic dilatation has a higher perforation risk than standard balloon dilatation due to the higher pressures and larger balloon size.[5] The risk can be minimised by always starting at the smallest balloon size (30 mm) for the initial dilatation.[6] Per oral endoscopic myotomy (POEM) is a newer treatment for achalasia, with some evidence for its consideration alongside surgical myotomy and pneumatic dilatation.[7] POEM has its own perforation risk.

All other modalities of oesophageal intubation including nasogastric tube placement, transoesophageal echocardiogram, and inadvertent oesophageal placement of an endotracheal tube can result in oesophageal perforation.[4] In contrast to some guidelines advocating blindly pushing through a food bolus, caution should be exercised in performing this manoeuvre unless it is known for certain that the distal lumen is not obstructed by a stricture, either benign or malignant. Pushing a food bolus distally should ideally only be done if the endoscope can pass the bolus and confirm there is no distal obstruction, although often this is not possible.

Mortality rates have improved over the years, but iatrogenic perforation of the oesophagus can still be a life-threatening condition. A case review of 75 patients with iatrogenic perforation reported a not insubstantial mortality rate of 19%. Prevention is the best solution, with continued efforts to increase awareness and training likely to reduce the incidence.[8]

SPONTANEOUS PERFORATION OF THE OESOPHAGUS

Boerhaave's syndrome is characterised by barogenic trauma in an otherwise normal oesophagus, leading to immediate and gross gastric content contamination of the mediastinum and often of the pleural cavity. The ensuing chemical and septic mediastinitis can precipitate a rapid deterioration in the patient's condition. The actual degree of damage to the oesophagus and ensuing contamination can vary considerably. The disruption of the oesophageal wall is associated with a sudden increase in intra-abdominal pressure. In most cases this is related to vomiting or retching, although weightlifting, parturition, defecation, the Heimlich manoeuvre, and status epilepticus have all been implicated in the past. The fact that vomiting is common but oesophageal perforation is not suggests as yet unrecognised anatomical or pathological abnormalities may exist. In apparent 'spontaneous perforation', an underlying cause such as malignancy, peptic ulceration, or infection is discovered in up to 20% of cases. Eosinophilic oesophagitis can also predispose to oesophageal perforation, spontaneously after vomiting to dislodge an impacted food bolus, or after endoscopic intervention.[9] The mechanism of a spontaneous perforation differs from that of a Mallory–Weiss tear, as the forces resulting in the latter are shearing in nature as opposed to the barogenic force in a perforation.[10]

The most common location for a spontaneous perforation is just above the oesophagogastric junction in the left posterolateral position. The perforation usually occurs in a solitary location, 1–8 cm long, with the disruption longer on the mucosal side than the adventitial side. In cases where the pleura is disrupted, this can occur at the time of the barogenic event or subsequently as a result of gastric acid erosion, exacerbated by intrathoracic pressure.

PENETRATING INJURIES

Penetrating injuries of the oesophagus are rare but associated with significant morbidity and mortality. The overwhelming majority of penetrating injuries to the oesophagus are associated with significant injury to the surrounding tissues and organs. The oesophageal injury can be overlooked at the time of initial presentation when the management of more immediately life-threatening vascular, cardiac, or lung injuries takes precedence. However, a delay in identifying and managing such oesophageal injuries increases the morbidity and mortality from the injury.[11–13] Injury should be suspected in any gunshot or knife wound to the cervical or mediastinal regions. The degree of disruption is dependent on the type of weapon involved and the velocity of any projectile. High-velocity projectiles will cause far greater damage due to the cavitation effect while lower velocity projectiles might result in more limited injury. The injury severity can be graded according to the American Association for the Surgery of Trauma.

Penetrating injuries from within are much less common, with causes including ingestion of sharp objects, fish or meat bones, and swallowed dentures (Fig. 16.1). The mechanism of penetrating injuries from within more often follows a pattern similar to iatrogenic or spontaneous perforation.

BLUNT TRAUMA

Blunt trauma that causes significant injury to the oesophagus is rare. The mechanism is almost exclusively high-impact trauma such as road traffic collisions and it is often associated with more immediately life-threatening injuries of the airway, heart, or lungs. The cervical oesophagus is at risk from severe flexion-extension of the neck or from impact of the neck or upper chest on the steering wheel. The fixed points of the oesophagus at the cricoid, carina, and pharyngo-oesophageal junction are most susceptible to rapid deceleration traction laceration. Barogenic damage can occur after a sudden rise in intra-abdominal pressure from compression against a closed glottis. Secondary injury to the oesophagus can occur following interruption of vascular supply.

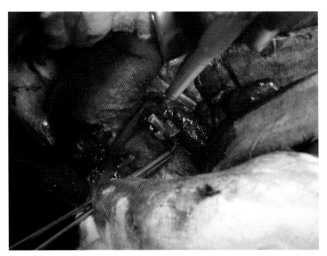

Figure 16.1 Full-thickness oesophageal perforation secondary to swallowed dentures.

Blast injuries to the oesophagus are exceedingly rare. There are few reports in the literature.

CLINICAL PRESENTATION

The clinical features depend upon the cause, site, and time from injury. Iatrogenic injuries ought to be recognised at the time of the event or confirmed shortly afterwards with appropriate investigation. The presentation of patients with spontaneous perforation or blunt trauma-related injury can be tenuous. The classical Mackler's triad in spontaneous perforation of vomiting, chest pain, and subcutaneous emphysema is actually an uncommon presentation. It was present in only 7 of 51 patients (14%) in one large case series.[14,15] As a result, the diagnostic error on spontaneous perforation is high, with only 5% of cases diagnosed at presentation. This can lead to diagnostic delays of greater than 12 hours[16] (Box 16.1). As time passes, the critical condition of the patient further obscures relevant clinical features and the pursuit of incorrect investigations can make the diagnosis even more elusive.

Depending on the aetiology and amount of contamination, pain may be severe, constant, retrosternal or epigastric, distressing, exacerbated by movement and poorly relieved by narcotics, or relatively mild. Dysphagia and odynophagia are common. Patients can be tachypnoeic and may sit up to splint their diaphragm. Abdominal pain or tenderness are not uncommon and can lead to a negative laparotomy, although this is less likely with computed tomography (CT) imaging. Subcutaneous emphysema takes time to develop; mediastinal emphysema precedes this and may be visible on a plain chest radiograph. With time the negative intrathoracic pressure draws air, food, and fluid into the mediastinum and pleural cavities. Chemical and microbial pleuromediastinitis develops. Pyrexia ensues, with the sympathetic nervous system response leading to pallor, sweating, peripheral circulatory shutdown, tachycardia, tachypnoea, and overt haemodynamic shock. This worsens as the systemic inflammatory response gives way to sepsis. Within 24–48 hours cardiopulmonary embarrassment and collapse develop as a consequence of overwhelming bacterial mediastinitis and septic shock. The combination of chest pain and shock may inappropriately, but all too commonly, lead to a cardiology

> **Box 16.1 Common misdiagnoses for spontaneous perforation of the oesophagus**
>
> **Medical**
> • Myocardial infarction
> • Pericarditis
> • Spontaneous pneumothorax
> • Pneumonia
> • Oesophageal varices/Mallory-Weiss tear
>
> **Surgical**
> • Peritonitis
> • Acute pancreatitis
> • Perforated peptic ulcer
> • Renal colic
> • Aortic aneurysm (dissection/leak)
> • Biliary colic
> • Mesenteric ischaemia

> **Box 16.2 Typical chest radiograph findings in spontaneous perforation of the oesophagus**
>
> • Pleural effusion
> • Pneumomediastinum
> • Subcutaneous emphysema
> • Hydropneumothorax
> • Pneumothorax
> • Collapse/consolidation

referral. Survival is dependent on treating sepsis, providing organ support as required, and evacuating contamination from the mediastinal and pleural cavities at the earliest possible opportunity.[17]

Systemic effects are less common when the cervical oesophagus is damaged, with neck pain, torticollis, dysphonia, cervical dysphagia, hoarseness, and subcutaneous emphysema predominating.

Penetrating oesophageal trauma manifests in the same pattern but a high index of suspicion based on the likely tract of the insult is essential for diagnosis. Any deep penetrating transcervical or transmediastinal injury, especially gunshot derived, should be deemed suspicious for oesophageal trauma. In contrast, blunt trauma rarely causes oesophageal injury, but in high-impact events a high index of suspicion should be exercised and injury actively excluded.

INVESTIGATIONS

PLAIN RADIOGRAPHY

The typical findings on plain chest radiography are subtle and dependent on the site and the time interval following the insult. These are documented in Box 16.2 and Fig. 16.2. A plain abdominal radiograph may help to exclude a perforated intra-abdominal viscus.[16]

COMPUTED TOMOGRAPHY

Urgent CT is the first-choice imaging modality and should not be delayed when the diagnosis is suspected. With the

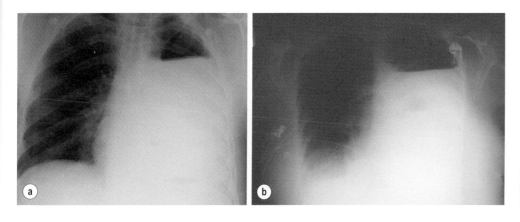

Figure 16.2 Typical chest radio-graph findings of intrapleural oe-sophageal perforation.

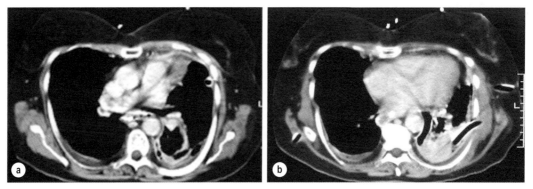

Figure 16.3 Computed tomography appearances of spontaneous oesophageal perforation. (a) Left pleural hydropneumothorax. (b) Left basal intercostal chest drain in the same patient as in (a).

advent of modern scanners, CT with intravenous contrast should be sensitive enough to identify the site of an oesophageal perforation, although some radiologists still prefer to also administer oral contrast.[18] In an intubated patient, the sensitivity of CT for spontaneous perforation is increased by placing a nasogastric tube just past the cricopharyngeus to run in a small amount of contrast media, although in practice this is now rarely performed (Fig. 16.3).[19] It is useful to evaluate images with a radiologist who specialises in (upper) gastrointestinal radiology if at all possible. CT is especially helpful in multi-trauma and critically ill patients with an atypical presentation.

In combination with complex interventional radiology, CT has also revolutionised the management of intrathoracic collections. It plays a vital role in assessing the progress of patients, be that after non-operative or operative management.

CONTRAST RADIOGRAPHY

Oral water-soluble contrast radiography ascertains the site, the degree of containment, and the degree of drainage of the perforation (Fig. 16.4). Aqueous agents are rapidly absorbed, do not exacerbate inflammation, and have minimal tissue effects. However, false-negative results in 27–66% and the limited applicability to a collapsed, unwell patient have downgraded their usefulness. In assessing healing of a perforation, the author would advocate the use of dilute barium to ascertain the presence or absence of any ongoing leak if water-soluble contrast studies were negative.

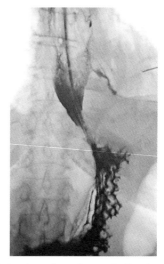

Figure 16.4 Contrast swallow demonstrating free extravasation of contrast media after oesophageal perforation during balloon dilatation of achalasia.

UPPER GASTROINTESTINAL ENDOSCOPY

Endoscopic assessment by an experienced endoscopist excludes the diagnosis if normal, influences management if underlying pathology is discovered, and facilitates the placement of a nasojejunal tube to allow enteral feeding (Figs. 16.5 and 16.6). Endoscopy can be performed in the sickest of patients, in the critical care unit, or in theatre, when other injuries or instability of the patient preclude radiological assessment.

It is often safest to perform endoscopy in suspected spontaneous perforation under a general anaesthetic with the patient intubated. This can allow for positive-pressure ventilation to reduce the risk of cardiorespiratory embarrassment by air insufflation into the mediastinum and pleural spaces. This risk is minimised by introducing the endoscope without insufflation and using suction to drain fluid from any cavity. It is important to be prepared for rapid chest decompression if chest drains are not already in situ. Otherwise endoscopy should be performed with an anaesthetist present and ready to intubate should the patient become unstable.

✅ In a retrospective review of 55 trauma patients, Horwitz et al. demonstrated 100% sensitivity and 92.4% specificity for upper gastrointestinal endoscopy in confirming oesophageal perforation, and although injuries were infrequent (prevalence 3.6%), no injuries were missed and the examination was safe.[20] In a similar study of 31 patients, endoscopy had a sensitivity of 100% and a specificity of 96% with no associated morbidity.[21] Endoscopy has also been used to examine the oesophagogastric anastomosis post-oesophagectomy without additional morbidity.[20–23]

OTHER INVESTIGATIONS

Thoracocentesis of gastric contents is diagnostic – a pH of less than 6.0, a high amylase, or microscopic squamous cells in the fluid can also confirm oesophageal perforation. Swallowed or injected oral/nasogastric dyes, such as methylene blue, may be diagnostically useful if a communicating drain is in situ. Dye staining can, however, be troublesome in the operative field if surgery is subsequently required.

MANAGEMENT

The rarity and severe consequences of inappropriate treatment have limited the ability to evaluate management options. Published observational case series often span many years, many centres, many surgeons, and many techniques. Survival is dependent on managing sepsis and controlling mediastinal and pleural infection, so surgery remains mandatory when gross contamination is present. Non-operative treatment has become standard for iatrogenic trauma where contamination is more limited and delay in diagnosis is uncommon. Patients require a multidisciplinary approach

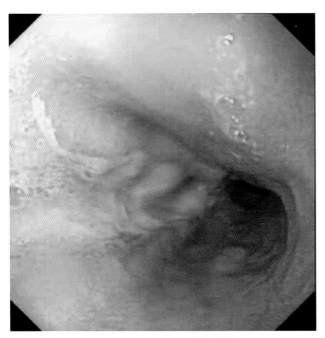

Figure 16.5 Endoscopic appearance of full-thickness spontaneous oesophageal perforation.

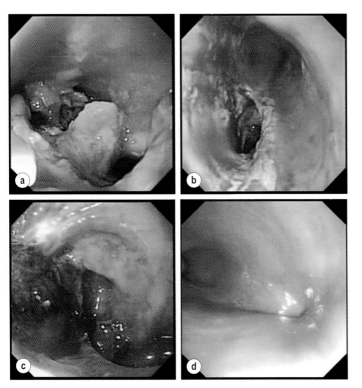

Figure 16.6 Endoscopic appearance of iatrogenic perforation. (a) Food bolus with false iatrogenic lumen alongside. (b) Appearance after food bolus removed. (c) Contained mediastinal cavity. (d) 6 weeks later following conservative management a small pit remains.

> ### Box 16.3 Initial resuscitation in spontaneous oesophageal perforation
>
> - Control of airway and supplementary oxygen
> - Large-bore intravenous access and intravenous fluid resuscitation
> - Intravenous broad-spectrum antibiotics and antifungals
> - Intravenous proton pump inhibitors
> - Strictly nil by mouth
> - Urethral catheterisation and fluid balance monitoring
> - Early anaesthetic and critical care involvement
> - Intercostal chest drainage (possibly bilaterally)
> - Nasogastric tube (placed under endoscopic or radiological guidance)
> - Enteral feeding access (nasojejunal tube or feeding jejunostomy)
> - Multidisciplinary approach with low threshold for aggressive/operative intervention

> ### Box 16.4 Criteria for non-operative management of oesophageal perforation
>
> - Perforation contained by mediastinal pleura
> - No solid food contamination of mediastinal or pleural spaces
> - Drainage of contrast back into the oesophagus on contrast swallow
> - No symptoms or signs of mediastinitis
> - Perforation through an oesophageal malignancy
> - Tolerance to pleural or mediastinal contamination with appropriate drainage

with input from intensive care, radiology, physiotherapy, dieticians, and rehabilitation services. Hospitals lacking these specialist facilities or the versatile surgical cover necessary to deal with the oesophagus by abdominal or left or right thoracic operative approaches should transfer these patients. This should occur at the earliest opportunity after stabilisation, as deterioration can be rapid and unpredictable.[4,24,25]

All patients with an oesophageal perforation can be critically ill. The immediate priorities are the establishment of a secure and adequate airway, stabilisation of cardiovascular status, analgesia, broad-spectrum antibiotics, antifungals, and antisecretory medication. Regular reassessment is obligatory, as an initially stable patient can rapidly decompensate. An early anaesthetic review is recommended. Box 16.3 documents the initial resuscitation.

NON-OPERATIVE MANAGEMENT

Non-operative, endoscopic, and minimally invasive operative management have all been shown to be safe and feasible in carefully selected patients who have either been diagnosed with minimal contamination and no mediastinitis or with a contained perforation. It may also be considered in those with a delayed diagnosis who have demonstrated tolerance. Non-operative treatment is not 'conservative'. Patients require intensive observation and a low threshold for intervention, with 20% of patients requiring aggressive surgical salvage.

Non-operative treatment comprises observation in a critical care environment with patients kept nil by mouth and preferably fed enterally, if necessary via a feeding jejunostomy. A nasogastric tube should be placed under endoscopic and/or radiological assistance past the perforation to decompress the stomach and to limit refluxate, especially in distal oesophageal perforations. Contrast radiology, endoscopy, and CT are used to monitor the status of the perforation. Collections should be drained. The timing of investigations is guided by the clinical condition of the patient, but weekly contrast or CT studies are not unreasonable. All patients should be given broad-spectrum intravenous antibiotics, and antifungal and antisecretory agents.

Iatrogenic cervical perforations are usually contained and thus managed non-operatively with percutaneous drainage of collections where necessary. Any resulting oesophagocutaneous fistulas heal rapidly in the absence of

distal obstruction. Operative prevertebral lavage, primary closure, and drainage via a left lateral incision anterior to the sternocleidomastoid is occasionally required and is well tolerated by even critically ill patients.

Criteria have been developed to aid the selection of suitable patients for non-operative management.[4,15,26] These are detailed in Box 16.4. Other factors requiring consideration include control of the perforation, excluding underlying oesophageal disease, absence of septic shock, and the ability to change the management strategy promptly if required. Case series applying these criteria demonstrate a mortality rate between 0% and 24%, but numbers are small and results are skewed by both selection and publication bias.

ADJUNCTS TO NON-OPERATIVE MANAGEMENT

An endoluminal approach can be used to support patients undergoing non-operative management and can replicate some of the principles of open surgery. This is pertinent in patients where the benefits of surgical exploration are outweighed by the risk and the ultimate outcome (in advanced or perforated cancer, for instance), or in patients in whom the defect is small, clean, and easily dealt with at the time of injury. All endoscopic approaches are technically difficult and should not be attempted by inexperienced operators unable to deal with the consequences of their actions. The mediastinitis, cardiorespiratory compromise, and sepsis accounts for mortality in these patients and not the actual underlying defect. Any endoluminal therapy should not be viewed as the sole definitive solution: ongoing active management is required. In many situations where endoluminal stents or clips have been used, it is apparent that the perforation would have healed with the above non-operative measures and without the endoluminal adjunct. This has to be borne in mind, especially when stents themselves can cause significant complications, including erosion and bleeding.

Closure: clips and sealants

Endoclips are well established in closing small, clean defects after endoscopic mucosal resection or submucosal dissection for early cancer and there are a few reports of endoscopic suturing.[27,28]

✓✓ In the absence of significant contamination, small iatrogenic perforations may be closed immediately using endoclips in addition to supportive non-operative treatment.[29] Endoclipping 'en face' in the oesophagus is challenging and should only be attempted by highly skilled endoscopists. It is also debatable whether this significantly alters the clinical course over a simple non-operative approach.

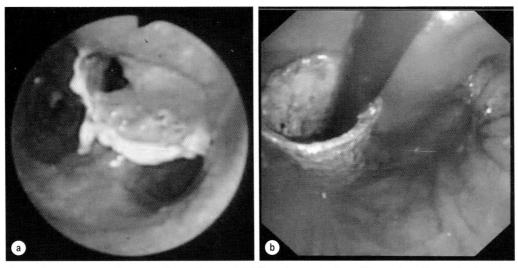

Figure 16.7   Endoscopic appearance of a septically eroded stent. (a) Bronchoscopic view of the carina with proximal stent erosion. (b) J-view of distal stent clearly lying in the proximal stomach, allowing free reflux into the airways.

There are a limited number of case reports of through-the-scope and over-the-scope clipping of spontaneous oesophageal perforation, but this cannot be recommended in the face of gross contamination.[30,31]

Diversion: stents

Self-expanding stents have been used to seal oesophageal perforations, chronic fistulas, and even postoperative anastomotic leaks.[32] Stents were not designed for use in a normal oesophagus. Migration rates approach 30% and concerns have been raised in terms of extending the defect through pressure necrosis and through the trauma of their subsequent removal.[33] Publication bias means that failure and the consequences of failure remain unknown. There is considerable variation in the timing of stent placement and number of stents used. It is evident that the majority of cases also involve aggressive non-operative management.[33–36] It is therefore difficult to attribute successful outcomes to the stent placement alone. One prospective stenting study lists 10 patients with a Boerhaave's perforation.[37] Stent migration was high (11 out of 33) and there was a 50% complication rate (bleeding/stent fracture/impacted stent) if stents were not removed before 6 weeks.

There is insufficient evidence to support the routine use of oesophageal stents in oesophageal perforations. The author suggests that their use is selective and should always be viewed as a temporary solution.

In patients whose physical condition precludes more aggressive treatments and those in whom resection is not deemed suitable, stents do offer a serious alternative. If utilised, then the stent should be removed within 4–6 weeks to avoid long-term complications since the biggest concern is septic erosion into the surrounding structures. This situation does not appear to be represented well in the literature, although a recent review suggested a 4% risk of erosion with a 20% mortality (Fig. 16.7).[37,38]

Drainage: repeated endoscopy

Endoscopic drainage and lavage of contained mediastinal perforations or even endoscopic placement of a vacuum sponge drainage system has been used for liquid contamination. This is certainly a newer approach, but labour intensive and not suitable for gross contamination.[39] A simpler alternative is to place a nasogastric tube into the cavity and apply low-pressure suction. This tube can gradually be withdrawn over time, allowing the cavity to heal from the distal extent proximally. Success in such patients may again simply reflect patients who would have done well with more simple non-operative treatment.[40,41]

Combined endoscopic/radiologic procedures

Interventional radiology can be used to site drains in loculated collections but can also be used in conjunction with endoscopy to place T-tubes through a defect to encourage enterocutaneous fistula formation and healing. This can be of use when surgery is too high risk or when defects persist despite other adequate non-operative measures.

✓✓ Evidence for the temporary use of covered, self-expanding metal or plastic stents as a primary treatment to seal a spontaneous perforation is limited.[38,39] Stents may have a place to control a postoperative leak and iatrogenic perforation in a highly select group of patients, although in the author's own institution excellent outcomes have been achieved without regular recourse to stents.[23]

OPERATIVE MANAGEMENT

Open surgery

Surgery is advocated if the patient has overt signs of sepsis, shock, gross contamination, an obstructing pathology, retained foreign body, major caustic injury, or has failed non-operative management. Virtually all gunshot wounds require surgery. The primary objective of surgical intervention is to restore oesophageal integrity and prevent further soiling. Thorough debridement, drainage, and lavage are more important for survival than the type of repair.[17] A feeding jejunostomy should be fashioned to facilitate enteral feeding, usually following thoracotomy once the patient can be turned into a supine position. Management of the patients by a multidisciplinary team is again emphasised. Underlying pathology should be dealt with. Spontaneous perforation of the oesophagus carries a considerable mortality risk and a long in-hospital recovery period should the patient survive.

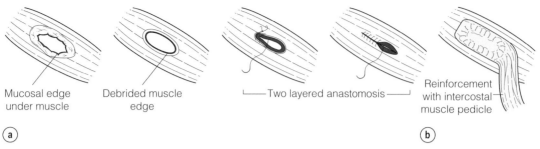

Mucosal edge under muscle

Debrided muscle edge

Two layered anastomosis

Reinforcement with intercostal muscle pedicle

(a)

(b)

Figure 16.8 (a) Primary closure and buttressing of the suture line. (b) Intercostal muscle flap.

A posterolateral thoracotomy on the side of the perforation is used to approach the oesophagus. This is most commonly on the left in the seventh or eighth intercostal space. Solid debris is removed and the pleural cavity thoroughly cleaned. The mediastinal pleura is widely incised to expose the injury. Necrotic, devitalised tissue is debrided. A longitudinal myotomy is made as the mucosal injury is usually longer than the muscular one and the oesophagus repaired.[42]

✔ Success with one surgical technique over another probably reflects the expertise and experience of the individual centre rather than a true outcome difference.

Primary repair with or without reinforcement

A single- or two-layered, primary repair can be fashioned using 2/0 or 3/0 interrupted absorbable sutures with or without a small-diameter bougie (40–46 F) in situ (Fig. 16.8). However, primary repair is associated with a significant leak rate (20–50%) and should be reserved for those operated on rapidly with demonstrably healthy tissue and limited soiling.[43] There is circumstantial evidence that reinforcing the suture line with an onlay patch of nearby tissues (such as omentum, pleura, lung, pedicled intercostal muscle grafts, gastric fundus, pericardium, or diaphragm) may reduce the leak rate (Fig. 16.9).[44] Appropriate drains should be placed around the repair in view of the high leak rates with primary repair.

T-tube repair

The concept of repair over a T-tube is to form a controlled oesophagocutaneous fistula.[45] A large-diameter (6–10 mm) T-tube is placed through the tear with the limbs lying beyond the boundaries of the perforation. The oesophageal wall is closed loosely around the tube with fine interrupted, absorbable sutures (Fig. 16.10). The author suggests considering anchoring the tube to the diaphragm as aortic erosion due to sepsis and pressure necrosis is possible.[46] The tube is externalised and secured. At least one further drain is placed around the repair. Apical and basal intercostal chest drains are sited. Healing is monitored by clinical examination, contrast radiology, and CT scans. The T-tube is left until a defined tract is established, with the majority removed endoscopically at around 6 weeks.

✔ In view of the high leak rate for primary repairs, the T-tube technique can be recommended for all patients.[15,46]

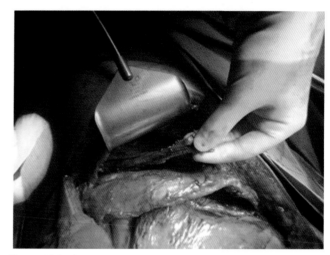

Figure 16.9 Intraoperative photograph of a raised intercostal muscle flap.

Resection

Oesophageal resection in the presence of a perforation is a major undertaking with an extremely high mortality. It is reserved for damage to a diseased oesophagus or in cases of extensive oesophageal trauma. This has even been performed in this setting as a minimally invasive approach.[47] If contamination is minimal then immediate reconstruction would be appropriate, but a delayed approach may also be taken with limited differences in outcome.[48] The use of non-definitive exclusion and diversion techniques is mostly historical but may occasionally be useful, such as in extensive caustic injuries.

Minimally invasive surgery: laparoscopic/thoracoscopic

Distal, clean, and immediately recognised iatrogenic perforations may be amenable to laparoscopic (transperitoneal) repair and drainage by surgeons used to working around the hiatus. This requires advanced laparoscopic skills in specialist centres with appropriate facilities.[49] Equally, selected cases can be managed thoracoscopically, most likely for washout and drainage, or for repair of the defect.[50–54]

Surgical repair over a stent

In view of the high leak rate of primary repair, some authors advocate a surgical repair over a stent (sutured transluminal or externally to prevent migration). This theoretically expedites a return to enteral nutrition;[55] however, the potential significant complications of stents remain, particularly the placement of a foreign body at the site of sepsis.

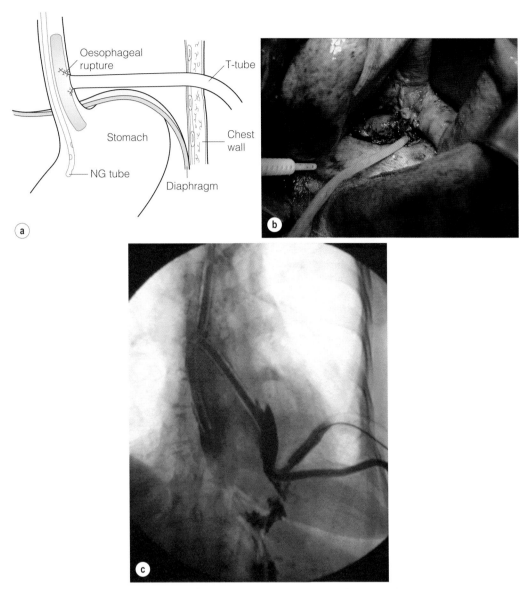

Figure 16.10 (a) Diagrammatic representation of T-tube repair of a spontaneous oesophageal perforation with the T-tube in situ. (b) Operative photograph. (c) Contrast radiological image of the same patient as in (b); note the additional intercostal chest drain with small contrast leak directly into this drain.

MANAGEMENT OF PENETRATING INJURIES

CERVICAL

Contained cervical perforations may be managed non-operatively irrespective of any delay. Repair should be undertaken when uncontained or in those requiring exploration for another reason. This is likely in any injury where the path traverses platysma or through the mediastinum.

THORACIC

Virtually all transthoracic gunshot wounds will require surgical exploration. Life-threatening cardiovascular, pulmonary, and tracheobronchial injuries take precedence. Specialist advice and input should be sought, but the majority of the oesophageal injuries will be able to be dealt with using the techniques described previously.[56] The overall mortality of penetrating thoracic oesophageal injuries is hard to ascertain but lies between 15% and 27% (lower for cervical trauma at 1–16%).[57] The morbidity arises mostly from associated spinal and airway trauma for cervical injuries, and from cardiorespiratory damage in thoracic trauma.

MANAGEMENT OF UNDERLYING PATHOLOGY

Patients who sustain a perforation of a malignant stricture constitute a difficult group to manage. Every effort should be made to prevent perforation during staging endoscopic procedures. Dilatation of malignant strictures causing dysphagia should only be considered for dilatation after careful consideration of the symptoms and alternatives, and counselling of the patient. Evidence shows that perforation through a malignancy renders the disease incurable. Any attempt at resection would therefore be palliative and surgical mortality in this context is high.[26,58,59] Those who have a perforation through a malignancy, or known inoperable disease, or who are unfit for surgery should be managed non-operatively. In this situation the use of a sealing palliative stent is appropriate. In patients where the perforation is separate to the malignancy, most authors recommend resection with a view to control of contamination and potential cure.[48,58]

✔ In the presence of oesophageal cancer, the priority is to determine if the lesion was operable before the perforation, and only if the perforation is separate to the underlying malignancy should consideration be given to performing an emergency subtotal oesophagectomy.

Iatrogenic perforation of achalasia is uncommon (1–5%) and usually managed non-operatively or endoscopically as these lesions are usually small, clean, immediately recognised, and well contained. Other pathologies such as peptic stricture, infections, or treatments such as radio/chemotherapy can also predispose to perforation. Specific operative intervention may be required and, despite reduced contamination, the associated surgical mortality is increased. The indications for operative management are the corollary of those documented in Box 16.4.

PARAOESOPHAGEAL SURGERY AND PROCEDURAL INJURIES

Direct oesophageal trauma is most commonly sustained during antireflux or hiatal hernia surgery, both open and laparoscopic, but the risk is low, of the order of 0–1.3%.[60,61] The risk increases with an intrathoracic approach, previous hiatal surgery, and suturing of the wrap to the oesophagus. The majority of injuries are recognised and repaired immediately with buttressing using the fundoplication wrap. Drainage is advised and it may also be appropriate to form a feeding jejunostomy or to place a nasojejunal tube until the repair is deemed safe by contrast radiology. The mortality of unrecognised and uncontained perforations approaches 20%. Trauma can also be sustained directly during thoracic and spinal surgery (< 0.5% of procedures), endotracheal intubation, nasogastric insertion, and surgical tracheostomy. In ventilated patients, the clinical features of an injury may be concealed. Indirect trauma can occur through pressure necrosis or devascularisation, although the rich vascular supply of the thoracic oesophagus makes this extremely uncommon.

MANAGEMENT ALGORITHM

✔✔ Diagnostic delay beyond 24 hours is associated with a poor outcome, a finding confirmed by a recent meta-analysis by the Benign Esophageal Perforation Collaborative.[62]

Even when managed promptly and aggressively, perforation of the oesophagus, especially Boerhaave-type disruption, carries a significant mortality rate. Reports to the contrary reflect selection bias. A management algorithm based on the therapeutic strategies outlined by the literature is demonstrated in Fig. 16.11. This is for guidance only and cases should be dealt with individually. Personal experience and expertise may well determine the best management.

Scoring systems attempting to stratify patients with oesophageal perforation have as of yet an unproven role in determining management decisions.[63] A UK-wide study to identify differences in practice is in set up and is likely to confirm variation in practice. It is unlikely that these data will be able to inform clinical practice, but the data could be used to inform future research proposals.

NON-PERFORATED SPONTANEOUS INJURIES OF THE OESOPHAGUS

Full-thickness oesophageal perforation contained by the mediastinal pleura is termed 'intramural rupture'.[64] This can occur spontaneously or secondary to instrumentation, food impaction, or coagulopathies. Non-operative treatments with or without endoscopic adjuncts are usually successful as the perforation is contained, but a minority may require surgical intervention.

'Black oesophagus syndrome' or acute oesophageal necrosis is extremely rare. This is circumferential mucosal and submucosal necrosis that ends sharply at the oesophagogastric junction in the absence of a caustic injury, most commonly presenting with upper gastrointestinal bleeding.[65,66] The most likely cause is vascular insufficiency from venous thrombosis as part of a 'two-hit' traumatic phenomenon associated with systemic hypotension. It has also been associated with thrombotic disorders. Diagnosis is endoscopic and treatment expectant with a low threshold for surgical resection, as the condition can rapidly progress to perforation. Mortality is high, often secondary to the underlying cause.

CAUSTIC INJURIES

Serious ingestion of a caustic substance is uncommon but devastating. Ingestion by children is more common, almost exclusively accidental, and usually associated with mild injuries.[67] Ingestion by adults is more often deliberate, although increasing cases are related to inadvertent consumption of caustic substances decanted into soft drinks bottles. Injuries in adults are more often severe and potentially life-threatening or life changing.

Most caustic substances can be grouped into acids or alkalis. Dangerous acids are readily available as toilet cleaners (hydrochloric acid), battery fluid (sulphuric acid), and in metalworking (phosphoric and hydrofluoric acids). In addition to local effects, ingestion of phosphoric or hydrofluoric acid leads to effects on metabolic calcium and magnesium levels through systemic absorption, which can cause refractory cardiac dysrhythmias. Specialist poisons advice is recommended and emergency personnel should take precautions, as even dermal exposure is hazardous. Strong alkalis are also readily available as cleaners and bleaches, although most household agents are only mild caustic agents.

There are two important misconceptions about caustic injuries. Firstly, that tissue penetration by acids is minimised by coagulative necrosis whereas alkalis more rapidly penetrate transmurally through liquefactive necrosis. Although pathologically correct, this is clinically irrelevant as the ingestion of any strong caustic agent in sufficient quantity will inflict a potentially fatal oesophageal or gastric injury. Furthermore, there is evidence to suggest that strong acid ingestion is

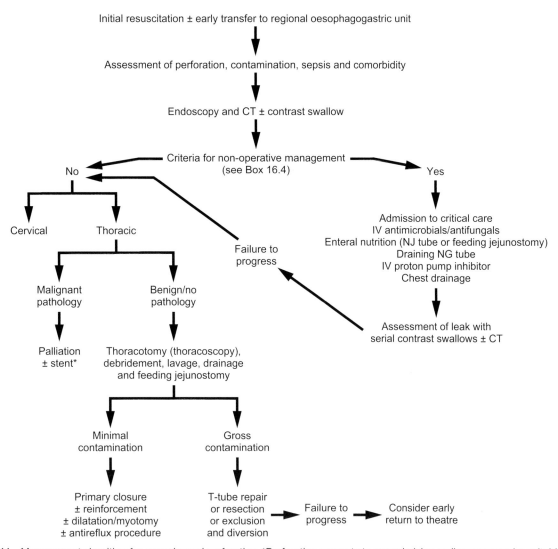

Figure 16.11 Management algorithm for oesophageal perforation. *Perforation separate to an underlying malignancy may be suitable for resection. *CT*, Computed tomography; *IV*, intravenous; *NG*, nasogastric; *NJ*, nasojejunal.

associated with greater systemic effects, a higher perforation rate and a higher mortality than alkali ingestion.[68] Secondly, acid ingestion causes gastric damage whereas alkali ingestion causes oesophageal injury. Although commonly cited, there is no evidence to support this.[69,70]

The severity of any caustic injury to the oesophagus or stomach is related to the corrosive properties, concentration, amount, viscosity, and duration of contact with the mucosa. Intentional caustic ingestions are associated with larger quantities of agent and are therefore more likely to result in severe injuries. In contrast, the amount ingested accidently by children is usually small.

CLINICAL PRESENTATION

Presentation can be varied and confusing. Clinical features are dependent on the substance and the time since ingestion. In accidental ingestion, symptoms and signs may not have developed due to rapid presentation. The absence of oral burns or pharyngo-oesophageal symptoms does not exclude more distal injury, as the caustic agent may have passed rapidly through the mouth and pharynx. In deliberate

---

Box 16.5 Acute symptoms and signs suggesting caustic injury of the oesophagus

- Refusal to eat or drink in children
- Facial oedema/burns
- Oropharyngeal pain
- Hypersalivation/drooling
- Stridor/hoarse voice
- Dyspnoea
- Dysphagia/odynophagia
- Chest pain
- Nausea and vomiting
- Epigastric pain/tenderness
- Haematemesis

---

ingestion the clinical features may be 'underplayed' by the patient. The clinical features of a caustic injury of the oesophagus are documented in Box 16.5.

Most patients survive to reach hospital unless aspiration has occurred. Glossopharyngeal burns cause oedema that may threaten the airway and prevent clearance of secretions with drooling and hypersalivation. Injury to the epiglottis and larynx leads to stridor and a hoarse voice. Dyspnoea is uncommon unless aspiration has occurred. Oropharyngeal burns can range from mild oedema and superficial erosions to extensive mucosal sloughing and necrosis. Acid burns form a black eschar whereas alkali burns look grey and dull. Oesophageal injury is suggested by dysphagia, odynophagia, retrosternal, or pleuritic chest pain. Gastric injury is manifested by epigastric pain, nausea, anorexia, retching, vomiting, and haematemesis. Patients may present shocked or in respiratory distress.

INVESTIGATION AND MANAGEMENT

The immediate priorities are establishment of a secure airway, stabilisation of cardiovascular status, and relief of pain. Severe oropharyngeal burns or respiratory compromise related to ingestion or subsequent vomiting may require early tracheal intubation and general anaesthesia. Similarly, any change from presentation of a patient's voice or ability to manage secretions should lead to prompt securing of the airway. Concurrent eye or facial burns should be irrigated with prompt ophthalmology and plastic surgery specialist involvement. Oral intake is prohibited. Gastric lavage, induced emesis, nasogastric aspiration, and the use of neutralising chemicals are contraindicated. Where possible the ingested agent and amount swallowed should be identified. Regional poison centres can then provide information regarding the properties of specific agents.

✓✓ Endoscopy and CT both have roles in determining optimum management for caustic ingestion and predicting systemic complications, death, and likelihood of subsequent stricture formation.[68,71-73] Endoscopy is considered the gold standard for staging of the burn (Fig. 16.12).

The severity of the injury is graded using a system similar to that for skin burns (Table 16.2). Differentiation between grades can be difficult, particularly for second- and third-degree burns, with implications for management. Consequently, some patients benefit from repeated evaluation (Table 16.3).[74] There has been interest in the use of oesophageal endosonography to assess depth of necrosis and damage to the muscle layers, but this currently offers no advantage over conventional endoscopic assessment.[75]

✓ All patients require admission and endoscopy by a skilled endoscopist as soon as the patient is stable, preferably within 24 hours of ingestion, to assess the stage of the oesophageal injury. A nasoenteric tube may be placed for early nutritional support. This can also act as a partial stent to prevent strictures, although if left in for too long without further endoscopic assessment of the need for a dilatation, can result in long strictures around the tube.[69,70,76]

CT assessment of caustic injury has also been demonstrated to have a role and a grading classification has been proposed (Table 16.4).[71,77] In adults, some centres have switched to a CT-based algorithm.[78] CT should also be used

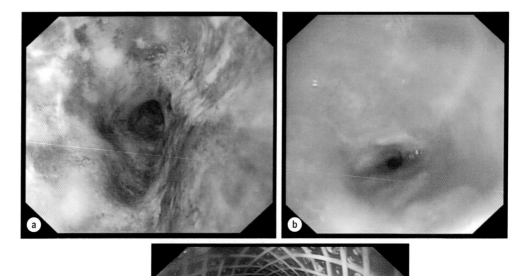

Figure 16.12 Endoscopic appearances of a caustic injury to the oesophagus. (a) Acute grade 3a alkali injury. (b) Appearance after 8 weeks with pinhole stricture. (c) A year later and refractory stricture treated by placement of a stent.

Table 16.2   Depth of oesophageal burn

Depth of Burn	Degree of Burn	Endoscopic Findings
Superficial	1	Mucosal oedema
Transmucosal with or without involvement of the muscularis	2a	Superficial ulcers, bleeding, exudates
	2b	Deep ulcers – focal or circumferential
Full thickness with or without adjacent organ involvement	3a	Full-thickness focal necrosis
	3b	Extensive necrosis

Table 16.3   Endoscopic staging of oesophageal caustic injury

Finding	First Degree	Second Degree	Third Degree
Bleeding	Hyperaemia only	Mild/moderate bleeding	Moderate/severe bleeding
Oedema	Mild	Moderate	Severe
Mucosal loss	None	Mucosal ulceration or blistering	Deep ulcers
Exudate	None	Present with or without pseudomembrane	Present with or without pseudomembrane
Appearance if endoscopy delayed	None	Granulation tissue	Eschar

Table 16.4   Computed tomography staging of oesophageal caustic injury

Grade 1	Normal
Grade 2	Wall and soft tissue oedema, increased wall enhancement
Grade 3	Transmural necrosis with absent wall enhancement

if perforation is suspected. In practice, the endoscopic and CT appearances will be complimentary, and in combination with the patient's clinical status will dictate the management.

Most caustic injuries are managed non-operatively. The use of steroids and antibiotics during the acute phase remains controversial, with conflicting evidence regarding their benefits.

✓✓ Methylprednisolone forms part of the treatment protocol of many units, particularly in children with burns of endoscopic grade 2b or greater.[79] Research continues into its use for the prevention of strictures in view of conflicting results from previous prospective randomised controlled trials in children about its benefit.[80,81]

Patients with severe burns who are most at risk of stricture formation also represent the highest perforation risk and steroids may mask clinical symptoms. The recommendation in adults is to avoid their administration during the initial management of a caustic injury.[78]

✓ Antibiotics should be reserved for those with proven infection, perforation, or aspiration, and in these cases the author suggests the additional use of antifungal agents.[82]

There are a few interesting animal-based research projects looking at other stricture-preventing medical treatments such as ibuprofen after oesophageal caustic injuries, but these have not yet been tried in a human population.[83]

Asymptomatic patients with unintentional ingestion but no oropharyngeal burns and normal or minor oesophageal findings may be discharged once they are able to take oral fluids. Intravenous fluids, analgesia, nutritional support, and antisecretory agents should be given to all other patients. Patients with endoscopic grade 1 and 2a injuries should be admitted and observed with clear fluids then diet reintroduced gradually over 24–48 hours. Endoscopy or contrast radiology studies should be arranged for 6–8 weeks after discharge to assess for strictures. Suicidal/intentional injury patients require psychiatric assessment prior to discharge. It is reasonable to observe patients with grade 2b and 3 burns, continuing nasojejunal feeding, and if there is no evidence of progression to perforation then clear fluids can be introduced from 48 hours. Be aware that the perforation risk is present for at least 7 days. Those who present with a perforation or deteriorate will require an emergency oesophagogastrectomy as the stomach is almost always injured. The author does not believe that laparoscopy has a role in assessing gastric viability. Immediate reconstruction with a substernal colonic interposition graft can be performed if there is minimal local contamination and stable patient physiology. More commonly, oesophagostomy and delayed reconstruction when the patient is nutritionally, physically, and mentally optimised is preferred. It is reasonable to consider resection in patients with extensive circumferential mucosal injuries in view of the problem of refractory strictures and the long-term cancer risk. The mortality for these caustic injuries is 13–40%, with the majority of deaths occurring in the adult suicidal group.[70] Mortality mainly stems from respiratory complications and delay in the aggressive surgical treatment of transmural necrosis. There is no place for 'conservative' treatment of a severe caustic oesophageal or gastric injury.

LONG-TERM COMPLICATIONS AND OUTCOMES

Oesophageal strictures develop in 5–50% of patients, 95% of which are distal and can be graded according to the

Table 16.5 The Marchand classification of oesophageal strictures

Circumferential	Length	Consistency	Grade
Incomplete	Short	Fibrotic	1
String-like circumferential	Short	Elastic	2
Complete	≤ 1 cm	Fibrotic	3
Complete	> 1 cm	Superficial fibrosis, easily dilated, non-progressive	4a
Complete	> 1 cm	Deep fibrosis, tubular, progressive, not easily dilated	4b

Marchand classification (Table 16.5).[84] Strictures are more likely to occur in initial grade 2B or worse injuries. Gastric scarring and deformity can lead to functional gastric problems as well as gastric outlet obstruction symptoms if scarring occurs at the pylorus or pre-pyloric regions. Most oesophageal strictures can be managed by serial Savary–Gilliard bougie or balloon dilatation.[85] Many such oesophageal strictures are long and so Savary–Gilliard dilatation might be preferred. Gastric stenoses can be managed with repeated balloon dilatation.

The procedure-related perforation incidence is less than 1%, but for safety the author advises allowing approximately 6 weeks after injury before attempting dilatation. Barium studies can be considered to diagnose strictures prior to repeat endoscopy. Antisecretory medication or even surgery may be required if reflux occurs after dilatation. Young patients with long grade 3 or 4 strictures are likely to require a lifetime of repeated dilatations with a cumulative risk of iatrogenic perforation and ultimately of cancer. In these patients, other options should be considered. Surgical options are to bypass or resect the obstructive segment or to perform a stricturoplasty. Bypass avoids dissection through mediastinal fibrosis, and a retrosternal or subcutaneous route for the neo-oesophagus may avoid a thoracotomy. However, retaining the damaged oesophagus retains the long-term cancer risk and can lead to problems related to secretions and bacterial overgrowth. Thoracotomy, resection, and colonic reconstruction (due to concurrent gastric damage) is therefore preferable. An alternative is an oesophageal stricturoplasty using a vascularised graft of colon, but again this retains the cancer risk. There is interest in the use of removable or absorbable stents for refractory strictures but evidence for their efficacy is limited.[86] There is also limited evidence for the use of endoscopic triamcinolone acetonide injection into the strictured segment to augment dilatation.[87]

CANCER RISK

Squamous malignant transformation of a caustically damaged oesophagus occurs in around 16%, a risk 1000 times that of the general population but with a long latent period for malignant change of between 15 and 40 years. Surveillance may be impractical with such a long latent period and the risk is not proportional to the severity of the injury. Early elective resection before transformation eliminates the risk, with low associated mortality in younger patients. In older patients, simply an awareness of the risk by clinicians and patients should lead to earlier diagnosis and an increase in the number of curative resections where deemed appropriate.

MANAGEMENT ALGORITHM

An algorithm for the management of caustic injuries of the oesophagus is detailed in Fig. 16.13.

INGESTION OF FOREIGN BODIES

The oesophagus is the most common site for impaction of ingested foreign bodies within the gastrointestinal tract, accounting for 75% of cases.[88] By far the majority occur in children under the age of 10 years, with coins, toys, crayons, and batteries being the commonest objects swallowed.[89] In adults, food boluses (predominantly meat) or impaction of food-related bone fragments are more common. This is especially the case in edentulous patients due to decreased palatal sensation. Cases involving other objects occur in people with mental or psychiatric difficulties, or related to drug and alcohol abuse, and in those seeking secondary gain such as prisoners. Most upper gastrointestinal units are aware of a number of recurrent offenders. Most foreign bodies impact in the cervical oesophagus, but impaction can occur at any of the physiological narrowings: the cricopharyngeus, the aortic arch, the left main bronchus, and the oesophago-gastric junction. Benign pathology accounts for some cases (e.g. Schatzki rings, peptic strictures, and eosinophilic oesophagitis). In contrast, malignant strictures are uncommonly associated with impaction due to the long development phase, but there are significant food bolus impaction rates associated with palliative treatments of malignant oesophageal lesions such as self-expanding metal stents.

CLINICAL PRESENTATION

In over 90% there is a clear history of ingestion associated with retrosternal pain or acute dysphagia at the level of the impaction and thus a rapid diagnosis.[90,91] In young children and uncooperative adults the diagnosis may not be so clear-cut. Suspicious symptoms in children are refusal of feeds, gagging, and choking, but some cases may remain concealed for months or even years. Chronic aspiration or reflux may represent long-standing impaction. A high index of suspicion is required for psychiatric patients with features suggestive of foreign body ingestion. Respiratory symptoms occur in 5–15%, especially in children and in cervical impaction, leading to coughing, wheezing, stridor, and dyspnoea. In adults, acute impaction in the cervical oesophagus can cause tracheal obstruction, leading to the so-called 'café coronary' or 'steakhouse syndrome'. Typically, sharp object ingestion (e.g. fish bones) can cause a persistent foreign body sensation despite easy passage through the oesophagus

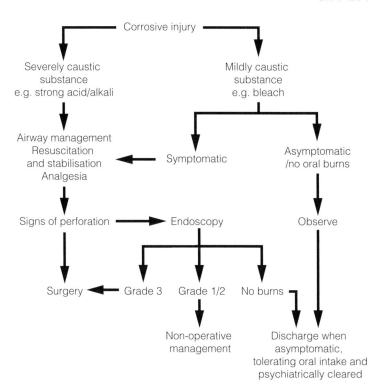

Figure 16.13 Management algorithm for caustic oesophageal injuries.

without impaction. Retrosternal pain and dysphagia are the commonest symptoms in adults with an impacted food bolus. Physical signs are usually limited unless impaction causes obstruction leading to drooling or perforation leading to neck swelling, erythema, tenderness, subcutaneous emphysema, or systemic effects. Long-standing impaction may lead to recurrent aspiration, empyema of the lung, perioesophagitis, oesophageal stenosis, or fistulation into the airways or major vessels.

If objects pass into the stomach without injury to the oesophagus, there are likely to be minimal symptoms unless the offending material causes obstruction to gastric emptying at the level of the pylorus or attempting to traverse to D1–D2 duodenal junction.

DIAGNOSIS

Plain radiographs may localise both radio-opaque and non-radio-opaque objects and are useful if perforation is suspected (Fig. 16.14). Both anteroposterior and lateral projections should be obtained, as objects may not be visible if overlying the vertebrae. This also helps to distinguish whether objects are in the digestive or tracheobronchial tract. In young children and infants, extensive plain radiography may be required to confirm or refute the diagnosis of a swallowed radio-opaque foreign body. Even in the absence of symptoms or physical signs a potential history of ingestion should prompt the use of radiography, as in one study 17% of asymptomatic children with a history of coin ingestion had an impacted oesophageal coin.[92] CT scans can more reliably identify the location of an impacted object and confirm the number of objects more accurately than plain imaging in cases of multiple ingestion. The rapid availability of CT in most centres is another reason why CT has superseded contrast swallows in this respect. CT is also the preferred modality for clarification regarding ingestion of non-radio-opaque

objects such as wood, aluminium, glass, and plastics. The use of hypertonic contrast media and barium should be avoided.

✔✔ Flexible endoscopy is the investigation of choice. It has been used safely for many decades and allows for immediate therapeutic intervention in 95%.[93,94] It can be performed in the endoscopy department or in the emergency theatre, particularly if airway compromise is a potential issue.

MANAGEMENT

✔✔ The majority of ingested foreign bodies will pass through the gastrointestinal tract uneventfully, with 10–20% requiring endoscopic removal due to impaction and around 3% requiring surgical removal.[91,93,94]

The indications for urgent intervention are:

1. Airway compromise.
2. Absolute dysphagia with aspiration risk.
3. Oesophageal or gastric impaction of a sharp object or button battery.
4. Oesophageal impaction of greater than 24 hours' duration.

The passage of a foreign body through the oesophagus does not always indicate success, as objects over 5–6 cm long or more than 2 cm in diameter are unlikely to pass through the pylorus or around the duodenal curves. Once the object is impacted, endoscopic removal may be difficult. Delivery of objects back through the oesophagogastric junction once in the stomach at times can also prove troublesome, even with the use of endoscopic overtubes. As such, expeditious retrieval while they remain in the oesophagus is advised. Similarly, although the majority of ingested sharp objects entering the stomach will traverse the gastrointestinal tract

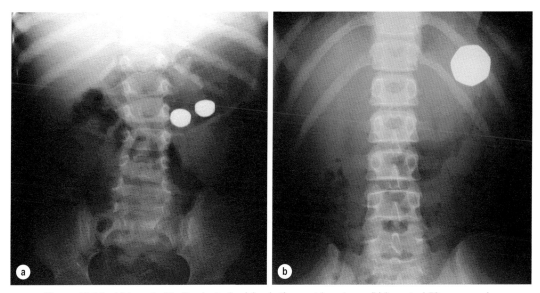

Figure 16.14 (a) Ingested button batteries lying in the gastric antrum. (b) Ingested 50-pence coin.

without incident, the perforation risk (up to 35%) suggests that retrieval, if safe, should be attempted.

In all other situations, individual management strategies depend on the symptoms, objects, and expertise of the receiving speciality, which includes paediatricians, surgeons, gastroenterologists, and psychiatrists.

✔ Observation of up to 24 hours is reasonable in asymptomatic patients with oesophageal or gastric coins or similar round, smooth objects, as many of these will pass spontaneously.[94,95]

A number of techniques to dislodge food boluses without recourse to endoscopy have been reported. Proteolytic agents (e.g. papain) that dissolve the food bolus may cause oesophageal trauma and are dangerous if aspirated and they are not recommended. Effervescent agents, such as carbonated drinks, and intravenous glucagon, which causes smooth muscle relaxation, were thought to help disimpact the food bolus, but there is no good evidence to support their use.[96,97] Failure to progress through the gastrointestinal tract or symptomatic deterioration should prompt surgical review. Therapeutic flexible endoscopy is as successful in object removal as rigid endoscopy but with a significantly lower complication rate (5% vs 10%) and avoids general anaesthesia in the majority of cases. In a minority of patients, the type of object, number of objects, or the inability of the patient to cooperate may dictate that general anaesthesia is required. Rigid endoscopy is still useful for impaction in the pharynx as the view and access are superior but should be abandoned for distal obstructions. Patience is important in endoscopic removal and is rewarded with a high success rate (around 95%).[93] Failure is most likely to occur with long (> 10 cm) or complex objects such as dental prostheses.

Smooth objects may be disproportionately difficult to retrieve. A variety of graspers, snares, magnets, and baskets may be required and it is useful to practise with the proposed grasper on a duplicate foreign body prior to the actual procedure. Expert endoscopic assistance can also prove invaluable. Coins should be orientated sideways to aid passage through the cricopharyngeus and sharp or pointed objects may require an overtube or endoscopic hood for safe

removal or manipulation to allow 'blunt end first' removal. Food impactions tend to occur in the distal oesophagus and are usually accompanied by underlying pathology. Eosinophilic oesophagitis is of interest as a predisposing factor to acute dysphagia and food impaction. This is especially relevant as the oesophageal mucosa is thin, friable, and easily traumatised by instrumentation – as such, dilatation should be avoided. Otherwise, flexible endoscopy allows relief of the impaction and diagnosis of any underlying pathology with concurrent mucosal biopsy.

Removal of the food bolus may again be achieved using a variety of techniques and tools. Larger boluses may require piecemeal removal, using an overtube if repeated intubation is required. Once the endoscope has been passed distal to the bolus then the bolus may be gently pushed into the stomach, but this technique should never be performed 'blindly' to avoid causing a perforation of a previously undiagnosed stricture. Definitive treatment such as dilatation of a peptic stricture may be performed after successful retrieval. If the aetiology of any underlying stricture is unclear, it is better to clear the obstruction and obtain biopsies to avoid the risks of perforating a malignant stricture.

'Disc' or 'button' batteries are easily ingested by children. Electrical discharge or release of the alkaline contents, once impacted, can lead to local damage, necrosis, and perforation. As such, urgent extraction is required if lodged within the oesophagus, and plain radiographs are helpful for localisation. However, if the battery has passed on to the stomach and duodenum, then 80–90% will pass without complication. Observation with serial radiography is used to monitor progression, reserving endoscopic or surgical intervention if the battery fails to progress out of the stomach within 48 hours, if the patient develops symptoms of intestinal injury, or if the battery fragments and there is evidence of mercury toxicity. Surgery may be necessary when endoscopy fails for large objects, for objects embedded in the oesophageal wall, or when there has been an associated or iatrogenic perforation. The surgical approach depends not only on the site and severity of the injury, but also associated inflammation and any underlying oesophageal pathology. Deliberate narcotic packet ingestion is a particularly taxing scenario. Endoscopic removal should not be attempted as successful

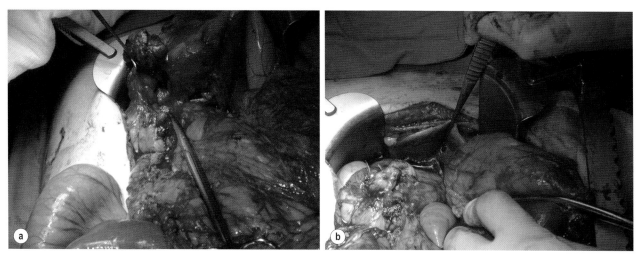

Figure 16.15   (a) Giant D1 ulcer. (b) Repair with antrectomy and closure of the anterior wall of the duodenum onto the fibrotic ulcer base.

retrieval is outweighed by the risk of rupture.[94] Most packets will pass safely through the bowel, but urgent surgery is indicated in cases where there is failure to progress, obstruction, or rupture, in conjunction with medical support for absorption of relevant contents.

DIFFICULT GASTRODUODENAL PERFORATIONS

The overwhelming majority of gastroduodenal perforations are related to peptic ulcer disease. Management of simple perforation is covered in Chapter 12. More complex perforations occur in 1–2% of all perforated ulcers, the majority in the context of giant peptic ulcers and in malignant perforations. It is generally agreed that giant ulcers are comprised of those with a diameter of greater than 2 cm, although a formal global definition has not been agreed. Mortality from giant ulcers is much higher and so the methods employed in closure are much more important. The decreasing incidence of such perforations in most countries makes experience of dealing with them limited. The published evidence base is therefore poor. Senior assistance or second opinions can prove invaluable. The incidence of malignancy in giant ulcers (duodenal or gastric) is higher and so needs to be considered at the time of diagnosis.

✔✔ Omental patch repair is sometimes possible even in the context of giant ulcers. Outcomes from patch repair and emergency resection have recently shown no difference in one case series and one meta-analysis.[98,99]

In the event that a perforated gastroduodenal ulcer cannot be closed with an omental (or falciform ligament) patch alone or as an adjunct to primary closure, options for closure include using an omental plug or jejunal serosal patch. Consideration should be given to more formal gastric decompression with a venting gastrostomy or duodenal decompression with a lateral (T-tube or Foley catheter placed in D2) or retrograde duodenostomy (Foley passed back up from proximal jejunostomy). Nutrition can be achieved by creation of a surgical feeding jejunostomy or insertion of a nasojejunal feeding tube. Copious

washout and placement of abdominal drains are mandatory around the site of repair.

Several diversion and exclusion techniques are also described, including stapling across the antrum without resection with formation of a gastrojejunostomy or Roux-en-Y reconstruction. Biliary diversion is still required in this scenario. If formal resection is required (antrectomy or subtotal gastrectomy with or without resection of D1) and standard duodenal stump closure is not feasible, then suturing the open duodenum (D1) to the capsule of the pancreas (Nissen closure) should be considered (Fig.16.15). Formal resection with immediate reconstruction should only be considered after close consideration of the patient's physiology and in discussion with the anaesthetist. With ongoing instability or physiological derangement, surgery should be limited to damage-control measures, with reconstruction postponed to later date once the patient's physiology has stabilised.

Endoscopic placements of stents at the time of surgery in cases of failed surgical closure are also reported but cannot be recommended as standard practice. Stents themselves have significant potential risks including erosion, downstream migration, and obstruction.

Management of perforated gastric cancer is also a situation best decided on a case-by-case basis. It is rare for a known patient with gastric cancer to present with a perforation during their staging or treatment process. In most cases, there is not a previous known diagnosis and the malignant nature of the perforation is only suspected at the time of surgery. Even then, operative suspicions need corroboration by formal histology. Frozen section is often not available or appropriate in the setting of emergency surgery. In the acute setting, with a physiologically unwell patient, expeditious surgery is required. Mortality from a primary resection in gastric cancer is particularly high.[100–102] A biopsy and then patch repair with copious lavage is likely the preferred option. In addition to the considerations of performing a resection in a patient who is physiologically unwell, a radical lymphadenectomy in the context of peritonitis is considerably demanding. Good longer term outcomes can be achieved with elective resection once the patient has recovered and the case discussed in the multidisciplinary setting.

CONCLUSION

Specialist oesophagogastric emergencies represent a wide variety of insults, leading to a wide spectrum of challenging injuries and conditions. Even minor injuries can be ultimately fatal if not recognised expediently and managed appropriately from the start. This is especially the case in oesophageal injury given the fragility of the oesophageal wall, the lack of oesophageal serosa, the proximity of vital organs, the inaccessibility, the lack of early symptoms and signs, and the potential rapid evolution of mediastinitis and sepsis. These difficult cases are relatively rare and most surgeons will deal with only a handful in their career. Consequently, cases are best managed by specialist units. Outcomes can be improved through prevention where possible, for example through safe and thorough training in therapeutic endoscopy, avoiding unnecessary procedures, better labelling of caustic substances, and development of smaller button batteries, and education.

Key points

Oesophageal perforation

- Urgent CT and flexible endoscopy are the diagnostic investigations of choice.
- Diagnostic delay leads to poorer outcomes.
- Between 75% and 90% of iatrogenic perforations occur distally and underlying pathology is common.
- Perforation of an oesophageal cancer renders these lesions incurable.
- Non-operative management is suitable for clean or contained perforations.
- Surgery remains the mainstay of treatment for gross contamination.

Oesophageal trauma

- Penetrating oesophageal trauma is easily missed with serious injuries to surrounding viscera.
- CT scanning and flexible endoscopy are the investigations of choice.

Caustic injury

- In suspected caustic ingestion, investigation is mandatory.
- Flexible endoscopy within 24 hours of ingestion and urgent CT should be used to assess the oesophagus.
- Most strictures can be managed by serial Savary–Gilliard bougie or balloon dilatation.
- Reconstructive surgery should be considered in young patients with refractory strictures, also bearing in mind the long-term cancer risk.

Ingestion of foreign bodies

- For ingestion of a foreign body flexible endoscopy is both the investigation and treatment option of choice.
- The majority of ingested foreign bodies will pass uneventfully.
- Observation of up to 24 hours is reasonable in asymptomatic patients with round, smooth objects.

Difficult gastroduodenal perforations

- Mortality from giant ulcers can be high so senior advice or assistance is invaluable.
- Omental patch repair, emergency resection and several other techniques have been described that could include gastric or duodenal decompression.

 References available at http://ebooks.health.elsevier.com/

KEY REFERENCES

[23] Dent B, Griffin SM, Jones R, et al. Management and outcomes of anastomotic leaks after oesophagectomy. Br J Surg 2016;103:1033–8. PMID: 27146631.

[29] Paspatis GA, Arvanitakis M, Dumonceau JM, Barthet M, Saunders B, Turino SY, et al. Diagnosis and management of iatrogenic endoscopic perforations: European society of gastrointestinal endoscopy (ESGE) position statement - update 2020. Endoscopy 2020 Sep;52(9):792–810. https://doi.org/10.1055/a-1222-3191. Epub 2020 Aug 11. PMID: 32781470.

The updated European guidelines recommend that if the expertise is available and the type of perforation suitable, immediate endoscopic closure of small iatrogenic perforations limits mediastinal or peritoneal contamination.

[38] Kamarajah SK, Bundred J, Spence G, Kennedy A, Dasari BVM, Griffiths EA. Critical appraisal of the impact of oesophageal stents in the management of oesophageal anastomotic leaks and benign oesophageal perforations: an updated systematic review. World J Surg 2020;44(4):1173–89. https://doi.org/10.1007/s00268-019-05259-6. PMID: 31686158.

[39] Rausa E, Asti E, Aiolfi A, Bianco F, Bonitta G, Bonavina L. Comparison of endoscopic vacuum therapy versus endoscopic stenting for esophageal leaks: systematic review and meta-analysis. Dis Esophagus 2018;31(11). https://doi.org/10.1093/dote/doy060. PMID: 29939229.

Oesophageal perforations can be managed successfully without stents; although stents have been used to treat perforations, the overall quality of the evidence in support of their use is poor, while initial comparisons potentially favour better results with newer vacuum therapy.

[62] Vermeulen BD, van der Leeden B, Ali JT, Gudbjartsson T, Hermansson M, Low DE, et al. Siersema PD; Benign Esophageal Perforation Collaborative Group. Early diagnosis is associated with improved clinical outcomes in benign esophageal perforation: an individual patient data meta-analysis. Surg Endosc 2020 Jul 17. https://doi.org/10.1007/s00464-020-07806-y. Epub ahead of print. PMID: 32681374.

This meta-analysis of 25 studies with almost 1 000 patients evaluated a diagnostic delay beyond 24 hours and confirmed that this increases mortality, the need for intervention, and hospital length of stay.

[68] Poley JW, Steyerberg EW, Kuipers EJ, et al. Ingestion of acid and alkaline agents: outcome and prognostic value of early upper endoscopy. Gastrointest Endosc 2004;60:372–7. PMID: 15332026.

[71] Chirica M, Bonavina L, Kelly MD, et al. Caustic ingestion. Lancet 2017;389:2041–52. PMID: 28045663.

[72] Cutaia G, Messina M, Rubino S, Reitano E, Salvaggio L, Costanza I, et al. Caustic ingestion: CT findings of esophageal injuries and thoracic complications. Emerg Radiol 2021 Mar 8. https://doi.org/10.1007/s10140-021-01918-1. Epub ahead of print. PMID: 33683517.

[73] Bruzzi M, Chirica M, Resche-Rigon M, Corte H, Voron T, Sarfati E, et al. Emergency computed tomography predicts caustic esophageal stricture formation. Ann Surg 2019;270(1):109–14. https://doi.org/10.1097/SLA.0000000000002732. PMID: 29533267.

Endoscopy has been proven a safe and effective technique for evaluating caustic injury while more recent evidence highlights a role of CT for guiding management.

[91] Alberto A, Ferrari D, Carlo Galdino Riva, Toti F, Bonitta G, Bonavina L. Esophageal foreign bodies in adults: systematic review of the literature. Scand J Gastroenterol 2018;53(10–11):1171–8. https://doi.org/10.1080/00365521.2018.1526317.

[93] Li ZS, Sun ZX, Zou DW, et al. Endoscopic management of foreign bodies in the upper-GI tract: experience with 1088 cases in China. Gastrointest Endosc 2006;64:485–92. PMID: 16996336.

[94] Birk M, Bauerfeind P, Deprez PH, Häfner M, Hartmann D, Hassan C, et al. Removal of foreign bodies in the upper gastrointestinal tract in adults: European Society of Gastrointestinal Endoscopy (ESGE) Clinical Guideline. Endoscopy 2016;48(5):489–96. https://doi.org/10.1055/s-0042-100456. Epub 2016 Feb 10. PMID: 26862844.

These studies and guidelines, based on observational or cohort studies (no randomised trials available), illustrate retrosternal pain as the most common symptom, sharp objects (particularly fish and chicken bones) as the most common foreign body, with the cervical oesophagus the most frequent site of impaction, and flexible endoscopy the therapeutic modality of choice; surgery is only required in 3.4%.

[98] Chan KS, Wang YL, Chan XW, Shelat VG. Outcomes of omental patch repair in large or giant perforated peptic ulcer are comparable to gastrectomy. Eur J Trauma Emerg Surg 2019 Oct 14. https://doi.org/10.1007/s00068-019-01237-8. Epub ahead of print. PMID: 31612272.

[99] Zhu C, Badach J, Lin A, Mathur N, McHugh S, Saracco B, et al. Omental patch versus gastric resection for perforated gastric ulcer: systematic review and meta-analysis for an unresolved debate. Am J Surg 2021;221(5):935–41.

This meta-analysis comprised nine retrospective, non-randomised studies dating back several decades, but included the more recent single-centre, retrospective study from Singapore of 110 patients with ulcers larger than 20 mm; both the single-centre study and the meta-analysis demonstrated no difference in outcome between patch repair and emergency gastrectomy, although both papers conclude the need for a randomised study.

17 Obesity and assessment for metabolic surgery

Carel le Roux | Moath Saleh Al Saqaaby

INTRODUCTION

World Health Organization (WHO) statistics reveal that 1.9 billion adults (39%) above 18 years of age were overweight, an estimated 650 million adults (13%) worldwide were obese in 2016, and 39 million children under 5 years of age were overweight or obese in 2020[1] (Figs. 17.1 and 17.2).

Medical management with caloric restriction, diets, and drug therapy do not provide sustained long-term weight loss in many patients. Metabolic surgery is currently the best treatment that provides long-term weight loss maintenance and comorbidity control.[2] In the Swedish Obese Subjects (SOS) intervention study, at 10 years follow-up the surgical group had 16% weight loss compared to 1.6% weight gain for patients managed conservatively.

> Metabolic surgery is the best treatment for obesity that provides long-term weight loss and maintenance. The SOS intervention study demonstrated that at 10-year follow-up, the surgical group had 16% weight loss compared to 1.6% weight gain for patients managed conservatively.[2]

The first metabolic procedures such as jejuno-ileal bypass and vertical banded gastroplasty have now been superseded by the most commonly performed procedures, namely Roux-en-Y gastric bypass (RYGB), vertical sleeve gastrectomy (VSG), laparoscopic adjustable gastric banding (LAGB), and biliopancreatic diversion (BPD) (with or without a duodenal switch [DS]). Techniques have also now evolved from open to laparoscopic techniques. The overall 30-day mortality rates after metabolic surgery can be as low as 0.3% in experienced high-volume centres, making it safe as well as highly effective.[3]

PATHOPHYSIOLOGY OF OBESITY AND OBESITY-RELATED DISEASES

Obesity is a risk factor for many obesity complications:

- Type 2 diabetes mellitus (T2DM) and micro- and macro-vascular complications
- Dyslipidaemia
- Hypertension
- Cardiovascular disease
- Non-alcoholic fatty liver disease (NAFLD)
- Non-alcoholic steatohepatitis (NASH)
- Obstructive sleep apnoea (OSA)
- Asthma
- Musculoskeletal pain and function
- Gastro-oesophageal reflux disease (GORD)
- Polycystic ovary syndrome (PCOS) symptoms
- Infertility
- Urinary incontinence
- Cancer, e.g. breast, endometrial, colon, oesophageal, hepatocellular
- Psychosocial functioning.

We now understand that obesity and its related complications are metabolic diseases involving complex gut–brain–endocrine (GBE) and adipocyte–brain–endocrine interactions.

The GBE axis is fundamental for energy homeostasis. Enteroendocrine cells (EECs) sense luminal factors, such as absorbed nutrients, via sensory transporters and various cell membrane receptors.[4] EECs are activated to secrete gut hormones such as oxyntomodulin (OXM) and glucagon-like peptide 1 (GLP-1), which alert the central nervous system (CNS) that nutrients are in the gut lumen via endocrine (circulation or lymphatics) or paracrine (activation of enteric, vagal and spinal afferent sensory neurons via local receptors) mechanisms. This signalling pathway activates metabolic control centres in the hindbrain and hypothalamus to control energy homeostasis, resulting in responses such as reduced food intake, increased energy expenditure (OXM), increased satiety, insulin release, and glucose homeostasis, slowing gastrointestinal (GI) motility, gut secretions, and nutrient utilisation.[5]

✅ It is now understood that metabolic surgery is not purely weight loss surgery. Metabolic surgery results in anatomical alterations that produce complex physiological interactions involving signalling between the gut and the brain, as well as adipocytes and the brain.

Adipose tissue consists of brown adipose tissue (involved in non-shivering thermogenesis) and white adipose tissue (which stores cholesterol and triglycerides [TGs], and acts as an endocrine and immune organ). An increase in the fat mass associated with obesity results in adipocyte and adipose tissue dysfunction, termed adiposopathy (or 'sick fat').[6] White adipocytes produce immune factors such as leptin and adiponectin (which has anti-inflammatory and antidiabetic properties); growth factors; adipocytokines such as IL-6 and tumour necrosis factor (TNF); and enzymes such as 11β-hydroxysteroid dehydrogenase. These contribute to inflammation and have a significant effect on obesity-related

248

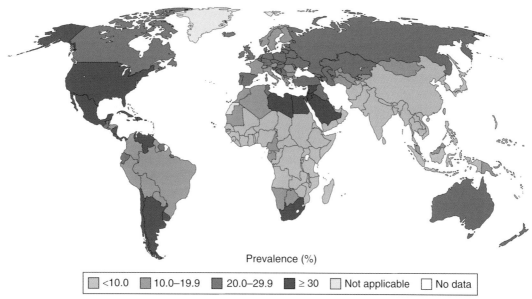

Figure 17.1 WHO statistics of global obesity prevalence.[1] These statistics are reflected in the Health Survey for England (HSE) 2014 statistics, which showed that a very high proportion (61.7%) of adults were overweight or obese, with prevalence showing an upward trend (see Fig. 17.2).[55] Obesity prevalence appears to be increasing in England, Scotland, and Wales, but interestingly not Ireland or Northern Ireland.[55]

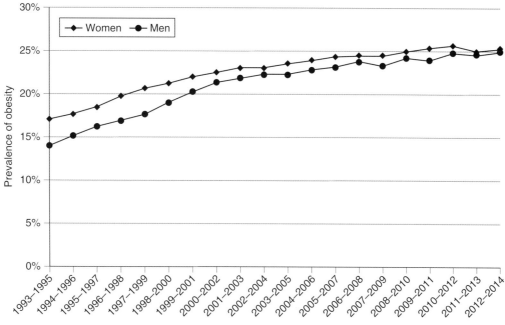

Figure 17.2 Health Survey for England 1993–2014: prevalence of obesity among adults aged 16+ years.[55]

complications. Metabolic surgery has been shown to result in favourable effects on these factors.[7,8] Understanding the mechanisms of metabolic surgery has significantly furthered our knowledge of the pathophysiology of obesity and its related comorbidities.

THE MECHANISMS OF ACTION AND RATIONALE FOR METABOLIC PROCEDURES

Metabolic procedures were originally developed as purely mechanically restrictive and/or malabsorptive procedures.

However, the contribution of restriction and malabsorption has been shown to be minimal. We now understand that they are metabolic procedures involving complex GBE and adipocyte–brain signalling that regulates appetite, satiety, weight, glucose metabolism, and other immunological processes.[5]

WEIGHT LOSS POST METABOLIC SURGERY

RYGB and VSG are the most commonly performed procedures and cause a 25–35% total body weight loss and maintenance.[9,10] The mechanisms underlying this include reduced food intake and increased energy expenditure.

FOOD INTAKE

After metabolic surgery, in contrast to low-calorie diets, patients report decreased pre-meal hunger and increased satiety.[11] Various components of the GBE axis can explain this reduction in food intake.

Gut hormones

Gut peptides are secreted from EECs that reside within the intestinal epithelium and are often referred to as satiety hormones. Metabolic surgery can increase the number of gut peptide-expressing EECs (e.g. L cells),[12] and therefore postprandial gut peptide secretion (e.g. GLP-1, GLP-2, and peptide YY [PYY]). Patients with the highest postprandial levels of satiety hormones lose the most weight post RYGB.[13] Changes in nutrient concentrations (higher in the distal segments) and faster delivery to the distal ileum post RYGB give stimulus to EECs to release these 'satiety' hormones, resulting in increased satiety, reduced food intake, and sustained weight loss.[14] In VSG, faster gastric emptying has been used to explain the rise in satiety hormones.[15] Both PYY and GLP-1 act at the arcuate nucleus (ARC) additively to suppress food intake[16,17] but also via vagal afferents terminating at the nucleus tractus solitarius (NTS) to signal satiety. GLP-1 also slows gastric emptying, inhibits glucagon release, and acts on the pancreas to secrete insulin (incretin effect).[18]

Neural mechanisms

Vagus signalling

The vagus nerve is an important regulator of food intake and body weight. Vagal afferents can be activated by the paracrine action of gut hormones in response to ingested nutrients or by mechanical stretch from the volume of food ingested.[19] The enteric nervous system may also activate spinal afferents and gut vagal afferents in response to gut hormones, as seen in rodents.[20] Post RYGB there is evidence that vagal signalling may play a role in satiation, reduction in signalling of ghrelin, reduction in meal size, and altered food preferences.[5] After LAGB, vagal signalling may reduce food intake and weight loss by reducing hunger and inducing satiation via neural mechanisms.[21] After VSG, hyperexcitation of NTS synapses and increased glutamate release due to vagal signalling may be the mechanism for reducing food intake, as suggested from rodent studies.[22]

Hypothalamic signalling and surgery

Vagal afferents synapse in the NTS of the dorsal vagal complex of the brain stem[23,24] and the NTS integrates and relays vagal signals to the ARC of the hypothalamus.[25] Many gut peptides influence energy homeostasis through ARC pro-opiomelanocortin (POMC) and agouti-related peptide (AgRP) neurons and neuropeptides, showing a clear association between the GBE axis and control of feeding behaviour after metabolic surgery.

Gut microbiota

After RYGB, the gut microbiota ratio observed in patients is reversed, with a reduced *Firmicutes:Bacteroides* ratio,[26] as well as increased Gammaproteobacteria[27] and *Escherichia coli*.[28] When the gut microbiota from mice post RYGB was transferred to germ-free mice, their body weight and body fat decreased.[29] Microbial fermentation of polysaccharides into short-chain fatty acids (SCFAs) may explain this observation.[29] SCFAs and bacterial antigens interact with EECs and stimulate gut hormone production associated with reduction in food intake in mice.[30] After surgery in humans some gut microbes have been directly linked to improvement of weight, metabolic status, and energy intake, while *Faecalibacterium prausnitzii* gut species have been correlated with a reduction in inflammation.[31]

Bile acids

Total plasma bile acids (BAs) are higher after RYGB,[32] BPD,[33] and VSG,[34] but not LAGB,[35] and their levels negatively correlate with postprandial glucose levels.[36] BAs are commonly suggested as mediators of the early metabolic beneficial effects of bariatric surgery, which is based on the consistent finding after bypass metabolic surgery that circulating BAs are increased in both fasting and postprandial conditions.[33,37] After RYGB, BAs are also found to positively correlate with several other metabolically active peptides, including adiponectin, PYY, and GLP-1.[11,36] BAs remain high for 3–4 years post-surgery and could play a role in intestinal hypertrophy, gut hormone secretion (GLP-1 and PYY) through G-protein–coupled receptor TGR5, lipid and glucose metabolism, as well as contribute to changes in gut flora.[38,39]

CHANGES IN FOOD PREFERENCE AND FOOD REWARD

Hedonic hunger is reduced after RYGB, with increased intake of fruit and vegetables and no fixation on energy-dense sweet and fatty foods; similar changes in food preferences are seen after VSG.[21] Both VSG and RYGB lead to an increase in gut hormones GLP-1 and PYY, which may have effects on central gustatory pathways related to feeding and reward: altered quality of tastants, palatability, and hedonic properties of sweet and fat stimuli.[40] Conditioned food avoidance rather than conditioned food aversion appears to be the main underlying mechanism for the changes observed in humans and rodents.

ENERGY EXPENDITURE

Studies assessing energy expenditure after metabolic surgery show varying results on total energy expenditure,[21] but have consistently demonstrated that diet-induced energy expenditure is increased after RYGB when compared with controls. BAs are increased after RYGB[41] and may modulate energy expenditure through their actions on brown adipose tissue or skeletal muscle.[38] The precise mechanism causing increases in diet-induced thermogenesis after RYGB is yet to be elucidated.[21]

COMPLICATIONS IMPROVEMENT OR RESOLUTION

Metabolic surgery has also been shown to result in obesity-related complication improvement or resolution.

The main mechanisms for this complication resolution after surgery include:

- Changes in eating behaviour and weight loss
- Gut hormones
- BA kinetics
- Adipocyte-derived factors
- Anatomical factors.

CHANGES IN EATING BEHAVIOUR AND WEIGHT LOSS

Metabolic surgery-induced weight loss alone has positive effects on complications such as functional impairment from arthritis. Caloric restriction results in reduced liver fat and improved hepatic insulin sensitivity,[42] while weight loss leads to improved peripheral insulin sensitivity improving T2DM, NASH, NAFLD, and metabolic syndrome. The quantity and type of food (e.g. fats, carbohydrates, proteins, vitamins, etc.) can influence adipose tissue function, dyslipidaemia, and atherosclerotic risk.[43] Weight loss also has cancer-protective effects by reducing the release of adipokines from adipose tissue including, growth factors, hormone production, and inflammatory cytokines (e.g. TNF-alpha, C-reactive protein [CRP], interleukins),[44] thus reducing cell proliferation and oxidative stress.[5]

GUT HORMONES

GLP-1 contributes to improved glycaemic control and has been associated with increased insulin secretion, increased insulin synthesis with beta-cell proliferation and improved beta-cell function,[42,45,46] as well as weight loss-induced improvements in insulin sensitivity. Both GLP-1 and PYY contribute to improvements in dyslipidaemia.[43] The improvements in insulin resistance post metabolic surgery lead to a reduction in sex hormone-binding globulin and IGF-1, which reduces cancer cell proliferation.[5]

BILE ACID KINETICS

BAs stimulate GLP-1. They affect insulin resistance by increasing energy expenditure in brown adipose tissue.[38] BAs also have beneficial effects on dyslipidaemia including reduced very low-density lipoprotein (VLDL) secretion, TG accumulation, and reduced hepatic TG production.[5,47]

ADIPOCYTE-DERIVED FACTORS

Adipocytokines (such as IL-6, TNF-alpha) secreted from adipose tissue are known to induce a low-grade inflammatory state associated with insulin resistance and dyslipidaemia.[8] Reduced CRP levels post RYGB suggest reductions in inflammation, which may help improve whole-body insulin sensitivity[48] and dyslipidaemia. In rodents, when nutrients enter the jejunum post duodenal-jejunal bypass (DJB) surgery they are sensed by receptors that release leptin, which reduce glucose levels[49] and reduce atherosclerosis and catecholamine release, decreasing blood pressure as well as having anticancer effects.[5] Increased adiponectin may also reduce hepatic inflammation and fibrosis through suppression of hepatic stellate cells,[50] improving NASH and NAFLD.

ANATOMICAL FACTORS

Operations such as BPD utilise a longer biliopancreatic limb (BPL) and produce greater reduction in insulin resistance, suggesting that the length of the BPL could be an influencing factor[51] in T2DM resolution.

RATIONALE FOR METABOLIC SURGERY

Obesity kills and the metabolic complications of obesity result in more than 2.8 million deaths and 35.8 million life-years of ill health each year worldwide.[52] The economic implications of obesity and obesity-related diseases and the burden on national health costs are substantial.[53] There is also an economic impact on the patient, who is more likely to suffer with the social stigma of obesity and more likely to be unemployed or take sick leave for obesity-related illness.

Metabolic surgery results in long-term weight loss, lifestyle/quality of life improvements, reduced mortality (30.7% lower after surgery compared to conservative management in the SOS study), and either improvement or complete resolution of complications, for example T2DM, hypertension, dyslipidaemia (mainly hypertriglyceridemia and low high-density lipoprotein (HDL) cholesterol level, but not hypercholesteremia), cardiovascular disease, OSA, certain cancers, NASH, and NAFLD.[2,54,55] There is also improvement in the microvascular (retinopathy, nephropathy, and neuropathy) and macrovascular (cardiovascular, cerebrovascular, and peripheral vascular disease) complications of T2DM. Surgery produces statistically significant reductions in myocardial infarction, stroke, atherosclerotic cardiovascular events, and overall mortality compared to conservative management.[56,57] This equates to fewer medications, fewer hospital visits, fewer hospital admissions, fewer visits to the General Practitioner (GP), and improved productivity. Consequently, the costs of laparoscopic metabolic surgery are fully recovered after 2.1 years.[58] Metabolic surgery itself has low morbidity and mortality. Given the huge economic and health impact that it has on patients, the rationale for surgery is clear.

✔✔ Metabolic surgery reduces mortality compared to conservative management and improves the comorbidities associated with obesity.[2,54,55]

INDICATIONS FOR METABOLIC SURGERY

Table 17.1 shows the National Institute of Health and Care Excellence (NICE) criteria for obesity by body mass index (BMI), used by many international associations.[59] However, NICE acknowledges that BMI is not a direct measure of adiposity and that waist circumference (WC) is a useful additional tool, particularly in patients with a BMI < 35 kg/m² (Table 17.2).

✔✔ NICE acknowledges that there are various problems with BMI-based criteria: BMI is not a direct measure of adiposity, it can be less accurate in muscular adults, and certain patient groups may have low BMIs but may have comorbidity risk factors that are of concern at lower BMIs.[59]

However, NICE criteria on the suitability for metabolic surgery for adults continue to be based on BMI criteria endorsed by the International Federation for the Surgery of Obesity and Metabolic Disorders (IFSO), National Institutes of Health (NIH), and several other organisations:

- BMI of > 40 kg/m².
- 35 kg/m² + significant complication (e.g. T2DM, hypertension, hyperlipidaemia OSA, obesity hypoventilation syndrome [OHS], Pickwickian syndrome, NAFLD, NASH, pseudotumour cerebri, GORD, asthma, functional disability).

Table 17.1 Body mass index categories (NICE criteria)

Classification	BMI (kg/m^2)
Underweight	< 18.5
Normal	18.5–24.9
Overweight	25–29.9
Obese I	30–34.9
Obese II	35–39.9
Obese III/morbid obesity	≥ 40
Patient with obesity and a high BMI value*	> 50

*Not part of NICE criteria.
BMI, Body mass index; *NICE*, (UK) National Institute of Health and Care Excellence.

Table 17.2 Health risks using waist circumference

BMI	Waist circumference		
	Low	High	Very high
Overweight	No increased risk	Increased risk	High risk
Obesity I	Increased risk	High risk	Very high risk

For men, waist circumference (WC) if < 94 cm is low, 94–102 cm is high, and > 102 cm is very high. For women, WC < 80 cm is low, 80–88 cm is high, and > 88 cm is very high.
BMI, Body mass index.

- All appropriate non-surgical measures have been tried but have failed to achieve or maintain adequate, clinically beneficial weight loss for at least 6 months.
- The person has been receiving or will receive intensive management in a specialist obesity service.
- The person is generally fit for anaesthesia and surgery.
- The person commits to the need for long-term follow-up.
- As a first-line option (instead of lifestyle interventions or drug treatment) for adults with a BMI > 50 kg/m^2 in whom surgical intervention is considered appropriate.

Metabolic surgery is now part of the treatment paradigm for T2DM patients with a BMI between 30 and 35 kg/m^2 when diabetes cannot be adequately controlled by optimal medical treatment.[10,60]

However, the International Diabetes Federation Taskforce on Epidemiology and Prevention suggests that surgery should be considered as an alternative treatment option in patients with a BMI between 30 and 35 kg/m^2 when diabetes cannot be adequately controlled by optimal medical regimens, especially in the presence of other major cardiovascular disease risk factors; and that in Asian patients as well as some other ethnicities of increased risk, BMI action points may be reduced by 2.5 kg/m^2.[10,60] Several associations now recognise that these patients should be considered for metabolic surgery, particularly if they have T2DM or metabolic syndrome, with one meta-analysis demonstrating improved glycaemic control and T2DM remission rates, and lower haemoglobin A1C (HbA1c), BMI, arterial hypertension,

and dyslipidaemia after surgery compared to medical treatment in patients with BMI < 35 kg/m^2.[61] Metabolic surgery has now been incorporated into the treatment algorithm for diabetes. There is currently insufficient evidence to recommend any particular operation for a particular condition or surgery for patients with BMI < 30 kg/m^2.[62]

There are several problems with BMI as it can be less accurate in muscular adults. Other patient groups may have low BMIs, but may have risk factors that are of concern at lower BMIs.[59] The original BMI criteria for surgery were issued in the NIH Consensus Development Conference Statement (March 1991) and developed by consensus of surgeons, physicians, and psychologists based on risk–benefit evidence. At this time surgery used the open technique and surgical risk was much higher than it is today. The ideal assessment tool has been elusive, although future criteria may incorporate WC, waist:hip ratio, complications/functional assessments, and body composition technologies.[62] As bariatric surgery becomes accepted as metabolic surgery, the criteria may also change to reflect this, with suggestions that the criteria should be lowered to BMI 35 kg/m^2 or BMI 30 kg/m^2 with coexisting complications.[63]

Metabolic surgery should only be considered in children/adolescents after exclusion of genetic and syndrome causes, and in centres that can offer specialist multidisciplinary paediatric bariatric services. The patients should have a BMI > 40 kg/m^2 (or 99.5th percentile for respective age) and at least one complication, have undergone a minimum of 6 months supervised weight loss under a paediatric weight loss clinic, have skeletal and developmental maturity, the ability to commit to medical and psychological assessment, and commitment to postoperative multidisciplinary treatment.[64] In patients over 60 years old, the aim of surgery is to improve quality of life as it is unlikely to affect lifespan, and therefore the risk:benefit ratio must be considered carefully before considering surgery in this age group.

Contraindications for surgery include: pregnancy, current drug or alcohol abuse, uncontrolled psychiatric illness (e.g. uncontrolled psychosis, severe personality disorder, severe learning disability), portal hypertension, diseases threatening life in the short term, absence of period of medical management, lack of understanding of the risk:benefit ratio, expected outcomes, alternatives and lifestyle changes required with metabolic surgery, and patients who are unable to self-care or have family who can do so.[62,64] In the management of T2DM, surgery is contraindicated if the patient has secondary diabetes, is antibody positive (anti-GAD or ICA), has C-peptide levels < 1 ng/mL, or is unresponsive to a mixed meal challenge.[64] Patients should also undergo the usual preoperative assessment to identify other non-obesity–related complications that may preclude surgery, e.g. Crohn's disease is a relative contraindication.

THE SPECIALIST METABOLIC SURGERY UNIT

A specialist metabolic surgery unit should provide a complete holistic multidisciplinary patient pathway from assessment, preoperative and perioperative care through to follow-up and any postoperative emergency care. Specialist units usually have several referring hospitals and primary care practices serving a large population. There are several multidisciplinary guidelines on what is required of a service from British Obesity and Metabolic Surgery Society (BOM-MS),[65] the IFSO,[64,66] and the American Society for Metabolic and Bariatric Surgery (ASMBS).[62]

There is evidence supporting a relationship between surgical volume and outcome (although an element of publication bias may exist). Schauer et al.[67] identified the learning curve for RYGB as 100 cases. Another study compared metabolic surgery performed at low-volume (< 50 cases per year), medium-volume (50–100 cases per year), and high-volume (> 100 cases per year) hospitals and found that those with more than 100 cases annually were associated with statistically significant reductions in length of stay, morbidity, and mortality, as well as costs. In patients older than 55 years, in-hospital mortality was threefold higher at low-volume compared with high-volume hospitals.[68] High-volume hospitals also have a lower rate of overall postoperative complications, which they attributed at least in part to formalisation of the structures and processes of care. Higher volume centres also have more income to support infrastructure, including staffing and facilities.

✔✔ Evidence suggests that higher volume centres (> 100 cases/year) have better outcomes in terms of length of stay, morbidity, and mortality than low-volume centres (< 50 cases per year).[68]

Such studies suggested that there needed to be a definition of what constitutes a properly trained bariatric surgeon and a bariatric unit. IFSO suggests three types of bariatric unit: Primary Bariatric Institutions (PBI), Bariatric Institutions (BIs), and Centre of Excellence Bariatric Institutions (COEBIs). PBIs are units just starting out in the care of bariatric patients and have very basic criteria (Box 17.1).[66] Additionally, consultant surgeons starting bariatric surgery at PBIs are required to meet certain requirements (e.g. laparoscopic general surgery training, completion of bariatric training course, testimonials by mentors, maintenance of a database, and commitment to lifetime follow-up). PBIs are advised not to undertake surgery on the patients with a BMI > 50 kg/m^2 in their first 1–2 years or until they have performed at least 50 procedures, or undertake revisional and complex procedures until the unit fulfils BI criteria. Some of the additional criteria for BIs include: ensuring that the director of metabolic surgery has at least 5 years' experience in the field and is capable of performing advanced metabolic procedures successfully; adequate facilities for morbidly and patients with a BMI > 50 kg/m^2; be a member of a national bariatric society; and availability of interventional radiologists as required. Surgeons must have advanced laparoscopic skills, have performed at least 50 procedures, and be capable of performing revisional surgery and surgery on patients with a BMI > 50 kg/m^2. COEBIs must additionally have performed 100 procedures (including revisional), provide an education programme for all staff, offer support groups for patients, and have lifetime follow-up for at least 75% of patients. Surgeons must be involved in accrediting less experienced surgeons, amongst other things.

The American Society of Metabolic and Bariatric Surgeons (ASMBS) have produced similar Centre of Excellence criteria for both the hospital and surgeon. However, there is evidence that creating centres of excellence has little or no impact on patient outcome.[69] The Society of American

> ### Box 17.1 Basic requirements to ensure a unit is fully equipped to undertake metabolic surgery*
>
> Basic requirements include:
> - Surgeons performing metabolic surgery have the appropriate certification, training, and experience
> - All members of the MDT and necessary allied specialities should be accessible and adequately experienced/qualified
> - A clearly documented institutional weight limit (to include equipment in outpatients/radiology/theatre, as well as manual handling and ward care)
> - 24-hour access to a bariatric surgeon and bariatric anaesthetist on call
> - Adequate basic equipment and facilities on the ward
> - Appropriately equipped operating theatres
> - Adequate biochemical and radiological facilities
> - On-site access for every patient to level 2 critical care services if required
> - Appropriate equipment to manage a transfer (including transfer ventilators)
> - Clear pathways for inter-hospital transfer
> - Records are kept of the adverse events that occur during the management of the patients
> - Adequate audit and clinical governance must be undertaken, including key quality indicators.
>
> *Adapted from International Federation for the Surgery of Obesity and Metabolic Disorders (IFSO) and British Obesity and Metabolic Surgery Society (BOMMS) guidelines.

Gastrointestinal and Endoscopic Surgeons (SAGES) have produced additional guidelines for 'credentialling' bariatric surgeons. All of these schemes are currently voluntary.

In the UK,[65] the service has been divided into bariatric units and bariatric centres, the combination of which form bariatric networks. A bariatric unit must have more than three consultant bariatric surgeons as well as adequate anaesthetic, dietician, and specialist nurse cover. Each surgeon should operate on at least 40 cases a year (although a lower volume is acceptable in a new unit at the outset). An established unit would be expected to have four bariatric surgeons to ensure adequate on-call cover, two full-time dieticians, and specialist nurses. Units are also expected to provide at least gastric banding, gastric bypass, and sleeve gastrectomy. Only basic revisional surgery should be carried out. They must also meet the basic criteria outlined in Box 17.1.

Bariatric centres are expected to perform at least five operations a week, with each consultant performing at least two operations a week – although there is flexibility dependent on the experience of the surgeon. A higher quality service is expected with an ideal volume of 300–400 cases a year, which may take several years to achieve. Bariatric centres should also be capable of performing more complex surgery (e.g. patients with a BMI > 50 kg/m^2, patients with multiple comorbidities, procedures such as DS, and revisional surgery). At the present time, there is no formal accreditation or 'credentialling' process in the UK for bariatric surgeons. However, this may be introduced in the foreseeable future. NICE does recommend that bariatric surgeons should be members of a recognised bariatric association (e.g. British

Obesity & Metabolic Surgery Society [BOMSS]) and audit their outcome data using a database (e.g. the National Bariatric Surgery Registry). It is also expected that centres have 24/7 consultant bariatric cover, including within 30 minutes of an emergency hospital presentation.

THE MULTIDISCIPLINARY TEAM

✓ A multidisciplinary team (MDT) is vital to deliver a safe and successful bariatric service.

The MDT should include:
- Specialist metabolic surgeons
- A bariatric nurse specialist
- A specialist bariatric dietician
- Specialist physicians with an interest in and commitment to metabolic medicine and the perioperative needs of patients undergoing metabolic surgery (a 'bariatric physician')
- Psychologist(s) and/or psychiatrists with experience in eating disorders
- Senior anaesthetist(s) with commitment to and experience of anaesthesia for metabolic surgery.

There should be standard referral pathways with categories of access to metabolic surgery (urgent, expedited, or standard)[70] as well as allied specialties integral to the care of patients, including a gastroenterologist or hepatologist, endocrinologist, diabetologist, cardiovascular and respiratory physician, a plastic surgeon for postoperative body contouring as required, and an eating disorder specialist.

A significant amount can be learnt from how good MDTs function for the management of patients with cancer. The key is that each member of the MDT has a defined role that is complementary to other members. Not all patients will need to see all members of the MDT and this will be guided by whether they have metabolic and/or psychological complications. All patients should be assessed and counselled by a surgeon and/or a physician, who will be responsible for their long-term weight loss maintenance. The surgeon should provide accurate, evidence-based, unbiased information regarding treatment options, including the risks and benefits of proposed surgical options. They should give adequate postoperative advice with respect to recovery, diet, realistic weight loss goals, and alarm symptoms (such as vomiting or severe abdominal pain) requiring urgent emergency department review. Written patient information sheets[71] for each intervention should help this process and the MDT should have clear protocols, including contacts for telephone advice for both the patient and professionals from other hospitals in the case of an emergency.

All patients should see a specialist dietician and/or specialist nurse, and this assessment should include advice on how to reduce post-surgical nutritional deficiencies. An anaesthetic preoperative evaluation is often required with respect to risk assessment. Patients able to achieve four metabolic equivalents (METs, a physiological measure of the energy cost of physical activity) are generally thought to be physically suitable for surgery. Patients with class III obesity

and those with cardiorespiratory comorbidity will require anaesthetic and/or a cardiorespiratory physician preoperative assessment. An appropriate specialist should assess patients with other complications, which have not been optimised, prior to undertaking surgery.

With respect to how the MDT functions, this varies worldwide, but there should be a focus on preoperative staging of the disease, planning how to limit surgical morbidity during the perioperative period, managing patients in the first few months after surgery, and then longer term planning on how to maintain patients in remission of the diseases that warranted surgical intervention in the first instance. MDT members can contribute significantly by focusing on prevention of nutritional or psychological side-effects of the operations while optimising the metabolic control afforded by surgery. Surgeons often chair the MDT, as they remain responsible for the short-, medium-, and long-term complications of the operations. However, the ultimate focus of the MDT has to be on keeping patients in long-term remission of their disease or in a state of optimal control.

A bariatric service must offer education, guidance, and counselling and motivational support throughout the treatment process. Patients should be aware of who is providing this support and how they can access it when required. Some units may offer a support group as part of both their preoperative counselling and postoperative follow-up care, while others employ social media or e-learning.

THE ROLE OF WEIGHT-MANAGEMENT PROGRAMMES

The aim of weight-management programmes (Fig. 17.3) is to reduce weight and improve obesity-related complications. General practitioners find that the advice to 'exercise more and eat less' is not usually successful in the long term.[72] Weight assessment and management clinics (WAMCs)[71,73] ideally provide a more extensive non-surgical weight-management service for weight loss or maintenance of weight loss, including:

- dietary interventions (structured eating plans, meal replacements, diets with a 600-kcal deficit, low-fat diets, low-calorie diets (900–1200 kcal/day), very low-calorie diets of 800 kcal/day or less);
- physical activity programmes (e.g. at least 30 minutes of moderate to high-intensity exercise 5 or more days/week with goal to be 300 minutes per week, including strength training two to three times per week,[10] with up to 60–90 minutes per day to avoid weight regain);
- behavioural and psychosocial interventions (e.g. cognitive behavioural therapy techniques such as goal setting, self-monitoring, stimulus control, a slower rate of eating, ensuring social support/assertiveness/reinforcement of change, cognitive restructuring, and relapse prevention with strategies for dealing with weight gain).

The addition of pharmacological agents that can achieve 10–25% weight loss in subgroups of patients needs to be employed. The most recent NICE guideline[59] states that very low-calorie diets should not be used routinely and only as part of a multicomponent weight-management strategy for people who need to lose weight rapidly (e.g. prior to

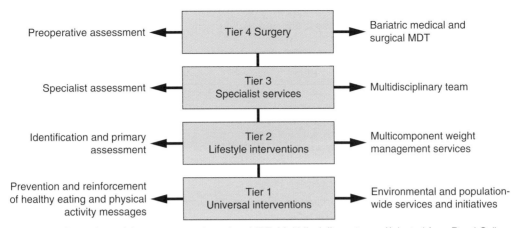

Figure 17.3 The clinical pathway for weight-management service. *MDT*, Multidisciplinary team. (Adapted from Royal College of Surgeons England. Weight assessment and management tier services – Commissioning guide 2014.[71])

knee-replacement surgery) and should not last longer than 12 weeks. It is vital that any diet is nutritionally complete and patients must understand how they can maintain weight loss in the longer term. The programme may be individualised or utilise group interventions. Similar to the success of supervised exercise programmes in patients with chronic limb ischaemia, such supervised weight-loss interventions are successful.[73] Due consideration should be given to how to manage patients after the very low-calorie diets come to an end, as weight regain usually follows if further interventions are not put in place. Drug treatment may be considered if the target weight loss is beyond 10%.

Most patients will not biologically respond to diet and exercise to achieve more than 10% weight loss. Blaming the patient for failing treatment is unjustified and such patients should be offered the opportunity of referral for medication or metabolic surgery.

In the UK, WAMCs are part of Tier 3 services[74] (see Fig. 17.3), whether they are in primary or secondary care and are commissioned by Clinical Commissioning Groups (Tier 1 and 2 services are commissioned by the local authority and Tier 4 services are commissioned centrally).[59,71,74] They are usually run by GPs or bariatric physicians who are part of the MDT. Community GPs will refer patients to a Tier 3 WAMC if patients require significant weight loss to address specific diseases and supervised lifestyle weight-management programme or self-directed dieting have failed the patient. Lifestyle weight-management programmes are part of Tier 2 community-based initiatives, with the aim to reduce food intake and increase exercise. There is evidence that commercially provided Tier 2 weight-management services (e.g. Weight Watchers/Slimming World) are more clinically effective and cost effective than primary care-based services led by specially trained staff.[75]

Generally, the indications for referral to a WAMC are the same as those for surgery. However, patients presenting with weight regain after surgery, nutritional deficiency due to surgery, or requiring revisional surgery may also be referred to the service even if their BMI is below 35 kg/m^2.[60,74] Children and adolescents should be referred to paediatric specialist services. Patients who are pregnant and some who have poorly controlled psychiatric illness should not be referred, but re-referred when appropriate.[73] There is no fixed time period for patients to remain in WAMCs prior to

being referred for surgery. However, the process can often take several months. Many patients do not require surgery after going through the WAMC service and have significant comorbidity improvement; however, if a patient has successfully lost weight with non-surgical approaches then bariatric surgery can still be considered as an appropriate method for long-term weight loss maintenance. Equally, patients with BMI > 50 kg/m^2 who are interested in surgery should not be denied effective surgical management by being forced to have repeated lifestyle modification attempts unless the patient can achieve more than 15% weight loss with non-surgical interventions.[74]

The WAMC should have an MDT,[74,76] including at least a bariatric physician, a nurse specialist, a dietician, and a psychologist, with easy access to psychiatry and physiotherapy services. Some institutions also have a surgeon involved in their weight-management service and there is significant overlap with the bariatric surgery MDT. At the WAMC, patients have comorbidities associated with obesity assessed. WC can also be an important marker of risk and can help guide treatment modalities (Table 17.3). Most obese patients have been shown to prefer their healthcare provider to be 'very direct/straightforward' and were 'extremely comfortable' discussing their weight.[77] However, patients with higher BMIs prefer their provider to 'discuss weight sensitively'. The uptake and success of weight-management programmes is lower in men and the use of techniques such as 'masculinisation' of advice regarding exercise, using humour, and focusing nutrition advice on portion size, alcohol intake, and emotional influences may be helpful in some settings to improve outcome.[73,78]

The patient's feelings and expectations, and willingness and confidence to make changes should be assessed sensitively. Patient education is key. Patients must understand the importance of lifestyle modification, their eating behaviours, the importance of reduction in ultra-processed food intake,[79] and increased exercise in order to lose weight. Furthermore, adequate preoperative education including eating behaviours, psychological factors, and appropriate information on metabolic surgery can lead to patients opting for surgery, as well as helping patients to change from one operation to another.[80] Such education facilitates patient choice and is likely to improve patient compliance and, therefore, outcome.

Table 17.3 NICE guidance on how body mass index and waist circumference can help guide management

BMI classification	Waist circumference Low	High	Very high	Comorbidities present
Overweight	1	2	2	3
Obesity I	2	2	2	3
Obesity II	3	3	3	4
Obesity III	4	4	4	4
1	General advice on healthy weight and lifestyle			
2	Diet and physical activity			
3	Diet and physical activity; consider drugs			
4	Diet and physical activity; consider drugs; consider surgery			

BMI, Body mass index.

The patient should be screened for hormonal (e.g. hypothyroidism) or known genetic causes for weight gain if there is clinical suspicion. All obesity-related complications (as aforementioned) should be investigated (often there is no prior diagnosis) and optimised as soon as they are identified, without waiting for weight loss.[59] This serves the additional purpose of preparing them for surgery if required.[62] Ascertaining psychological factors that may be a barrier to engagement and compliance is also important. Additionally, some psychotropic medications can cause weight gain.

Patients are not expected to lose a set amount of weight prior to referral for surgery. Weight loss during a supervised diet is likely to predict the patient's biological ability to lose weight but may not predict outcome after surgery. Often these preoperative diets were used to determine whether patients were motivated or compliant, but as the biological mechanisms through which surgery works are being understood, it is becoming clearer that preoperative psychological factors do not predict long-term weight loss outcomes. Preoperative weight loss of at least 5% can reduce operative time and potentially operative risk by making surgery technically easier (e.g. a smaller liver volume following milk or very low-energy diets),[81,82] although this does not necessarily equate to a reduction in postoperative complications.[81] However, having a BMI > 55 kg/m² is one of the leading causes for complications and death after RYGB, so in this patient cohort weight loss preoperatively is desirable.[83]

✔✔ Preoperative weight loss of at least 5% can reduce operative time and potentially operative risk, although this does not necessarily equate to a reduction in postoperative complications,[81] except in patients with a BMI > 55 kg/m², when it is believed to reduce postoperative mortality.[83]

The current practice if adequate weight loss is achieved in patients without comorbidity or in whom comorbidity has been optimised is to refer these patients back to the GP. This may be appropriate, but if sufficient control of the disease is not achieved or an appropriate long-term plan is not in place, then referring patients back prematurely may result in poorer long-term disease remission. Patients who are unsuitable for surgery but have ongoing complex obesity-related comorbidity might be kept in an obesity clinic. Those who are identified during assessment to be engaged,

knowledgeable about the surgery/risks/benefits, motivated, realistic, and physically 'fit' with full optimisation of complications are referred on for surgery. They must also understand the long-term nutritional requirements and lifelong follow-up.[62] Surgery is taken up by less than 1% of patients with obesity that could benefit from it.[84]

MULTIDISCIPLINARY ASSESSMENT OF PATIENT SUITABILITY FOR METABOLIC SURGERY

A multidisciplinary assessment of patients, using validated risk assessment tools, is essential when selecting and preparing patients for metabolic surgery. This assessment should identify indications and contraindications to surgery, optimise management of medical complications prior to surgery, educate the patients about operative choices and risks of the procedures, and ensure that patients have realistic expectations. The assessment should include a full history including psychosocial evaluation, examination, blood tests and appropriate investigations (Table 17.4).

RISK ASSESSMENT

The overall mortality and morbidity of bariatric surgery is low. However, patients with multiple or complex complications of obesity are at higher risk. A risk assessment needs to assess existing complications and whether they are reversible, the patient's age and health status, as well as their functional state if surgery is not undertaken and compare this to the risk of postoperative morbidity and mortality. The responsibility for this lies with all the members of the MDT.

✔✔ Patients must undergo risk stratification prior to surgery. There are several validated scoring systems. In the Edmonton Obesity Staging System (EOSS), high scores predict increasing mortality due to obesity-related complications.[85] However, it is important to note that high scores should not necessarily preclude surgery and patients with a high score may derive the most benefit from surgery.

To ascertain the level of risk and stratify patients' suitability for surgery various risk assessment tools have been

Table 17.4 Preoperative checklist for metabolic surgery

History and examination (obesity-related comorbidities, cause of obesity, weight/BMI, weight-loss history, commitment, exclusions related to surgical risk)

Routine bloods (fasting glucose and lipids, U&Es, LFTs, urine dipstick; clotting, G&S, FBC)

Nutrient screening (iron studies, vitamin B₁₂, and folic acid (RBC folate, homocysteine, methylmalonic acid optional), and 25-vitamin D (vitamins A and E optional); consider more extensive testing in patients undergoing malabsorptive procedures based on symptoms and risks)

Cardiorespiratory evaluation with sleep apnoea screening (ECG, chest X-ray, echocardiography if cardiac disease or pulmonary hypertension suspected; DVT evaluation if clinically indicated)

GI evaluation (*Helicobacter pylori* screening in high-prevalence areas; gallbladder evaluation and upper GI endoscopy if clinically indicated)

Endocrine evaluation (*HbA1c/FPG*) with suspected or diagnosed prediabetes or diabetes; fasting plasma glucose; thyroid-stimulating hormone (TSH) symptoms or increased risk of thyroid disease; androgens with PCOS suspicion (total/bioavailable testosterone, DHEAS, D4-androstenedione); screening for Cushing's syndrome if clinically suspected (1 mg overnight dexamethasone test, 24-hour urinary-free cortisol, 11 pm salivary cortisol)

Clinical nutrition evaluation by dietician

Psychosocial-behavioural evaluation

Document medical necessity for metabolic surgery

Informed consent

Provide relevant financial information (not relevant to NHS currently)

Continue efforts for preoperative weight loss

Optimise glycaemic control

Pregnancy counselling

Smoking cessation counselling

Verify cancer screening by primary care physician

BMI, Body mass index; *DHEAS*, dehydroepiandrosterone sulphate; *DVT*, deep vein thrombosis; *ECG*, electrocardiogram; *FBC*, full blood count; *G&S*, group and save; *GI*, gastrointestinal; *HbA1c*, haemoglobin A1C; *LFT*, liver function test; *PCOS*, polycystic ovary syndrome; *RBC*, red blood cell; *U&E*, urea and electrolytes.
Based on Mechanick et al.[62]

Table 17.5 The Obesity Surgery Mortality Risk Score (OS-MRS)

1 point for each of:	Class A (0–1 points) low risk
Male	
Age ≥ 45 years	Class B (2–3 points) medium risk
BMI ≥ 50 kg/m²	
Hypertension	Class C (4–5 points) high risk
Known risk of DVT/PE	

This score has been validated in gastric bypass, where mortality was 0.2% in class A patients and 2.4% in class C patients.[124] It has also been shown to predict postoperative complications after laparoscopic metabolic procedures.[125]

Table 17.6 The Edmonton Obesity Staging System (EOSS)

0	No apparent risk factors	e.g. blood pressure, serum lipid, and fasting glucose levels within normal range, physical symptoms, psychopathology, functional limitations and/or impairment of wellbeing related to obesity
1	Presence of obesity-related subclinical risk factors	e.g. borderline hypertension, impaired fasting glucose levels, elevated levels of liver enzymes, mild physical symptoms (e.g. dyspnoea on moderate exertion, occasional aches and pains, fatigue), mild psychopathology, mild functional limitations, and/or mild impairment of wellbeing
2	Presence of established obesity-related chronic disease	e.g. hypertension, type 2 diabetes, sleep apnoea, osteoarthritis), moderate limitations in activities of daily living and/or wellbeing
3	Established end-organ damage	e.g. myocardial infarction, heart failure, stroke, significant psychopathology, significant functional limitations, and/or impairment of wellbeing
4	Severe (potentially end-stage) disabilities from obesity-related chronic diseases	e.g. severe disabling psychopathology, severe functional limitations, and/or severe impairment of wellbeing

Adapted from Padwal et al.[85]

developed and validated. The most extensively validated tool is the American Society of Anaesthesiologists (ASA) score, which is used to ascertain anaesthetic risk. Several validated scores exist to assess surgical risk, including the Obesity Surgery Mortality Risk Score (OSM-RS; Table 17.5), the EOSS (Table 17.6), and the King's Obesity Staging Score (KOSS; Table 17.7).

The KOSS helps the clinician in treatment choice in patients with obesity to choose either surgery or other modalities, and also to identify and stratify obesity-related complications that can be downstaged by metabolic surgery.[86,87]

The EOSS has surpassed OSM-RS as being a more comprehensive scoring system taking into account the severity of obesity-related comorbidity and is currently the preferred scoring system of BOMMS. High scores in both EOSS and OSM-RS are a strong predictor of increasing mortality,

which is independent of BMI, metabolic syndrome, or increased WC.[85,88] According to the NSBR 2014 report,[89] although the majority of patients operated on are EOSS stage 2 before surgery, the proportion of patients classified in stages 3 or 4 has increased substantially between 2006

Table 17.7 Applied modified 'King's Obesity Staging Score criteria for assessment of obesity

Criteria	Stage 0	Stage 1	Stage 2	Stage 3
	'Normal health'	'At risk of disease'	'Established disease'	'Advanced disease'
Airways	Normal	Snoring	Requires CPAP	Cor pulmonale
Body mass index (kg/m^2)	< 35	35–40	40–60	> 60
Cardiovascular	< 10%	10–20%	Heart disease	Heart failure
Diabetes	Normal	Impaired fasting glycaemia	Type 2 diabetes	Uncontrolled type 2 diabetes
Economic	Normal	Expensive travel/clothes	Workplace discrimination	Unemployed due to obesity
Functional	Can manage three flights of stairs	Manages one or two flights of stairs	Requires walking aids or wheelchair	House bound
Gonadal	Normal	PCOS	Infertility	Sexual dysfunction
Health perceived	Normal	Low mood or QoL	Depression or poor QoL	Severe depression
(Body) Image	Normal	Dislikes body	Body image dysphoria	Eating disorder with purging (drug use or vomiting)
Junction gastroesophageal	Normal	Heartburn	Oesophagitis	Barrett's oesophagus
Kidney	Normal	Proteinuria	GFR < 60 mL/min	GFR < 30 mL/min
Liver	Normal	Raised LFT/NAFLD	NASH	Liver failure
Medication				

BMI, Body mass index; *CPAP*, continuous positive airway pressure; *GFR*, glomerular filtration rate; *LFT*, liver function test; *NAFLD*, non-alcoholic fatty liver disease; *NASH*, non-alcoholic steatohepatitis; *PCOS*, polycystic ovary syndrome; *QoL*, quality of life.
Adapted from Aylwin et al.[91] and Abdelaal et al.[92]

and 2013 – the proportion of women classified as stage 4 rose from 1% to more than 16%; the proportion of men classified as stage 4 rose from 5% to more than 20%. Stage 4, therefore, does not preclude surgery – it may in fact be this group that derives the most benefit from surgery. Giving higher weighting to certain comorbidities, for example T2DM, may make the score a better prognostic tool.[85] It has also been validated in the context of postoperative outcome, with postoperative complication rates after metabolic surgery of 0% for EOSS 0, 1.6% for EOSS 1, 8.2% for EOSS 2, and 22.4% for EOSS 3.[90] The authors of this study concluded that patients should be recommended for obesity surgery when their EOSS stage is 2 to prevent impairments associated with metabolic disease and to reduce the risk of postoperative complications.

The KOSS uses the mnemonic ABCDEFGHIJKLM and incorporates BMI and functional status into a scoring system (Table 17.7).[91,92]

It can be used to identify and stratify obesity-related complications that can be 'downstaged' by treatment in a similar way to how surgery is often used to downstage cancer. As with the other scores, it focuses on health gain and not purely weight loss, and may be an easier tool to use to track health improvements in patients.

It is important to be aware of these scoring systems, understanding their advantages and limitations to make a decision on which one to use in clinical practice. Furthermore, certain factors have been associated with poor outcome after bariatric surgery (e.g. male, age > 50 years, open technique, chronic renal failure, congestive heart failure, and peripheral vascular disease)[76,93] and such factors should be incorporated into the ideal scoring system.

IDENTIFYING AND OPTIMISING OBESITY-RELATED COMORBIDITIES

DIETETIC ASSESSMENT

All patients should have a nutritional assessment, including protein, vitamins, minerals, and micronutrient measurements, with any deficiencies being corrected before any bariatric surgical procedure.[76] Preoperative lab work should include nutrient screening with iron studies, vitamin B$_{12}$ and folic acid (red blood cell folate [RBC folate], homocysteine, methylmalonic acid optional), and 25-vitamin D (vitamins A and E optional); consider more extensive testing in patients undergoing malabsorptive procedures based on symptoms and risks.[10] Whole-blood thiamine levels may be considered in patients prior to bypass procedures (RYGB and biliopancreatic diversion with DS).[10] Vitamin A, parathyroid hormone, phosphate, zinc, selenium, and copper levels can be assessed more selectively due to cost considerations.[94] This is not only important to mitigate the harmful effects of deficiencies in these nutritional factors, but also to optimise nutritional status prior to procedures that result in micronutrient malabsorption. Of note, patients taking proton pump inhibitors and/or metformin have a higher prevalence of vitamin B$_{12}$ deficiency.[95]

RESPIRATORY ASSESSMENT: OSA, ASTHMA, AND PULMONARY ASSESSMENT

Up to 38% of patients assessed for bariatric surgery may have undiagnosed OSA.[96] Patients with OSA must be optimised preoperatively.

Up to 38% of patients assessed for metabolic surgery may have undiagnosed OSA.[96] The STOP–BANG screening tool (Snoring, Tired, Observed apnoeas, high blood Pressure, BMI > 35 kg/m^2, Age > 50 years, Neck circumference (> 43 cm [17 in] for males, > 41 cm [16 in] for females), male Gender; where yes to five or more questions indicates a high risk of OSA and warrants further investigation with polysomnography) is recommended by the Society of Bariatric Anaesthetists.[97] If OSA or OHS is diagnosed, the patient should be started on appropriate management. Those already diagnosed should be allowed to use their own continuous positive airway pressure (CPAP) machines on the ward as necessary.

All patients should also have a chest radiograph and patients with intrinsic lung disease or disordered sleep patterns should have a formal pulmonary evaluation, including arterial blood gas measurement.[62]

SMOKING

Smoking is a known risk factor for poor wound healing, impaired health, and anastomotic ulcer.[98]

In a retrospective review of the National Surgical Quality Improvement Program (NSQIP) database, Haskins et al. found that smoking within the year before vertical sleeve gastrectomy (VSG) was associated with increased 30-day morbidity and mortality risk, compared with nonsmokers.[99]

Structured cessation programs are more effective than general advice, which is more effective than usual care. All smokers must be advised to stop smoking at any time before metabolic surgery, even if it is within 6 weeks before surgery,[100] and appropriate referral made for a long-term solution.[10,76]

METABOLIC AND ENDOCRINE ASSESSMENT

Type 2 diabetes mellitus

Patients with elevated preoperative HbA1c are more likely to have postoperative hyperglycaemia, which is independently associated with reduced remission of T2DM, acute renal failure, and wound infections.[101] Glycaemic control should be optimised preoperatively using the usual hospital management algorithm, which may include dietary modification, exercise, nutritional therapy, and drug treatment as required. Reasonable targets for preoperative glycaemic control, which may be associated with shorter hospital stays and improved metabolic procedure outcomes, include an HbA1c value of 6.5–7.0% (48–53 mmol/mol) or less and peri-procedure blood glucose levels of 80–180 mg/dl. More liberal pre-procedure targets, such as an HbA1c of 7–8% (53–64 mmol/mol), are recommended in patients with advanced microvascular or macrovascular complications, extensive complications, or longstanding diabetes in which the general goal has been difficult to attain despite intensive efforts.[10,62] However, UK commissioning guidelines state that inability to achieve glycaemic control should not be a bar to or delay referral for metabolic surgery. Patients with HbA1c more than 8% (> 64 mmol/mol) or uncontrolled diabetes should be referred back to a diabetologist for optimisation. High preoperative C-peptide levels have been associated with T2DM remission rates following RYGB and may be a good marker for patient selection in the future.[102]

In T2DM patients, glycaemic control should be optimised preoperatively to a HbA1c of 6.5–7.0% (48 mmol/mol; 7.8–8.6 mmol/L) and a fasting blood glucose level of 110 mg/dL (6.1 mmol/L). Patients may be considered for surgery at higher HbA1c levels of 7–8% (53 mmol/mol–64 mmol/mol) estimated average glucose (8.6–10.2 mmol/L) if they have advanced microvascular or macrovascular complications, extensive comorbid conditions, or long-standing poorly controlled diabetes despite all efforts.[62]

Additionally, a personal or family history of hypoglycaemia, as well as symptoms of hypoglycaemia (exercise- or meal-related shakiness, sweating, palpitations, blurred vision, difficulty concentrating, unexplained near-syncope, syncope, or seizures) should be ascertained, prompting preoperative endocrinology review.[76] If preoperative hyperinsulinaemic hypoglycaemia is diagnosed, patients should be considered for gastric banding, which would not be expected to further enhance incretin secretion and hyperinsulinaemia.[76]

Thyroid function

Thyroid function tests are usually routinely done, but some authors suggest that only patients who are high risk for or exhibit symptoms of thyroid disease require thyroid function tests with serum thyroid-stimulating hormone (TSH) level.[62] Patients diagnosed with hypothyroidism should be managed appropriately with medical treatment. In patients on thyroid hormone replacement or supplementation, TSH levels must be monitored after metabolic procedures and medication dosing adjusted, as dose reductions are more likely with weight loss but can increase with malabsorption after DS. Oral liquid forms of levothyroxine may be considered in those patients with difficulty swallowing tablets after metabolic procedures. Oral liquid or softgel forms of levothyroxine may be considered in patients with significant malabsorption after DS in whom adequate TSH suppression to normal ranges is difficult after metabolic procedures.[10]

PSYCHOLOGICAL ASSESSMENT

Preoperative psychological assessment is important for good outcomes and aiding compliance. The presence of more than two psychiatric/mental health disorders and eating disorders increases the risk of postoperative problems, such as reduced weight loss maintenance.[64]

Currently, there is no single robust assessment tool that assesses all psychosocial domains pre-metabolic surgery. Hartmann-Boyce et al. investigated behavioural techniques and modes of delivery as they impact obesity interventions. They note that most behavioural interventions do not use the wide variety of behaviour change strategies available but focus on goal setting and action planning as well as self-monitoring and feedback.[103] In a 2015 systematic review, the Master Questionnaire, a 56-item true/false questionnaire, was identified as the only tool that assessed patients on multiple eating behaviour domains in patients with obesity.[104] As a screen for binge eating, the Binge Eating Scale (BES) demonstrates good sensitivity (94%).[104,105] The presence of two or more psychiatric/mental health disorders and eating disorders (such as binge eating) increases the risk of problems after metabolic surgery, which may result in poorer long-term benefits of surgery, such as weight loss maintenance.[64] Therefore, a thorough preoperative psychological assessment can identify potential behavioural, nutritional, familial, and personality factors that may require additional interventions to improve the success of surgery. Consideration should be given to crisis interventions, psychological support, psychotherapy,[106] as well as those at risk of suicide in the long term. This assessment may be structured using the acronym BEST:[107]

- **B**iological factors – family history, relevant comorbidity.
- **E**nvironmental factors – eating behaviour, exercise, effects of obesogenic environment.
- **S**ocial/psychological factors – psychotropic medication, abuse, psychiatric comorbidity.
- **T**iming of weight loss intervention – stressors.

Patients must be screened for psychopathology such as schizophrenia, bipolar disorder, personality disorder, anxiety and depression, self-harm, substance misuse or dependence, and eating disorders. After RYGB, high-risk groups should stop drinking alcohol due to impaired alcohol metabolism and risk of alcohol misuse postoperatively.[108] Some patients may need to have their management optimised prior to being reassessed for surgery (e.g. those with untreated or unstable mental health conditions, active alcohol or substance misuse, an active eating disorder, self-harm in the past 12 months, dementia, current non-adherence to treatment, and a recent significant life event, e.g. bereavement or a relationship breakdown).[71]

Validated screening tools should be used to identify pathology that may require psychiatric input or potentially contraindicate surgery. The SCOFF Eating Disorder Screening Tool[87] is a validated tool for eating disorders.

CARDIOVASCULAR ASSESSMENT

Fasting lipids should be checked in all patients and optimised. Not only are they associated with cardiovascular complications, but high preoperative TG levels are also associated with NASH and low HDL levels with NAFLD.[109] NASH and NAFLD should be investigated in patients with dyslipidaemia. The effect of weight loss on dyslipidaemia is variable and incomplete; therefore, lipid-lowering medications should not be stopped unless clearly indicated.[10] Although WC measurements provide additional information regarding the risk of cardiometabolic disease, it is of very little value in patients with a BMI > 35 kg/m².

✅ Fasting lipids should be checked in all patients and optimised. Patients with dyslipidaemia should be assessed for NASH and NAFLD.

All patients should also have an electrocardiogram if indicated prior to surgery. Further cardiological investigations should be required only if patients have risk factors, signs, or symptoms of cardiovascular disease, with referral to a cardiologist as necessary.[62] There are few data on interventions to reduce cardiovascular risk in metabolic surgery patients, although standard care involves optimising the management of blood pressure, dyslipidaemia, and glucose control.[76] Continuation of beta-blocker treatment may reduce cardiac events and improve mortality in patients.[110] If a beta-blocker after metabolic surgery is needed, a hydrophilic compound like atenolol may be preferred.[111]

GASTROINTESTINAL ASSESSMENT

Liver function tests (LFTs) should be performed in all patients. Those with elevated LFTs or GI symptoms should undergo further investigations – which may include a viral hepatitis screen, imaging studies (e.g. abdominal ultrasound), contrast studies, or endoscopy. Routine evaluation of the metabolic surgical patient with an abdominal ultrasound is not recommended, except in those patients requiring an investigation for symptomatic biliary disease and elevated liver enzymes, or non-alcoholic fatty liver.[112] Liver biopsy may be done during surgery to confirm any suspected diagnosis of liver disease (predominantly NASH, NAFLD, or early cirrhosis with normal blood results). Considering (NAFLD) age, WC, serum alanine aminotransferase (ALT), serum TGs, aminotransferase-to-platelet ratio, and ultrasound and transient elastography all have some predictive value, there are no reliable noninvasive pre-surgical predictors of disease severity or progression.[113–115] Fasting lipids should be checked in all patients and optimised. Patients with dyslipidaemia should be assessed for NASH and NAFLD. Cirrhosis can lead to poor outcomes after metabolic surgery, including necessitating a liver transplant, and it is vital to diagnose and stage cirrhosis preoperatively if clinically evident.[116]

The risk of metabolic surgery in patients carefully selected with Child–Pugh class A liver cirrhosis is not prohibitive, but caution and additional surveillance should be undertaken as their overall risk for perioperative complications and mortality is increased.[117,118]

Preoperative screening for *Helicobacter pylori* before metabolic surgery may be required in high-prevalence areas, with some studies suggesting preoperative diagnosis correlates with anastomotic ulceration and perforation, although others refute this.[62] *H. pylori* may be implicated in the development of gastritis, peptic ulcer, and gastric carcinoma.[119–121] Screening for *H. pylori* is recommended for this reason in patients undergoing gastric bypass procedures.[94]

Preoperative weight loss (e.g. using a preoperative milk diet) for liver shrinkage is encouraged. All patients should also have renal function tests, particularly if they have hypertension or diabetes, with referral to a nephrologist if significant renal disease exists.[76] Patients with renal disease can also have fluid overload contributing to increased weight and may have an increased risk of infection, particularly if undergoing gastric banding.[122] It is important to verify that cancer screening will be done as per usual protocols or by primary care physicians pre-procedure.

GYNAECOLOGY ASSESSMENT

✅ All female patients should be advised against pregnancy for 12 months postoperatively due to the increased risk of fetal malnutrition secondary to maternal malnutrition, and also be counselled regarding postoperative contraception.[62] Bioavailability of oral contraceptives may be reduced post metabolic surgery, and alternate methods of contraception need to be considered.[111] Additionally, oestrogen therapy (both contraception and hormone-replacement therapy) should be discontinued before surgery to reduce deep vein thrombosis (DVT) risk.[62]

Patients with class III obesity and those with high risk scores need to undergo rigorous preoperative assessment with anaesthetic input. The consenting process should include the operative options, potential benefits, risks/complications, perioperative mortality, long-term implications of surgery such as vitamin supplementation, and the need for long-term follow-up.[59] Of interest is the ASMBS Guideline, which suggests that consent should include the experience of the surgeon with the specific procedure offered and whether the hospital has an accredited metabolic surgery programme. Such accountability may become more commonplace as surgeon-specific outcome reporting becomes standard.

CONCLUSION

Obesity has become a global pandemic associated with high economic, health, and psychosocial costs. Metabolic surgery works via complex physiological mechanisms to alleviate this burden as part of an appropriate treatment algorithm. Appropriate patient selection and preoperative work-up is vital to the long-term success of metabolic surgery.

Key points

- Obesity and its related complications have become a global pandemic increasing in incidence.
- Currently, metabolic surgery is the best treatment that results in sustained weight loss maintenance and remission of complications. However, best medical therapy with metabolic surgery may be considered the best modality in the future.[123]
- The pathophysiology of obesity and its complications involves complex physiological mechanisms involving GBE and adipocyte–brain–endocrine interactions.
- Metabolic surgery ameliorates these by changes in eating behaviour and weight loss, gut hormones, BA kinetics, adipocyte-derived factors, and anatomical factors.
- The rationale for metabolic surgery is based on a cost benefit, with significant socioeconomic and health benefits.
- Indications for surgery are based on NICE/NIH/IFSO criteria using BMI and obesity-related complications.
- A specialist bariatric/metabolic unit should be able to provide preoperative, postoperative elective, and emergency care, as well as meeting basic criteria including adequate surgical volume and training of staff.
- All bariatric/metabolic units should have a fully staffed MDT.
- WAMCs have the vital role of weight loss, management of complications, and assessment of suitability for surgery.
- All patients must undergo rigorous risk assessment prior to surgery.
- All obesity-related complications should be identified preoperatively and optimised prior to surgery.

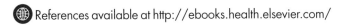 References available at http://ebooks.health.elsevier.com/

KEY REFERENCES

[2] Sjöström L, Lindroos AK, Peltonen M, et al. Lifestyle, diabetes, and cardiovascular risk factors 10 years after bariatric surgery. N Engl J Med 2004;351:2683–93. PMID: 15616203.
This paper reports results of the 10-year follow-up of the Swedish Obese Subjects Study. It demonstrates that bariatric surgery produces sustained long-term weight loss, lifestyle improvement, and risk factor improvement in comparison to conservative management.

[54] Sjöström L, Narbro K, Sjöström CD, et al. Effects of bariatric surgery on mortality in Swedish obese subjects. N Engl J Med 2007;357:741–52. PMID: 17715408.
This paper reports the mortality statistics of the 10-year follow-up of the Swedish Obese Subjects Study. It demonstrates that bariatric surgery significantly reduces mortality compared to conservative management.

[59] National Institute for Health and Care Excellence (NICE). Obesity: Identification, assessment and management. 2014. Clinical Guideline [CG189] https://www.nice.org.uk/guidance/cg189.
This NICE guideline outlines diagnostic, assessment, and management criteria for obesity. It discusses the BMI criteria for bariatric surgery and its limitations.

[60] Dixon JB, Zimmet P, Alberti KG, et al. Bariatric surgery: an IDF statement for obese type 2 diabetes. Diabet Med 2011;28(6):628–42. PMID: 21480973.
A consensus document from a working group of diabetologists, endocrinologists, surgeons, and public health experts recommending that bariatric surgery can be considered an appropriate treatment for people with T2DM and obesity not achieving treatment targets with medical therapies, especially in the presence of other major comorbidities. Bariatric surgery was considered an effective, safe, and cost-effective therapy for obese T2DM.

[61] Müller-Stich BP, Senft JD, Warschkow R, et al. Surgical versus medical treatment of type 2 diabetes mellitus in nonseverely obese patients: a systematic review and meta-analysis. Ann Surg 2015;261:421–9. PMID: 25405560.
This systematic review evaluated surgical versus medical T2DM treatment in patients with a BMI < 35 kg/m². Metabolic surgery was superior to medical treatment for short-term remission of T2DM and comorbidities.

[62] Mechanick JI, Youdim A, Jones DB, et al. Clinical practice guidelines for the perioperative nutritional, metabolic, and nonsurgical support of the bariatric surgery patient – 2013 update: cosponsored by American Association of Clinical Endocrinologists, the Obesity Society, and American Society for Metabolic and Bariatric Surgery. Obesity 2013;21:S1–27. PMID: 23529939.
These are comprehensive, evidence-based guidelines on the perioperative care of a bariatric surgery patient, including criteria for optimising glycaemic control and postoperative care.

[64] Fried M, Yumuk V, Oppert JM, et al. Interdisciplinary European Guidelines on metabolic and bariatric surgery. Obes Surg 2014;24:42–55. PMID: 24081459.
Comprehensive European evidence-based guidelines on perioperative care, including the importance of psychological support.

[68] Nguyen NT, Paya M, Stevens CM, et al. The relationship between hospital volume and outcome in bariatric surgery at academic medical centers. Ann Surg 2004;240:586–94. PMID: 15383786.
This study demonstrates a relationship between hospital volume and outcomes, suggesting that high-volume centres (~100 cases) have reduced morbidity, mortality, and length of stay.

[81] Alami RS, Morton JM, Schuster R, et al. Is there a benefit to preoperative weight loss in gastric bypass patients? A prospective randomized trial. Surg Obes Relat Dis 2007;3:141–5; discussion 145–6. PMID: 17331803.
This study demonstrated that although preoperative weight loss reduced perioperative time, it did not affect major complication or conversion rates, or have any bearing on the resolution of comorbidities.

[85] Padwal RS, Pajewski NM, Allison DB, et al. Using the Edmonton Obesity Staging System to predict mortality in a population-representative cohort of people with overweight and obesity. CMAJ (Can Med Assoc J) 2011;183:E1059–66. PMID: 21844111.
This study demonstrated that the EOSS predicted increased mortality and that it could be used to assess obesity-related risk and prioritise treatment.

[96] Rasmussen JJ, Fuller WD, Ali MR. Sleep apnea syndrome is significantly underdiagnosed in bariatric surgical patients. Surg Obes Relat Dis 2012;8:569–73. PMID: 21925966.
This study demonstrated that 38% of patients with sleep apnoea syndrome presenting for bariatric surgery were previously undiagnosed. It highlights the importance of diagnosing, assessing, and managing this condition prior to surgery.

18 Bariatric operations and perioperative care

Shaw Somers

SELECTION OF PROCEDURE

PATIENT CHOICE

Patients need to have a reasonable knowledge of the concepts of appetite, satiety, and weight-loss maintenance. An understanding of healthy diet, portion sizes, and eating behaviour is mandatory to successful long-term efficacy of bariatric surgery.

Patients should also have an understanding of the main procedures and their pros and cons.

✔✔ Patients should discuss their own clinical situation with the multidisciplinary team (MDT) and chose a procedure based upon their specific needs and expectations. While the patient should actively choose their procedure, the MDT manages the process. Guidance may be required if the patient chooses an option that the MDT considers clinically inappropriate.[1]

Counselling of procedure risks is especially pertinent to bariatric surgery. Patients must understand the impact of the major complications of each procedure, with emphasis on the relevance to their own life circumstances (e.g. gastric band slippage, gastric sleeve leak).

The importance of regular follow-up to long-term outcomes cannot be overemphasised. Patients must be aware of their obligations to their own health following a bariatric procedure and be fully 'signed-up' to comply with long-term review.

SURGICAL FACTORS INFLUENCING SELECTION

Previous surgery may impact on the technical feasibility of bariatric surgery. Previous gastric surgery (e.g. fundoplication) may prevent placement of a gastric band or accurate gastric sleeve formation. Previous intestinal surgery or known small-bowel adhesion disease may preclude any form of intestinal bypass.

Intestinal disease, such as Crohn's disease or extensive colitis, may render any form of bypass surgery intolerable and unwise. Those patients who have lost significant small intestinal length would also be unwise to consider intestinal bypass for weight loss.

A diagnosis of hiatal hernia does not preclude bariatric surgery. Most bariatric surgeons would repair the hiatus around a suitable oesophagogastric bougie and then proceed with whichever procedure was planned. Anterior repair is preferred for modest defects, while larger hiatal defects are repaired 'fore and aft' to prevent oesophageal kinking at the oesophagogastric junction (OGJ).

Gallstones are common among the obese population. Many bariatric surgeons would counsel for a possible cholecystectomy to remove stones and ensure duct clearance before undertaking a bariatric procedure, as gastric band patients with severe cholecystitis may risk infection of the gastric band. Patients with a gastric bypass who suffer small gallstones passing into the common bile duct are faced with a dilemma of access for stone extraction.

OPEN VERSUS LAPAROSCOPIC?

The vast majority of modern bariatric surgery is undertaken laparoscopically. Even those that have undergone a prior open abdominal procedure can expect a successful laparoscopic revision procedure.

GENERAL PREOPERATIVE CARE

FAMILIARITY WITH THE 'PATIENT PATHWAY' AND PREOPERATIVE EXPECTATION SETTING

Patients should be carefully counselled regarding their proposed procedure. They should understand the preoperative preparation required, the pre-assessment process and optimisation of comorbidities, and the sequence of events on the day of surgery. This will help allay anxiety and fear regarding the procedure. A careful explanation of the immediate postoperative experience and subsequent early postoperative dietary rehabilitation is useful. Finally, patients should be aware of the expectations for weight loss and dietary tolerance for their procedure.[1]

Patients should also be counselled regarding potential complications and their signs and symptoms. They should also have a contact number in case of emergency, and instruction on where to present and what information to relate to attending doctors.

NUTRITIONAL REPLETION

Despite being obese, many patients can harbour vitamin or mineral deficiency, which must be identified and addressed before surgery is undertaken. Specifically, vitamin B group, vitamins C and D, iron, and folate can be assessed and normalised with dietetic advice and supplementation.[2]

CONSENT FOR SURGERY

The process of patient consent is especially important in bariatric surgery. While many patients will have undergone careful counselling and assessment through the Tier 3–4 process, it cannot be assumed that they understand the personal implications of their surgery and the complications that may arise. It is the operating surgeon's responsibility to ensure that consent is both informed and appropriate to the individual. Many centres will utilise a detailed procedure-specific consent form that would list both general and procedure-specific risks and complications. Ideally, patients should be given a consent form for their chosen procedure to read and sign at home.[3]

STABILISATION OF COMORBIDITIES

Patients should undergo a structured assessment by a physician as part of the multidisciplinary management of their perioperative care. Optimisation of any comorbidity is essential to optimal outcomes from surgical intervention.[4]

1. *Obstructive sleep apnoea (OSA):* Patients should ideally have been screened for this during their initial referral or Tier 3 work-up. A minimum period of 6 weeks continuous positive airway pressure (CPAP) therapy is recommended before undertaking surgery in a newly diagnosed OSA sufferer. Adequate CPAP therapy is vital to reduce pulmonary hypertension and right heart strain in the preoperative period.[5]
2. *Type 2 diabetes mellitus:*

   ✓✓ Patients with less-than-optimal control should have a diabetic review before surgery. Blood glucose and HbA1c levels must be optimised to reduce risk in the perioperative period. However, it is accepted that those patients with significant insulin resistance will require bariatric surgery to gain better glycaemic control.[6]

1. *Ischaemic heart disease and hypertension:* Optimisation of drug therapy is important to minimise preoperative risk of infarction or stroke. Cardiological advice should be sought in such patients.[4]
2. *Depression:* Many patients present for bariatric surgery with depressive illness on medication. Generally, their medication can be continued immediately postoperatively. However, contact with their psychiatrist or general practitioner should be sought to clarify the past psychiatric history and medication requirements.
3. *Non-alcoholic fatty liver disease (NAFLD):* The majority of patients presenting for bariatric surgery will have an enlarged fatty liver. This can progress to NAFLD with varying degrees of fibrosis and eventually cirrhosis. Patients with deranged liver function tests should be investigated to exclude gallstones as well as NAFLD. Preoperatively, patients should undergo a very low-calorie diet for at least 2 weeks to effect 'liver shrinkage'. This is usually achieved by a low-carbohydrate diet, or a milk diet.[7]
4. *Pre-habilitation fitness:* Enhancement of patient fitness can be achieved by structured exercise regimes and the encouragement of physical activities in daily life. This has been shown to improve exercise tolerance and recovery following surgery.[4]

ENHANCED RECOVERY AFTER BARIATRIC SURGERY

A variety of schemes have been devised in order to provide a streamlined patient pathway with high-quality perioperative care, designed to achieve a fast-track service. These have many features in common with other enhanced recovery pathways, but require some bariatric-specific points for this patient population.[8]

DAY OF SURGERY

Most patients are admitted on the day of surgery. This requires thorough pre-assessment, as well as screening of preoperative blood tests and investigations by an anaesthetist to prevent cancellation. Blood crossmatch is rarely required for elective primary surgery, although many centres will hold a group and save specimens for 'stapled' cases or revision surgery.

Venous thromboembolism (VTE) prophylaxis must be prescribed for bariatric patients. NHS hospitals have 'in house' protocols for patients of all sizes and these should be applied to all bariatric cases.

Patients should be advised to bring their own CPAP machine to hospital for use postoperatively. This will be optimally adjusted for the individual patient's use.

Patients are encouraged to walk to the operating theatre if at all possible to avoid issues with handling and bed management. The patient is then asked to self-position on the theatre table and is anaesthetised in-situ.

REQUIREMENT FOR HIGH-DEPENDENCY UNIT/HICARE

Patients with severe OSA, complex surgery, or complicated surgery, or the complex comorbid patient will require a greater degree of postoperative monitoring and intervention. These are best managed in a high-dependency unit (HDU)/HiCare setting.

GENERAL CONSIDERATIONS FOR SURGERY

EQUIPPING THE SERVICE

STAFF

Many bariatric surgical units are self-contained services. A minimum of two surgeons, a specialist nurse, a specialist dietician, and a psychologist should make up the surgical team. This allows for availability of appropriate skills and facilitates 24/7 cover for bariatric patients. The availability of a bariatric physician to assist the preoperative management of severe comorbidities would be advantageous.

FURNITURE

Clearly, patients with high body weight need appropriate furniture. This applies to all points in the patient pathway. Chairs, couches, beds, and theatre tables need to be of an appropriate weight rating for the individual patient. Specifically designed furniture is now available for all shapes and sizes of patients, and it is therefore inappropriate to subject a patient to risk of harm by 'bodging' together furniture items to accommodate them. Table lateral extension pieces and footplates are particularly valuable.

SURGICAL KIT

The vast majority of bariatric patients can be managed using standard laparoscopic equipment. Careful port positioning and a willingness to move ports, or use extra ports, gives better access than struggling with 'difficult' ports or long instruments.

A choice of laparoscope should be available. Most surgeons would prefer 30-degree angled scopes, but for difficult cases a long 45-degree scope is useful.

Availability of 'open' kit

In the rare instance of conversion to open surgery, the availability of suitable mechanised retraction systems is vital to access and efficient operating.

PATIENT HANDLING AND POSITIONING

Patients should be encouraged to move themselves whenever possible. Once anaesthetised, trained personnel should undertake patient handling utilising appropriate aids such as Hover mattresses, slides, and support equipment.

Surgeons differ in their patient position preference. Both supine and split leg configurations have their pros and cons. If a patient is supine on the table, a foot board should be employed to minimise patient slippage when placed steeply head-up to assist access.

SURGICAL APPROACH

Access to the obese patient's peritoneal cavity is best achieved using an optical system in the left upper quadrant (LUQ). Occasionally, a veress needle may be used to gain initial insufflation in patients who have had previous surgery. Insufflation pressures of 14–16 mmHg may be required to lift a heavy abdominal wall away from internal organs. The siting of operative laparoscopic ports is critical to ensure efficient and torque-free operating. These should be planned in advance, but the position modified in light of findings at initial laparoscopy (e.g. a massive liver). Generally, one should avoid ports close to the costal margin, liver, or umbilicus.

Many surgeons require the placement of an orogastric tube/bougie for accurate surgical technique. It is important to consider the appropriate size for this before surgery. For laparoscopic adjustable gastric banding (LAGB) or Roux-en-Y gastric bypass (RYGB), one would consider a 34-Fr tube, for a vertical sleeve gastrectomy (VSG) 36–40-Fr.

ANAESTHETIC CONSIDERATIONS

Bariatric anaesthesia has evolved with bariatric surgery. Such is the prevalence of obesity, the skill set required to manage patients with obesity is now required for all anaesthetists and surgeons, irrespective of specialty.

PREOPERATIVE

Anaesthetic assessment should be part of the initial bariatric assessment pathway. Assessment of baseline respiratory function, ventilatory competence, and airway access can be made at an early stage. Planning for management of the patient with a difficult airway can be undertaken, including assessing the need for nasal fibre-optic intubation or awake intubation.

PERIOPERATIVE

Specific anaesthetic issues are best covered in anaesthetic reference texts. Crucial to safe surgery is maintenance of patient relaxation, patient positioning, safe and accurate passage of orogastric tubes, and avoidance of fluid overload.

Box 18.1 Postoperative analgesic regimen

- Diclofenac PR 75 mg bd or ibuprofen syrup 400 mg tds
- Paracetamol 1 g qds IV
- Oramorph 5–10 mg 4-hourly prn for breakthrough pain

Bd, Twice daily; *IV*, intravenously; *PR*, rectally; *prn*, as required; *qds*, four times daily; *tds*, three times daily.

POSTOPERATIVE

Following wound closure, patients are awakened from anaesthesia in a specific and controlled manner. Patients should be fully reversed from their neuromuscular blockade to enable full respiratory effort and, if required, specific reversal agents should be given (e.g. sugammadex). The patient should be moved across to a bariatric bed and positioned sitting bolt upright before extubation (never supine).

Close observation should be undertaken for the first 6 hours with constant SaO_2 monitoring. If the patient is known to suffer from OSA, their usual mask and machine should be employed to give CPAP.

Patients are normally encouraged to take oral fluids when awake, starting with 60 mL water hourly and, if well tolerated, progress to free fluids after 6 hours. Sloppy diet starts from the first postoperative day.

Mobilisation to a bariatric chair when awake is to be encouraged and opiate-sparing analgesia is generally employed (see Box 18.1), with nonsteroidal anti-inflammatory drugs (NSAIDs) given regularly. No urinary catheter is used unless indicated.

POSTOPERATIVE MANAGEMENT OF SIGNIFICANT COMORBIDITIES

TYPE 2 DIABETES MELLITUS

Diabetic bariatric patients should be managed with great care. While the expectation is for rapid postoperative control of glycaemia, blood sugar levels can be volatile and should be actively kept below 10 mmol/L. In patients with poor preoperative control, or with high preoperative insulin requirements, a sliding-scale insulin regimen is commonly employed in the perioperative period. When oral intake is established, metformin should be restarted as a crushed tablet dosage two or three times daily. Most patients should stay on at least one metformin 500 mg daily. It is not recommended to restart insulin upon discharge unless oral medication fails to control hyperglycaemia.

Patients should be directed to visit their local diabetic team to monitor blood glucose, and oral hypoglycaemic requirements on at least a weekly basis in the first month.

HYPERTENSION

Postoperatively, there is an acute resolution of hypertension that can persist for many days. However, it is unnecessary to restart antihypertensives until the blood pressure starts to rise in the weeks following surgery as premature therapy can cause hypotension and dizziness.

OBSTRUCTIVE SLEEP APNOEA

Patients with diagnosed OSA should restart nocturnal CPAP therapy on the first postoperative night. Treatment should continue until retesting confirms resolution of OSA.

THE OPERATIONS

Bariatric surgery is a rapidly and continually evolving field. Over the past 50 years, procedures have become obsolete and new ones proposed. As we learn more about the physiology of the gut and its control, more specific procedures have been designed to effectively diminish appetite, enhance satiety, and reduce calorie intake. We have started to depart from the notion of restriction and malabsorption as the modus operandi of these interventions (see Chapter 19).

The vast majority of bariatric procedures are now undertaken laparoscopically. If an open approach is mandated or becomes necessary, the technical procedure goals should not be changed.

GENERAL PRINCIPLES

Most common bariatric procedures require dissection of the angle of His and exposure of the left crus in part or all. It is therefore essential to have a good working knowledge of the anatomy of this region, the local relations, and blood supplies.

Liver retraction is required at some point in the majority of bariatric procedures and is usually achieved using a xiphisternal hook-type retractor, or a laparoscopic conformable retractor. Fan blade-type retractors are still occasionally used. Some authors describe using suture retraction of the liver but this can be capricious, especially if the liver is bulky and fatty.

Few patients require extra-long ports or instruments. Although these are available, their extra length can be unwieldy, and unless essential for access, they can impede rather than improve technical feasibility.

ADJUSTABLE GASTRIC BANDING

The procedure for LAGB is detailed below.[9] See Fig. 18.1.

- Position a laparoscopic stack at the patient's left shoulder.
- The patient is anaesthetised supine, moving to a 45-degree head-up tilt with a slight tilt towards the surgeon standing on the right. Antibiotic prophylaxis is given.
- Visual access LUQ 5-mm port with a 0-degree 5-mm laparoscope. General laparoscopy, note size, and state of liver. 15-mm L mid-zone port, 5-mm L lateral and 5-mm R lateral (Fig. 18.2a).
- Liver retraction; shepherd's crook style at xiphisternum, confirming flexible via far R lateral port.
- Passage of a 34-Fr orogastric tube to the mid-stomach, decompress.
- Retract the liver and identify the hiatus. Inspect for hiatal hernia. If in doubt, explore the hiatus anteriorly and repair the anterior crura with one or two non-absorbable sutures. Assess the size of the band required to suit the patient. Open the selected adjustable gastric band (AGB) kit and prime the band and port with sterile saline.
- Mobilise the hiatal fat pad from the stomach to expose the angle of His and OGJ.
- Open the lesser omentum to visualise the right crus. At the point where a transverse band of fat traverses the inferior part of the right crus, divide the peritoneum and

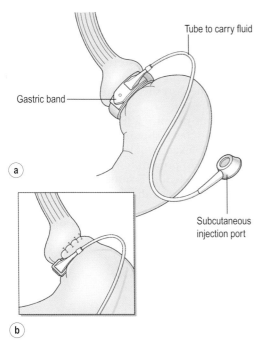

Figure 18.1 A gastric band showing small 'virtual' pouch of stomach below the (a) oesophagogastric junction and (b) gastro-gastric tunnelling sutures.

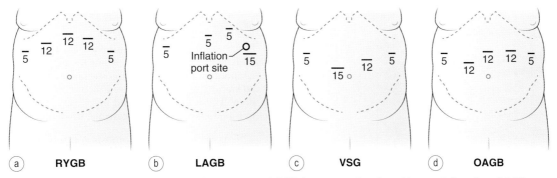

Figure 18.2 (a–d) Laparoscopic port positions for bariatric surgery. *LAGB,* Laparoscopic adjustable gastric banding; *OAGB,* one anastomosis gastric bypass; *RYGB,* Roux-en-Y gastric bypass; *VSG,* vertical sleeve gastrectomy.

gently insert graspers behind the oesophageal bundle to emerge just anterior to the left crus. This should be achieved with no more than gentle finger pressure. Some surgeons prefer to use a 'finger'-type dissector for this manoeuvre. The grasper is then 'parked' behind the oesophagus while the AGB is inserted into the abdomen through the 15-mm port and 'parked' in the LUQ. The tail of tubing is then grasped at its end and pulled through the retrogastric tunnel. The AGB tubing is then gently fed through the tunnel until the AGB body is sitting within the tunnel behind the OGJ. The band is then locked and checked.

- Most surgeons will 'fix' the AGB by creating a gastro-gastric tunnel. This is usually achieved by taking a number of suture bites of fundus lateral to the AGB and suturing this above the band to the stomach pouch distal to the OGJ or the left crus. This is thought to prevent migration of the gastric wall up through the AGB (band slippage).

- The AGB tubing is again grasped at its free end and tunnelled through one of the LUQ 5-mm ports, then subcutaneously to emerge at the 15-mm port site for attachment and implantation of the adjustment port. The adjustment port should be fixed to the external oblique fascia with loose non-absorbable sutures to prevent 'flipping'. The wounds are closed and dressed.

VERTICAL SLEEVE GASTRECTOMY

The procedure for VSG is detailed below.[10] See Fig. 18.3.

- Position a laparoscopic stack at the patient's left shoulder.
- The patient is anaesthetised supine, moving to 45-degree head-up tilt with a slight tilt towards the surgeon standing on the right. Antibiotic prophylaxis is given. Some surgeons prefer to operate between the patient's legs with the patient in a modified Lloyd-Davies position.
- An optical 12-mm port with a 0-degree scope gains abdominal access. General laparoscopy is performed and the liver size and texture noted. Further ports are inserted as shown in Fig. 18.2b. The number and size of ports vary between surgeons, but the author typically uses two 12-mm and two 5-mm ports. Typically the surgeon will then swap to an angled-view scope. In large patients a long 45-degree scope is ideal.

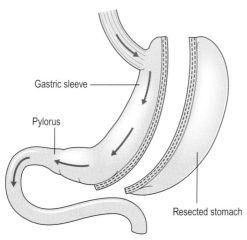

Figure 18.3 Sleeve gastrectomy.

(Figure labels: Gastric sleeve; Pylorus; Resected stomach)

- Liver retraction is performed, and the oesophageal hiatus assessed. A minimum bougie size of 34 Fr is inserted to the distal stomach to decompress the stomach and to guide the stapling for the creation of the sleeve. Some authors recommend a larger bougie to prevent narrowing and stricture of the sleeve. This issue has been reviewed and reported from the American BOLD database.[10]

- If in doubt about the presence of a hiatal hernia, explore the hiatus anteriorly and repair the anterior crura with one or two non-absorbable sutures.

- The greater curve is devascularised and mobilised from 4 cm proximal to the pylorus to the OGJ using either harmonic dissection or bipolar sealing electrocautery.

- The hiatal fat pad is then mobilised and the angle of His taken down. The bare area of stomach is mobilised from the left crus to expose this from its base to the crural arch.

- Thus prepared, the gastric sleeve can then be created by firing consecutive staplers from 5 cm proximal to the pylorus up to the OGJ along the bougie. Staples must be applied loosely adjacent to the bougie, never tight. Care must be taken when stapling adjacent to the OGJ, and sufficient slack given to avoid 'catching' the distal oesophagus in the staples. This is thought to predispose an early leak. Once divided, the resected stomach is carefully removed via one of the 12-mm port sites. This may require dilatation of the port site and steady traction to withdraw the specimen.

- Some surgeons perform a leak test of the gastric sleeve, but this has not been shown to decrease the incidence of complications. Fixation of the sleeve has been advised by some surgeons to prevent torsion or kinking. The lateral aspect of the staple line is sutured to the cut edge of the greater omentum, or if the pancreas can be avoided, the retroperitoneum.

- Port sites are then closed, with fascial sutures to the extraction site.

ROUX-EN-Y GASTRIC BYPASS

PRINCIPLES

✓ The basic principles of a gastric bypass include a small gastric pouch and variable length limbs of the Roux-en-Y reconstruction[11] (see Fig. 18.4).

The gastric pouch size varies, but consensus has been reached that a longer thin pouch is better than either a micropouch or a larger pouch.[12,13]

✓✓ Gastric bypass limb lengths have been investigated both experimentally and clinically.[14] The biliopancreatic (BP) limb has been shown to determine long-term weight loss, and a minimum length of 50 cm is suggested. Many surgeons use 80 cm to 1 m; in super-obese patients 150 cm can be considered. The Roux limb should be at least 1 m in all patients; in super-obese or diabetic patients, 1.5 m can be considered.

The gastrojejunal anastomosis is often checked for leaks, either by the instillation of methylene blue down an orogastric tube while the Roux limb is gently occluded distal to the anastomosis, or a less messy alternative is to position the patient flat, install saline into the LUQ, then inflate the

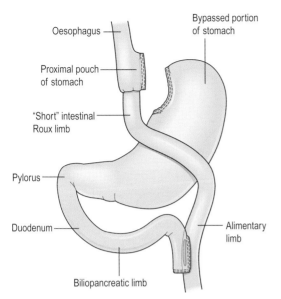

Oesophagus

Bypassed portion
of stomach

Proximal pouch
of stomach

"Short" intestinal
Roux limb

Pylorus

Duodenum

Alimentary
limb

Biliopancreatic limb

Figure 18.4 Gastric bypass showing a short vertical lesser curve-based gastric pouch with a Roux-en-Y jejuno-jejunostomy.

pouch and gastrojejunostomy (GJ) with 50 mL of air via an orogastric tube. Mesenteric windows should be closed with non-absorbable sutures.[15]

ACCESS

- Position a laparoscopic stack at the patient's left shoulder.
- The patient is anaesthetised supine, moving to 45-degree head-up tilt with a slight tilt towards the surgeon standing on the right. Antibiotic prophylaxis is given. Some surgeons prefer to operate between the patient's legs with the patient in a modified Lloyd-Davies position.
- Abdominal access is gained via an optical 12-mm port with a 0-degree scope in the LUQ. General laparoscopy is performed and the liver size and texture noted. Further ports are inserted as shown in Fig. 18.2a. The number and size of ports vary between surgeons, but the author typically uses three 12-mm and two 5-mm ports. Typically the surgeon will then swap to a 30-degree angled-view scope.
- Before embarking on the gastric bypass there should be an inspection of the upper stomach and small intestine to ensure that a bypass is feasible.

There are two methods for performing gastric bypass, pouch first and Roux first.

POUCH-FIRST APPROACH

This is usually performed from between the patient's legs, with the patient in a steep head-up position throughout.

- Liver retraction is performed and the oesophageal hiatus assessed. The hiatal fat pad is mobilised and the angle of His taken down.
- At a point at least 5 cm distal to the OGJ, the lesser curve fat is dissected from the gastric wall to form a tunnel to the lesser sac. A 'blue' width 45-mm staple cartridge is inserted and the stomach stapled perpendicular to the lesser curve. The stomach is then stapled vertically to the angle of His using one or two 60-mm 'blue' width staples. This creates a small gastric pouch of approximately 20 mL volume.

- The transverse colon is lifted superiorly, and if the greater omentum is bulky it is split in the midline using harmonic dissection or bipolar sealing diathermy. The duodenojejunal (DJ) flexure is identified, and the small bowel measured for a distance of between 50 cm and 1 m. The loop is then lifted over the transverse colon to the gastric pouch. A small access hole is made in the anti-mesenteric border of the loop, and the cartridge of a 'blue' width stapler inserted. A corresponding access hole is made in the most dependent part of the gastric pouch staple line (usually at the junction of the first and second staple firings).
- The stapler anvil is inserted into the gastric pouch and a short 20-mm linear GJ formed, the access hole being closed in one or two layers of absorbable suture around a 34-Fr orogastric tube. Some surgeons use a 25-mm circular stapler inserted through the small intestine, with the anvil introduced via an orogastric 'tail' passed through the mouth (Orvil system, Medtronic). An alternative is to hand sew the anastomosis with two layers of continuous absorbable suture around a 34-Fr orogastric tube.[16,17]
- Once the GJ is formed, the small bowel loop is divided with a linear stapler proximal (i.e. BP limb side) to the GJ. The BP limb is then anastomosed to the Roux limb between 1 m and 1.5 m distal to the GJ with a 45-mm linear stapler.
- The stapler access hole is closed with absorbable suture, and the mesenteric window closed with non-absorbable suture. The mesenteric window between the Roux limb and the transverse mesocolon (Petersen defect) is closed with a non-absorbable suture to complete the procedure.

ROUX-FIRST APPROACH

This is usually performed in two phases, with the patient supine and legs together. The surgeon stands at the patient's right shoulder to create the Roux-en-Y loop, then at the patient's right hip for the gastric pouch phase.

The greater omentum is split in the midline using harmonic dissection or bipolar sealing diathermy. The DJ flexure is identified, and the small bowel measured for a distance of between 50 cm and 1 m. It is then divided with a 'white' width stapler. The BP end is marked with a suture. The Roux end is then grasped and a further 1–1.5 m measured distally. The BP end is then sutured to this point and the two small bowel loops stapled together with a 'white' width 45-mm staple. The stapler access hole is then closed with absorbable suture, and the mesenteric window closed with non-absorbable suture. The end of the Roux limb is marked with a suture.

A gastric pouch is formed as per the pouch-first approach and the GJ created using the pre-formed Roux limb by either linear stapler, or circular stapler, as above. The Petersen defect is then closed to complete the procedure.

ONE ANASTOMOSIS ('MINI') GASTRIC BYPASS[18]

This variation of the gastric bypass has been variously named, indicating an uncertainty regarding its true nature. However, authorities agree that the term 'mini' is inappropriate for a procedure that is a major intervention, with potential risks for long-term malnutrition.[19,20]

The one anastomosis gastric bypass (OAGB) is technically more straightforward than a Roux-en-Y approach. However,

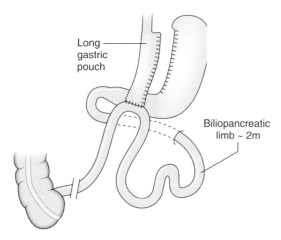

Figure 18.5 One anastomosis gastric bypass.

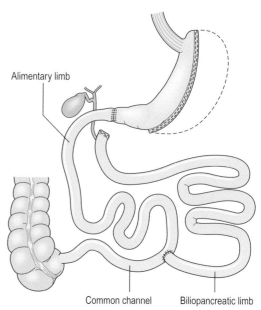

Figure 18.6 A sleeve gastrectomy/biliopancreatic diversion with a duodenal switch ('duodenal switch').

the analogy with a Polya-type gastrectomy reconstruction is valid, as are the medium- and longer term pitfalls of the latter, such as bile reflux and potential long-term risk of neoplasia.

The principles of this approach (Fig. 18.5) are to create a long, narrow gastric pouch, which is anastomosed to an undivided loop of small intestine 2 m distal to the DJ flexure. This creates a much longer BP limb, which is thought to mediate a greater neuroendocrine response and genuine malabsorption.

ACCESS

- Position a laparoscopic stack at the patient's left shoulder.
- The patient is anaesthetised supine, moving to 45-degree head-up tilt with a slight tilt towards the surgeon standing on the right. Antibiotic prophylaxis is given. Some surgeons prefer to operate between the patient's legs with the patient in a modified Lloyd-Davies position.
- An optical 12-mm port gains abdominal access with a 0-degree scope in the LUQ, somewhat lower than for the Roux-en-Y techniques. General laparoscopy is performed and the liver size and texture noted. Further ports are inserted as shown in Fig. 18.2d. The number and size of ports vary between surgeons, but the author typically uses three 12-mm and two 5-mm ports. Typically the surgeon will then swap to a 30-degree angled-view scope.
- Before embarking on the gastric bypass, there should be an inspection of the upper stomach and small intestine to ensure that a bypass is feasible.

Liver retraction is performed and the oesophageal hiatus assessed. The hiatal fat pad is then mobilised and the angle of His taken down. At a point at least 10 cm distal to the OGJ, the lesser curve fat is dissected from the gastric wall to form a tunnel to the lesser sac. A 'blue' width 45-mm staple cartridge is inserted and the stomach stapled perpendicular to the lesser curve. A minimum 38-Fr bougie is then passed down to the transverse staple line and the stomach is then stapled vertically to the angle of His using two or three 60-mm 'blue' width staples. This creates a long, narrow gastric pouch of approximately 50 mL volume.

- The omentum and transverse colon are then lifted and the DJ flexure is identified. The jejunum is then measured 2 m from the DJ flexure and this loop is brought up to the gastric pouch. The apex of this loop is then anastomosed

to the gastric pouch by either hand sewing with two layers of continuous suture, or a vertical posterior stapling with a blue 45-mm linear cartridge with suture closure of the access hole. There are descriptions of 'hitching' sutures to prevent bile reflux into the gastric tube, but their use is controversial.[18] The procedure is concluded with a leak test of the GJ.

- Closure of the mesenteric window is not considered routine in this technique.

TRUE MALABSORPTIVE OPTIONS

BILIOPANCREATIC DIVERSION[21]

This is a 'classic' malabsorptive procedure championed by Dr Scopinaro in Genoa.[21] It has largely been superseded by modern non-resective laparoscopic versions.

Essentially, the technique involves division of the stomach horizontally in the mid-body. The distal stomach is resected and the duodenum stapled. The ileum is divided 1.5 m from the ileocaecal valve and the distal end anastomosed to the gastric remnant with a wide GJ. The distal end of the BP limb is then anastomosed to the ileal limb between 75 cm and 1 m from the ileocaecal valve. The mesenteric windows must be closed.

DUODENAL SWITCH[22]

In this version of the BPD operation, the stomach is resected vertically in the form of a loose VSG (at least 40-Fr orogastric bougie) (Fig. 18.6). This is performed as per the description above, with similar port positions. Once the sleeve is formed, the greater curve devascularisation is carried distally past the pylorus to the point where the duodenum is in contact with the pancreas. The duodenum is then mobilised from its adhesions to the bile duct and transected 3–4 cm distal to pylorus with a blue 60-mm staple cartridge.

The ileocaecal valve is then identified and the small bowel divided 1.5–2 m proximally with a 'white' stapler cartridge.

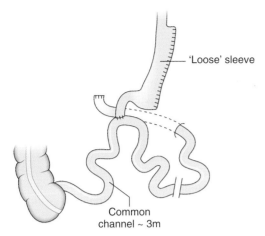

Figure 18.7   A single anastomosis duodeno-ileostomy.

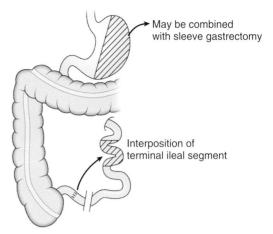

Figure 18.8   A jejuno-ileal interposition.

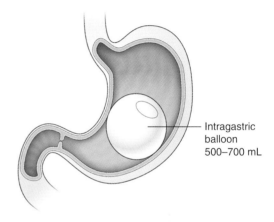

Figure 18.9   An intragastric balloon.

The divided end of the BP limb is anastomosed to the ileal limb between 75 and 100 cm from the ileocaecal valve with a stapled small-bowel anastomosis as described above. Attention should be paid to the direction of flow and closure of the mesenteric window.

The procedure is completed with a two-layer hand-sewn duodeno-ileostomy. This anastomosis is leak tested.

SLEEVE AND DUODENAL ILEOSTOMY[23]

A simplified version of the duodenal switch has been proposed by Cottam et al. and Torres et al.[23] This is essentially analogous to the OAGB, but utilises the whole gastric sleeve with distal division of the duodenum some 3–4 cm from the pylorus, as per the duodenal switch procedure (Fig. 18.7).

A loop of ileum is then measured 2–3 m from the ileocaecal valve and anastomosed end-to-side with the duodenum using a two-layer continuous absorbable suture technique. This is leak tested to complete the procedure.

ILEAL INTERPOSITION[24]

In this technique, a 60-cm segment of distal ileum is isolated and the remaining ileum reconstituted. The isolated segment is then interposed with antegrade motility just distal to the DJ flexure (Fig. 18.8). Care must be taken with closure of the mesenteric windows and orientation of the intestine.

GASTRIC PLICATION[25]

This procedure has been popularised in Eastern Europe and the Middle East due to the absence of stapling and relatively low cost. The stomach is dissected and prepared as per the sleeve gastrectomy. A series of non-absorbable plicating sutures are then placed from fundus to antrum to create a plicated narrow stomach.

ENDOSCOPIC APPROACHES[26]

It is inevitable that patients unwilling to undergo abdominal surgery will accept the growing number of endoscopic options available to assist weight loss. While not always the domain of the surgeon, a knowledge of these techniques is required to assist in the management of such patients considering revision surgery, or the management of complications arising from these techniques.

INTRAGASTRIC BALLOON[27]

A growing number of implantable intragastric balloons are available. These are mainly fluid filled and cause gastric irritation and delayed emptying. They are associated with early nausea and gastric spasm, which settles after 1–2 weeks. The patient is sedated and, following an endoscopy, the un-inflated balloon is introduced into the upper stomach and inflated with 500–700 mL water containing 10 mL methylene blue (Fig. 18.9). The latter is included so that in the event of a leak with balloon deflation, the patient will be aware of passing green urine and can notify their doctor. The balloon can then be removed before any possibility of migration through the pylorus.

Fluid-filled intragastric balloons are generally scheduled for endoscopic removal between 6 and 12 months after insertion. A special endoscopic needle-tip cannula is advanced into the balloon to aspirate the fluid. The deflated balloon is then grasped and withdrawn transorally.

A number of 'swallowable' gas-filled balloons are available that appear to act slightly differently by floating on gastric contents to stimulate the gastric fundus.

ENDOBARRIER[28]

This device is a short, barbed duodenal stent from which a sleeve of plastic extends distally 60 cm along the proximal

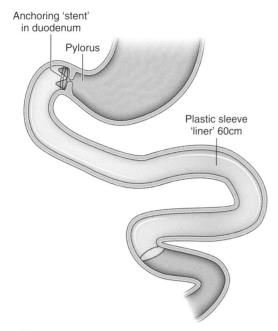

Figure 18.10 An endoscopic duodenojejunal liner.

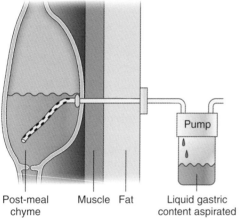

Figure 18.11 Aspiration gastrostomy.

jejunum (Fig. 18.10). The device requires radiologically assisted endoscopic placement and removal, usually under general anaesthetic, and is implanted for a maximum of 6 months. Complications such as duodenal perforation or bleeding have been reported, in addition to distal migration and impaction-obstruction.

ENDOSCOPIC PLICATION[29]

Utilising a new generation of endoscopic suturing, it is possible to achieve a greater curve plication from the internal aspect of the stomach. This approach is gaining popularity with patients unwilling to have 'surgery'.

ASPIRATION GASTROSTOMY[30]

This is essentially the placement of a wide-bore percutaneous gastrostomy using a semi-rigid tube. After a meal, the patient drinks some water and the percutaneous endoscopic gastrostomy (PEG) is aspirated to remove food before it passes through the pylorus for digestion (Fig. 18.11).

MANAGEMENT OF EARLY POSTOPERATIVE COMPLICATIONS

Elective bariatric surgery is safe and thankfully rarely complicated.[31] Patients treated according to enhanced recovery after bariatric surgery (ERABS) protocols should easily manage early discharge with minimal functional impairment.

Technically difficult procedures, procedures that require multiple staple firings, and revision surgery are all more likely to suffer technical problems. A high index of suspicion is required to diagnose any problems early and institute appropriate treatment.

Identification of a patient in difficulty can be challenging. Measurement of CRP > 100 mg/dL on postoperative day 1 is predictive of a complication.[32] Patients complaining of ongoing pain, tachycardia, tachypnoea, or fever should not be discharged. Regular observations should be used to identify a trend in observations. If suspicion exists for the presence of a complication, then investigation should be undertaken.

Computed tomography (CT) scan with oral contrast can be done if the expertise exists to accurately 'read' scans in a morbidly obese patient, and the patient will fit in the scanner. Faced with an unwell postoperative patient and in the absence of any likely helpful investigations, most experienced bariatric surgeons would take their patient back to theatre for an exploratory laparoscopy and upper gastrointestinal endoscopy under general anaesthesia. This will allow prompt diagnosis and treatment of any surgical complication. A clear laparoscopy will reassure the surgeon and point towards a non-technical complication.

BLEEDING

Bariatric surgery requires little tissue dissection, so 'raw' surfaces are minimised. Vessels to be divided are managed with modern haemostat dissectors, so bleeding is rare. However, rough grasping of recently divided vessels may cause a burst bleed from the ends of sealed vessels.

Staple line bleeding is reduced by the incorporation of staple line reinforcement materials.[33] Attention must be paid to selecting a suitably wide staple height to accommodate the gastric wall without undue crushing.

LEAK

Leakage from anastomosis or staple lines is the bête noir of bariatric surgery.[34] This may occur as a technical error in construction, or from tissue failure, and is more common with revision or difficult surgery. Leakage may occur immediately (often due to technical error) or delayed (due to failure of tissue or healing). Patients will usually describe feeling unwell and present with tachycardia, tachypnoea, and LUQ pain on deep inspiration.

✓✓ Investigation with water-soluble contrast swallow is rarely helpful, while CT with oral contrast only marginally more so. Most experienced surgeons would take a patient with a suspected leak back to theatre for endoscopy and laparoscopy under GA. Confirmation of a leak allows adequate peritoneal toilet and appropriate drainage.[34]

Management of specific leaks requires careful judgement by an experienced team. Maintenance of nutrition is vital in such patients, as it may take some time for sepsis to resolve and the leak to heal.

INTESTINAL OBSTRUCTION[35]

This complication almost exclusively occurs in patients with an intestinal component to their surgery. While rare, small-bowel obstruction can be a calamitous postoperative complication.

Obstruction at the jejuno-jejunostomy is usually due to malconstruction of this anastomosis. Complete small-bowel obstruction with vomiting and colic is rare. More commonly, obstruction of the BP limb leads to pain and gastric distension. This is usually diagnosed on chest X-ray in a distressed postoperative patient with LUQ discomfort. Failure to recognise this may lead to gastric perforation. Re-operation with revision of the jejuno-jejunostomy is often required.

Internal herniation can occur even after closure of potential defects. Opinion varies as to the need for closure of all mesenteric defects, but consensus is building that 'windows' should be closed.[15]

Internal herniation presents with abdominal pain, distension, and sometimes vomiting. Obstruction of the alimentary limb is late in the process, so vomiting is often absent, with BP limb obstruction the predominant feature. CT scan will usually diagnose this problem, and prompt surgical intervention will avert disaster.

EARLY ACUTE GASTRIC BAND SLIPPAGE

This rare but important complication[36] leads to pain and intolerance of oral intake in the gastric band patient. It is due to a posterolateral prolapse of the fundus proximally 'up' through the band causing incarceration and, if left untreated, proximal gastric strangulation. Diagnosis is by plain X-ray to identify the gastric band position and water-soluble contrast swallow. Immediate deflation, followed by prompt laparoscopic repositioning or removal of the band, is required.

OUTCOMES OF BARIATRIC SURGERY

Outcomes have been demonstrated to be better from centres with high volume. Surgical risk in over 15 000 patients was assessed using data from the Michigan Bariatric Surgery Collective. These showed that the risk of serious complications was reduced from 4% to 1.9% in centres performing more than 300 procedures and individual surgeons performing more than 250 procedures.[37]

An increasing number of case series illustrate the risks in the learning curve for gastric bypass surgery and the need for defined mentoring.[38]

The UK National Bariatric Surgery Registry has compulsorily collated data from NHS bariatric units since 2010. This has provided a clear insight into the short-term results of bariatric procedures in the UK. The data are shown in Tables 18.1 and 18.2.[31]

Worldwide, there are increasing data confirming the role of surgically induced weight loss in the improvement of comorbidities as well as the prevention of their development. While trials of various procedures have attested differing efficacy of one procedure over another, the basic fact remains that all bariatric operations can induce significant weight loss in the prevention and improvement of comorbidities. This has been tested against 'best medical intervention' in a number of settings and bariatric surgery has proven itself superior in efficacy.[39–41]

Table 18.1   Primary operations: 30-day outcomes, financial years 2013–2018

Analysis by procedure	30-day outcomes The most common 30-day complication of primary bariatric surgery reported in the NBSR was bleeding. Primary surgery for adults: 30-day complications; operation in financial years 2013–2018				
			30-day complication		
30-day outcomes		No	Yes	Unspecified	Rate
	Roux-en-Y gastric bypass	704	164	18 236	18.9%
Bleed	OAGB/MGB	54	0	1 461	0.0%
	Sleeve gastrectomy	508	76	13 257	13.0%
	Roux-en-Y gastric bypass	800	76	18 228	8.7%
Obstruction	OAGB/MGB	55	0	1 460	0.0%
	Sleeve gastrectomy	417	0	13 424	0.0%
	Roux-en-Y gastric bypass	808	57	18 239	6.6%
Leak	OAGB/MGB	54	0	1 461	0.0%
	Sleeve gastrectomy	540	43	13 258	7.4%
	Gastric band	89	2	4 408	2.2%
Re-operation	Roux-en-Y gastric bypass	522	7	18 575	1.3%
	OAGB/MGB	55	0	1 460	0.0%
	Sleeve gastrectomy	479	1	13 361	0.2%

MGB, Mini gastric bypass; *NBSR*, National Bariatric Surgery Registry; *OAGB*, one anastomosis gastric bypass.

Table 18.2 Primary operations: postoperative in-hospital mortality and operation, financial years 2013–2018

Operation and kind of postoperative complication		Primary surgery for adults: postoperative complications; operations in financial years 2013–2018			
		Complication reported			
		No	Yes	Unspecified	Rate
Cardio-vascular complications	Gastric band	4 075	2	422	0.05%
	Roux-en-Y gastric bypass	17 930	43	1 131	0.24%
	OAGB/MGB	1 484	1	30	0.07%
	Sleeve gastrectomy	13 086	28	727	0.21%
	All	**36 575**	**74**	**2 310**	**0.20%**
Other complications	Gastric band	4 034	30	435	0.74%
	Roux-en-Y gastric bypass	17 509	448	1 147	2.49%
	OAGB/MGB	1 470	18	27	1.21%
	Sleeve gastrectomy	12 774	303	764	2.32%
	All	**35 787**	**799**	**2 373**	**2.18%**
In-hospital mortality	Gastric band	4 497	0	2	0.00%
	Roux-en-Y gastric bypass	19 061	9	34	0.05%
	OAGB/MGB	1 510	2	3	0.13%
	Sleeve gastrectomy	13 817	5	19	0.04%
	All	**38 885**	**16**	**58**	**0.04%**

MGB, Mini gastric bypass; *NBSR*, National Bariatric Surgery Registry; *OAGB*, one anastomosis gastric bypass.

✔✔ Data from the maturing Swedish Obese Subjects (SOS) study show long-term benefit in terms of survival and quality of health.[42] The results are maintained out to 15 years.

Future answers may come from the ongoing By-Band-Sleeve study, one of the largest randomised controlled trials of bariatric surgery in the world.[43]

Key points

- Bariatric procedures are an evolving field of upper gastrointestinal surgery.
- The mechanism of action of each procedure is incompletely understood (see Chapter 19).
- There is no 'perfect procedure'; every bariatric operation will 'fade with time'.
- The choice of procedure is a match between patient expectation and known effects.
- The therapeutic environment and postoperative care pathway is key to success.
- Gastric banding remains a viable procedure for motivated patients.
- Gastric bypass has withstood scientific scrutiny and remains one of the most reliable and durable procedures. OAGB is gaining popularity.
- Sleeve gastrectomy is attractively simple in concept, but has limitations in durability.
- More complex procedures are for special indications and for specialist units.

🌐 References available at http://ebooks.health.elsevier.com/

▶ RECOMMENDED VIDEOS

- General bariatric – http://www.ibcclub.org/videos/ https://www.websurg.com/search/?search_q=bariatric#
- Gastric Band – https://www.websurg.com/MEDIA/?noheader=1&doi=vd01en1624e
- Sleeve gastrectomy – https://www.youtube.com/watch?v=KM6UQzMwbWU
- Gastric bypass – https://www.websurg.com/MEDIA/?noheader=1&doi=vd01en4464 https://www.websurg.com/MEDIA/?noheader=1&doi=vd01en2948
- OAGB – https://www.youtube.com/watch?v=SKglIeUodNw
- Duodenal Switch – https://www.websurg.com/MEDIA/?noheader=1&doi=vd01en3574
- Sleeve and duodenal ileostomy procedure – https://www.youtube.com/watch?v=uSjsbPfg-eM

KEY REFERENCES

[1] Neff KJ, Olbers T, le Roux CW, Bariatric surgery. The challenges with candidate selection, individualizing treatment and clinical outcomes. BMC Med 2013;11(1):8. PMID: 23302153
A comprehensive summary of preoperative issues in bariatric surgery.

[6] Dixon JB, Zimmet P, Alberti KG, et al. Bariatric surgery: an IDF statement for obese Type 2 diabetes. Diabet Med 2011;28:628–42. PMID: 21480973
The International Diabetes Federation is the umbrella organisation for 200 national diabetes associations in 160 countries. The working group for this statement reviewed the literature from 1991 to 2010 on diabetes and bariatric surgery before a consensus conference in Brussels in December 2010. This paper details recommendations on clinical practice and future research.

[14] Mahawar KK, Kumar P, Parmar C, et al. Small bowel limb lengths and Roux-en-Y gastric bypass: a systematic review. Obes Surg 2016;26(3):660–71. PMID: 26749410
This systematic review concludes that a range of 100–200 cm for a combined length of BP or alimentary limb gives optimum results with RYGB in most patients.

[31] Welbourn R, Small P, Finlay I, et al. Consultant outcomes publication extract from the national bariatric surgery Registry. 2017. Available from: http://www.bomss.org.uk/wp-content/uploads/2017/03/Bariatric-Surgery-Clinical-Outcomes-Publication-for-2015-16.pdf
The Clinical Outcomes Publication extract is an annual publication of outcomes from bariatric surgery in the NHS. The figures indicate the safety of bariatric surgery in the UK.

[34] Kim J, Azagury D, Eisenberg D, et al. ASMBS position statement on prevention, detection, and treatment of gastrointestinal leak after gastric bypass and sleeve gastrectomy, including the roles of

imaging, surgical exploration, and nonoperative management. Surg Obes Relat Dis 2015;11(4):739–48. PMID: 26071849

A comprehensive guide to the investigation and management of leaks after bariatric surgery.

[39] Dixon JB, O'Brien PE, Playfair J, et al. Adjustable gastric banding and conventional therapy for type 2 diabetes: a randomized controlled trial. JAMA 2008;299:316–32. PMID: 18212316

This is the only randomised controlled trial that compares banding to medical therapy for new-onset diabetics in the body mass index range 30–40 kg/m².

[40] Schauer PR, Bhatt DL, Kirwan JP, et al. Bariatric surgery versus intensive medical therapy for diabetes – 3-year outcomes. N Engl J Med 2014;370(21):2002–13. PMID: 24679060

This randomised trial showed that bariatric surgery led to better glycaemic control and quality of life at 3 years than medical management alone.

[41] Mingrone G, Panunzi S, De Gaetano A, et al. Bariatric–metabolic surgery versus conventional medical treatment in obese patients with Type 2 diabetes: 5-year follow-up of an open-label, single-centre, randomised controlled trial. Lancet 2015;386(9997):964–73. PMID: 26369473

This randomised trial showed that surgery is more effective than medical treatment for the long-term control of obese patients with type 2 diabetes.

[42] Sjöström L. Review of the key results from the Swedish Obese Subjects (SOS) trial – a prospective controlled intervention study of bariatric surgery. J Intern Med 2013;273(3):219–34. PMID: 23163728

A summary of the highlights from this ground-breaking and insightful study.

19 Follow-up and late complications of bariatric surgery

Brijesh Madhok | Kamal Mahawar | Richard Welbourn

INTRODUCTION

The evidence base for bariatric surgery (BS) has increased considerably over the last 10 years, with a number of large non-randomised[1] and randomised studies[2,3] documenting its superiority over the best available medical therapy for the management of obesity and related comorbidities. The last Cochrane review of randomised controlled trials (RCTs) showed that BS resulted in better weight loss and comorbidity improvement compared to non-surgical interventions.[4] More recently, a meta-analysis of seven RCTs with at least 2 years' follow-up found that remission of type 2 diabetes mellitus (T2DM) was observed in 52.5% of patients undergoing BS compared to 3.5% on medical management after 2 years.[5] There are, however, differences in outcomes depending on the surgical procedure. A recent systematic review[6] of five RCTs comparing 5-year outcomes of sleeve gastrectomy (SG) and Roux-en-Y gastric bypass (RYGB), the two most commonly performed bariatric procedures worldwide, found both to be effective for weight loss and resolution of obesity-related comorbidities, but RYGB was associated with significantly better 5-year weight loss outcomes.

✓✓ Surgery results in greater improvement in weight loss outcomes and obesity-associated comorbidities compared with non-surgical interventions, regardless of the type of procedure used.[4–6]

The Swedish Obese Subjects (SOS) study[1] compared outcomes in 2010 patients undergoing BS – 376 gastric banding (GaB), 1369 vertical banded gastroplasty (VBG), and 265 RYGB – and 2037 receiving conventional medical treatment in a controlled, non-randomised study. The mean changes in body weight over 2, 10, 15, and 20 years were -23%, -17%, -16%, and -18% in the surgery group compared to 0%, 1%, -1%, and -1% in the control group, respectively. In addition, the surgery group had a hazard ratio (HR) of 0.76 for overall mortality compared with the control group (95% CI 0.59–0.99; $P = 0.04$). More recent publications from the SOS study have reported a significant decrease in the risk of heart failure (HR 0.65, 95% CI 0.54–0.79; $P < 0.001$)[7] and longer life expectancy at 3 years (95% CI 1.8–4.2; $P < 0.001$)[8] in the surgery group compared to the control group. In the 1980s, VBG was very common, but this is now rarely performed. SG is now the commonest procedure worldwide (46% of procedures) followed by RYGB (38.2%), one anastomosis gastric bypass (OAGB) (7.6%) and GaB (5.0%).[9]

✓✓ The landmark SOS study found that BS for severe obesity is associated with long-term weight loss (> 20 years) and decreased overall mortality. In comparison, the average weight change in the control group was less than ±2%.[1]

FOLLOW-UP AFTER BARIATRIC SURGERY

The importance of adequate lifelong follow-up after BS cannot be overstated. A National Institute for Health and Care Excellence (NICE)-accredited commissioning guidance recommended[10] that Weight Assessment and Management Clinics should ensure that patients recognise the need for lifelong follow-up before a referral for BS can be made.

QUALITY OF AVAILABLE FOLLOW-UP DATA

There is a paucity of level 1 data on the long-term durability, complications, and re-operation rates after BS, which makes healthcare planning difficult.[11] At the same time, several RCTs comparing SG with RYGB have now reported 5-year outcomes[6] and two RCTs have even reported 10-year outcomes – one comparing metabolic surgery (RYGB or biliopancreatic division [BPD]) with conventional medical therapy,[12] and another comparing GaB with RYGB.[13]

Although a number of non-randomised studies report on longer term outcomes after BS, the majority are compromised of the poor numbers available for follow-up. This introduces follow-up bias. A recent systematic review examining 10-year outcomes after all bariatric procedures included 57 datasets with only two RCTs – one GaB versus medical therapy and another GaB versus RYGB.[14] The quality of most studies was reported to be 'low', with many gaps in the data. Also, there are few data on the long-term cost-effectiveness of surgery. For all these reasons, it is not possible yet to distinguish between those patients for whom surgery should be positively recommended, as opposed to those who are eligible for surgery according to agreed thresholds. More randomised studies with adequate 5-year, 10-year, and even longer follow-ups could answer these questions.

It is further recognised that there is significant variation in reporting methods and the definition of outcomes measured. This poses problems for attempts of systematic synthesis of data in meta-analyses. The bariatric community has responded to these challenges by attempting to standardise reporting of outcomes[15] after BS and develop a core outcome set that should be used in every large RCT. At the same time, to power any individual study adequately to answer all of these potential outcome measures is not an easily surmountable challenge.

FRAMEWORK FOR FOLLOW-UP

Although it is generally agreed that BS patients need lifelong follow-up, there is a complete lack of robust evidence to inform the frequency and nature of the possible interventions. It is further unclear whether the responsibility should lie with the bariatric team or the general practitioner (GP).

Lack of patient education, adherence to lifelong follow-up, and provision of healthcare funding for follow-up are further challenges that need to be overcome. Recent guidelines[16,17] by national societies on follow-up and monitoring of patients after BS are driven by clinical experience and some scientific evidence.

In the UK, the recommendations by NICE[18] form the framework for follow-up after BS (Box 19.1). NICE lays the responsibility for the follow-up during the first 2 years with the bariatric team and for lifelong annual follow-up thereafter with primary care, as part of a shared care model of chronic disease management. These guidelines are an aspiration, given the current preparedness of primary care for bariatric patient care. Also, since a range of serious issues requiring specialist expertise can develop over the course of the lifetime after surgery, it is important that a workable shared care chronic disease model is developed between BS teams and primary care.[10]

GUIDELINES FOR FOLLOW-UP

The NHS England Obesity Clinical Reference Group commissioned a multi-professional group to undertake the daunting task of developing post-BS follow-up guidelines. The group, which also had patient representation, published[19] its recommendations along with the strength of the evidence. Four different shared clinical models were proposed and examined. The common features included annual review, the ability for a GP to refer back to the specialist centre, and submission of follow-up data to the national database. The group recommended that:

1. 'All multidisciplinary bariatric surgery teams should follow-up patients at regular intervals post-surgery and offer a minimum of 2 years follow-up.'
2. All patients should have 'routine monitoring of blood tests' (Grade A evidence). The exact nature and frequency of such monitoring as enumerated in the British Obesity and Metabolic Surgery Society (BOMSS) guidelines[16] is based on clinical judgement rather than more robust scientific evidence.
3. 'Gastric band patients should have annual follow-up indefinitely' (Grade C evidence). This is challenging since most GPs have not been taught to do band adjustments. However, GPs could use the annual visit as a prompt to refer a patient to the surgical team for advice on band adjustment.
4. 'Patients should have lifelong monitoring to ensure optimum nutrition is maintained' (based on NICE recommendation). This recommendation reinforces the need for bariatric teams to work with GPs to make local protocols for which tests are needed and red flags that would alert GPs to refer patients back.

A PRAGMATIC SOLUTION

Despite the lack of level 1 evidence, the arbitrary 2-year follow-up led by the BS multidisciplinary team (MDT) of surgeon, physician, dietician, specialist nurse, mental health professional, and others seems appropriate since weight loss in most patients will have reached a plateau by then and therefore be in a 'steady state'. During the 2 years, joint care with GPs is also appropriate, in preparation for care being mainly under the GPs after this time. Annual follow-up visits with bariatric teams and subsequently with GPs should be used to review existing medications as well as to look for potential signs of long-term nutritional or surgical complications.[10]

✔ Regular follow-up after BS is required to achieve good outcomes and early diagnosis of complications. Patients should have regular review by the bariatric MDT at least for the first 2 years after surgery, and then annually by the GP as part of a shared care approach.[10,19]

OUTCOMES AFTER BARIATRIC SURGERY

WEIGHT LOSS OUTCOMES

There is robust evidence to suggest that BS results in sustainable weight loss in the long term. A recent systematic review looking at 5-year outcomes from five RCTs concluded that both RYGB and SG result in sustained weight loss.[6] This meta-analysis found a significantly greater percentage of excess weight loss (%EWL) following RYGB compared with SG (65.7% vs 57.3%, $P < 0.001$).

✔✔ All current bariatric operations result in significant weight loss even at 5 and 10 years. Long-term data after OAGB are lacking.[6,14]

Box 19.1 NICE recommendations regarding follow-up after bariatric surgery

- Bariatric surgery is a treatment option for people with obesity if the person commits to the need for long-term follow-up
- Surgery for obesity should be undertaken only by a multidisciplinary team that can provide regular postoperative assessment, including specialist dietetic and surgical follow-up
- Offer people who have had bariatric surgery a follow-up care package for a minimum of 2 years within the bariatric service. This should include:
  - Monitoring nutritional intake (including protein and vitamins) and mineral deficiencies
  - Monitoring for comorbidities
  - Medication review
  - Dietary and nutritional assessment, advice, and support
  - Physical activity advice and support
  - Psychological support tailored to the individual
  - Information about professionally led or peer-support groups
- After discharge from bariatric surgery service follow-up, ensure that all people are offered at least annual monitoring of nutritional status and appropriate supplementation according to need following bariatric surgery, as part of a shared care model of chronic disease management

DIABETES OUTCOMES

There is a wealth of data from high-quality studies showing a durable effect of BS on T2DM. A recent meta-analysis[5] of seven RCTs found that the chance of remission of T2DM was significantly higher after BS compared with medical management after at least 2 years' follow-up (risk ratio [RR] 10, 95% CI 5.5–17.9, $P < 0.001$). Another recent systematic review and meta-analysis[6] examining 5-year outcomes reported that the resolution of T2DM was 37.4% and 27.5% after RYGB and SG, respectively. The difference was not significant, probably because the individual RCTs were not powered to evaluate the differences in diabetes resolution rates.

More recently, a smaller RCT compared 10-year outcomes in patients with obesity and T2DM who underwent metabolic surgery (RYGB or BPD) or received conventional medical therapy.[12] The 10-year remission rates for T2DM were significantly higher in the surgical group.

Late relapse of T2DM may be seen in up to a third of patients after initial successful remission.[20] However, this should not be seen as a 'failure' of BS, as these patients still benefit from improved glycaemic control with fewer anti-diabetic medications and reduced risk of other comorbidities secondary to T2DM. A recent RCT reported that RYGB was significantly more effective than medical therapy in inducing remission of albuminuria and early-stage chronic kidney disease (CKD) in patients with T2DM and obesity.[21]

Bariatric surgery is more effective than intensive medical therapy in the long-term control of T2DM in patients who also suffer from obesity[5,6]

OTHER COMORBIDITY OUTCOMES

BS has been shown to improve multiple obesity-related comorbidities such as hypertension (HTN), obstructive sleep apnoea (OSA), non-alcoholic fatty liver disease (NAFLD), gastro-oesophageal reflux disease (GORD) and Barrett's oesophagus (with RYGB), dyslipidaemia, and ischaemic heart disease (IHD). A recent RCT[2] showed significant improvement in blood pressure (BP) control and remission of HTN 3 years after RYGB compared to patients only on medical therapy.

Two recent systematic reviews found that BS was effective in reducing nocturnal hypoxaemia in patients with OSA.[22,23] Fakhry et al. published a systematic review[24] reporting significant improvement in all stages of NAFLD following BS. Adil et al. reported significant regression of Barrett's oesophagus and improvement in GORD after RYGB.[25]

A recent systematic review[26] of large population-based cohort studies including 269,818 patients who underwent BS and 1,270,086 control patients found that BS significantly reduced all-cause mortality ($P < 0.001$) and cardiovascular mortality ($P < 0.001$). BS was also associated with a reduced incidence of several comorbidities such as T2DM ($P = 0.010$), HTN ($P < 0.001$), dyslipidaemia ($P = 0.010$), and IHD ($P = 0.001$).

Bariatric surgery improves and reduces the incidence of various obesity-related diseases such as hypertension, dyslipidaemia, ischaemic heart disease, and NAFLD, and significantly reduces all-cause mortality[24,26]

LONG-TERM COMPLICATIONS AFTER BARIATRIC SURGERY

Many patients develop long-term surgical complications after BS. This is in addition to the nutritional complications that these patients are at high risk of developing, and other complications of massive weight loss such as gallstones and loose skin. Complications associated with commonly performed bariatric procedures with an approximate incidence and the options available for management are shown in Table 19.1.

LONG-TERM COMPLICATIONS AFTER SLEEVE GASTRECTOMY

Five- to 10-year follow-up data with SG are now being reported. It is becoming apparent that some patients will present with symptoms of GORD unresponsive to medical management, a second large group will need further surgery either due to inadequate weight loss or weight regain, and a third smaller group will present with mechanical problems with the gastric sleeve.

GASTRO-OESOPHAGEAL REFLUX DISEASE

GORD has a strong link with SG, most likely due to the changes in anatomy and physiology.[27] A recent systematic review including 10,718 patients from 46 studies found that 19% of patients experience postoperative GORD, 23% develop de novo GORD, and 4% of all patients require revision to RYGB due to severe acid reflux.[28] Another recent systematic review reported the pooled prevalence of Barrett's oesophagus after SG to be 11.6% ($P < 0.001$), and the risk of oesophagitis increased by 13% every year after SG.[29] At the same time, proximal migration of gastric cardia, where the intestinal metaplasia is commonly seen, after SG can lead to diagnostic confusion with Barrett's oesophagus. Adequately designed endoscopic studies are, therefore, needed to draw firm conclusions.

Both persistent and de novo GORD are common after SG, with a theoretical risk of developing Barrett's oesophagus. About 4% of patients may require revision to RYGB due to symptoms of GORD that persist despite optimal medical management.[28,29]

STRICTURE

Patients with stricture or stenosis of the sleeve usually present with intermittent vomiting often associated with difficulty in consuming solid foods. Diagnosis is easily confirmed by a contrast study or endoscopy. A number of management options – endoscopic dilatation, laparoscopic sero-myotomy, or wedge resection – have been described and may be successful. A conversion to RYGB with the formation of a pouch above the stricture is however the best treatment option for these patients and guaranteed to bring relief.[30]

TWIST OR KINK

Patients with SG can develop a number of other mechanical problems with the sleeve, such as a twist or kink, with a functional hold-up. Patients present with persistent regurgitation

Table 19.1 Long-term surgical complications after commonly performed bariatric procedures

Procedure	Complication	Approximate incidence (%)	Management
Sleeve gastrectomy	Reflux oesophagitis	10.0–20.0	PPIs and/or conversion to other bariatric procedure
	Stricture	0.2–0.3	Endoscopic dilatation, laparoscopic sero-myotomy or wedge resection, or conversion to other bariatric procedure
	Twist or kink	0.2–0.3	Conversion to other bariatric procedure
Gastric bypass (RYGB and OAG)	Internal hernia	1.0–3.0 (RYGB) 1.0 (OAGB)	Reduction of hernia and closure of spaces
	Anastomotic stricture	2.0–5.0	Dilatation or revision
	Reactive hypoglycaemia	1.0–2.0	Medical management, very occasionally reversal of RYGB or conversion to sleeve gastrectomy
	Marginal/anastomotic ulcer	3.0–5.0	PPIs ± sucralfate, stop smoking, exclude gastrinoma, revision of anastomosis
Gastric band	Band slippage	3.0–11.0	Repositioning or removal
	Gastric pouch and/or oesophageal dilatation	4.0–19.5	Deflation with gradual refilling or band removal
	Band erosion	0.9–11.2	Endoscopic or laparoscopic removal
	Port/tubing complications	5.3–17.5	Port replacement/tube shortening
	Reflux oesophagitis	0–19.7	Band deflation ± PPIs or band removal

GORD, Gastro-oesophageal reflux disease; *PPI*, proton pump inhibitor; *RYGB*, Roux-en-Y gastric bypass.

and/or vomiting. The diagnosis is usually easily established on a contrast study that shows hold-up at the incisura angularis, despite there being a way through on endoscopy. Conversion to RYGB is usually successful.

LONG-TERM COMPLICATIONS AFTER GASTRIC BYPASS (RYGB AND OAGB)

The four major long-term surgical complications after RYGB or OAGB are an internal hernia, anastomotic stricture, reactive hypoglycaemia, and marginal ulcers at the gastrojejunostomy anastomosis. There is also the additional risk of gastro-oesophageal reflux after OAGB, which is managed in much the same way as GORD after SG.[31]

INTERNAL HERNIA

Herniation of the small bowel through internal defects created during either GB method is a recognised complication with an incidence that may be cumulative over time. If not diagnosed promptly, it can lead to massive gut infarction with disastrous consequences. Internal hernias usually become symptomatic years after surgery when the patient has lost some weight with the consequent opening of potential internal spaces. Many patients will have recurrent colicky abdominal pain long before the diagnosis is made by laparoscopy.

A recent systematic review of six observational studies (*n* = 10,031) and two RCTs (*n* = 2609) suggested that closure of mesenteric defects in RYGB may be associated with lower risks of internal herniation and re-operation for small-bowel obstruction (SBO) compared with non-closure of the defects.[32] Although less common as there is only one defect, internal herniae can also happen after OAGB. Until robust evidence develops, the authors recommend closure of Petersen's space in these patients too.

There is no high-quality evidence to guide the closure technique, but a non-absorbable running suture or clips (in one or two layers) is recommended. The use of glue should be regarded as investigational at present.

✔ Closing internal spaces at the time of RYGB and OAGB reduces the risk of internal hernia and re-operation for SBO compared with non-closure.[32]

ANASTOMOTIC STRICTURE

Strictures can develop at both gastrojejunal and jejunojejunal anastomoses. Gastrojejunostomy strictures appear to be commoner with the use of circular staplers[33] and lend themselves easily to endoscopic diagnosis and management. Unresponsive ones may need a surgical revision of the anastomosis. Jejuno-jejunostomy strictures, in contrast, are uncommon and may be difficult to diagnose in the earlier stages until the patient presents with a bowel obstruction, which may be closed loop obstruction. Treatment involves refashioning of the anastomosis. A stricture of the gastrojejunal anastomosis with OAGB will need conversion to a Roux-en-Y configuration.

REACTIVE HYPOGLYCAEMIA

Severe hypoglycaemia with neuroglycopaenic symptoms is mainly seen after GB, and rarely after SG. A recent study[34] found that 11.6% of the 1138 RYGB patients reported at least one episode of severe hypoglycaemia after a mean delay of 25.5 months. The annual incidence rate was 2.5% in the first year, 3.7% in the second year, and reducing to 1.5% in the third year. The exact aetiology remains uncertain but probably includes a combination of late dumping, beta-cell hyperfunction, and an exaggerated incretin response. Diagnosis can be challenging and relies on confirming Whipple's triad (low serum glucose with associated symptoms or signs that are immediately relieved by increasing the serum glucose level). Dietary modifications are the cornerstone of treatment. Pharmacotherapy using acarbose, diazoxide, calcium channel blockers, or octreotide is often successful.[35] Very unusually, surgical intervention such as feeding using a gastrostomy tube or gastric bypass reversal may be required.

MARGINAL ULCER

Approximately 3.0–5.0% of GB patients develop marginal ulcers. Although the majority will present within 1–2 years, they can occur many years later. Typically, patients have persisting epigastric pain, with or without nausea and vomiting. Smoking, non-steroidal inflammatory drugs, *Helicobacter pylori* colonisation, and ischaemia of the gastric pouch seem to be associated with an increased incidence of marginal ulcers.[36] The diagnosis is by endoscopy. Treatment with high-dose proton pump inhibitors (PPIs) with or without sucralfate, in conjunction with smoking cessation advice, usually results in prompt healing. It is important that patients undergo a check follow-up endoscopy to ensure healing, as some ulcers do not heal on medical management. An underlying gastro-gastric fistula should be sought with a contrast X-ray swallow when an ulcer fails to heal.

✔ It is important to ensure healing of a marginal ulcer after GB by performing a check endoscopy. Persistent ulceration may be due to an underlying gastro-gastric fistula or could result in one.

Ulcers that persist despite all conservative measures need to be excised with a revision of the gastrojejunostomy and in the case of OAGB, conversion to RYGB. Many units eradicate *H. pylori* before RYGB and give a PPI perioperatively to reduce the risk of marginal ulcer.[37] Although there is no randomised evidence that this is effective, there is some evidence to suggest that the incidence of marginal ulcers after GB is inversely proportional to the length of pouch and the duration of prophylaxis, leading to some surgeons now recommending PPI prophylaxis for prolonged periods after surgery.

LONG-TERM COMPLICATIONS AFTER GASTRIC BAND

A systematic review[38] of 17 studies involving a total of 9706 GaB patients and 1974 patients available 10 years after surgery observed a median long-term complication and re-operation rate of 42.7% (range 5.9–52.9%) and 36.5% (range 7.2–66.1%), respectively. Approximately 22.9% (range 5.4–54.0%) of patients had their GaB removed, most commonly for complications. Another study[39] of long-term results with 897 GaB over a period of 18 years found that 56.0% of patients suffered long-term complications and 41.6% of bands were removed for complications, weight regain, or intolerance. The percentage of patients with inadequate weight loss and weight regain increased from 18.4% at 2 years to 43.0% at 10 years and >70.0% beyond 15 years.

✔ Even in specialist centres,[14] GaBs are associated with a high complication and re-operation rate in the long term. This is probably why the procedure has decreased in popularity in recent years in almost all parts of the world.

Some of the common long-term complications of GaB are discussed later. In addition, a large number of GaB patients undergo band removal for poor metabolic response, including dissatisfaction with weight loss or 'band intolerance', loosely used to describe unhappiness with results or quality of life with a GaB.

GASTRIC BAND SLIPPAGE

A slipped GaB is much more common during the early postoperative phase prior to the formation of a fibrous capsule around the band, but it can also happen years later. A RCT published in 2016[40] found that the slippage rate was significantly higher (10.3% vs 3.6%, P = 0.005) in the absence of fixation gastro-gastric sutures.

✔ GaB is more likely to slip in the absence of fixation gastro-gastric sutures.[40]

Patients usually present with a combination of recent-onset vomiting, regurgitation, and dysphagia. A history of chronic regurgitation and dysphagia some time after surgery is usually indicative of an enlarged pouch rather than slippage. An abnormal phi angle, the 'O sign', inferior displacement of the superolateral GaB margin, and the presence of an air–fluid level above the GaB have been described as important radiological signs. Sometimes it can be difficult to differentiate slippage from pouch formation, and the duration and acuteness of symptoms then remain the only practically useful discriminators. Pain is usually not an accompanying feature of any of the GaB complications, but in the case of slippage might indicate infarction of the prolapsed stomach. Clinically, persistent vomiting, regurgitation, and dysphagia, despite an empty band, should raise suspicion of a slipped band. Urgent band removal leads to prompt relief.

ENLARGED GASTRIC POUCH

Approximately 4.0–5.0% of patients[41] develop an enlarged gastric pouch above the band with consequent hold-up of food and delayed emptying, regurgitation, and vomiting. This is usually a result of either eating too quickly or the band being too tight. Diagnosis usually requires a contrast study that shows an enlarged pouch with a displaced band, often in conjunction with delayed pouch emptying. In milder cases, deflation of the band via the subcutaneous access port followed by cautious refilling later is all that is needed, as well as patient education about eating patterns. In more severe and recurrent cases, the band needs to be removed. In one randomised study[42] it was found that placement of the band at the oesophagogastric junction was associated with a lower incidence of pouch formation and slippage in comparison to retrogastric placement, but samples were too small to draw any meaningful conclusions.

GASTRIC BAND EROSION

Erosion of the GaB into the lumen of the stomach is reported in approximately 3.2% of patients[14] and is probably related to either an over-restricted band or infection. Patients usually present with loss of satiety, abdominal pain and/or vomiting, or recurrent infection of the port or tubing several years after primary surgery. Erosion can be suspected on contrast studies or CT scanning, but an endoscopy is required for confirmation. The band must be removed. This is better done using a hybrid endoscopic/laparoscopic approach, provided the buckle of the band has eroded into the stomach. A laparoscopy is still needed for division of tubing and removal of the port. Sometimes one needs to wait for a few months to allow for the band to erode completely before attempting the hybrid approach. Complete surgical removal is only recommended if endoscopic treatment has failed and may be difficult due to adhesions.

POUCH AND TUBING COMPLICATIONS

Approximately 10–15% of GaB patients will develop complications such as leakage or kinking of the tube, a tilted or inaccessible port, or infection.[14] Most of these are easily resolved by local re-operation with or without a change of the port and/or shortening of the tube.

GASTRO-OESOPHAGEAL REFLUX DISEASE

A number of patients may develop symptoms of acid reflux in the long term. Reduction in the fill volume and medical management with PPIs is all that is usually required, but persistent unresponsive GORD may need band removal.

NUTRITIONAL COMPLICATIONS AFTER BARIATRIC SURGERY

Deficiency of certain vitamins and minerals is common in the general population, and obesity itself predisposes to the problem.[43] In addition, BS can lead to a further reduction in the intake and absorption of many micronutrients. Best practice guidelines from the American Society for Metabolic and Bariatric Surgery (ASMBS)[17] and BOMSS[16] recommend routine supplementation with a range of vitamins and minerals, and periodic monitoring to ensure the adequacy of the supplementation regimen (Tables 19.2 and 19.3).

Although the need for vitamin and mineral supplementation in bariatric patients is accepted, there is much debate on the exact dose and route of administration for each trace element for different bariatric procedures.

Table 19.2   Recommendations regarding nutritional supplementation after different bariatric procedures

Supplement	Guideline	SG	GB	GaB	BPD/DS
Multivitamin/mineral tablet	ASMBS: Multivitamin/mineral tablet containing iron, folic acid, and thiamine (Grade B, Level 2)	2 tablets daily	2 tablets daily	1 tablet daily	2 tablets daily
	BOMSS: Multivitamin/mineral tablet containing thiamine, iron, selenium, 2 mg copper, and 15 mg zinc (GPP)	1 tablet daily	1 tablet daily	1 tablet daily	1 tablet daily
Calcium and vitamin D	ASMBS: Calcium Citrate 1200–1500 mg/day (Grade B, Level 2)	Yes	Yes	Yes	Yes 1800–2400 mg/day
	ASMBS: Vitamin D (at least 2000 to 3000 units/day titrated to levels > 30 ng/mL) (Grade A, Level 1)	Yes	Yes	Yes	Yes
	BOMSS: Ensure good dietary intake of calcium and supplement only indicated if rise in serum PTH (GPP) BOMSS: 2000–4000 units/day vitamin D (Grade D, Level 4)	Yes	Yes	No	Higher doses may be required
Vitamin B$_{12}$	ASMBS: Vitamin B 12,350–1000 µg/daily orally or 1000 µg/monthly parenterally as needed (Grade B, Level 2)	Yes	Yes	Yes	Yes
	BOMSS: Vitamin B$_{12}$ injection 1 mg 3-monthly	Yes	Yes	No	Yes
Iron	ASMBS: Males and no history of anaemia – 18 mg elemental iron Menstruating women – 45–60 mg elemental iron daily (Grade A, Level 1)	Yes	Yes	No	Yes
	BOMSS: 36–66 mg elemental iron daily Additional, 50–100 mg in women who are menstruating (Grade B, Level 2)	Yes	Yes	No	Yes

ASMBS, American Society for Metabolic and Bariatric Surgery; *BOMSS*, British Obesity and Metabolic Surgery Society; *BPD/DS*, biliopancreatic diversion with duodenal switch; *GaB*, gastric banding; *GB*, gastric bypass; *GPP*, good practice point; *SG*, sleeve gastrectomy.

Table 19.3 Recommendations regarding monitoring after different bariatric procedures

Monitoring recommendation	Guideline	SG	GB	GaB	BPD/DS
Frequency of visits	ASMBS: Initial, interval until stable, once stable (months) BOMSS: Nothing specific for each procedure but generally recommends follow-up at 3, 6, and 12 months, and annually after that	1, 3–6, 12	1, 3–6, 12	1, 1–2, 12	1, 3, 6
Full blood count	ASMBS: At each visit BOMSS: (3, 6, and 12 months in the first year, and then annually)	Yes Yes	Yes Yes	Yes Only annually	Yes Yes
Urinary calcium	ASMBS: 24-hour urinary calcium excretion at 6 months and then annually BOMSS: No recommendation	Yes	Yes	Yes	Yes
Haematological and bone health parameters	ASMBS: Folic acid, iron studies, vitamin D, parathyroid hormone BOMSS: Urea + electrolytes, liver function tests, ferritin, folic acid, calcium, vitamin D, parathyroid hormone (3, 6, and 12 months in the first year and annually thereafter)	– No	– Yes	– No	– Yes
Vitamin B_{12}	ASMBS: Vitamin B_{12} (annually) BOMSS: 6 and 12 months in the first year and then annually. No need to monitor if patient is on intramuscular injections	Yes Yes	Yes Yes	Yes No	Yes Yes
Vitamin A	ASMBS: Vitamin A (initially and 6–12 monthly thereafter) BOMSS: Monitor as follows	No Measure if steatorrhoea or symptoms of night blindness	Optional Measure if steatorrhoea or symptoms of night blindness	No Measure if steatorrhoea or symptoms of night blindness	Yes Every 3 months in first year and then annually if stable
Zinc, copper, and selenium	ASMBS: Evaluation with 'specific findings' BOMSS: Monitor as follows – Check zinc levels if unexplained anaemia or hair loss Check copper levels if unexplained anaemia or poor wound healing	No Monitor annually	Yes Monitor annually	No Monitor annually	Yes Monitor annually
Selenium	ASMBS: Selenium evaluation with 'specific findings' BOMSS: Check selenium levels if unexplained anaemia, metabolic bone disease, chronic diarrhoea, or unexplained cardiomyopathy	No No	Yes Monitor annually	No No	Yes Monitor annually
Thiamine	ASMBS: Thiamine evaluation with 'specific findings' BOMSS: As clinically appropriate	Yes Yes	Yes Yes	Yes Yes	Yes Yes
Vitamins E and K	ASMBS: Insufficient evidence to recommend routine screening BOMSS: Monitor vitamin E in unexplained anaemia, neuropathy. Consider vitamin K deficiency if excessive bruising/coagulopathy	– As clinically appropriate	– As clinically appropriate	– As clinically appropriate	– Monitor annually
Lipid profile	ASMBS: Lipid evaluation every 6–12 months based on risk and therapy BOMSS: Monitor in those with dyslipidaemia	Yes Yes	Yes Yes	Yes Yes	Yes Yes

ASMBS, American Society for Metabolic and Bariatric Surgery; BOMSS, British Obesity and Metabolic Surgery Society; BPD/DS, biliopancreatic diversion with duodenal switch; GaB, gastric banding; GB, gastric bypass; SG, sleeve gastrectomy.

Table 19.4   Incidence of common nutritional deficiencies after bariatric surgery

Complication	Incidence (%)
Hypoalbuminaemia	3.0–18.0
B_1 deficiency	≤ 49.0
B_{12} deficiency	19.0–35.0
Vitamin D deficiency	25.0–73.0
Iron deficiency	17.0–45.0
Zinc deficiency	12.0–91.0
Copper deficiency	3.8–18.8
Hair loss	30.0–50.0
Neurological complications	≤ 1.1

Similarly, although there is a consensus that patients with symptoms of nutritional deficiency should be promptly investigated and treated, there is less clarity on the need to screen for asymptomatic deficiencies. For example, BOMSS[16] recommends routine annual monitoring of serum copper and zinc levels after RYGB, but ASMBS[17] does not. A systematic review concluded that the cost of routine monitoring of serum copper levels might not be justified for adequately supplemented, asymptomatic patients who have undergone RYGB.[44] Another systematic review concluded that clinically relevant zinc deficiency is rare after RYGB, and routine monitoring is unnecessary unless patients develop specific symptoms.[45]

It is also not known if the cost of regular monitoring of levels of different vitamins and minerals is justified in asymptomatic patients taking recommended supplementation. The overall effect of patient adherence to all the recommended supplementation on the subsequent development of deficiencies is also not known.

SUPPLEMENTATION AND MONITORING AFTER SLEEVE GASTRECTOMY

In contrast to GaB, the SG can affect the absorption of some trace elements through its effect on the size of the gastric surface, acid production, and production of intrinsic factor. This means that these patients have a higher requirement for supplements than those undergoing a GaB (Table 19.2). BOMSS recommends annual monitoring of full blood count (FBC), renal and liver function tests, ferritin, folic acid, calcium, vitamins D and B_{12}, parathyroid hormone, zinc, and copper for these patients, while selenium and other micronutrients are reserved for those with symptoms suggestive of these deficiencies (Table 19.3).

SUPPLEMENTATION AND MONITORING AFTER RYGB

RYGB reduces calorie intake, causing little if any protein-calorie malabsorption. However, as the operation diverts food away from the duodenum and proximal jejunum, absorption of the vitamins and minerals predominantly absorbed there is affected. The need for supplementation and monitoring is hence greater than for either GaB or SG. This is also reflected in the guidance from ASMBS and BOMSS (Table 19.2). BOMSS recommends annual monitoring of

the FBC, renal and liver function tests, ferritin, folic acid, calcium, vitamins D and B_{12}, parathyroid hormone, zinc, copper, and selenium for these patients, while vitamin A, E, and K only if there are symptoms and signs to suggest deficiency (Table 19.3). Although there are currently no specific recommendations for OAGB patients, it seems reasonable to recommend the same supplementation and monitoring regimen for them as for patients undergoing RYGB, until more data emerges.

SUPPLEMENTATION AND MONITORING AFTER GASTRIC BANDING

During the time of weight loss, intake is necessarily less, on a background of pre-existing vitamin deficiency. Therefore BOMSS[16] recommends one 'complete' over-the-counter multivitamin and mineral tablet daily only for GaB patients.

In addition, folic acid 5 mg daily is recommended before conception and for the first 12 weeks of pregnancy. Thiamine replacement is also recommended for those with prolonged vomiting, and vitamin D and/or iron if required. BOMSS recommends that FBC, renal, and liver function tests, and serum ferritin and folate levels are monitored annually in the long term routinely. Specific symptoms should be investigated on their own merits.

SUPPLEMENTATION AND MONITORING AFTER BILIOPANCREATIC DIVISION ± DUODENAL SWITCH

A substantial part of the mechanism of weight loss after BPD/DS is probably malabsorption due to a large amount of bypassed small bowel. Therefore, BPD/DS is also associated with significant malabsorption of a number of micronutrients. This is reflected in increased recommended supplementation and monitoring protocols (Tables 19.2 and 19.3).

COMMONLY ENCOUNTERED NUTRITIONAL PROBLEMS

All members of bariatric MDT must be familiar with the common long-term nutritional problems that may arise in their patients and how to manage them. Estimates of the incidence of some common nutritional complications seen with BS are shown in Table 19.4. A recent systematic review found the current evidence to be very limited, and most studies were of 'low' quality.[46] In practice, there is significant variation in these rates depending on the procedure, the supplementation protocol, patient compliance, and the monitoring strategy.

PROTEIN-CALORIE MALNUTRITION

This can happen irrespective of weight loss after any bariatric procedure, but is more common after malabsorptive procedures such as BPD/DS or distal gastric bypasses with longer than standard limb lengths. It is rare after standard RYGB, OAGB with a 150-cm biliopancreatic limb, SG, or GaB, when it usually indicates some other complication. For example, PCM after standard RYGB could be caused by an anastomotic stricture. After SG it may indicate a twist, kink, or stricture. After GaB it may indicate a chronically tight GaB, gastric pouch formation, or chronic slippage.

NEUROLOGICAL COMPLICATIONS

Vitamin B_{12}, thiamine (B_1) and copper deficiency can lead to devastating neurological complications after BS and are more likely after procedures that re-route the small bowel. A recent study reported that of the 38 patients with neurological complications, 53% had experienced surgical complications and gastrointestinal symptoms including vomiting.[47] The majority of the patients were deficient in vitamin B (74%), and most commonly vitamin B_1 (47%).

✔ Neurological complications are rare after BS and usually indicate a micronutrient deficiency. Vitamin B_{12}, thiamine, and copper constitute the most frequent deficiencies associated with neurological problems.[47]

However, even purely gastric procedures can be associated with these complications. Early diagnosis is important, as delays in treatment may be associated with significant morbidity and even mortality.

ANAEMIA

Up to 15% of patients can develop iron-deficiency anaemia (IDA) after BS in the absence of any overt blood loss. The exact incidence varies but it is generally agreed that patients undergoing BPD/DS are at the highest risk, followed by OAGB, RYGB, SG, and GaB. Pre-menopausal women and patients with pre-operative iron deficiency are at higher risk.[48] Although iron deficiency is the most common cause of anaemia, deficiencies of vitamin B_{12}, folic acid, and copper can also cause anaemia and should be investigated depending on the supplementation regimen and the response to treatment with iron. Needless to say, all patients with IDA should also be asked about any overt bleeding and/or sinister symptoms. The ASMBS therefore recommends evaluation for other age-appropriate causes (Grade D).

HAIR LOSS AND DERMATOLOGICAL COMPLICATIONS

Although hair loss is common after BS, it is usually self-limiting. A recent systematic review reported the incidence to be as high as 57% (95% CI 42–71%) and young women are especially at higher risk.[49] It is usually a consequence of rapid weight loss and is self-limiting. Low serum levels of zinc, folic acid and ferritin are common in patients who have suffered hair loss. Dermatological manifestations and skin changes may also suggest zinc, niacin (vitamin B_3), vitamin A, or other micronutrient deficiency.[50]

✔ Hair loss is common after BS and is usually self-limiting. Severe hair loss and/or dermatological manifestations may suggest zinc, folic acid, or ferritin deficiency.[49] Deficiencies of niacin (vitamin B_3), selenium, biotin, iron, vitamin A, etc. may also be associated with skin rash or hair loss.[50]

BONE HEALTH

Patients with obesity have a higher prevalence of vitamin D deficiency, and BS may further compromise intake or absorption of vitamin D and/or calcium. Current guidelines universally recommend supplementation with vitamin D and calcium in these patients to prevent bone depletion. Although several authors have suggested a potential link

between RYGB and osteoporotic fractures,[51] and SG and reduced bone mineral density,[52] it is currently a matter of debate.

WEIGHT REGAIN

Some weight regain is common after any BS, but up to a quarter of patients may experience significant weight regain, which can be associated with deterioration in the quality of life and obesity-related conditions such as T2DM and HTN.[53] A recent systematic review of 11 studies on RYGB and 5 on SG found several inadequacies in the reported literature but concluded that weight regain appeared to be higher after SG compared to RYGB.[54] A large multicentre study with a 5-year follow-up of 9617 patients reported that 35.1%, 14.6%, and 3% after SG, RYGB, and OAGB, respectively, may experience significant weight regain.[55] The quantity and quality of follow-up and successful adoption of lifestyle changes are thought to improve weight loss and prevent weight regain.[56]

DEFINITIONS

There are no standard, accepted definitions of insufficient weight loss or weight regain in BS. Surgeons (and many patients) focus on parameters of weight – initial weight loss and weight regain – since these are easy to measure in the clinic. Some authors have used the proportion of patients who do not lose half of their excess weight as a definition of insufficient weight loss. A recent systematic review found 23 different definitions of insufficient weight loss and only 21 of the 77 studies provided a definition of weight regain, emphasising the need for consensus.[57]

✔✔ Attempts to define good response, and primary and secondary poor responders after BS have so far proved difficult.[57]

In the future, payers might demand clearer definitions. These are also needed for the comparison of different revisional surgery options for insufficient weight loss or weight regain after an individual bariatric procedure. It is also important to avoid the term 'failure' with respect to insufficient weight loss, as patients may take this to refer to their own behaviour.

CAUSES OF WEIGHT REGAIN

There are two broad groups: technical problems with the operation, and other or patient factors. Examples of the former include a gastro-gastric fistula in RYGB and tubing leakage or a dilated gastric pouch in GaB. Examples of patient factors include the return of appetite and loss of early satiety with RYGB and SG. Two recent systematic reviews reported that an imbalanced diet and maladaptive eating behaviour may also contribute to weight regain.[58,59] This may be due to possible physiological/metabolic adaptation to the hormonal changes that are thought to contribute to the initial weight loss.[60] However, in a very small sample size it has been shown that the postprandial secretion of glucose-dependent insulinotropic polypeptide (GIP) and glucagon-like peptide 1 (GLP-1) was lower in those with significant weight regain after RYGB compared to those maintaining weight loss.[61] It is also possible that some patients may be genetically predisposed to weight regain. In carriers of a fat mass and obesity-associated (FTO) gene variant, weight regain was more common and occurred sooner after surgery.[62] An attractive goal of genetic research, therefore, is to predict those who will respond better to some operations than others.

✓ Eating habits, lifestyle, psychological factors, technical factors, physiological adaptation, and genetic factors all play a role in significant weight regain after BS.[58–60]

Mental health factors that predispose to weight regain are poorly understood. Further psychosocial problems such as relationship breakdown and addiction transfer (alcoholism and substance abuse) can become apparent after surgery and could lead to weight regain.

MANAGEMENT OF WEIGHT REGAIN

Patients with weight regain who wish to have further treatment should be assessed fully by the bariatric MDT and include an assessment of barriers to weight loss by a mental health professional. Surgical technical problems should be ruled out by contrast examinations or endoscopy.

✓ Patients with significant weight regain should undergo a thorough dietetic, psychological, and surgical assessment for the reasons behind it in a multidisciplinary setting.

Management options include dietary/psychological counselling, pharmacotherapy, and revisional surgery. These need to be considered on a case-by-case basis after discussion within the MDT.[63] In the future, new pharmacotherapeutic agents will likely be available that could be used in conjunction with or instead of revision surgery.[64]

REVISIONAL BARIATRIC SURGERY

DEFINITION

A review by the ASMBS[65] used the term re-operative BS for all related re-operations carried out after a bariatric procedure. This included conversion to a different bariatric procedure, further surgery for complications management, and adjustment of the original procedure to improve outcomes. Other surgeons[66] have suggested the term revision be used for operations to correct or modify the original bariatric procedure (such as re-sleeve, resection of a dilated gastric pouch after RYGB, alteration of limb lengths, replacement GaB), and reserve conversion where the original procedure is changed to a different procedure (SG/RYGB after GaB or RYGB after OAGB). Many others, and probably the majority, loosely use the term revisional BS to include modifications of a bariatric procedure as well as conversion to a different bariatric procedure.

✓ There is currently no consensus on the definition of revisional BS, and some use the all-encompassing term 're-operative bariatric surgery'.[65] Many surgeons loosely use the term 'revisional bariatric surgery' to indicate modifications to a bariatric procedure or its conversion to a different procedure.

JUSTIFICATION FOR A PAYER TO PROVIDE A REVISIONAL PROCEDURE

Although cost-effectiveness data to support a second or third bariatric procedure for patients who have not responded to their first procedure are lacking, it can be argued that there is a strong moral imperative for carefully considered conversion or adjustment surgery. In support of this, revisional joint-replacement surgery is routinely funded, as is an escalation of anti-diabetic therapy when diabetes control with one treatment is suboptimal. As most patients considering conversion will have lost some weight, the consent process needs to include discussion of the higher risks and lower benefits compared to the primary procedures.[67] For this reason, some advocate centralising conversion surgery to high-volume surgeons and centres.

PATIENT SELECTION AND INDICATIONS

There are no RCTs of revisional BS. Therefore patients need to be guided by the expertise of their surgical team about the options available. The first consensus statement of 70 international experts on revisional BS was recently published.[68] Experts recommended a preoperative nutritional and psychological evaluation, endoscopy, and contrast series before revisional surgery. Expected weight loss with a new bariatric procedure should be calculated from the original weight before primary surgery so that expectations are properly managed. The MDT process should include nutritional assessment and correction of any deficiencies, especially if the patient is malnourished after a previous malabsorptive procedure.

✓ Nutritional and psychological factors should be addressed and endoscopy and contrast series should be undertaken before any revisional BS for poor weight loss or weight regain.[68]

There are many cohort studies of successful weight loss or maintenance with GaB or SG conversion to RYGB done for technical complications. A simple removal of GaB usually leads to weight regain and recurrence of comorbidity. There are few long-term data comparing the available options.

REVISIONS AFTER GASTRIC BANDING

RYGB, SG, OAGB, single-anastomosis duodeno-ileal bypass with sleeve gastrectomy (SADI-S), and BPD/DS have all been described for conversions after GaB with satisfactory further weight loss, but RYGB and SG remain the commonest options. In a systematic review of revisional surgery after GaB including 36 studies with a total of 2617 patients, 60.5% of the conversions were to RYGB and the rest to SG. Both procedures were found to be safe, with a pooled morbidity of 13.5% and a mortality of 0.0004%, with no difference between the two groups.[69] There are no reported differences in complication rates between conversion performed in one or two stages, but an erosion should be allowed to heal first and it is preferable to wait for a stretched stomach from a band slippage to recover. A recent systematic review of 25 studies did not find any significant difference between leak rates following one- or two-stage conversion to SG or RYGB.[70]

✔ For conversion of GaB to SG or RYGB, one- and two-step conversions were found to be equally safe in a systematic review.[70] However, there is a potential for selection bias in this review of observational studies.

REVISIONS AFTER SLEEVE GASTRECTOMY

Re-sleeve, RYGB, OAGB, SADI-S, and BPD/DS are all described for the conversion of SG for weight regain or other complications such as GORD, and there are few comparative data. A recent large French nationwide study reported 10-year outcomes from 224,718 SGs, indicating a revision rate of 4.7%, 7.5%, and 12.2% at 5, 7, and 10 years post-procedure, respectively.[71] The previous history of GaB was associated with a higher risk of revision ($P < 0.001$). The main reasons to revise SG were persistence of obesity (87%) and GORD (5.2%), and the most common revision procedure was RYGB (75.2%) and re-sleeve (18.7%).

A recent systematic review concluded OAGB to be safe and effective as a revisional procedure following SG.[72] The most common reason for revision was noted to be inadequate weight loss or weight regain, but the results were combined for revisional surgery after other procedures including GaB and VBG, making it difficult to draw conclusions following revisions, specifically after SG. There are also data suggesting that a conversion to RYGB brings excellent relief from GORD symptoms but does not yield much further weight loss.[73] There are also reports of successful conversion to SADI-S, especially from countries where OAGB is not yet approved.[74]

✔ The need for revisional surgery after SG appears to increase with time. Re-sleeve, RYGB, OAGB, SADI-S, and BPD/DS have all been used for revisions after SG, with few level 1 data to establish the superiority of one over the other.[72,74–76] RYGB is probably the best revisional option for patients with significant GORD following SG, whereas OAGB or SADI-S might be more appropriate for further weight loss and comorbidity resolution.

REVISIONS AFTER RYGB

Surgically it is challenging to convert RYGB to another operation, and occasionally it may be reversed. A systematic review of 799 patients in 24 studies having conversions or adjustments after RYGB identified five studies of conversion to distal RYGB (DRYGB), five of revision of the gastric pouch/anastomosis, six of adding a GaB, two of conversion to BPD/DS, and six of endoluminal adjustment procedures (i.e. StomaphyX).[77] The mean excess body mass index (BMI) loss was 54.0% and 52.2% after DRYGB up to 1 and 3 years, respectively, 43.3% and 14.0% after gastric pouch/

anastomosis revision, 47.6% and 47.3% after GaB revision, and 63.7% and 76.0% after BPD/DS. Endoluminal procedures resulted in excess BMI loss of 32.1% with up to 1-year follow-up; longer term data are unavailable for these at present. In this review, gastric pouch/anastomosis revision was associated with the lowest major complication rate at 3.5% and DRYGB with the highest at 11.9%. Mortality (0.6%) was seen only in the DRYGB group.

Recently, the only revisional procedure that reached a consensus of the experts was lengthening the biliopancreatic limb for inadequate weight loss or weight regain after RYGB or OAGB.[68]

OUTCOMES OF REVISIONAL BARIATRIC SURGERY

Although there are very few studies reporting on longer than 5-year results, current evidence suggests that revisional surgery is required after all operations for a variety of reasons and is effective for weight loss and resolution of obesity-related comorbidities in the short term.[71,75,78,79]

COST-EFFECTIVENESS AND ECONOMIC BENEFITS OF BARIATRIC SURGERY

There are a number of cost-effectiveness analyses indicating that the upfront cost of BS for severe and complex obesity is recouped within 3–4 years after the operation, with substantial cost savings thereafter. A recent systematic review with a meta-analysis of 61 studies reported that compared to no/conventional treatment, BS has direct cost savings over a lifetime scenario.[80] There are limited data on the cost-effectiveness of revisional surgery, and there are no data for body-contouring procedures to deal with loose skin. The cost of follow-up and supplements adds to the overall burden on healthcare systems, but there are substantial wider benefits to society that are not included in standard methods of calculating cost-effectiveness. These include improved mortality and lower risk of cancer (particularly in females).

A systematic review of occupational outcomes after BS found that those undergoing surgery were 3.24 ($P = 0.01$) times more likely to return to work than non-surgical controls and experienced significant reductions in the mean number of annual sick days.[81] Remarkably, the pooled analysis suggested that 26.4% of unemployed patients were able to return to work after BS.

✔✔ Those undergoing BS are more likely to return to work than non-surgical controls and experience significant reductions in the mean number of annual sick days.[81]

BS is associated with reduced all-cause mortality and an increased quality of life. It further reduces the incidence of cardiovascular diseases and leads to remission or improvement in conditions such as T2DM, HTN, dyslipidaemia, and sleep apnoea. As expected, this translates into healthcare savings: in a systematic review in 2015 of 11 studies on 37,720 patients, it was found that the average number of medications per patient decreased from 3.9 ± 1.86 before surgery to 1.75 ± 1.85 after surgery, with a 49.8% reduction in total cost of medications after a follow-up of 6–72 months.[82] A recent study with data from the UK National Bariatric Registry (NBSR) on 1847 patients with obesity and T2DM on insulin observed significantly higher rates of cessation of insulin at 5 years after surgery compared to best medical therapy, thus resulting in a cost saving of £4229 per patient.[83]

✅ A systematic review[82] showed that the average number of drugs per patient decreased from 3.9 ± 1.86 before BS to 1.75 ± 1.85 after surgery, with a 49.8% reduction in the total cost of drugs after a follow-up of 6–72 months.

A UK Health Technology Assessment programme report published in 2009 found that for patients with a BMI ≥ 40 kg/m^2, the incremental cost-effectiveness ratios for surgery ranged from £2000 to £4000 per quality-adjusted life-year (QALY) gained over 20 years. This was well below the £20 000 per QALY threshold for cost-effectiveness used by NICE. For patients with diabetes and a BMI of 30–39 kg/m^2, the incremental cost-effectiveness ratio fell to £1367 per QALY gained. That means that if a decision-maker is willing to pay £20 000 for an additional QALY, the probability of surgery being cost effective over 20 years is 100%.[84] These figures show that BS has the same cost-effectiveness as public health interventions such as smoking cessation and prescribing statins for primary prevention of cardiovascular disease – both remarkably effective public health strategies.[85]

✅ Although there is an upfront cost to BS, it is well below the typical threshold of £20 000–£30 000 used by NICE for approving a treatment.

FUTURE ROLE OF BARIATRIC SURGERY

The World Health Organization (WHO) now recognises obesity as a noncommunicable disease, with a huge global burden affecting 603.7 million adults and even worse 107.7 million children worldwide in 2015.[17] BS is the only intervention remotely effective in the longer term at inducing and maintaining weight loss for those with severe and complex obesity, although some new data are emerging on the effectiveness of medical management in the short to medium term.[86] Currently accepted criteria for BS were agreed some 25 years ago. Over this period, aided by the revolution of minimally invasive surgery, the safety of BS has improved enormously. Surgical mortality is now rare and most large studies report mortality of 1:500–1:1000. Bariatric operations are being simplified and undertaken by even less invasive means, leading to the possibility that mortality and morbidity could decrease even further. Thus, SG has seen a meteoric rise[9] as a stand-alone procedure, rates of OAGB have increased, and several endoscopic procedures are being enthusiastically evaluated.[87]

Therefore, it is perhaps surprising that, in the complete absence of effective public health measures to stem the rising tide of severe and complex obesity, there is so little uptake of BS by healthcare systems worldwide. In developed health services, it is made available to only a fraction (much less than 1%) of those who might benefit. Updated NICE guidelines published in 2014 were the first in the world to lower the BMI

eligibility threshold for T2DM to be considered for surgery to 30 kg/m^2.[18] This guidance also used the phrase 'expedited assessment' to push for patients with T2DM diagnosed within 10 years, if they have a BMI of 35 kg/m^2 or more, to be referred to the BS team. Despite these changes, there has been no corresponding increase in surgery in the UK.

One of the ongoing and future challenges therefore, if BS is to become increasingly commissioned and accepted as mainstream, is to dispel the myth that BS is dangerous and improve its perception by the public and healthcare workers. Adding the word 'metabolic' to describe the effects of the surgery could be a step in the right direction.[85]

As more pharmacotherapeutic agents[86] become available, it is likely that surgery will be done in combination with medication, in the same way that cancer surgery is often preceded or followed by chemotherapy. Large-scale RCTs of surgery and medication that include cost-effectiveness will be needed to establish which patients would benefit.

The quality of the surgical evidence should continue to improve as large-scale, multicentre, pragmatic, funded RCTs are performed. RCTs without funding lack independent data collection (therefore risking bias) and do not have the logistic ability to capture long-term (10 years and more) comprehensive follow-up data, because of the considerable financial and staffing resource required to do this. In the UK a large, pragmatic, multicentre RCT – 'By-Band-Sleeve' – is comparing head to head the three commonest procedures (RYGB, GaB, and SG), and has recently completed recruitment of 1341 patients.[88] National registries, where patients are purposefully identified, can plug the gap between RCTs and what happens to the whole operated population, but only if funding enables sufficient follow-up (grade B evidence).

Bariatric/metabolic surgery is now a recognised speciality. It is possible that in the future its role could be extended to those with metabolic syndrome without obesity. The future will see the development of endoscopic and surgical procedures that maximise metabolic benefits with no or minimal weight loss.

✅ It is anticipated that BS will assume a greater role in the management of selected individuals with T2DM, class 1 obesity, and metabolic syndrome.

Surgeon factors can improve outcomes, and initiatives such as the Metabolic and Bariatric Surgery Accreditation and Quality Improvement Program (MBSAQIP) and the Swedish registry SOREG (Scandinavian Obesity REGistry) lead the way in advancing self-regulation and improving outcomes. In the UK, annual individual consultant mortality reporting is a similar process, via data submitted to the National Bariatric Surgery Registry. This has already produced national reports of clinical outcomes reporting and reports on individual consultant mortality have been continuously reported annually since 2014.[89] With better data capture and enhanced compliance from the bariatric community and hospitals, this data set can become an extremely useful resource for healthcare planners and practitioners of BS.

✅ Increasing uptake and accuracy of national surgery registries will help improve the quality and expand the role of BS in the treatment of various obesity-associated diseases.

Key points

- BS is associated with long-term significant weight loss and a reduction in all-cause mortality. An important UK RCT to look at in the future would be the By-Band-Sleeve Trial, which has recently finished recruitment of 1341 patients.
- Placement of gastric band close to the oesophagogastric junction with a small gastric pouch and fixation using gastro-gastric sutures are associated with lower slippage rates. Gastric bands are associated with high re-operation rates, even in the specialist centres.
- Sleeve gastrectomy produces durable weight loss but is associated with new-onset GORD in approximately 20% of patients. Some patients need conversion to Roux-en-Y gastric bypass for symptoms of GORD unresponsive to medical management, and yet others need conversion to OAGB or SADI-S for further metabolic benefit. There is some evidence that SG may predispose to the development of Barrett's oesophagus.
- Closure of internal spaces at the time of RYGB or OAGB reduces the incidence of internal hernia.
- Bariatric surgery patients need lifelong follow-up similar to many chronic disease patients. These patients need supplementation with a range of micronutrients and annual haematological monitoring for the rest of their life.
- Eating habits, lifestyle, psychological factors, technical factors, physiological adaptation, and genetic factors all play a role in significant weight regain after BS. Where possible, these should be addressed before any revisional BS for these indications.
- Increasing uptake and accuracy of national surgery registries will help expand the role of BS in the treatment of various obesity-associated diseases.

References available at http://ebooks.health.elsevier.com/

KEY REFERENCES

[1]   Sjostrom L. Review of the key results from the Swedish Obese Subjects (SOS) trial - a prospective controlled intervention study of bariatric surgery. J Intern Med 2013;273(3):219–34
   The SOS study is the first long-term (> 20 years) prospective, controlled trial to provide information on the effects of BS. Compared with usual care, BS was associated with a long-term reduction in overall mortality and decreased incidence of T2DM, myocardial infarction, stroke, and cancer.

[4]   Colquitt JL, Pickett K, Loveman E, Frampton GK. Surgery for weight loss in adults. Cochrane Database Syst Rev 2014;8:CD003641
   This Cochrane systematic review showed that surgery results in greater improvement in weight loss outcomes and weight-associated comorbidities compared with non-surgical interventions, regardless of the type of procedure used.

[5]   Khorgami Z, Shoar S, Saber AA, Howard CA, Danaei G, Sclabas GM. Outcomes of bariatric surgery versus medical management for type 2 diabetes mellitus: a meta-analysis of randomized controlled trials. Obes Surg 2019;29(3):964–74
   A meta-analysis of seven RCTs showed a superior and persistent effect of BS versus medical management for inducing remission of T2DM. Compared with medical management, patients with RYGB had better glycaemic control and improved levels of high-density lipoproteins and triglycerides.

[6]   Sharples AJ, Mahawar K. Systematic review and meta-analysis of randomised controlled trials comparing long-term outcomes of Roux-en-Y gastric bypass and sleeve gastrectomy. Obes Surg 2020;30(2):664–72
   A recent meta-analysis of five RCTs comparing long-term outcomes of RYGB and SG. Both RYGB and SG result in sustained weight loss and comorbidity control at 5 years. RYGB resulted in greater %EWL, improved dyslipidaemia, and a lower incidence of postoperative GORD.

[14]   O'Brien PE, Hindle A, Brennan L, et al. Long-term outcomes after bariatric surgery: a systematic review and meta-analysis of weight loss at 10 or more years for all bariatric procedures and a single-centre review of 20-year outcomes after adjustable gastric banding. Obes Surg 2019;29(1):3–14
   A systematic review of 57 studies, of which 33 were eligible for a meta-analysis examining long-term (> 10 years) outcomes after BS. All current procedures result in substantial and durable weight loss, with re-operation being common after all procedures. More long-term follow-up data are required after OAGB/MGB and SG.

[24]   Fakhry TK, Mhaskar R, Schwitalla T, Muradova E, Gonzalvo JP, Murr MM. Bariatric surgery improves nonalcoholic fatty liver disease: a contemporary systematic review and meta-analysis. Surg Obes Relat Dis 2019;15(3):502–11
   A meta-analysis of 21 studies suggested that BS should be considered as a treatment of NAFLD. BS improves steatosis and steatohepatitis in the majority of patients and improves or resolves liver fibrosis in up to 30% of patients.

[26]   Wiggins T, Guidozzi N, Welbourn R, Ahmed AR, Markar SR. Association of bariatric surgery with all-cause mortality and incidence of obesity-related disease at a population level: a systematic review and meta-analysis. PLoS Med 2020;17(7):e1003206
   An important meta-analysis of 18 large-scale population-based studies showed that BS was associated with a reduced rate of all-cause mortality and cardiovascular mortality. BS was strongly associated with reduced incidence of T2DM, HTN, dyslipidaemia, and IHD.

[28]   Yeung KTD, Penney N, Ashrafian L, Darzi A, Ashrafian H. Does sleeve gastrectomy expose the distal esophagus to severe reflux?: a systematic review and meta-analysis. Ann Surg 2020;271(2):257–65
   A meta-analysis of 46 studies found that the increase of postoperative GORD after SG was 19% and de novo reflux was 23%. The long-term prevalence of oesophagitis was 28% and BE was 8%. Four percent of all patients required conversion to RYGB for severe reflux.

[29]   Qumseya BJ, Qumsiyeh Y, Ponniah SA, et al. Barrett's esophagus after sleeve gastrectomy: a systematic review and meta-analysis. Gastrointest Endosc 2021;93(2):343–52 e2
   A recent meta-analysis of 10 studies with follow-up up to 10 years after SG reported the pooled prevalence of Barrett's oesophagus to be 11.6%. Most cases were observed after 3 years of follow-up, and the risk of oesophagitis increased by 13% each year after SG.

[32]   Hajibandeh S, Hajibandeh S, Abdelkarim M, et al. Closure versus non-closure of mesenteric defects in laparoscopic Roux-en-Y gastric bypass: a systematic review and meta-analysis. Surg Endosc 2020;34(8):3306–20
   A meta-analysis of six observational studies and two RCTs showed that closure of mesenteric defects in RYGB may be associated with lower risks of internal herniation and re-operation for SBO compared with non-closure of the defects.

[40]   Le Coq B, Frering V, Ghunaim M, et al. Impact of surgical technique on long-term complication rate after laparoscopic adjustable gastric banding (LAGB): results of a single-blinded randomized controlled trial (ANOSEAN Study). Ann Surg 2016;264(5):738–44
   A multicentre RCT including 706 procedures reported that use of the gastro-gastric suture significantly reduced the rate of re-intervention for band retrieval or repositioning at three years.

[57]   Bonouvrie DS, Uittenbogaart M, Luijten A, van Dielen FMH, Leclercq WKG. Lack of standard definitions of primary and secondary (non)responders after primary gastric bypass and gastric sleeve: a systematic review. Obes Surg 2019;29(2):691–7
   A systematic review of 112 studies found that the recent literature regarding definitions of weight loss outcomes is highly inconsistent, and concluded that to compare the literature international consensus is required.

[81]   Sharples AJ, Cheruvu CV. Systematic review and meta-analysis of occupational outcomes after bariatric surgery. Obes Surg 2017;27(3):774–81
   A meta-analysis of 10 studies found the overall evidence to be limited, but suggested those undergoing surgery are more likely to return to work than non-surgical controls. Three of the studies demonstrated significant reductions in the mean number of annual sick days.

INDEX